A Textbook of Neuroanatomy

Dedication

To my father, Antonios,
my mother, Garifalia, and
my sister Oursikía
for their contribution to my education
MAP

To my wife, Roseann,
my daughter, Jen, and
my mother, Mary
LPG

XXV
The brain within its groove
Runs evenly and true;
But let a splinter swerve,
'T were easier for you
To put the water back
When floods have slit the hills,
And scooped a turnpike for themselves,
And blotted out the mills!

Emily Dickinson

A Textbook of Neuroanatomy

Maria A. Patestas

Associate Professor of Anatomy
Department of Anatomy
Des Moines University
Des Moines, Iowa

Leslie P. Gartner

Professor of Anatomy
Department of Biomedical Sciences
Baltimore College of Dental Surgery
Dental School
University of Maryland at Baltimore
Baltimore, Maryland

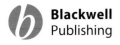
Blackwell
Publishing

BLACKWELL PUBLISHING
350 Main Street, Malden, MA 02148-5020, USA
108 Cowley Road, Oxford OX4 1JF, UK
550 Swanston Street, Carlton, Victoria 3053, Australia

First published 2006 by Blackwell Publishing Ltd

Library of Congress Cataloging-in-Publication Data

Patestas, Maria A.
   A textbook of neuroanatomy / Maria A. Patestas and Leslie P. Gartner.
      p.   cm.
Includes bibliographical references and index.
   ISBN 1-4051-0340-X (paperback : alk. paper)
   1. Neuroanatomy.   I. Gartner, Leslie P.   II. Title.
QM451.G285 2004
611.8–dc22   2003026897

A catalogue record for this title is available from the British Library.

Set in 9/11.5pt Palatino
by Graphicraft Limited, Hong Kong
Printed and bound in India
by Replika Press Pvt. Ltd

For further information on
Blackwell Publishing, visit our website:
http://www.blackwellpublishing.com

Contents

Preface

This *Textbook of Neuroanatomy* was written with the student in mind in full knowledge of the apprehension with which he or she faces the prospect of learning a subject matter that frequently intimidates the student population. The material appears daunting, not only due to its very nature of being associated with polysyllabic words, but also because there are so many eponyms and synonyms for the myriad of terms that are necessary for the proper description of the nervous system. The good news is that neuroanatomy is simply being maligned by its nefarious reputation, for it is a logical, relatively benign subject, whose comprehension does not require Einsteinian brilliance, but merely a willingness to learn the meaning of a large fistful of new words and the ability to read a map and follow it from one place to another. In order to help the student easily achieve the goal of learning neuroanatomy we made this textbook complete, concise, yet easy to read, and well illustrated with many schematic diagrams to expound upon the concepts being discussed. Presenting the material in a relevant context will make the learning experience simpler, more enjoyable, and more memorable.

We envisioned writing a book that was accessible and clear—one that students would not have to wade through in order to discern key information of human neuroanatomy. We have also highlighted the interrelationships between systems, structures, and the rest of the body as we go through the various regions of the brain. We think a broad understanding of neuroanatomy, supported with a basic understanding of its physiology, is critical so that students do not get bogged down memorizing structures but instead learn the principles. This conceptual basis of the "big picture" helps establish the foundation for future studies in the health sciences and for the logic that helps drive it.

The text is divided into two sections. The first nine chapters provide an overview of neuroanatomy that introduces terms, and should be viewed as the vocabulary lessons which are necessary evils in the mastering of a new language. For no matter how well one understands the grammar of a foreign language, it is the possession of a rich vocabulary that permits one to communicate with speakers of that tongue. The second part of this textbook, Chapters 10–23, utilizes the vocabulary of the first part to detail information concerning the various pathways and discrete systems that act in concert to perform the myriad of functions of the human nervous system.

Special features include:

- chapter opening outlines that provide a quick overview of the chapter content and organizational logic;

- clinical cases open each chapter, setting the stage for the relevance of that chapter's context;
- key points in the chapter are highlighted in the text;
- clinical case questions indicate the relevance of the chapter opening case at key points in the chapter—the answers appear on the related website;
- summary tables within each chapter function as study guides to assist students in learning and memorizing;
- clinical considerations sections indicate the medical conditions relevant to the chapter topics;
- synonym/eponym tables help organize the many possible terms for each vocabulary word;
- a follow-up to each clinical case is given at the end of each chapter and discusses the opening case, helping tie together the text and its medical application;
- questions to ponder at the end of each chapter reinforce the relevance of the material, with the answers to even questions given on the website and the answers to odd questions appearing at the end of the book;
- an accompanying website includes all the illustrations, the even answers for questions to ponder, and all the answers for clinical case questions. It also features animations of key processes and links to useful sources. The site can be found at www.blackwellpublishing.com/patestas. An instructor's CD-ROM version is also available.

ACKNOWLEDGMENTS

We would like to thank the many individuals who helped us bring this project to fruition, including our editors at Blackwell Publishing: Nancy Whilton, our publisher, who signed and oversaw the publishing process; Elizabeth Frank, our assistant editor, who managed the flow and review of multiple drafts; our desk editor, Jane Andrew, who scrutinized the fine detail; and our production editors Rosie Hayden, Sarah Edwards, and Cee Pike, who ably managed the complex physical construction of this project. Our artist, Todd Smith, worked closely with us to ensure a first-rate art program, and Dr Scott Thompson wrote the clinical cases that begin and close each chapter.

Additionally, we would like to thank the many reviewers who commented on the manuscript in its development. Dr Robert Sikes, in particular, was an invaluable reviewer, who provided specific and thorough comments on many draft chapters, and the entire art program. We also would like to acknowledge the many helpful comments made by the reviewers: Stephen Lahr, Curt Anderson, Melody Harrison,

Lyn Turkstra, Angela Ciccia, Denise Johnson, Min Yu, John Stein, Mohammad Jamali, Robert Berry, and Judy Schotland. Their help was instrumental in the crafting of this book. And finally, we would like to thank our respective families for all the time we took away from them in the writing of this textbook.

While we appreciate all of the assistance that we received from our editors and colleagues, the responsibility for errors, omissions, and shortcomings is ours. In view of that fact, we welcome criticisms and suggestions for improvement of this text.

Maria A. Patestas (maria.patestas@dmu.edu)
Leslie P. Gartner (lgartner@umaryland.edu)

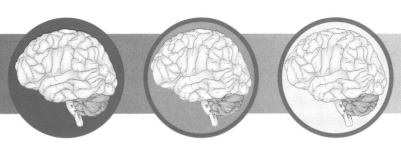

PART 1

General Principles of the Nervous System

CHAPTER 1

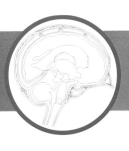
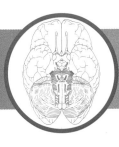
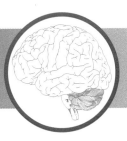

Introduction to the Nervous System

CELLS OF THE NERVOUS SYSTEM

CENTRAL NERVOUS SYSTEM

PERIPHERAL NERVOUS SYSTEM

QUESTIONS TO PONDER

The human nervous system is an extremely efficient, compact, fast, and reliable computing system, yet it weighs substantially less than most computers and performs at an incredibly greater capacity. It has the capability of performing tasks that are far beyond the abilities of any computer yet devised. The present textbook deals mostly with the anatomy of the central nervous system, and in case the reader wonders why we study neuroanatomy, we should remember that it is our central nervous system more than anything else about us that makes us what we are, human beings.

The nervous system is subdivided, *morphologically*, into two compartments, the **central nervous system (CNS)**, the brain and the spinal cord, and the **peripheral nervous system (PNS)**, which emanates from and is a physical extension of the CNS. The PNS is composed of cranial and spinal nerve fibers and ganglia. *Functionally*, the nervous system is also subdivided into two components, the **somatic nervous system**, which is under the individual's conscious control, and the **autonomic nervous system**, which controls the myriad of activities in conjunction with the voluntary nervous system. The autonomic nervous system is a tripartite organization, in that it has a **sympathetic**, a **parasympathetic**, and an **entreric** component. Simply stated, the first initiates the "flight or fight" response, the second is concerned with the body's vegetative activities, whereas the enteric nervous system is involved in regulating the process of digestion. It must be understood, however, that the interplay of these three systems maintains **homeostasis**. The autonomic nervous system acts upon three cell types to perform its functions, these are cells of glands, smooth muscle, and cardiac muscle. Moreover, the nervous system has two other functional components, **sensory** and **motor**. The sensory component collects information and transmits it to the CNS (and is therefore called **afferent**), where the information is sorted, analyzed, and processed. Generally speaking, the motor component delivers the results of the analysis away from the CNS (and is therefore called **efferent**) to the effector organs, i.e., muscles and glands, resulting in a response to the stimulus.

Discussion of the topics of neuroanatomy requires that the student be familiar with some of the specialized terminology of the subject matter. One of the problems that students have in studying neuroanatomy is that there is a plethora of terms applied to the same or similar structures. It is important, therefore, to begin the discussion of this subject matter by listing and defining in Table 1.1 some of the terminology the student will encounter.

CELLS OF THE NERVOUS SYSTEM

Neurons

Neurons are the functional units of the central nervous system

The functional unit of the nervous system is the **neuron**. There are several types

Terms	Definition
Arcuate	Arc-like, resembles a segment of a circle
Bilateral	On both sides
Brainstem	Originally this term referred to the entire brain with the exception of the telencephalon; most neuroanatomists refer to the medulla oblongata, pons, and mesencephalon as the brainstem
Caudal	Toward the tail (proceeding to a lower position; the opposite of rostral)
Column	A large bundle (also funiculus) of ascending or descending nerve fibers, composed of several different fasciculi (e.g., dorsal column of the white matter of the spinal cord)
Commissure	A bundle of nerve fibers that run horizontally, connecting the right and left sides of the central nervous system (e.g., anterior commissure)
Contralateral	The opposite side (e.g., in many instances the right side of the brain receives information from and controls the left side, *contralateral*, of the body
Cortex	The periphery of a structure; the opposite of medulla
Decussation	The level in the central nervous system where paired fiber tracts cross from one side of the body to the other (e.g., pyramidal decussation)
Exteroceptor	A sensory receptor that provides information to the central nervous system concerning the external environment
Fasciculus	A bundle (also tract) of ascending or descending nerve fibers within the central nervous system (e.g., fasciculus cuneatus)
Fiber	A long, thin structure; refers to an axon or a collection of axons
Fovea	A depression or a pit (e.g., fovea centralis of the retina)
Funiculus	A large bundle (also column) of ascending or descending nerve fibers, composed of several different fasciculi (e.g., dorsal funiculus of the white matter of the spinal cord)
Ganglion	A collection of nerve cell bodies in the peripheral nervous system (although it is used occasionally in reference to a collection of nerve cell bodies in the central nervous system, e.g., basal ganglia)
Glomerulus	Structures with a spherical configuration (e.g., synaptic glomeruli in the olfactory bulb)
Infundibulum	A funnel-like structure (e.g., infundibulum of the hypohysis)
Interoceptor	A sensory receptor that provides information to the central nervous system concerning the internal environment
Ipsilateral	The same side (e.g., in some instances the right side of the brain receives information from and controls the right side, *ipsilateral*, of the body)
Lamina	A layer of a specific material such as the layering of nerve cell bodies in the spinal cord
Myelin	A fatty substance that surrounds certain axons; composed of spiral layers of the cell membranes of Schwann cells (in the peripheral nervous system) and of oligodendroglia (in the central nervous system)
Neurite	A collective term for axons and dendrites
Neuropil	A complex of axons, dendrites, and processes of neuroglia that form a web-like network between nerve cell bodies of the gray matter
Nucleus	Core; in a cell it is the region of the cell that houses the chromosomes; in the central nervous system it is a collection of nerve cell bodies
Operculum	A cover or lid (e.g., parietal operculum of the cerebrum that overhangs and partially masks the insula)
Peduncle	A massive collection of nerve fiber bundles that connect the cerebrum and the cerebellum to the brainstem
Perikaryon	The cell body of a neuron (i.e., a neuron without its dendrites and axon); also referred to as soma
Plexus	The interwoven arrangements of nerve fibers that serve a specific region (e.g., brachial plexus)
Project	When one group of nerve cells relay their information to a second group of nerve cells, it is said that the first group "projects" to the second group (e.g., the hippocampal formation projects to the hypothalamus)
Proprioceptor	Sensory nerve endings in muscles, joints, and tendons that inform the central nervous system concerning the position and movements of the regions of the body in space (e.g., muscle spindle)
Raphe	A seam or midline structure (e.g., raphe nuclei of the reticular formation)
Rostral	Toward the nose (proceeding toward a higher position; the opposite of caudal)
Tract	A bundle (also fasciculus) of ascending or descending nerve fibers within the central nervous system (e.g., tractus solitarius)

Table 1.1 ● Common terms in neuroanatomy.

of neurons (detailed in Chapter 3) but they all have similar structures and functions. Neurons are capable of receiving, conducting, and transmitting impulses to each other as well as to muscle cells and cells of glands. Usually, neurons receive information at processes known as **dendrites** and transmit information along their single **axon**. Thus dendrites conduct information toward the cell body, whereas axons conduct information away from the cell body. Neurons usually communicate with each other as well as with other cells at **synapses**, where neurotransmitter substances are released from the axon terminal of the first neuron and bind to receptor molecules on the surface of the second neuron (or muscle/gland cell). Neurons may also communicate with each other via gap junctions, intercellular pores that permit the movement of small secondary messenger molecules from the cytoplasm of one cell into the cytoplasm of the neighboring cell, initiating a requisite response in the target cell.

Neuroglia

Neuroglia constitute several categories of non-neuronal cells, namely microglia, macroglia, and ependymal cells

Additional cells, known as **neuroglia**, constitute several categories of non-neuronal supporting cells. Those in the central nervous system are known as macroglia, ependymal cells, and microglia. The first two are derived from cells of the neural tube, whereas microglia are macrophages whose origins are monocyte precursors of the bone marrow.

Ependymal cells form a simple cuboidal epithelium that lines the central canal of the spinal cord and the ventricles of the brain. Additionally, these cells also participate in the formation of the choroid plexus, vascular tufts of tissue that manufacture cerebrospinal fluid. Macroglia is a collective term for the protoplasmic astrocytes, fibrous astrocytes, and oligodendroglia. **Protoplasmic astrocytes** support neurons in the gray matter, form a subpial barrier, and envelop capillaries of the CNS. **Fibrous astrocytes** are located in the white matter and appear to function in a similar fashion to protoplasmic astrocytes. Astrocytes also function in scavenging ions and neurotransmitter substances from the extracellular spaces. **Oligodendroglia** form myelin sheaths around axons and also surround dendrites and cell bodies of neurons in the CNS. Schwann cells are located in the PNS and they function in forming myelin around axons of the PNS. They also envelop unmyelinated axons.

CENTRAL NERVOUS SYSTEM

The central nervous system is composed of the large, anteriorly situated brain and smaller, cylindrically shaped spinal cord

The **central nervous system** is a complex, hollow tube, whose rostral end, the **brain**, is enlarged and folded in an elaborate manner, whereas its caudal end, the **spinal cord**, is a long, tubular structure (Fig. 1.1). The brain is housed in the cranial cavity and at the foramen magnum is continuous with the spinal cord, housed in the vertebral canal. The **dorsal** surface of the spinal cord is closer to the spinous processes of the vertebrae, whereas its **ventral** surface is closer to the bodies of the vertebrae. Since the CNS, as well as most of the body, is bilaterally symmetric, the **sagittal** (midsagittal, according to some) plane bisects it into right and left halves. Positioning toward the sagittal plane is considered to be the **medial** direction and away from the sagittal plane is the **lateral** direction.

Brain

The brain is subdivided into five regions: the telencephalon, diencephalon, mesencephalon, metencephalon, and myelencephalon

The **brain** is subdivided into five major regions, the largest being the **telencephalon**, which is composed of the cerebral hemispheres; the other regions are: the **diencephalon**, whose component parts are the epithalamus, thalamus, hypothalamus and subthalamus; the **mesencephalon**, consisting of the cerebral peduncles (tegmentum and crus cerebri) and the tectum (superior and inferior colliculi); the **metencephalon**, including the pons and cerebellum; and the **myelencephalon** (medulla oblongata). Frequently the medulla oblongata, mesencephalon, and the pons are collectively termed the **brainstem**. The lumen of the CNS is a narrow slit, the central canal, in the spinal cord, but is expanded into a system of **ventricles** in the brain and is filled with cerebrospinal fluid. Twelve pairs of cranial nerves emerge from the brain to supply motor, sensory, and parasympathetic innervation for the head and neck and much of the viscera of the body.

Spinal cord

The spinal cord is a cylindrical structure whose neurons are arranged in such a fashion that the motor functions are ventrally positioned and the sensory functions dorsally positioned

The **spinal cord** (Fig. 1.2) is a cylindrical aggregate of nervous tissue, where white matter surrounds a central cylinder of gray matter. The neurons of the spinal cord are arranged in such a fashion that those concerned with somatic motor function are located in the **ventral horn** and their axons leave via the ventral rootlets. These are accompanied by axons of the preganglionic sympathetic neurons, located in the **lateral horn** of the spinal cord in the thoracic and upper lumbar regions, and axons of preganglionic parasympathetic neurons located in the lateral horn of the sacral spinal cord. The **dorsal horn** of the spinal cord is the location where central processes of unipolar neurons of dorsal root ganglia enter the spinal cord via dorsal rootlets bringing sensory information to the CNS. **Interneurons** connect two neurons to each other (e.g., unipolar sensory neurons of the dorsal root ganglia to motor neurons of the ventral horn). Thus, interneurons have the capability of facilitating or inhibiting a motor response to a sensory stimulus. For example, if you prick your finger the reflex response is to pull the finger away from the offending stimulus; however, if a health professional sticks your finger for a blood test, the interneuron inhibits the withdrawal of the finger.

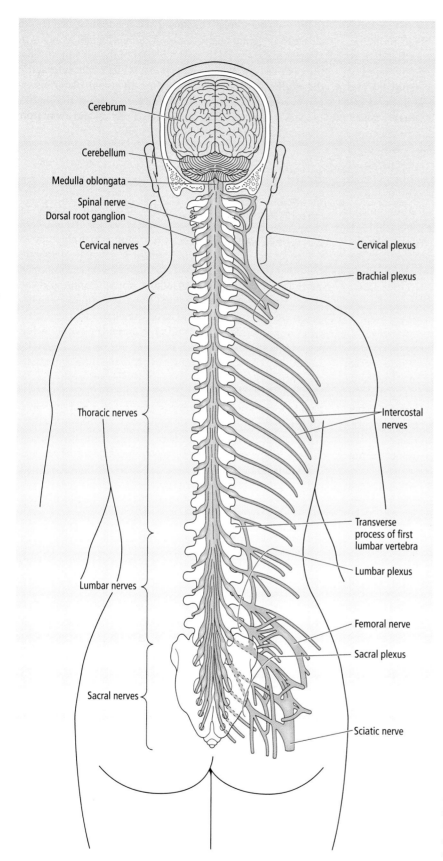

Cerebrum

Cerebellum

Medulla oblongata

Spinal nerve

Dorsal root ganglion

Cervical nerves

Cervical plexus

Brachial plexus

Thoracic nerves

Intercostal nerves

Transverse process of first lumbar vertebra

Lumbar plexus

Lumbar nerves

Femoral nerve

Sacral plexus

Sciatic nerve

Sacral nerves

Figure 1.1 ● The brain, spinal cord, spinal nerves, and major somatic plexuses. Note that the back of the skull as well as the spinal processes of the vertebrae have been removed and that the dura mater and the arachnoid have been opened up so that the spinal cord may be viewed in its entire length.

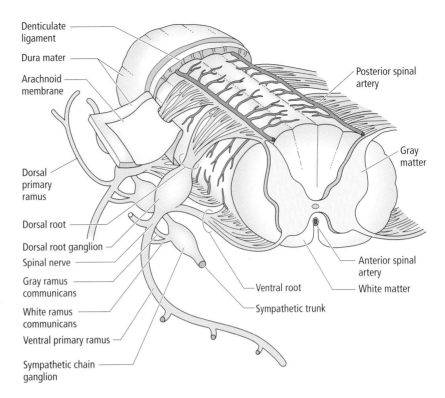

Denticulate ligament
Dura mater
Arachnoid membrane
Dorsal primary ramus
Dorsal root
Dorsal root ganglion
Spinal nerve
Gray ramus communicans
White ramus communicans
Ventral primary ramus
Sympathetic chain ganglion
Posterior spinal artery
Gray matter
Anterior spinal artery
White matter
Ventral root
Sympathetic trunk

Figure 1.2 ● The spinal cord, its meninges, spinal nerves, and sympathetic chain ganglia.

The white matter of the spinal cord is composed of ascending and descending tracts of nerve fibers that connect regions of the CNS to one another. Ventral and dorsal rootlets at each level of the spinal cord join each other to form the spinal nerves that leave the spinal cord at regular intervals, indicative of its segmentation. Attached to each dorsal root is a dorsal root ganglion, housing the soma of the unipolar (pseudounipolar) neurons.

Gray matter and white matter

Gray matter is composed of neuron cell bodies, clusters of which within the CNS are known as nuclei, whereas white matter is recognized by the presence of myelinated axons

The nerve cell bodies of the CNS are grouped into large aggregates, known as gray matter. Gray matter may be arranged in sheaths, as in the cerebral cortex, or as a smaller collection of nerve cell bodies, known as a **nucleus** (or occasionally, and technically incorrectly, a ganglion, e.g., basal ganglia). There are two major categories of neurons, those whose axons leave the CNS and **interneurons**, whose axons remain within the CNS. The first group, called **principal cells** by some neuroanatomists, are generally motoneurons (somatic or autonomic), whereas interneurons relay information from one (or one group) of neurons to a second (or second group) of neurons within the CNS (e.g., the interneuron of a reflex arc).

White matter is composed of processes of neurons, many of whose axons are wrapped in a myelin sheath, which in a living individual has a white color. These axons are collected into small bundles, known as **fasciculi**, or large bundles, called **funiculi**. Certain larger fiber bundles are named **tracts** or **capsules**, whereas axons that cross the midline to connect identical structures on opposing sides are known as **commissures**. Axons that travel up or down the CNS and cross the midline from one side to the other are said to **decussate** at the point of crossing over.

PERIPHERAL NERVOUS SYSTEM

The peripheral nervous system is a continuation of the CNS; it is composed of clusters of nerve cell bodies, known as ganglia, as well as of bundles of axons and central processes, known as nerves

The **peripheral nervous system** is composed of cranial nerves, spinal nerves, their associated ganglia, and nerve fibers of the autonomic nervous system. It must be understood that the PNS is in physical continuity with the CNS, in fact cell bodies of many of the nerve fibers (axons) of the PNS are located in the CNS.

Somatic nervous system

The somatic nervous system is composed of the 12 pairs of cranial nerves and their ganglia as well as of the 31 pairs of spinal nerves and their dorsal root ganglia

There are 12 pairs of cranial nerves, identified both by name as well as by Roman numerals I through XII. All cranial nerves, with the exception of the vagus (CN X), serve structures in the head and neck only. The vagus nerve has responsibilities in the head and neck, but also serves many of the thoracic and abdominal viscera, e.g., the heart and alimentary tract. Those cranial nerves that have sensory components possess sensory ganglia housing the cell bodies of unipolar neurons whose single process bifurcates into a central and a peripheral process. The central process of a unipolar neuron enters the brain, whereas its peripheral process goes to a sensory receptor. There are no synapses occurring in these sensory ganglia.

There are 31 pairs of spinal nerves (8 cervical, 12 thoracic, 5 lumbar, 5 sacral, and 1 coccygeal), attesting to the segmentation of the spinal cord (see Fig. 1.1). The cell bodies of sensory neurons (unipolar neurons) are located in the dorsal root ganglia (sensory ganglia). Again, it must be remembered that there are *no synapses* occurring in the dorsal root ganglia. The single process of each neuron bifurcates and the short central process joins other central processes to form dorsal rootlets that enter the spinal cord. The peripheral process goes to a sensory receptor, which, when stimulated, causes depolarization of the peripheral process; the wave of depolarization spreads to the central process, which transmits the stimulus either to an interneuron (in a three neuron reflex arc) or to a motoneuron (in a two neuron reflex arc, e.g., the patellar reflex). Although the above description is true for reflex arcs, it must be realized that in most instances the incoming information is transmitted to higher levels in the brain and is processed either cognitively or subconsciously, or both, rather than just relying on simple reflex phenomena. These motoneurons are multipolar neurons whose cell bodies are located in the ventral horn of the spinal cord and serve *skeletal muscle cells only*. Their axons leave via the ventral rootlets that join the dorsal rootlets to form the **spinal nerve**.

Each spinal nerve bifurcates to form a smaller **dorsal primary ramus** and a larger **ventral primary ramus**. Dorsal primary rami supply sensory and motor innervation to the back, whereas ventral primary rami supply the lateral and anterior portion of the trunk. Ventral rami that supply the

thorax and abdomen usually remain as separate nerves, whereas those of the cervical and lumbosacral regions join each other to form **plexuses** from which individual nerve bundles arise to serve the head, neck, and upper and lower extremities. Each spinal nerve receives sensory information from the skin of the segment, or **dermatome**, of the body that it serves. The entire body is mapped into a number of dermatomes; however, there are overlaps in the innervation, so that a single dermatome is supplied by more than one spinal nerve. Such overlaps prevent the total anesthesia of a particular dermatome if the dorsal rootlets of the spinal nerve supplying it are damaged.

Autonomic nervous system

The autonomic nervous system regulates the activities of smooth muscle, cardiac muscle, and glands, and is divided into three systems: the sympathetic, parasympathetic, and enteric nervous systems

The autonomic nervous system is a motor system, but unlike somatic motoneurons, it does *not* serve skeletal muscle cells, instead it innervates cardiac muscle cells, smooth muscle cells, and secretory cells of glands. Additionally, whereas a somatic motoneuron **directly** innervates its muscle cell (Fig. 1.3), in the autonomic nervous system the neuron whose cell body is located in the CNS (**preganglionic** or **presynaptic neuron**) synapses with a second neuron (**postganglionic** or **postsynaptic neuron**) located in a ganglion in the PNS. It is the axon of the *postganglionic neuron* that synapses with the cardiac muscle cell, smooth muscle cell, or secretory cell of a gland. Thus the autonomic nervous system is said to be a two cell system, and synapses *always occur* within an autonomic ganglion (Fig. 1.3). The axon of the preganglionic neuron is myelinated and is known as the **preganglionic fiber**. The axon of the postganglionic neuron is not myelinated, and is known as the **postganglionic fiber**.

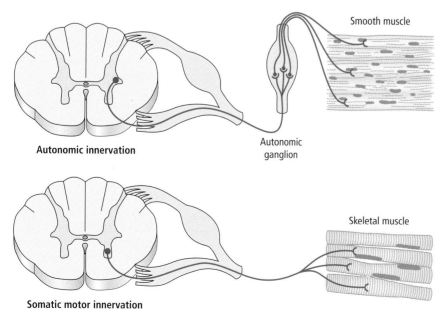

Figure 1.3 ● Diagram demonstrating the difference between autonomic innervation (top) and somatic motor innervation (bottom). Observe that two neurons are present in the autonomic supply, whereas a single motoneuron is present in the somatic motor system.

The autonomic nervous system is responsible for the maintenance of homeostasis, and is composed of three functional components: **sympathetic**, **parasympathetic**, and **enteric**. The sympathetic component prepares the body for "fight and flight," whereas the parasympathetic prepares the body for a vegetative state (e.g., digestion). The enteric nervous sytem is situated completely within the wall of the digestive tract and controls the entire process of digestion. Although the sympathetic and parasympathetic components of the autonomic nervous system modulate its activities, the enteric nervous system can function quite well on its own if the sympathetic and parasympathetic components are severed. Cell bodies of preganglionic sympathetic neurons are located in the lateral horn of the thoracic and upper lumbar spinal cord (T1 to L2,3), whereas those of the preganglionic parasympathetic neurons are located in the brain (and their axons travel with CN III, VII, IX, and X) and the lateral horn of the sacral spinal cord (S2–S4). Postganglionic cell bodies of sympathetic neurons are usually located near the spinal cord, within the **sympathetic chain ganglia**, or a little farther away, in collateral ganglia. The cell bodies of postganglionic parasympathetic neurons, however, are located in ganglia that are in the vicinity of the viscera being innervated.

The cell bodies of the sensory neurons that supply the viscera are located in the dorsal root ganglia of spinal nerves or in the sensory ganglia of cranial nerves, along with the somatic sensory neurons. However, their peripheral processes accompany the preganglionic autonomic fibers into their respective ganglia, but do *not* synapse in those ganglia. Moreover, these peripheral fibers continue to accompany the postganglionic autonomic fibers to the same destinations. In spite of their route, these sensory neurons are *not* considered to be a part of the autonomic nervous system. Sensory information relayed by these autonomic sensory nerves are not registered as part of the conscious experience, and even pain sensations are experienced as "referred pain" in somatic regions of the body (e.g., **angina pectoris**, where pain sensations arising in the heart muscle are experienced as pressure in the chest, back, and arm (regions served by the same segmental spinal nerve)).

QUESTIONS TO PONDER

1. What is the relationship between the central and peripheral nervous systems?

2. What is meant by the "fight or flight" response?

3. Why are there more oligodendroglia than neurons in the central nervous system?

4. What single characteristic is the major difference between microglia and the other neuroglia of the central nervous system?

5. What is the major difference between a two neuron reflex arc and a three neuron reflex arc, aside from the simplistic fact that one has an extra neuron associated with it?

CHAPTER 2

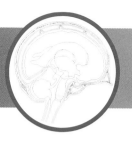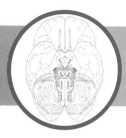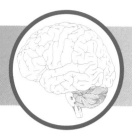

Development of the Nervous System

CLINICAL CASE

A 22-year-old woman presents to the emergency room. She is obviously pregnant and near term. There has been no prenatal care. A uterine ultrasound is performed that detects an abnormality. She is estimated to be 37 weeks pregnant. The obstetrician on call wishes to perform an emergency Caesarian section delivery because of the abnormality that was detected. This was performed without incident.

Examination of the newborn shows a fist-sized mass in the midline lumbosacral region. This protrudes above the skin surface and is dusky gray in appearance. The newborn has a normal cry and arms seem to move normally. Skin color is normal and temperature is normal. The legs do not move and are flaccid. There is deformity noted of the hips, ankles, and feet. Subsequent examination reveals a lack of cry or any physical response to sensory stimulation of the legs.

Embryogenesis, the development of the future individual, begins with the fusion of the male and female gametes, the spermatozoon and the oocyte, respectively. This occurs in the fallopian tube (oviduct). The process of fusion is known as **fertilization**, subsequent to which the fertilized ovum is referred to as a **zygote**, the very beginning of a new individual (Fig. 2.1). The mitotic activity of the zygote is responsible for the increase in the number of cells that will be required for the construction of the future individual as well as for the embryonic component of the supporting structures that will ensure the requisite nourishment for normal development and growth of the future embryo.

The normal development of the embryo is divided into a number of stages and the interested reader is referred to a textbook of human embryology. In the present textbook, human embryology is presented from the perspective of neuroanatomy and only those aspects of human development are presented that will assist the student in appreciating the complexity and beauty of how the nervous system progresses from an ill-defined cluster of cells to an amazingly intricate functional unit. In order for the reader to be able to grasp the manner in which this process occurs, it is advisable to show not only the development of the nervous system *per se*, but also that of the structures that envelop and surround the nervous system. Therefore, this chapter includes a description of early embryology, the development of the pharyngeal arches, formation of the face, and some of the molecular events that appear to govern this entire process.

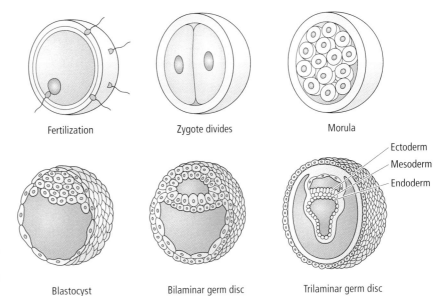

Figure 2.1 ● The early development of a human embryo. Fertilization, the fusion of the haploid sperm nucleus with the ovum's haploid nucleus, results in the formation of a diploid cell, known as a zygote. As the zygote undergoes mitosis, a solid cluster of cells is formed, the morula. Continued cell division and rearrangement of the newly formed cells results in the formation of a hollow sphere of cells, the blastocyst, whose cells form the bilaminar germ disc and later the trilaminar germ disc.

EARLY DEVELOPMENT

During early development the zygote undergoes mitotic division to form a cluster of cells, known as the morula, whose cells rearrange themselves to form the hollow blastocyst

The zygote undergoes a series of mitotic divisions, known as **cleavage**, which will result in the formation of a solid cluster of cells, where each cell is smaller than the original zygote. This cluster of cells resembles a mulberry, and hence is known as the **morula**. The cells of the morula secrete a viscous fluid that creates a central cavity by pushing the cells to the periphery until a hollow ball of cells is formed, known as the **blastocyst** (Fig. 2.1).

Although most of the cells of the blastocyst are at the periphery, a few of the cells are trapped inside, adhering to one of the poles of this hollow ball of cells. These trapped cells are the **embryoblasts (inner cell mass)**, whereas the peripherally positioned cells are the **trophoblasts**.

The embryoblasts will give rise to the **embryo** whereas the trophoblasts are responsible for the formation of the embryonic portion of the **placenta**.

Bilaminar germ disc

The bilaminar germ disc is composed of two cell layers: the epiblast and the hypoblast

The cells of embryoblasts rearrange themselves to form two layers, the **epiblasts** and the **hypoblasts**, and the embryo becomes known as the **bilaminar germ disc**. The epiblast is closer to the trophoblast cells than is the hypoblast, and the forming embryo is about 7–8 days old (Fig. 2.1). By this time it has reached the uterine cavity, where it burrows into the wall of the uterus. This process of **implantation** begins on the late sixth or early seventh day after fertilization and is completed on the eleventh day.

During the period of implantation some of the cells of the epiblast delaminate, forming a membrane over the remaining epiblast. This new layer of cells is composed of the **amnioblasts**, which will give rise to the **amniotic sac**, and the space between the amnioblasts and the epiblasts is known as the **amniotic cavity**.

Trilaminar germ disc

The trilaminar germ disc is responsible for the establishment of the three primary germ layers: the ectoderm, mesoderm, and endoderm

At about the fourteenth day post fertilization, at the anterior end of the bilaminar germ disc, a few cells of the epiblasts form desmosomal contacts with a few cells of the underlying hypoblast, thus forming the **prochordal plate**, which will be the future **buccopharyngeal membrane**. Approximately 1 day later a longitudinal furrow, the **primitive groove**, develops in the epiblast on the posterior aspect of the bilaminar germ disc, the anteriormost extent of which is deeper, and is referred to as the **primitive pit**. Bordering both sides of the primitive groove is an elevation of cells, the **primitive streak**, whereas the anterior border of the primitive pit is a small elevation of cells, the **primitive node (Hensen's node)**.

Formation of ectoderm, mesoderm, and endoderm

Cells of the epiblast undergo active mitosis along most of its surface and the newly formed cells migrate to the primitive streak. Here they enter the primitive groove and pass into the space between the epiblasts and the hypoblast, thus forming a new, intermediate layer of cells, the **mesoderm**. Some of these cells do not stop in the mesoderm space, but displace most of the original cells of the hypoblast, pushing the original cells of the hypoblast laterally. The cells of the hypoblast become incorporated into an extraembryonic region, known as the yolk sac. As this process is occurring, the epiblast is renamed the **ectoderm** and the new cell layer that replaces the hypoblasts is referred to as the **endoderm**. Thus, as a result of the conversion of the embryoblast of the blastocyst into the trilaminar germ disc, a process known as **gastrulation**, the embryo is composed of three layers (ectoderm, mesoderm, and endoderm), and is known as the **trilaminar germ disc** (Fig. 2.1). The entire embryo, at this time, is approximately 1 mm in length.

Cells of the mesoderm cannot penetrate the contact of the ectoderm and endoderm at the prochordal plate, but they can migrate around this region of adhesion, and some mesoderm cells will be located anterior to this structure. These cells are **cardiogenic cells**, and begin to form the future heart. An additional group of cells migrate from the primitive node into the primitive pit and proceed anteriorly, *en masse*, between the ectoderm and the endoderm until they reach the prochordal plate, where their progress is blocked. This pencil-shaped column of cells is known as the **notochordal process**, and it possesses special *inductive* capabilities. The notochord induces the cells of the ectoderm lying above it to proliferate and form the flat **neural plate**, the beginning of the primitive nervous system of the embryo.

NEURULATION

Neurulation is the process whereby the embryo internalizes its developing nervous system

Since, at this time the primitive nervous system is on the external aspect of the body, it has to be internalized. The process of internalization, known as **neurulation**, is accomplished by an alteration in cell shape and by increased mitotic activity, especially of the lateral edges of the neural plate. These activities begin to fold the neural plate into a longitudinal furrow, the **neural groove**, whose two walls are the **neural folds**. Further cell division and continued change in cell morphology cause the neural folds of the two sides to approximate and fuse with each other in the midline, forming the **neural tube** (Fig. 2.2). The process of fusion starts at the midcervical level and proceeds anteriorly (rostrally) and posteriorly (caudally) and is completed by the end of the fourth week of gestation. The final regions of the neural tube to be closed are the **anterior** and **posterior neuropores**. The cells of the neural tube just above the notochord differentiate to form the **floor plate**. These cells induce the differentiation of neuroblasts into motoneurons and establish the polarity of the neural tube.

Note that the clinical case at the beginning of the chapter refers to an embryonic abnormality detected during an ultrasound examination of the fetus.

1 Where is the lesion in relation to the innervation of the upper extremities?

2 Where is the lesion in relation to the motor innervation of the legs?

3 Where is the lesion in relation to the sensory innervation of the legs?

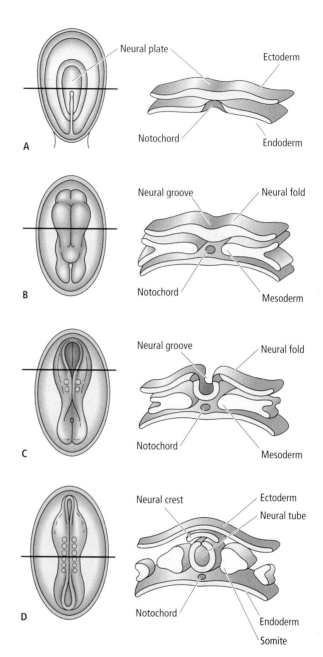

Figure 2.2 ● (A) The notochord is responsible for inducing the overlying ectodermal cells to form the neural plate. (B, C) As the embryo continues its development, it enters the stage of neurulation, the process whereby the forming nervous system is brought into the body by the formation of an intermediary neural groove, and finally a neural tube, the precursor of the brain and spinal cord. (D) Note that the neural crest, initially the lateral aspect of the neural plate, becomes separated as the neural tube is formed. Cells of the neural crest give rise to all of the ganglia of the peripheral nervous system as well as to numerous additional structures of the developing embryo.

Fusion of the lateral edges of the right and left sides of the central nervous system (CNS) is accompanied by fusion of the ectoderm, whose edges became approximated during neural tube formation. The simultaneous fusions permit a separation of the neural tube from the overlying ectoderm, and complete internalization of the nervous system. Incomplete fusion results in a relatively common developmental anomaly known as **spina bifida**. The nervous system, including the organs of special senses, originate from three sources: the **neural tube** (CNS, somatic motoneurons, and preganglionic autonomic neurons); the **neural crest** (see below); and the **ectodermal placodes** (lens of the eye, inner ear, pituitary gland, and contribution to the formation of somatic sensory ganglia of the cranial nerves).

Neural crest

The neural crest is a narrow strip of cells at either edge of the developing neural plate

As the edges of the neural folds meet each other, some of their cells do not participate in the formation of the neural tube, instead they form a narrow strip of cells, the **neural crest** (Fig. 2.2). The cells of the neural crest will migrate throughout the body to form almost the entire peripheral nervous system, including the enteric nervous system, dorsal root ganglia, sensory ganglia of the cranial nerves, all postganglionic autonomic neurons, as well as melanocytes, parenchymal cells of the suprarenal medulla (chromaffin and ganglion cells), Schwann cells and satellite cells of the peripheral nervous system, and most of the mesenchymal cells of the head and anterior neck. Therefore, most of the mesenchymal cells of this region are not derived from mesoderm, instead they are neuroectodermal in origin and are referred to as **ectomesenchyme**. Derivatives of the neural crest, neural plate, and ectodermal placodes are summarized in Table 2.1. The cells of the neural crest follow four general pathways marked by signaling molecules manufactured and released by neighboring cells. Examples of these molecules are retinoic acid, transforming growth factor, and fibroblast growth factor. These signaling molecules contact cell surface receptors of target cells, activating intracellular molecular systems that cause specific responses within those cells. Some of these responses activate cytoplasmic enzyme systems, whereas other responses include the activation of **transcription factors** that regulate specific gene expressions, each resulting in the activation of specific inductive processes necessary for the formation of the nervous system.

Paraxial mesoderm

The paraxial mesoderm lies lateral to the developing neural tube and becomes segmented into clustered blocks of tissue known as somites

The mesoderm lying lateral to the neural tube and notochord in the region of the future trunk is known as the **paraxial mesoderm**, and it becomes segmented into paired blocks of tissue, known as **somites** (Fig. 2.3). Each somite is composed of three elements. These are the **sclerotome**, responsible for the formation of two succeeding vertebrae and their intervening intervertebral disc; **myotome**, responsible for the formation of the muscle masses associated with that segment of the trunk; and **dermatome**, responsible for the formation of the dermis of the skin in its particular area of the trunk.

The region of the paraxial mesoderm lateral to the somites is known as the **intermediate mesoderm** and it forms the urogenital system. The most lateral aspect of the paraxial mesoderm, known as the **lateral plate mesoderm**, splits into

Neural crest	Neural plate	Ectodermal placodes
Neurons of: dorsal root ganglia; ganglia of CN V, VII, VIII, IX, and X; enteric plexuses; sympathetic ganglia; parasympathetic ganglia	Prosencephalon: cerebral hemispheres; basal nuclei; neurohypophysis	Sensory ganglia: CN V, VII, VIII, IX, and X
Satellite cells of: sensory ganglia; sympathetic ganglia; parasympathetic ganglia	Mesencephalon: cerebral peduncles; tegmentum; tectum	Lens of the eye
Glia cells of: enteric ganglia	Metencephalon: cerebellum; pons	Olfactory system: receptor cells; epithelium
Suprarenal medulla: chromaffin cells; neurons	Myelencephalon: medulla oblongata	Ear: organ of Corti; epithelium of membranous labyrinth
Carotid body parenchyma	Spinal cord	Adenohypophysis
Melanocytes; Schwann cells	All neurons of the CNS	Teeth: enamel
Head: most connective tissue elements; dentin, pulp, cementum; choroid, sclera	All oligodendroglia and astrocytes	
Meninges: dura, arachnoid, pia	Ependymal cells (including those covering the choroid plexus)	
Tunica media of: great vessels from heart	Optic nerve	
	Eye: retina	
	Epithelium of: ciliary body; ciliary processes; iris	

Table 2.1 ● Derivatives of the neural crest, neural plate, and ectodermal placodes.

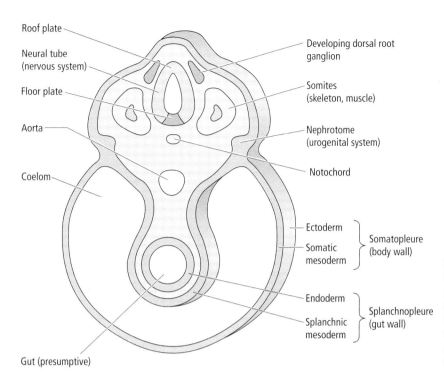

Roof plate
Neural tube (nervous system)
Floor plate
Aorta
Coelom
Gut (presumptive)
Developing dorsal root ganglion
Somites (skeleton, muscle)
Nephrotome (urogenital system)
Notochord
Ectoderm
Somatic mesoderm
} Somatopleure (body wall)
Endoderm
Splanchnic mesoderm
} Splanchnopleure (gut wall)

Figure 2.3 ● Cross-section through a developing human embryo during the process of neurulation. Note the presence of somites, gut, and intraembryonic coelom (body cavity). It is interesting to realize that the precursors of many of the future organ systems, such as the digestive, respiratory, urogenital, musculoskeletal, and nervous systems are being established at this early stage of development.

two sheaths and the intervening space between these two sheaths is known as the **coelom**, or body cavity (Fig. 2.3). The dorsal of the two sheaths of the lateral plate mesoderm becomes known as the **somatic mesoderm**, and together with its associated ectoderm this is referred to as the **somatopleure**. The ventral sheath is known as the splanchnic mesoderm and, together with its associated endoderm, is referred to as the **splanchnopleure**. The somatopleure gives rise to the body wall whereas the splanchnopleure forms the wall of the gut. The coelom becomes subdivided into the peritoneal, pleural, and pericardial cavities.

Segmentation of the paraxial mesoderm of the head is incomplete and, instead of forming somites, it is said to form about 18–20 pairs of **somitomeres**, somite-like structures that are responsible for the formation of the muscles of the head. The anteriormost seven pairs of somitomeres remain as unsegmented structures, whereas the posterior somitomeres become transformed into somites.

Pharyngeal arches

Pharyngeal arches are pairs of ectodermally covered mesenchymal thickenings responsible for the formation of much of the head and neck

As the neural tube becomes internalized, its anterior region, the future brain—whose development is detailed below—is developing so rapidly that it grows above and anterior to the prochordal plate, it overlies the cardiogenic region, and approximates the amniotic sac. The anterior end of the embryo, possibly to provide more room for growth, begins to bend in an inferior direction (**cephalic flexure**). As that occurs, the future heart becomes neatly tucked beneath the embryo, and the prochordal plate, now

referred to as the **buccopharyngeal membrane**, becomes positioned superiorly to the developing heart, separating the **stomadeum**, the primitive oral cavity, from the developing foregut (**pharynx**). Note that the stomadeum is in fact a space captured by the embryo from the amniotic cavity. The formation of the stomadeum is indicative of the initiation of the development of the face.

As the buccopharyngeal membrane degenerates during the fifth week of development and communication is established between the future oral cavity and the pharynx, the stomadeum deepens and begins to be surrounded by ectodermal-covered mesenchymal thickenings, the **pharyngeal arches** (previously named *branchial arches*). These bilaterally positioned arches develop in an anteroposterior direction. The first arch is the **mandibular arch**, the second is the **hyoid arch**, whereas successive arches are numbered 3, 4, and 6, with the notable absence of the fifth pharyngeal arch, which in humans is rudimentary. Between neighboring arches an external depression—the ectodermally lined **pharyngeal groove**—is encountered, with its anatomical counterpart on the inside, the **pharyngeal pouch**, an **evagination** of the endodermally lined pharynx.

Genetic influences of pharyngeal arch development

The connective tissue elements of the pharyngeal arches, especially those associated with the developing musculature, arise from somitomere mesoderm, whereas the majority of the mesenchyme, particularly in the anterior regions of the arches, arise from neural crest material. These neural crest-derived cells arise from the midbrain and the rhombomeres

Arch	Skeletal	Ligaments	Muscle	Nerve

Mandibular (I)	Meckel's cartilage
	Maxillae
	Mandible
	Malleus
	Incus
		Spheno-
		  mandibular
		Anterior
		  ligament of
		  malleus
			Muscles of mastication:
			  temporalis
			  masseter
			  medial and lateral
			    pterygoids
			  tensor veli palatini
			  tensor tympani
			  digastric (anterior
			    belly)
			  mylohyoid
				Trigeminal (CN V)

Hyoid (II)	Reichert's cartilage
	Hyoid bone:
	  lesser cornu
	  body
	Styloid process
	Stapes
		Stylohyoid	Muscles of facial
			expression:
			  stapedius
			  digastric (posterior
			    belly)
			  stylohyoid
				Facial (CN VII)

III	Hyoid bone:
	  greater cornu
	  body
			Stylopharyngeus	Glossopharyngeal
				(CN IX)

IV and VI	Thyroid cartilage
	Laryngeal cartilages:
	  cricoid
	  arytenoid
	  corniculate
	  cuneiform
			Pharyngeal muscles
			Pharyngeal constrictors
			Laryngeal muscles
				CN XI via the
				  pharyngeal branch
				  of CN X and the
				  pharyngeal plexus
				Recurrent laryngeal
				  branch of CN X

Modified from Hiatt, JL & Gartner, LP (2001) *Textbook of Head and Neck Anatomy*, 3rd edn. Lippincott, Williams & Wilkins, Baltimore.

Table 2.2 ● Pharyngeal arch derivatives and their innervation.

and, during early pharyngeal arch formation, express homeobox gene products (*Hoxb* genes) that reflect their sites of neural origin.

Pharyngeal arch derivatives (Table 2.2)

Each pharyngeal arch possesses its own vascular and neural supply as well as a supporting cartilaginous skeleton and associated skeletal muscles

Each pharyngeal arch possesses its own cartilage, nerve, vascular, and muscular components. The first two arches become developed to the greatest extent, whereas the last one is the most poorly developed. Only some of their derivatives will be discussed.

First pharyngeal arch (mandibular arch)

The first pharyngeal arch is responsible for the formation of the maxillary and mandibular arches and the muscles of mastication

The cartilage of the first (mandibular) arch is a horseshoe-shaped structure, known as **Meckel's cartilage**. Most of this cartilage will disappear, except for its anteriormost extent which participates in the formation of the **mental symphysis** and its posteriormost extent which gives rise to the **malleus** and **incus**, two of the three **ossicles** of the ear. The perichondrium of Meckel's cartilage becomes the **sphenomandibular ligament** and the **anterior ligament of the malleus**.

The ectomesenchyme of the first pharyngeal arch forms the muscles of mastication (temporalis, masseter, and lateral and medial pterygoid muscles), as well as the following muscles: the tensor veli palatini, tensor tympani, anterior belly of the digastric, and mylohyoid. Since these muscles are derived from the mandibular arch, they are innervated by the nerve of this arch, the **trigeminal nerve (CN V)**. The mandibular arch, as will be evident later in this chapter, is responsible for the formation of much of the face.

The development of the mandibular arch is dependent on the presence of the epidermally derived signaling molecule, **endothelin-1** (ET-1). This molecule probably functions in the facilitation of the interaction between the ectomesenchymal cells and the epithelial components of the arch, a process necessary for the development of structures that originate in the mandibular arch.

Second pharyngeal arch (hyoid arch)

The second pharyngeal arch overgrows the remaining arches and is responsible for the formation of the muscles of facial expression and part of the hyoid bone

The cartilage of the second or hyoid arch is known as **Reichert's cartilage**. Most of this cartilage will also disappear, but parts of it will be responsible for the formation of the **stapes**, the third ossicle of the ear, as well as the **styloid process**, and the lesser cornu and superior aspect of the body of the hyoid bone. Additionally, the **stylohyoid ligament** is derived from the perichondrium of Reichert's cartilage.

The muscles of facial expression take their origin in the hyoid arch mesoderm, along with the stapedius, stylohyoid, and the posterior belly of the digastric muscles. All of the above muscles are, therefore, innervated by the nerve of the second arch, the **facial nerve (CN VII)**.

The homeobox gene *Hoxa-2* is responsible for the normal development of the hyoid arch and its derivatives. In the absence of *Hoxa-2* the formation of second arch derivatives does not occur, instead first arch derivatives develop in the hyoid arch. The implication of this switch is that mandibular arch substances form by default and *Hoxa-2* gene products prevent the default condition from taking place.

Third pharyngeal arch

The third pharyngeal arch is responsible for the formation of the stylopharyngeus muscle and part of the hyoid bone

The cartilage of the third arch is unnamed, but it is responsible for the formation of the greater horn and the inferior half of the body of the hyoid bone. The only muscle to be derived from the mesoderm of the third arch is the stylopharyngeus muscle, innervated by the **glossopharyngeal nerve (CN IX)**, the nerve of the third arch.

Fourth and sixth pharyngeal arches

The fourth and sixth pharyngeal arches participate in the formation of the larynx and its muscular apparatus

The cartilages of the fourth and sixth pharyngeal arches are also unnamed. They participate in the formation of the skeleton of the larynx. It is believed that the muscles associated with the larynx and pharynx are derived from the mesenchyme of these arches. The innervation of these muscles is somewhat confusing, for they receive their nerve supply from the **pharyngeal plexus** (composed of fibers from CN IX, X, and XI). The nerves of the fourth and sixth arches, however, are the superior laryngeal and recurrent laryngeal branches of the vagus nerve (CN X), respectively.

Pharyngeal groove derivatives

Pharyngeal grooves are external depressions located between succeeding pharyngeal arches; the first pharyngeal groove forms the external ear canal, while the others disappear during development

Only the first pharyngeal groove, that between the mandibular and hyoid arches, gives rise to a definitive structure. This groove becomes deeper and approximates the first pharyngeal pouch, so much so, that only a thin membrane, the **pharyngeal membrane (closing plate)**, separates the groove from the pouch. This closing plate becomes the tympanic membrane whose external surface is covered by the ectodermal derivative of the first pharyngeal groove. The remainder of the first pharyngeal groove becomes the **external auditory canal**.

The subsequent pharyngeal grooves are submerged by the sudden spurt of growth experienced by the second pharyngeal arch, which grows in an inferior direction, to form the future neck. Occasionally, the submerged pharyngeal grooves do not become obliterated, and thus remain as **cervical sinuses**, which may result in the formation of cervical cysts.

The message for this sudden growth spurt arises from the epithelium covering the tip of the second arch. These ectodermal cells express BMP-7, sonic hedgehog, and fibroblast growth factor 8, which are responsible for the proliferation of the mesenchymal cells of the hyoid arch.

Pharyngeal pouch derivatives (Table 2.3)

Pharyngeal pouches are internal depressions located between succeeding pharyngeal arches

The **first pharyngeal pouch**, lying between the mandibular and hyoid arches, forms the Eustachian tube, the tympanic cavity, and the endodermal lining of the eardrum. The **second pharyngeal pouch** forms the palatine tonsils. The **third pharyngeal pouch** gives rise to the thymus and the inferior parathyroid glands. The **fourth pharyngeal pouch** forms the superior parathyroid gland, and perhaps part of the thymus, and the **fifth pharyngeal pouch** gives rise to the parafollicular cells of the thyroid gland.

Genetic and molecular aspects of development

Development of an embryo is controlled by a sequence of genetically controlled temporospatial phenomena

Development of the embryo requires a blueprint of spatial phenomena that occur at specific, predetermined periods of time, a process referred to as **patterning**. This blueprint is located in the nucleus of each cell, present in the chromosomes as a group of related genes. Various intra- and extracellular parameters cause the activation or suppression of these genes and in this fashion facilitate the normal sequence of growth and development.

Region	Pouch I level	Pouch II level	Pouch III level	Pouch IV level	Pouch V level
Roof		Pharyngeal tonsils			
Lateral walls	Tympanic cavity and lining of tympanic drum Mastoid air cells Auditory tube	Palatine tonsils and fossa	*Dorsal:* Inferior parathyroid *Ventral:* Thymus	*Dorsal:* Superior parathyroid *Ventral:* Thymus	Ultimobranchial body incorporated into the thyroid gland as parafollicular cells (secrete calcitonin)
Floor (pharyngeal endoderm related to pharyngeal arch)	Tongue (anterior two-thirds) Foramen cecum (rostral end of the thyroglossal duct)	Tongue (posterior one-third) Lingual tonsil	Tongue (part of the base)	Tongue (part of the base) Epiglottis	

* Modified from Hiatt, JL & Gartner, LP (1987) *Textbook of Head and Neck Anatomy*, 2nd edn. Lippincott, Williams & Wilkins, Baltimore.

Table 2.3 ● Derivatives of the pharynx and pharyngeal pouches.

Homeobox genes and growth factors

Homeobox genes control the temporal sequence of transcription factor synthesis

Genes code for the synthesis of specific proteins, many of which are enzymes that are responsible for the occurrence of specific events. Certain genes have been conserved through evolution and their study in lower organisms, such as the fruitfly, has provided information that is directly applicable to the developmental processes of higher organisms, including humans. A family of genes, known as the **homeobox genes**, code for the synthesis of **transcription factors**, proteins that bind to and regulate the expression of other genes.

The time sequence of the events controlled by products of these homeobox genes and by **growth factors** are essential for normal development because certain genes can be switched on only if some other genes have already been activated and if still other genes have not as yet been switched on. In other words, there are "windows of opportunity" for the occurrence of certain events and if that timeframe is missed then development will not proceed normally. Therefore, these homeobox genes become activated in a specific order, and their sequential expression establishes a pattern of developmental events. In order for development to progress in a normal manner, cells must interact with each other. These interactions may involve the physical contact of two cells or the release of a particular substance by one cell, referred to as the **signaling cell**, to act as a message for the other cell, known as the **target cell**.

Signaling molecules

Signaling molecules are released by signaling cells to convey a message to particular target cells that possess receptor molecules specific for the released signal

The substance that is released is known by various names, such as **signaling molecule**, **growth factor**, or **ligand**, and it reaches its target cell by traveling in the body fluids. Since the signaling molecule may meet a number of other cells, it is important that only the target cells become influenced by that particular molecule and this process is ensured by the presence of **receptor molecules** on the surfaces of cells. Usually, a specific receptor molecule recognizes only a particular signaling molecule. This is similar to a lock and key concept, where a specific lock can be opened only by a particular key.

If physical contact between cells is required, it is important that the two cells recognize each other. Cell recognition is also a function of a series of cell surface receptor molecules, some of which act as the keys and the others as locks. Usually several molecules are involved on each cell so as to ensure that only the intended target cell is influenced by the signaling cell.

Once the cell surface receptors come into contact with and bind the signaling molecule, or come into contact with the molecules on the signaling cell's surface, a sequence of intracellular events is initiated resulting in the regulation of a single gene or a series of genes of the target cell. The expression of these genes may cause the release of further signaling molecules, may alter the activities of the target cell, may prompt the target cell to differentiate into another cell type, may compel the cell to proliferate, or may direct the cell to undergo **apoptosis** and die. Each of these events is necessary for normal development to occur. The process whereby one cell causes its target cell to differentiate, that is become transformed into a different cell type, is known as **induction**.

It is interesting to note that the number of growth factors that regulate development are relatively small. The reason for the paucity of their number is that they act in combination with each other, and by simple permutations and combinations of just a few of these factors a tremendous number of signals may be generated.

EARLY DEVELOPMENT OF THE SPINAL CORD AND BRAIN

During its early development the neural tube is subdivided into three regions: the prosencephalon, mesencephalon, and rhombencephalon

Initially, the neural tube is composed of a single layer of columnar cells, known as **neuroepithelial cells**. Proliferation of these cells results in a thickened tubular structure whose cephalic region begins to form three enlargements: the **prosencephalon** (forebrain), **mesencephalon** (midbrain), and **rhombencephalon** (hindbrain). The caudal extent of the neural tube forms the **spinal cord**. As the three vesicles are developing, the **cephalic flexure** in the region of the mesencephalon and the **cervical flexure**, between the rhombencephalon and the future spinal cord, are also forming.

By the fifth week of gestation the prosencephalon is divided into two regions: the **telencephalon** with its two lateral swellings, the future cerebral hemispheres, and the **diencephalon**, whose optic vesicles are in the process of development. The rhombencephalon is also subdivided, by the **pontine flexure**, into two regions: the **metencephalon**, which will form the pons and the cerebellum, and the **myelencephalon**, which will develop into the medulla oblongata. These flexures provide increased space for the folding and three-dimensional organization of the brain.

The lumen of the developing CNS is subdivided into the ventricles of the brain and the central canal of the spinal cord. The **lateral ventricles** of the cerebral hemispheres communicate with the **third ventricle** of the diencephalon via the **interventricular foramina** (of Monro). The **fourth ventricle**, located in the rhombencephalon, communicates with the third ventricle via the **cerebral aqueduct** (of Sylvius) located in the mesencephalon.

Neuroepithelial cells

The neuroepithelial cells form a three-layered neural tube, composed of ventricular, intermediate, and marginal zones

As the **neuroepithelial cells** continue to proliferate, they establish a thicker wall composed of a pseudostratified epithelium, each of whose cells initially extends the entire thickness of the developing neural tube. As development progresses, some of these neuroepithelial cells remain adjacent to the lumen, whereas most cells migrate away from it, resulting in a three-layered neural

tube. The layer adjacent to the lumen is known as the **ventricular zone (ependymal layer)**, some of whose cells develop into **ependymal cells** that line the ventricles of the brain and the central canal of the spinal cord. The middle region of the developing neural tube is the **mantle layer (intermediate zone)**. The third layer of the developing neural tube, located the farthest from the lumen is the **marginal layer (marginal zone)**.

Since these neuroepithelial cells are quite long, initially they extend from the lumen of the neural tube to its periphery, spanning all three layers. Hence one may name regions of these cells according to the zone in which they are located. When a neuroepithelial cell is ready to undergo mitosis its nucleus migrates from the ventricular zone to the region of the cell occupying the marginal layer and the cell enters the S phase (DNA synthesis) of the cell cycle. Upon completion of the S phase, the nucleus returns to the ventricular zone, and the cell shortens and becomes round so that the cell is located completely in the ventricular zone. It is here that the cell divides to give rise to two daughter cells, which may remain in the ventricular zone or migrate to the mantle layer or into the marginal layer (Fig. 2.4).

There appear to be at least two types of neuroepithelial cells: those that can be stained for glial fibrillary acidic (GFA) proteins (GFA positive) and those that lack GFA proteins (GFA negative). GFA-negative cells give rise to an enormous number of daughter cells that eventually differentiate into **migratory neuroblasts** that are no longer able to divide. GFA-positive cells also give rise to an immense number of daughter cells that will differentiate into **glioblasts** and **ependymal cells**. Neuroblasts arise first and glioblasts and ependymal cells originate later. Neuroblasts migrate from the ventricular zone into the mantle layer where they differentiate into **neurons**. Glioblasts give rise to all macroglia (**astrocytes** and **oligodendroglia**), and **ependymal cells** line the ventricles of the brain and the central canal of the spinal cord.

As the neuroblasts are differentiating into neurons within the mantle layer they develop **axons** that grow into the marginal layer. Concomitantly, many glioblasts will migrate into the marginal layer, and those that become oligodendroglia form a protective cellular sheath around the developing axons, dendrites, and cell bodies within the mantle layer. Many of the axons will become myelinated by the oligodendroglia. Thus, in the spinal cord, the mantle layer is the future **gray matter**, whereas the marginal layer, composed of numerous myelinated axons and attendant neuroglia, becomes the **white matter**.

Myelination in the CNS begins around the sixteenth week of gestation and continues until the individual is about 3 years old, although recently it has been shown that in the frontal lobes of the brain this process may continue into the early twenties. It is interesting to note that there is a phylogenetic component to the sequence of myelination, in that the older pathways are myelinated before newer pathways; also motor roots of spinal nerves are myelinated before sensory roots.

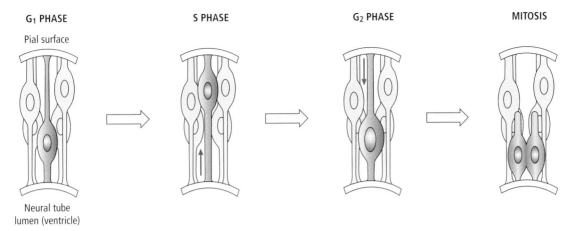

G₁ PHASE

Pial surface

S PHASE

G₂ PHASE

MITOSIS

Neural tube
lumen (ventricle)

Figure 2.4 ● Neuroepithelial cells are long cells that initially extend from the pial (marginal) to ependymal surface of the neural tube. As they enter the cell cycle to form new cells, their nuclei migrate along the length of the cell. G₁ phase: the nucleus is in the vicinity of the ventricular surface and begins to migrate to the pial surface. S phase: the nucleus is in the pial surface and at the end of the S phase the nucleus begins its return to the ventricular surface. G₂ phase: the nucleus reaches the ventricular surface and the cell begins to shorten. Mitosis (M phase): the cell divides to give rise to two daughter cells in the ventricular zone.

DEVELOPMENT OF THE SPINAL CORD

Basal plates, alar plates, and dorsal root ganglia

The basal plates and alar plates of the mantle layer are separated from each other by the sulcus limitans, a longitudinal furrow extending the entire length of the future spinal cord

The mantle layer increases in thickness in a disproportionate fashion, causing a ventral and dorsal thickening (**basal plate** and **alar plate**, respectively) of the entire length of the wall of the future spinal cord. These two thickenings are separated from each other by a longitudinal furrow, known as the **sulcus limitans**. The neuroblasts of the basal plate differentiate into motoneurons, responsible for the motor function of the spinal cord (**ventral gray column**), whereas neuroblasts of the alar plate differentiate into **interneurons**. Some of these interneurons will receive sensory information from primary sensory neurons (including those of the dorsal root ganglia). In the thoracic and upper lumbar regions (T1 through L2–L3) of the future spinal cord an intermediate thickening is discerned. Neuroblasts of this region will give rise to preganglionic sympathetic neurons (forming the **lateral gray column**) of the autonomic nervous system. It should be noted that various synonyms are in common use among neuroanatomists and some of these are given at the end of the chapter.

The central midline of the floor (**floor plate**) and roof (**roof plate**) of the neural tube has few, if any, neuroblasts, and is devoid of nerve cell bodies. However, neuronal processes will be present in these regions, conveying information between the two halves of the spinal cord.

Neurons of the **dorsal root ganglia** arise from cells of the neural crest. These neurons are responsible for delivering information from the sensory receptor organs to the spinal cord for processing.

Histodifferentiation of neuroblasts

Neuroblasts are more or less spherical cells that differentiate to form the various classes of neurons: unipolar (pseudounipolar), bipolar, and multipolar

Neuroblasts, which begin their differentiation as relatively spherical cells, form two processes at opposite poles. Usually, one of the processes, the **dendrite**, begins to arborize, whereas the other process, the **axon**, remains unbranched. The manner in which the axon and dendrite are established and modified, permits neurons to be classified as unipolar (pseudounipolar), bipolar, and multipolar (Fig. 2.5).

Unipolar (pseudounipolar) neurons are located in sensory ganglia. The two processes of each of these cells begin to grow toward and fuse with one another, forming a single process. This unified process then divides into two processes that grow in opposing directions. One of the processes, the **central process**, enters the dorsal horn of the spinal cord where it may terminate or ascend to higher levels. Collections of central processes form the dorsal roots of the spinal nerve. Collections of **peripheral processes** join the ventral root fibers to form the **spinal nerve**.

Bipolar neurons retain their two processes at opposing poles of the cell body. Dendrites of these cells collect information from the periphery of the body, whereas their axons deliver information to the CNS for processing. Bipolar neurons are associated only with the olfactory epithelium, cerebral cortex, retina, cochlear nucleus, and the vestibular nucleus.

Multipolar neurons instead of having only two processes, develop several. One of these is the axon, whereas the remainder are dendrites. Collections of axons of multipolar neurons of the basal plate grow through the marginal zone to form the ventral root of the spinal cord. As mentioned above, they join with collections of peripheral processes of unipolar neurons of the dorsal root ganglia to form the spinal nerve.

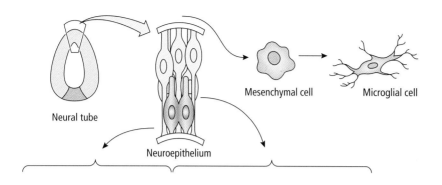

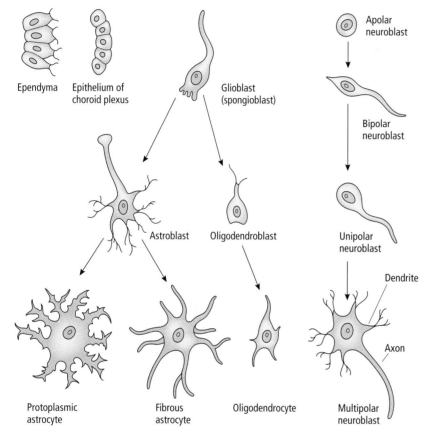

Figure 2.5 ● The origin of the developing cells of the CNS. Note that all of the cells are derived from the original neural tube, with the notable exception of the microglial cells, which are phagocytes of the CNS and originate from mesenchymal cells. Ependymal cells will line the ventricles of the brain as well as the central canal of the spinal cord; they also participate in the formation of the choroid plexus. Glioblasts will give rise to macroglia, namely the protoplasmic and fibrous astrocytes, as well as to oligodendrocytes; these cells are supporting cells of the CNS and, in the case of oligodendroglia, form myelin sheaths of CNS neurons. Neuroblasts are responsible for the formation of the neurons of the CNS.

Further differentiation of the basal and alar plates

Neuroblasts of the basal plate differentiate into multipolar neurons, whereas those of the neural crest-derived dorsal root ganglia differentiate into unipolar (pseudounipolar) neurons

As neuroblasts of the **basal plate** differentiate they become multipolar neurons whose axons grow not only into but through the marginal layer and pierce the external boundary of the neural tube. Collections of these axons travel together forming the **ventral rootlets** of the spinal cord. These ventral rootlets join others in their vicinity to form the **ventral root** of a spinal nerve.

At the same time, central processes of the unipolar neurons of the dorsal root ganglia pierce the external aspect of the neural tube at the **dorsolateral sulcus**, and enter the marginal zone or the alar plate. Central processes that enter the alar plate form synapses with the **interneurons** whose axons form synaptic contacts with motoneurons of the basal plate, and in this fashion form simple reflex arcs. Those that enter only the marginal layer travel to higher levels in the CNS. Many of these central processes travel *en masse* to reach their specific destinations. Collections of fibers going to the same destination are named accordingly.

As described above, collections of the peripheral processes of unipolar neurons join the ventral roots to form the mixed (motor and sensory) **spinal nerves**. Motor nerves effect muscle contraction or glandular secretion, whereas sensory nerves transmit information from outside or inside the body. Motor nerves propagate information that goes *away* from the CNS to a muscle (or gland) and are called **efferent nerve fibers**. Sensory nerves propagate information *toward* the CNS and are called **afferent nerve fibers**.

Development of modalities

A typical spinal nerve possesses all four functional components, known as modalities

Motor fibers of spinal nerves that innervate skeletal muscle are said to be **general somatic efferent (GSE)** fibers, whereas motor fibers that innervate smooth muscle, cardiac muscle, or glands are said to be **general visceral efferent (GVE)** fibers. Sensory fibers that bring information from the skin, skeletal muscle, tendons, and joints are called **general somatic afferent (GSA)** fibers, whereas those that bring information from the viscera (membranes, glands, and organs) are named **general visceral afferent (GVA)** fibers. The visceral components (GVE) belong to the **autonomic nervous system** (sympathetic and parasympathetic); however, GVA fibers are not autonomic fibers. A typical spinal nerve has all of these four functional components (also known as **modalities**). These modalities develop in specific regions along the alar and basal plates of the spinal cord, forming columns of recognizable gray matter along the length of the spinal cord, known as the GSA, GVA, GVE, and GSE columns.

It should be noted that GVE columns are present only in the thoracic, upper lumbar (L1–L3), and sacral levels (S2–S4). The regions of the GSE column responsible for motor innervation of the upper and lower extremities are quite extensive and are, therefore, divided into larger medial and smaller lateral motor columns. The medial motor columns are responsible for supplying the axial muscles, whereas the lateral columns serve the extremities. Similarly, in the alar compartment, the regions that receive information from the extremities are larger than the remaining areas. It should be noted that cranial nerves carry additional modalities that are discussed below.

As discussed above, during early embryogenesis, clusters of cells, known as **somites**, form on either side of the developing spinal cord. These somites form the skeletal muscles, skin (dermatomes), and connective tissue of the body. Skin and skeletal muscle derived from a particular somite are innervated by neurons arising from the segment of the spinal cord (and dorsal root ganglion) in its vicinity, giving rise to segmental innervation of the embryo that is conserved in the adult. Since, in the early embryo, the length of the vertebral canal equals the length of the spinal cord, the segment of the spinal cord is at the same level as the body segment. However, since growth in body length surpasses the lengthening of the spinal cord, in the adult the spinal cord is much shorter than the vertebral canal and thus (especially caudally), the body segment innervated lies farther away than it does in the embryo. The region of the vertebral canal that is devoid of spinal cord in the adult is occupied by the accumulation of dorsal and ventral rootlets, collectively known as the **cauda equina** (as well as the non-nervous pial filament, the filum terminale). The space occupied by these structures is an enlarged subarachnoid space, known as the **lumbar cistern**.

DEVELOPMENT OF THE BRAIN

During early development the brain is subdivided into three morphologically recognizable components: the prosencephalon, mesencephalon, and rhombencephalon

During early development the primary brain divisions —the rhombencephalon, mesencephalon, and prosencephalon (from caudal to rostral)—were established, as were the three flexures, the cephalic, cervical, and pontine flexures. Since the development of the rhombencephalon is similar to that of the spinal cord discussed above, the embryology of the brain will be detailed in the reverse order to permit a more logical approach to its study. Table 2.4 summarizes the adult structures derived from the three primary divisions (Fig. 2.6).

Myelencephalon

The posteriormost region of the developing brain is the myelencephalon

The **myelencephalon** gives rise to the medulla oblongata, the rostral continuation of the spinal cord. During the development of the myelencephalon, the pontine flexure arises, and appears to stretch the roof plate, which becomes a thin epithelial layer. The alar plates of the two sides move farther away from one another,

Table 2.4 ● Derivatives of the primary brain divisions.

Primary brain divisions	Derivatives of the divisions
Rhombencephalon (hindbrain)	
Myelencephalon	Medulla oblongata
	Inferior cerebellar peduncles
	Fourth ventricle (caudal aspect)
Metencephalon	Pons
	Cerebellum
	Middle and superior cerebellar peduncles
	Fourth ventricle (rostral aspect)
Mesencephalon (midbrain)	Cerebral peduncles
	Tectum
	Tegmentum
	Cerebral aqueduct (of Sylvius)
Prosencephalon (forebrain)	
Diencephalon	Epithalamus
	Thalamus
	Hypothalamus (caudal aspect)
	Third ventricle (caudal aspect)
Telencephalon	Cerebral hemispheres
	Cerebral cortex
	Corpus striatum
	Hypothalamus (rostral aspect)
	Third ventricle (rostral aspect)
	Lateral ventricles

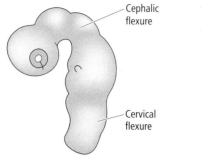

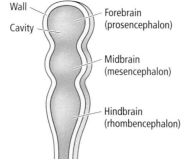

Human brain at 6 mm

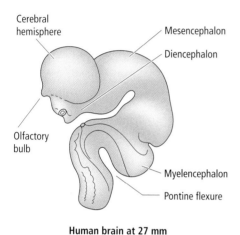

Human brain at 27 mm

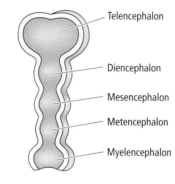

Figure 2.6 ● Three-dimensional representation of the human brain (left) and its longitudinal section (right; as if the brain were stretched out) at 6 and 27 mm of development. Note that the three primary brain divisions of the 6 mm embryo give rise to the five divisions of the 27 mm embryo.

and the intervening cavity of the hindbrain becomes the caudal aspect of the **fourth ventricle** (Fig. 2.7). The junction between the dorsal edge of the alar plates and the roof plate is known as the **rhombic lip**, composed of an inferior and a superior rhombic lip (located in the myelencephalon and metencephalon, respectively). Nuclei of cranial nerves VIII through XII as well as part of the nucleus of the trigeminal nerve (CN V) are formed from the alar (sensory neurons) and basal plates (motor neurons). Also, neuroblasts from the alar plate migrate ventrally to become the neurons constituting the **inferior olivary nuclei** (as well as the **nucleus gracilis** and **nucleus cuneatus**). Subsequent to the establishment of the nuclei fiber tracts will appear, the most pronounced of which are the **pyramids**.

Metencephalon

The nuclei of cranial nerves VI and VII as well as the remaining portion of cranial nerve V arise from the alar and basal plates of the **metencephalon**. Moreover, two important, large structures develop from cells migrating from the alar plates of the metencephalon. One group of cells migrates ventrally to form the **pontine nuclei**, whereas the other group migrates to the superior rhombic lip to form the **cerebellum**.

The rostral-most portion of the rhombencephalon is the metencephalon

Three groups of motoneurons develop from the **basal plates** of the metencephalon: the **somatic efferent** (gives rise to the nucleus of the abducent nerve), **general visceral efferent** (parasympathetic fibers for the facial nerve), and **special visceral efferent** (gives rise to the motor nuclei of the trigeminal and facial nerves, which will innervate muscles of branchiomeric origin, the first and second branchial arches).

Three groups of sensory nuclei develop from the **alar plates** of the metencephalon: the **somatic afferent** (neurons of the trigeminal and some neurons of the vestibulocochlear nerves), **general visceral afferent**, and **special visceral afferent**.

Cerebellum

The inferior aspect of the two rhombic lips thickens to form the right and left cerebellar plates that will fuse with one another to develop into the two cerebellar hemispheres

As neurons of the alar plate undergo intense mitotic activity, their proliferation causes an expansion of each rhombic lip (the dorsolateral aspect of the neural tube). As the inferior aspect of the rhombic lip forms a bulge in the wall of the fourth ventricle its superior aspect increases greatly in size, and these two thickenings are known as the **cerebellar plates**

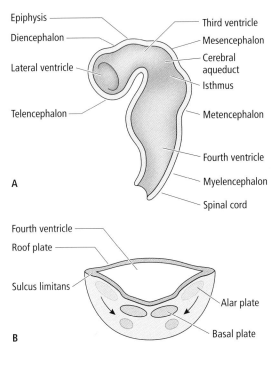

A

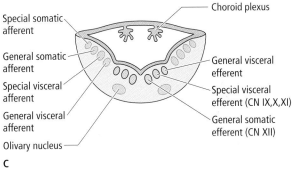

B

C

Figure 2.7 ● Diagrams of the developing nervous system. (A) Longitudinal section of the brain and spinal cord of an 11 mm embryo. (B) Transverse section of the myelencephalon of an early embryo depicting the alar and basal plates. The arrows indicate the migration of cells from the alar plates to form the future olivary nuclei. (C) Transverse section of a later stage of the myelencephalon depicting the development of nuclei from the alar and basal plates.

(Fig. 2.8). The cerebellar plates of the right and left side grow toward each other and fuse in the midline, each half forming the future cerebellar hemispheres. The inferior aspect of the cerebellar plates will become greatly reduced in size and remain as the roof over the ventricle; in the adult it forms the **vermis**. During the process of cerebellar formation, neuroblasts enter the marginal layer and form the cerebellar cortex. The huge number of cells that are being formed cause folding of the cortex into leaf-like structures called **folia**. Neuroblasts that remain in the mantle layer of the forming cerebellum also proliferate to form the **dentate** and **deep cerebellar nuclei**. Axons to and from the cerebellar cortex form very large tracts, such as the superior, middle, and inferior cerebellar peduncles and the corticopontocerebellar pathway.

Mesencephalon

The mesencephalon is the midbrain and surrounds the cerebral aqueduct (of Sylvius)

The **mesencephalon** is situated rostral to the pons and is the region of the midbrain flexure. Its wall becomes quite thick, obliterating much of the central lumen, which becomes a narrow cleft—the **cerebral aqueduct (of Sylvius)** connecting the third and fourth ventricles. The alar plates give rise to the **tectum**, composed of the **superior** and **inferior colliculi**, which are reflex centers for visual and auditory signals, respectively. Additionally, the alar plate is believed to give rise to the **periaqueductal gray**. The basal plate is responsible for the formation of the **tegmentum**, whose **red nucleus** and **substantia nigra**, along with the nuclei of the **oculomotor** and **trochlear nerves**, arise from its neuroblasts. With continued development of the cerebral cortex the ventral aspect of the mesencephalon thickens considerably, forming the **cerebral peduncles**, fiber tracts leading to and from the cerebral cortex.

Prosencephalon

The **prosencephalon** is the forebrain and is divided into two regions, the diencephalon and the prosencephalon.

Diencephalon

The diencephalon, the caudal part of the forebrain, gives rise to the epithalamus, thalamus, and hypothalamus

The three regions of the **diencephalon**—the epithalamus, thalamus, and hypothalamus—form as three separate bulges in the walls of the **third ventricle**. The habenular nuclei and the pineal body form the **epithalamus**. The largest portion of the diencephalon, the **thalamus**, is separated from the underlying hypothalamus by the hypothalamic sulcus, a transverse groove in the wall of the third ventricle. The close functional association of the thalamus with the cerebral cortex necessitates a synchronous developmental association between these two structures. As nuclei within the thalamus (medial and lateral geniculate bodies, as well as the medial, lateral, anterior, and ventral thalamic nuclei) increase in size, they bulge into the third ventricle, decreasing its size. Frequently, the nuclei of the right and left thalami fuse at a small region across the third ventricle, forming the **massa intermedia**. Nuclei within the **hypothalamus** form ventral to the hypothalamic sulcus. These nuclei will be responsible for monitoring and controlling various endocrine and autonomic functions. Additionally, a ventral evagination of the hypothalamus is responsible for the formation of the **median eminence** and the **infundibulum** (see below).

As the diencephalon develops, the roof of the third ventricle becomes extremely thin, so that it is formed only of a layer of ependymal cells and the vascular pia mater. This vascular roof invaginates into the third ventricle, forming the choroid plexus. Although choroid plexuses develop in all of

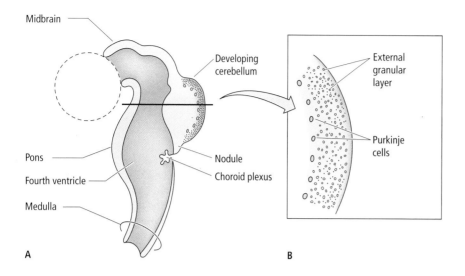

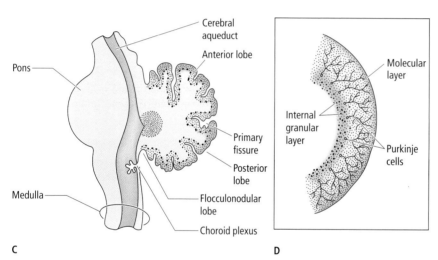

Figure 2.8 ● The developing cerebellum: (A, C) longitudinal sections at 6 and 17 weeks, respectively; (B, D) cellular morphology of the developing cerebellum at 6 weeks and shortly after birth. At 11 weeks the cerebellar plate forms and even Purkinje cell precursors are evident. By the twelfth week the right and left cerebellar hemispheres may be observed, separated from each other by the future vermis. By the seventeenth week of development, folia are apparent and the primary fissure is clearly recognizable.

the ventricles of the brain, their developmental process is identical to that occurring in the third ventricle and is not treated again during the discussions of the other ventricles. Concomitant with the development of this choroid plexus, three bulges become evident on the floor of the third ventricle, and these form the mammillary bodies, the infundibulum, and the optic chiasma.

Pituitary gland

The pituitary gland (hypophysis) is an important endocrine gland that develops from the diencephalon as well as from an evagination, Rathke's pouch, derived from the roof of the oral cavity

The **infundibulum** of the diencephalon is a downward evagination of the floor of the third ventricle. As the infundibulum grows down, it meets an ectodermal diverticulum of the oral cavity, known as **Rathke's pouch**. These two structures fuse with each other to form the **pituitary gland (hypophysis)**. The **neurohypophysis** (median eminence,

stalk, and pars nervosa) arises from the infundibulum, whereas the **adenohypophysis** (pars tuberalis, pars distalis, and pars intermedia) derives from Rathke's pouch (Fig. 2.9). A small colloid-filled cleft frequently remains as a vestige of the lumen of Rathke's pouch, in the pars intermedia.

Eye development

The nervous and pigmented layers of the retina of the eye develop from the evagination of the ventrolateral wall of the diencephalon

During the third week of gestation, the ventrolateral wall on each side of the future diencephalon gives rise to an **optic vesicle**. These hollow vesicles grow in a lateral direction, reach the basal lamina of the head ectoderm, and induce the ectoderm to form the **lens placode**, the precursor of the lens of the eye. The optic vesicle invaginates to form a two-layered structure, known as the **optic cup**, which gives rise to the nervous and pigmented layers of the retina; the connection between the optic cup and the forming brain becomes known

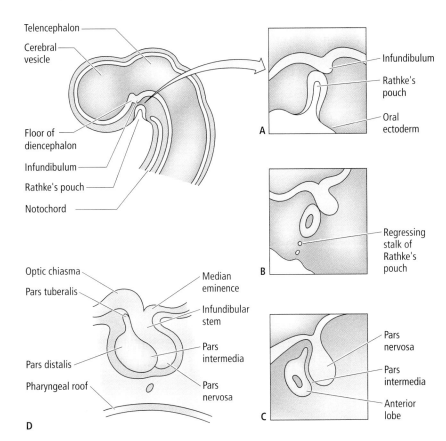

Figure 2.9 ● Development of the pituitary gland (hypophysis). Sagittal section of a 5-week-old embryo displaying the floor of the diencephalon with the beginning of the infundibulum and the roof of the stomadeum, showing its outpocketing, known as Rathke's pouch. (A) By the seventh week of development, Rathke's pouch contacts the infundibulum. (B) Around the ninth week of development, Rathke's pouch loses contact with the stomadeum. (C) Around the tenth week of development, cells of Rathke's pouch proliferate to form the adenohypophysis. (D) The formed pituitary.

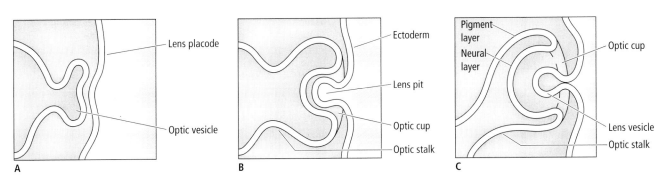

Figure 2.10 ● Development of the eye begins with the outgrowth of the diencephalon, known as the optic vesicle, around the time that the embryo is 4.5 mm long from crown to rump. (A) The optic vesicle induces the ectoderm to form the lens placode. (B) By the time the embryo is 5.5 mm long, the optic vesicle invaginates to form the optic cup and the lens placode differentiates to form the lens pit, which at this point is wide open to the outside. (C) The lens pit begins to form the lens vesicle around the time the embryo is 7.5 mm long and the optic cup forms a two-layered structure, the neural and pigment layers. The optic stalk, which will form the optic nerve, is also being established.

as the **optic stalk** (Fig. 2.10). As axons growing out of the developing retina increase the thickness of the wall of the optic stalk, its lumen becomes obliterated, and the optic stalk becomes known as the **optic nerve**. The optic nerves of the right and left sides join in the midline to form the **optic chiasma**, where axons arising from the medial half of each retina cross over to the opposite side.

As the rim of the optic cup, in contact with the lens placode, encircles the prospective lens to form the **iris**, a slight cleft (**choroid fissure**) remains, permitting the future central artery and vein of the retina access to the retina.

Telencephalon

The anteriormost portion of the prosencephalon, the telencephalon, is mainly responsible for the formation of the cerebral hemispheres

The rostral extent of the neural tube is the **telencephalon**, which extends from the diencephalon to the **lamina terminalis**, the anteriormost boundary of the neural tube. The telencephalon undergoes a tremendous growth spur, forming the two telencephalic vesicles that will overgrow much of the brain by developing into the two **cerebral hemispheres**.

The lumina of the telencephalic vesicles remain as the large, cerebrospinal fluid-filled lateral ventricles. These two ventricles will communicate with each other as well as with the third ventricle via the **interventricular foramen** (of Monro).

Growth of the telencephalic vesicles is asymmetric, in that the lateral expansion, forming the prospective **insula**, enlarges less than do the dorsal, posterior, and medial regions. In fact, some of these regions overgrow and cover the insula and, in the adult, they are named the temporal, frontal, and frontoparietal opercula. The anterior expansion is also slight, forming the future **olfactory bulb**. Continued growth of the telencephalic vesicles within the limited space of the cranial cavity is responsible for the folding of the developing cerebral cortex into elevations called **gyri** and intervening grooves, known as **sulci**. Some of the deeper grooves are named **fissures**; these separate lobes of the cerebral hemispheres from each other.

Major fiber tracts—the **optic chiasma**, **anterior commissure**, and the **corpus callosum**—develop in the region of the lamina terminalis. These fiber tracts connect similar areas of the right and left cerebral hemispheres to each other.

The superior aspect of the telencephalic vesicle, known as the **pallium**, is responsible for the formation of the **cerebral cortex**, a thin layer of gray matter covering the great mass of white matter of the cerebral hemispheres. Neuroblasts of the inferior aspect of the telencephalic vesicles undergo intense mitotic activity, forming a highly cellular region. Due to the large number of axons that pass through this cell-rich area, connecting the cerebral cortex to other regions of the brain and to the spinal cord, this area appears striated and is thus referred to as the **corpus striatum**. Many of these fibers join to form a major fiber tract, the **internal capsule**, that will isolate clusters of cells of the corpus striatum from each other; these cell clusters develop into the **lentiform nucleus** (putamen and globus pallidus) and the **caudate nucleus**.

CLINICAL CONSIDERATIONS

Spinal cord
The most common defect of the neural tube is incomplete fusion of the neural groove, resulting in **spina bifida cystica**. This involves a protrusion of the spinal cord tissue through a bony defect, so that a portion of the nervous tissue is visible on the individual's back as a cyst-like structure. There are various degrees of spina bifida, the worst of which involves mental retardation as well as paralysis below the level of the lesion. Although the cause of this anomaly is not known, there are several agents, such as an excess maternal intake of vitamin A and hyperthermia, that increase its incidence. Newer diagnostic methods, such as ultrasound examination during the eleventh and subsequent weeks of gestation, as well as measuring α-fetoprotein levels in the amniotic fluid, can indicate and detect the presence of spina bifida cystica.

Spinal dermal sinus is a condition that frequently displays the presence of a slight depression, similar to a dimple, in the midline of the sacral region of the back. This slight depression is indicative of the final fusion of the sacral spinal cord level, where the separation of the neural tube from the surface ectoderm was almost incomplete. In fact, occasionally a fibrous cord persists between the dura mater and the dermis just beneath the dimple.

Brain
Hydrocephalus is a condition where the ventricles of the brain or the subarachnoid spaces (in external hydrocephalus) accumulate an excessive amount of cerebrospinal fluid (CSF). In the neonate this is most frequently a result of occlusion of the cerebral aqueduct that hinders the flow of CSF from the third into the fourth ventricle. In very extensive cases, the continued manufacture of CSF by the choroid plexuses of the two lateral and third ventricles increases the fluid volume of the ventricles, resulting in enlargement of the head, reduction in the thickness of the bones of the cranium, and compression of the walls of the ventricles. Such compression may cause lamination of the cerebral cortex resulting in severe mental retardation. A type of hydrocephalus, known as **communicating hydrocephalus**, is caused by the **Arnold–Chiari malformation**. This anomalous condition is characterized by herniation of the

cerebellum and medulla into the foramen magnum, which impedes absorption of CSF, leading to the expansion of the ventricles with subsequent enlargement of the head. Arnold–Chiari malformation usually accompanies severe cases of spina bifida.

Anencephalus is due to the lack of fusion of the anterior neural groove. It is thus similar to spina bifida, in that the nervous tissue (in this case the brain) is open to the environment rather than being enclosed in the bony cranium. Usually the nervous tissue is directly continuous with the skin of the scalp. Frequently vascular agenesis accompanies this condition and much of the forming brain becomes necrotic a few weeks prior to birth.

Microcephaly is a condition with varied causes, such as maternal pelvic X-irradiation, a recessive genetic trait, or infection of the fetus with toxoplasmosis. As the name implies, microcephaly is characterized by a small head and small brain. The cerebral cortex is usually hypocellular with a resultant mental retardation and predisposition to motor disorders and seizures.

Agyri (lissencephaly) is characterized by the absence of fissures and sulci and an indiscriminate arrangement of neurons. This occurs as a result of decreased cellular activity and a consequent diminishing of brain growth.

Corpus callosum agenesis, an infrequent but interesting condition, is characterized by the absence of the corpus callosum, the major communicating pathway between the two cerebral hemispheres. Occasionally the condition is asymptomatic and individuals may be of average IQ. Frequently, however, mental deficiency and the occurrence of tremors and seizures are present.

Holoprosencephaly, defective development of the prosencephalon, may be of varying severity, extending from major malformation of the calvaria, forebrain, and midfacial skeleton to minor malformations involving these regions. The primary etiology of this condition is the consumption of alcohol during the first month or so of pregnancy. It should be stressed that even small quantities of alcohol consumed during this time and even a single instance of "binge" drinking may cause severe retardation and deformations of the midface. The association of alcohol consumption and holoprosencephaly is also referred to as the **fetal alcohol syndrome**.

SYNONYMS AND EPONYMS OF THE NERVOUS SYSTEM

Name of structure or term	Synonym(s)/ eponym(s)
Alar plate	Dorsolateral lamina
Basal plate	Ventrolateral lamina
Cerebral aqueduct	Aqueduct of Sylvius
Embryoblast	Inner cell mass
Floor plate	Ventral lamina
Hyoid arch	Second pharyngeal arch
Interventricular foramen	Foramen of Monro
Mandibular arch	First pharyngeal arch
Mantle layer	Intermediate zone
Marginal layer	Marginal zone
Mesencephalon	Midbrain
Pharyngeal arches	Branchial arches
Pharyngeal grooves	Branchial grooves
Pharyngeal membrane	Closing plate
Pharyngeal pouches	Branchial pouches
Primitive node	Hensen's node
Prosencephalon	Forebrain
Rhombencephalon	Hindbrain
Roof plate	Dorsal lamina
Unipolar neurons	Pseudounipolar neurons
Ventricular zone	Ependymal layer (matrix cell layer)

FOLLOW-UP TO CLINICAL CASE

This newborn has a myelomeningocele, generically known as **spina bifida**. A myelomeningocele is one of the disorders in a group of conditions known as neural tube defects, otherwise known as dysraphism. A neural tube defect can occur along any part of the developing CNS. When it affects the region that should eventually become the brain it is known as anencephaly, meaning the brain is literally absent. However, it most commonly affects the most caudal portion and becomes know as spina bifida. There is failure of closure and neurulation of the neural tube. This occurs during the first few weeks of gestation.

Spina bifida cystica refers to an open spinal defect where nervous tissue and/or meninges protrude from a defect in the vertebral column and are exposed to the outside environment on the surface of the back. A myelomeningocele is an open defect where the spinal cord and meninges are exposed and often form a tumor-like mass in the midline just above the buttock. **Spina bifida occulta** refers to a closed spinal defect where skin covers the defect, and the spinal cord and meninges are within the defective vertebral column. A closed spinal defect is obviously milder than an open one. An overlying cutaneous abnormality, such as a tuft of hair or hemangioma, or a subcutaneous lipoma (a benign fatty tumor) may betray an underlying closed spinal defect. Both give rise to neurologic deficits, though those with open spinal defects are already present at birth and tend to be severe. Neurologic deficits such as leg weakness, sensory deficits in the legs, and urinary incontinence can occur much later in a closed spinal defect. This can present any time from early childhood to adulthood. It often occurs secondary to a tethered cord syndrome (a low-lying conus medullaris related to anchoring of the spinal cord or filum terminale to surrounding tissues).

A myelomeningocele needs to be surgically repaired within 48 hours of birth. The mortality rate from infection or other complications would otherwise be near 100%. A downward herniation of the cerebellum through the foramen magnum is always present (Chiari II malformation). Hydrocephalus may also be present and both of these conditions may require surgery. Orthopedic malformations of the hip and/or feet often occur and may need to be corrected surgically.

Folic acid supplement very early in pregnancy decreases the incidence of neural tube defects, although the reason is unclear. The incidence is decreasing in the Western world, though it is still a common fetal malformation.

QUESTIONS TO PONDER

1. What is the importance of the transformation of the embryoblast of the blastocyst into the trilaminar germ disc?

2. What is the significance of Hensen's node?

3. What is the significance of homeobox genes?

4. What is the significance of the cellular arrangement of the developing neural tube?

5. What is the similarity between the development of the pituitary gland and the eye?

CHAPTER 3

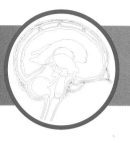
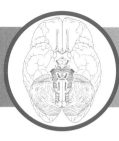
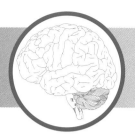

Histophysiology of the Nervous System

CLINICAL CASE

A 32-year-old man complains of numbness and tingling in his left arm which began 5 days ago. He has also noted some recent "staggering" when walking and he feels quite off balance. There is no dizziness or weakness. He knows of no precipitating event. He has no other complaints. Upon asking about past history, he recalls that about 3 years ago he had an episode of bilateral leg paralysis and poor sensation in the legs. This improved over the course of 2 months and his legs got back to normal. No specific etiology was found at that time. He has not followed up with a doctor.

Examination shows sensory loss and altered sensation to stimulation in the left distal upper extremity and hand. Finger movements in both hands show poor coordination, somewhat more so on the left, but there is no weakness found in the face, arms, or legs. Gait is mildly ataxic. He cannot walk heel to toe in a straight line. Reflexes in the arms are normal, and are brisk at the knees and ankles but not necessarily pathologically so. Neurologic exam is otherwise unremarkable.

Aside from the meninges, vascular supply, and minor connective tissue elements, the central nervous system (CNS) is composed only of cells. These are categorized into two types: **neurons**, which receive and transmit impulses, and **neuroglia**, which support and facilitate the proper functioning of the neurons. A collection of neurons within the CNS is referred to as a **nucleus** (not to be confused with the nucleus of a cell), whereas a collection of neurons in the peripheral nervous system (PNS) is known as a **ganglion**.

Neurons form **reflex arcs**, where information from the periphery is carried by a sensory neuron to the CNS, and is directly transmitted to a motoneuron for a motor response. This is the simplest reflex arc because it involves only two neurons. An example of a **two cell reflex arc** is the patellar reflex (knee jerk). Most reflex arcs are **three or more cell reflex arcs**, since they include a third neuron, the **interneuron**, interposed between the sensory neuron and the motoneuron. The reflex response associated with a three cell reflex may be overridden when the interneuron receives an input from higher centers of the brain that prevent it from transmitting the information from the sensory neuron to the motoneuron.

Neurons communicate with each other as well as with other target cells through specialized cell junctions, known as **synapses**. There are two types of synapse. They may be **electrical (gap junctions)**, where ions or small molecules may go from one cell into another cell by traversing small, contiguous channels present in the cell membranes of the two cells. The other type are **chemical**, where one cell releases ligands (e.g., neurotransmitters) into a narrow intercellular space, known as the synaptic cleft, and the ligand binds to receptors of the other cell's membrane, initiating the desired result.

Neuroglia are located both in the CNS and in the PNS. They act to support the neuron, both physically and nutritionally, to protect the neuron by forming an insulating sheath around it and its processes, as well as to isolate the neuron and its processes from the external milieu. It is interesting to note that the number of neuroglia far outnumber the number of neurons.

NEURONS

A neuron is composed of a cell body, also known as a soma or perikaryon, and one or more processes, known as dendrites and a single axon

The neuron has two regions, the **cell body (perikaryon, soma)** and neuronal processes called **dendrites** and **axons** (Fig. 3.1); a neuron may possess several dendrites but it has only a single axon. Dendrites and axons frequently possess a higher percentage of the neuron's cytoplasm than does the soma, due to the large number of dendrites per neuron as well as due to the, possibly, great length of the axon.

Soma

The soma houses the nucleus and many of the organelles of the neuron

The size and morphology of the cell body vary and are specific to the particular region of the nervous system. The most prominent feature of the **soma** is the **nucleus**, which is usually round to oval, centrally placed, and possesses a fine chromatin network and a well-defined nucleolus. The **cytoplasm** of the perikaryon is rich in **free ribosomes** and **rough endoplasmic reticulum** (RER), whose cisternae form numerous close, parallel configurations which, when viewed with light microscopy, stain dark blue with acidophilic stains and are frequently referred to as Nissl bodies. Protein synthesis occurs on both free ribosomes for use in the cytosol and on the RER for eventual packaging. The **Golgi complex** is usually near the nucleus and is responsible for the modification and packaging of the various proteins, enzymes, and chemical messenger molecules manufactured on the RER. Numerous profiles of **smooth endoplasmic reticulum** (SER) are also present in the neuronal cytoplasm. Many of these are located just deep to the plasmalemma as **hypolemmal cisternae**, believed to be responsible for the sequestering of calcium. The energy requirement of the neuron is met by the presence of numerous **mitochondria**, which are distributed throughout the cell body. As such, protein synthesis, respiration, and many of the essential cellular functions occur in this region of the cell (Fig. 3.2). The cell body is also rich in endosomes and lysosomes, as well as various types of vesicles that are being ferried to and from the processes.

The cell body also contains numerous **inclusions**, nonliving substances such as melanin pigments, lipofuscin, and lipid droplets. Melanin pigments are present in cells only in

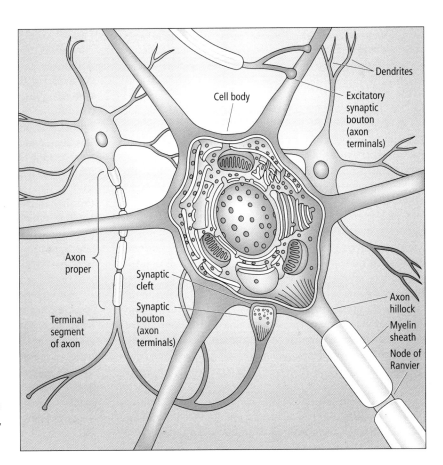

Figure 3.1 ● Diagram of a multipolar neuron. Note that the processes of other neurons make synaptic contacts with it. Synapses may be formed, as illustrated, with the soma or with the dendrites, although other types of synapses also occur.

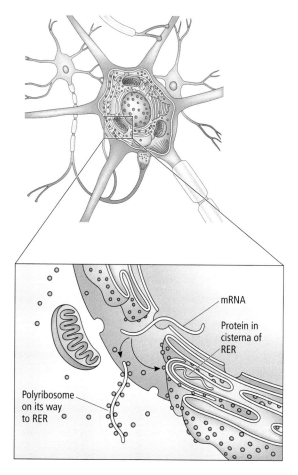

Figure 3.2 • Section of a multipolar neuron displaying a messenger RNA, transcribed from the DNA, leaving the nucleus, picking up ribosomes to form a polysome and proceeding to the rough endoplasmic reticulum (RER). On the surface of the RER the mRNA is translated and proteins, destined to be packaged into vesicles, are synthesized and funneled into the lumen of the RER.

certain locations, such as the locus cereus and the substantia nigra, but their function in these cells is not known. Lipofuscin is believed to be the indigestible remains of lysosomal activity and, since it is known to increase as a function of age, it is frequently referred to as "age pigment." Lipid droplets are present in the cytoplasm of neurons, and in other cells, as a form of energy reserve.

Cytoskeletal components of neurons consist of microfilaments, neurofilaments, and microtubules. **Microfilaments**, composed mostly of filamentous actin, are associated mainly with the cell membrane and aid in axon or dendrite elongation and in the movement of the plasmalemma. **Neurofilaments** are intermediate filaments that frequently become clumped during preparation for light microscopy, forming long filamentous threads known as **neurofibrils** (less than 2 μm in diameter). Neurofilaments assist in the regeneration and development of axons and dendrites. **Microtubules** are long, rigid, flexible structures that possess microtubule-associated proteins (such as MAP-2 in the cytoplasm and dendrites and MAP-3 in the axon). Microtubules provide a scaffold-like structure to maintain cell shape and aid in the transport of materials to and from the soma.

Dendrites

Dendrites are short, branching processes of neurons that may house some organelles and transmit impulses toward the cell body

Dendrites, whose proximal region may house organelles, such as RER, SER, mitochondria, and vesicles, are relatively short, branching extensions of the cell body. Each neuron may have a number of dendrites, each of which receives signals from specialized receptors, axons, or other neurons and transmits these signals *toward* the cell body. Often the surface of some dendrites is increased due to the presence of **dendritic spines**, permitting the presence of a greater number of synapses. Moreover, since dendrites are usually highly branched structures they may receive information concurrently from many different sources

Axons

Each neuron has only a single axon, which originates from the organelle-free region of the soma, known as the axon hillock, that appears unstained in light microscopic preparations

The axon is divided into three regions: the initial segment, the axon proper, and the axon terminals. The **initial segment** is the short transition (30–50 μm in length) between the **axon hillock** and the axon proper. A characteristic feature of the initial segment is the thickening on the axoplasmic aspect of the axolemma (axon membrane) that is believed to be indicative of the presence of voltage-gated sodium channels. The initial segment is the primary region of the axon responsible for the *initiation and propagation of action potentials.*

The **axon proper** is a long process (in some instances exceeding 100 cm in length), whose diameter, which may be as great as 15–20 μm, remains constant for much of its length. Axons may possess a **myelin** covering (see below) that begins at the axon proper and stops at the axon terminal. The myelin sheath is elaborated in discontinuous segments, and each myelinated segment is called an **internode**. The discontinuities of myelin between adjacent internodes are referred to as **nodes of Ranvier**. Occasionally the axon proper has branches, known as **collaterals**, that diverge from the main axon at right angles. At its terminus the axon may arborize, forming numerous **axon terminals** (also known as **bouton terminaux** and **end feet**), which permits a single axon to make synaptic contact (see below) with numerous other neurons (or muscle or gland cells). The axoplasm does not possess ribosomes or RER, although mitochondria, SER, vesicles, neurofilaments, and microtubules are present.

Material produced in the soma is transported, via the assistance of microtubules and their microtubule-associated proteins, to the axon for its use. Such transport is referred to as **anterograde transport**. Material, such as horseradish peroxidase, may be conveyed in the opposite direction, toward the cell body, and this process is referred to as **retrograde transport**. Collectively, anterograde and retrograde transports are referred to as **axonal transport**, a process that is dependent on the presence of the ATPase molecular motors dynein and kinesin. The former is responsible for retrograde

Transport type	Transport rate (mm/day)	Substance being transported
Anterograde (slow component a)	0.1–1.0	Tubulins, microtubule associated proteins, neurofilament proteins
Anterograde (slow component b)	1.0–10	Enzymes, proteins, clathrin, myosin, actin
Anterograde (fast, using **kinesin**)	50–500	Organelles (vesicles, mitochondria, secretory granules)
Retrograde (fast, using **dynein**)	200–300	Enzymes, proteins, lysosomes, horseradish peroxidase

Table 3.1 ● Axonal transport.

transport, whereas the latter functions in anterograde transport. Table 3.1 details the types and velocity of transport and the substances being transported. Axonal transport is essential for the health of the muscle cell or the gland that is being innervated. If this **trophic relationship** is interrupted, the muscle or gland atrophies.

Synapses

The synapse is a specialized intercellular junction that permits communication between neurons in the CNS or a neuron and an effector cell (another neuron, muscle cell, or gland cell) in the PNS

A **synapse** may be **electrical** with a synaptic cleft width of 2–4 nm or **chemical** with a synaptic cleft width of 20–30 nm. In an electrical synapse ions are exchanged via gap junctions, whereas in a chemical synapse **messenger molecules (ligands)** are housed in **synaptic vesicles** and are released into the synaptic cleft. These messenger molecules are of two types, namely **neurotransmitters** and **neuromodulators**, and they are released from the axon terminal to depolarize (or hyperpolarize) the membrane of the effector cell. Since electrical synapses are seldom present in mammals (except in the retina, cerebral cortex, and brainstem), only chemical synapses will be discussed in this textbook and the reader is referred to a textbook of histology or cell biology to become familiar with the structure of gap junctions.

There are several types of possible synaptic contacts within the CNS (Fig. 3.3), depending upon the regions of the neurons involved (e.g., axoaxonic, axosomatic, axodendritic, dendrodendritic), the most common being the axodendritic, where the axon of one neuron synapses with the dendrite of another neuron. In all chemical synapses the "message" travels across the synaptic cleft to the effector cell, giving rise to the terminology: presynaptic cell (the neuron releasing the messenger molecules) and postsynaptic cell (the effector cell). Thus there are three major functional components of a synapse, namely the **presynaptic membrane**, the **synaptic cleft**, and the **postsynaptic membrane**. These membranes are specialized so that the messenger molecules contained in the synaptic vesicles are released at the proper sites (**active sites**) on the presynaptic membrane, and so that they bind to receptor molecules located at specific sites of the post-

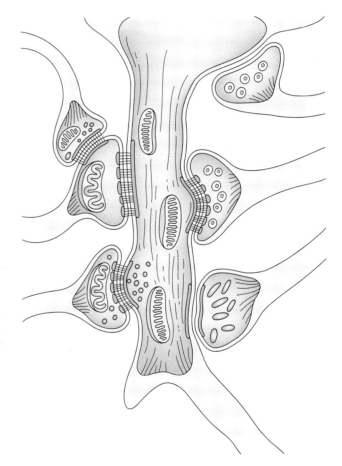

Figure 3.3 ● Synapses along a dendrite. Note that one of the axon terminals (terminal boutons, end-feet) has an axon terminal impinging on it, probably acting in an inhibitory capacity. (Modified from Williams, PL, ed. (1998) *Gray's Anatomy*, 38th edn. Churchill Livingstone, London; fig. 7.19b.)

synaptic membrane. When seen in electron micrographs, the cytoplasmic aspect of either one of these membranes frequently displays a filamentous electron density known as the **presynaptic density** or **postsynaptic density**. Depending on the arrangement of these submembrane densities, the synapses are said to be either **type I** or **type II** (Table 3.2). Type I synapses are also known as **asymmetric synapses** since their postsynaptic density is thicker than their

Characteristic	Type I synapse	Type II synapse
Submembrane density	Asymmetric (thin presynaptic and thick postsynaptic density)	Symmetric (thin presynaptic and thin postsynaptic density)
Synaptic vesicle morphology	Round (50 nm in diameter)	Flattened (15–40 nm)
Synaptic cleft width	30 nm	20 nm
Functional type	Excitatory	Inhibitory

Table 3.2 ● Types of synapses.

presynaptic density. Type II synapses are also referred to as **symmetric synapses** since the two densities are of equal thickness. Usually, type I synapses possess round synaptic vesicles whereas type II synapses possess flattened synaptic vesicles. Generally, type I synapses are excitatory, so that the membrane of the effector cell becomes depolarized, initiating an **excitatory postsynaptic potential (EPSP)**. Conversely, type II synapses are usually inhibitory, initiating an **inhibitory postsynaptic potential (IPSP)** so that the membrane of the effector cell becomes hyperpolarized, causing it to be less responsive to attempts at depolarization.

Axon terminal and presynaptic membrane

The axon terminal is the region that participates in synapse formation; the area of the plasmalemma of the axon terminal that contacts the synaptic cleft is known as the presynaptic membrane

The cytoplasm of the **axon terminal** is rich in cytoskeletal elements, such as microtubules, neurofilaments, spectrin, and microfilaments. Additionally, it also houses cisternae of SER, coated vesicles, occasional endosomes, a number of mitochondria, and numerous synaptic vesicles. **Synaptic vesicles** are membrane-bound vesicles whose membranes contain numerous unique integral proteins that assist in binding the vesicles to specific sites within the axon terminal. They contain chemical messengers (ligands, neurotransmitter molecules), ATP, and some proteoglycans, all of which are destined to be released into the synaptic cleft. Some of these synaptic vesicles are held in reserve away from the active site, whereas others are located at the active site.

The submembrane density on the cytoplasmic aspect of the **presynaptic membrane** is composed of globular to oblong electron-dense subunits that are arranged in a hexagonal array at the active site (Fig. 3.4). These oblong structures are protein complexes, known as **docking complexes**, which form a **presynaptic grid** whose interstices are just large enough to accept synaptic vesicles but prevent these vesicles from contacting the presynaptic membrane.

Most synaptic vesicles are held in reserve, away from the active site. However, some are bound (*docked*) to the docking complex so that when an action potential arrives at the axon terminal they are ready to fuse with the presynaptic membrane, open into the synaptic cleft, and release their messenger molecules.

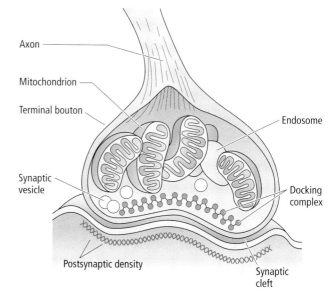

Figure 3.4 ● An axon terminal (terminal bouton) forming a synapse. Note that the synaptic vesicles are in close relationship with the docking complexes of the presynaptic membrane. The axon terminal also houses mitochondria and endosomes.

The arrival of an action potential at the presynaptic membrane opens **voltage-gated calcium channels** located at the active site (possibly as a part of the docking complex), permitting the influx of Ca^{2+} ions into the axon terminal (Fig. 3.5). The presence of Ca^{2+} ions permits the fusion of the membrane of the *docked* synaptic vesicle with the presynaptic membrane and the subsequent release of its messenger molecules into the synaptic cleft. Precise control of calcium availability is necessary to ensure that only the required amount of messenger molecules are released as the consequence of a single action potential.

The sequestering of Ca^{2+} ions is performed by at least three mechanisms:

1 A cytosolic protein binds Ca^{2+} ions in the vicinity of the presynaptic membrane.
2 Calcium storage vesicles located in the axon terminal possess Ca^{2+} pumps that remove Ca^{2+} ions from the end-foot cytosol.

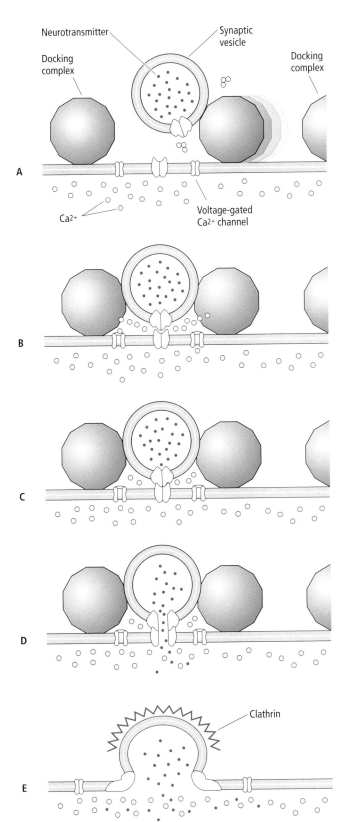

3   Na^+/Ca^{2+}-coupled transporters in the axon terminal membrane exchange extracellular Na^+ ions for cytosolic Ca^{2+} ions.

These three mechanisms act in conjunction with each other to control Ca^{2+} availability at the active site (Fig. 3.6).

Continued synaptic vesicle fusion with and incorporation into the presynaptic membrane would enlarge the axon terminal; therefore, the excess membrane is recaptured by the formation of **clathrin-coated pits**. The pits form clathrin-coated vesicles and the captured membranes are returned to the cytosol. They travel as **endocytic vesicles**, possibly along microtubule-marked pathways. These vesicles lose their clathrin coat before fusing with the elements of SER to be recycled in the formation of new synaptic vesicles.

Since the flow of Ca^{2+} ions into the axon terminal is very important for the release of the messenger molecules into the synaptic cleft, a method of diminishing its entry into the end-foot has evolved in mammals, a process known as **presynaptic inhibition**. This process occurs in areas where an axon forms a synapse with the axon terminal of another axon (Fig. 3.7). Hence, there are three neurons involved at this location:

1   The axon terminal of neuron A contacting the axon terminal of neuron B.
2   The axon terminal of neuron B that contacts neuron C.
3   The dendrite (or soma) of neuron C.

The axon terminal of neuron A releases a chemical messenger destined for Cl^- ion channels of the axon terminal of neuron B. The binding of the ligands opens Cl^- ion channels causing an influx of Cl^- ions into the axon terminal of neuron B, hyperpolarizing its presynaptic membrane and making it much more difficult to open its voltage-gated Ca^{2+} ion channels. This event makes it less likely that neuron B will be able to release its chemical messengers intended for neuron C, and it is this inhibition of the activity of neuron B that is referred to as presynaptic inhibition.

Synaptic cleft and postsynaptic membrane

The space located between the presynaptic membrane and the postsynaptic membrane is known as the synaptic cleft

The **synaptic cleft** is a 20–30 nm wide extracellular space between the presynaptic and postsynaptic membranes. This space contains diverse

Figure 3.5 ● Synaptic vesicles are held in reserve by docking complexes near the active sites of the presynaptic membrane. (A) Voltage-gated calcium channels of the presynaptic membrane are closed and the synaptic vesicle does not contact the presynaptic membrane. (B, C) The arrival of an action potential opens the voltage-gated calcium channels; the influx of calcium ions permits the proper alignment of the synaptic vesicle with the presynaptic membrane by inducing slight rearrangements of both the docking complexes and the synaptic vesicle. (D) Once aligned properly, the synaptic vesicle fuses with the presynaptic membrane, opens, and releases its contents into the synaptic space. (E) To prevent an increase in the area of the presynaptic membrane, the excess membrane is recaptured as clathrin-coated pits and the membranes are recycled in the cytosol. (Modified from Kingsley, RE (1996) *Concise Text of Neuroscience.* Williams & Wilkins, Baltimore; p. 96.)

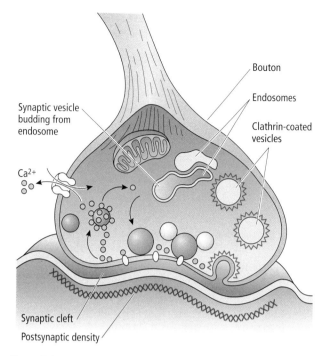

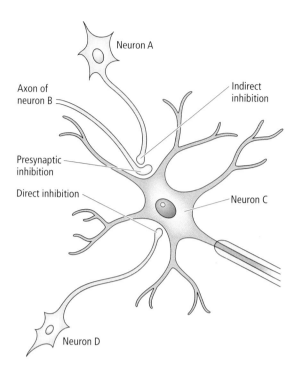

Figure 3.6 ● Some synaptic vesicles are formed in the soma and are transported into the axon terminal, whereas others are formed locally in the end-foot by budding from endosomes, and still others form via endocytosis of the presynaptic membrane. In order to prevent a constant release of neurotransmitters, the calcium level is reduced in the axon terminal by being actively exchanged for Na^+, by being sequestered in the smooth endoplasmic reticulum, as well as by being bound to cytoplasmic proteins. Furthermore, to maintain a constant size of the presynaptic membrane as it is enlarged by fusion of the synaptic vesicles with it, it is reduced by endocytosis via the formation of clathrin-coated vesicles that will then either join the endosomes or will form new synaptic vesicles.

Figure 3.7 ● Diagram depicting the difference between direct and indirect inhibition. Note that in direct inhibition, neuron D forms a synapse with the large multipolar neuron C, permitting transmission of information directly. In indirect inhibition, neuron A forms a synapse with the axon of neuron B and it is that other neuron that synapses with the large multipolar neuron C; thus the information is transmitted indirectly.

families of macromolecules, some of which appear to be filamentous and span the entire width of the synaptic cleft. Many of these macromolecules are believed to be the extra-cytoplasmic aspects of the various transmembrane proteins of the presynaptic and postsynaptic membranes, whereas others are molecules of the extracellular matrix. It has been demonstrated that many of these synaptic cleft proteins are necessary to maintain a rigorous alignment of the active sites of the presynaptic membrane with those regions of the post-synaptic membrane that house receptor molecules designed to bind the released chemical messengers. These chemical substances, released in predetermined quantities, known as **quanta** (as many as 20,000 molecules), cross the synaptic cleft and bind to specific receptor molecules of the postsynaptic membrane. Each synaptic vesicle contains one quantum of chemical messenger molecules, which is the minimum amount necessary to precipitate a single postsynaptic event (**depolarization** or **hyperpolarization**).

The **postsynaptic membrane** is a region of the effector cell plasmalemma that is modified to receive and react to the chemical messenger (ligand) released into the synaptic cleft. Binding of the ligand results in the opening of ion channels

with subsequent depolarization or hyperpolarization of the effector cell plasmalemma. The submembrane density of the postsynaptic membrane is connected, via thin filamentous material, to an abundance of intertwined cytoskeletal ele-ments, the subsynaptic **web**. The cytosol in the immediate vicinity of the subsynaptic web houses, among others, micro-tubules, microfilaments, SER and, frequently, RER along with numerous mitochondria. The cytosol also contains enzymes such as protein kinase C and calmodulin-dependent kinase II. The postsynaptic membrane houses two major types of receptors: ionotropic and metabotropic receptors.

1 **Ionotropic receptors** are ligand-gated ion channels and the chemical messengers that bind to them are known as **neurotransmitters**. The binding of a neurotransmitter alters the conformation of the protein constituting the ion channel, opening it and permitting the flow of ions through it. Thus, a neurotransmitter is a chemical messen-ger that has a *direct* effect on the ion channel and the effect is *rapid*.

2 **Metabotropic receptors** bind chemical messengers known as **neuromodulators** or **neurohormones**. These molecules also interact with a receptor molecule, causing a conformational change in its protein(s); however, this receptor molecule is not an ion channel. Instead, this receptor molecule interacts with other protein complexes,

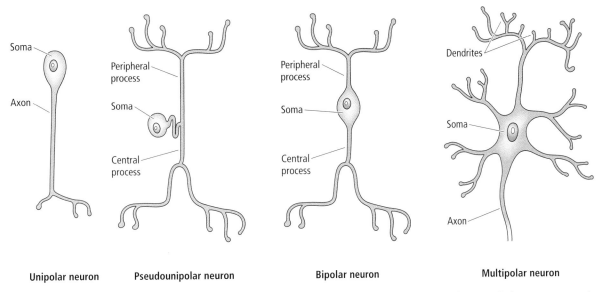

Figure 3.8 ● Neurons are classified into different categories depending on the number of processes they possess. Note that true unipolar neurons are rare in humans and that pseudounipolar neurons are also referred to as unipolar neurons.

such as **G-proteins**. G-proteins in turn interact with one of the cell's secondary messenger systems, thus modulating the metabolic activities of the effector cell. In this fashion the required response occurs as an *indirect* function of the coupling of the ligand to the receptor and the effect is *slow*.

The above two points are true in most instances, but there are exceptions. The following generalization should therefore be appreciated, namely that *neurotransmitters have a direct influence*, whereas *neuromodulators and neurohormones have an indirect influence* in effecting the desired result. It is also important to realize that the same chemical messenger may elicit different responses depending on the type of ionotropic or metabotropic receptor with which it is associated. The various types of neurotransmitters and neuromodulators are discussed in Chapter 4.

Classification of neurons

The number of processes a neuron possesses permits a classification of these cells into the following categories: unipolar, bipolar, multipolar, and pseudounipolar neurons (Fig. 3.8). **Unipolar neurons** are rare in vertebrates; they possess no dendrites, only an axon. **Bipolar neurons**, such as the ones in the olfactory mucosa, possess an axon and a dendrite, whereas **multipolar neurons**, such as the motoneurons of the spinal cord, have a single axon and two or more dendrites. An additional type of neuron, the **pseudounipolar neuron** (also referred to as **unipolar neurons** in vertebrates) start out, during embryogenesis, as bipolar neurons. The axon and dendrite of this neuron fuse into a single process that later bifurcates. Neurons of the dorsal root ganglia and the ganglia of cranial nerves are representatives of this category.

NEUROGLIA

The five types of neuroglia are the supporting cells of the central and peripheral nervous systems

There are five types of supporting cells associated with the nervous system, four in the CNS (astroglia, oligoden-droglia, microglia, and ependymal cells) and one in the PNS (Schwann cells) (Table 3.3). Neuroglia of the CNS are usually smaller and about 10 times more numerous than neurons.

Astrocytes are stellate-shaped cells with numerous, long processes that extend between and among the neurons and vascular elements occupying much of the extracellular spaces of the CNS. Their processes surround all neural elements and also form gap junctions with one another. Additionally, astrocytes form a **perivascular covering** around blood vessels as well as a **glial-limiting membrane** at the interface of the brain and pia mater. There are two types of astrocytes: **fibrous astrocytes**, located in white matter, and **protoplasmic astrocytes**, located in gray matter. Both types of astrocytes are characterized by the unique **glial fibrillary acidic protein** (GFAP) intermediate filaments contained in their cytoplasm. Astrocytes are believed to:

- provide physical and nutritional support to the neurons of the CNS;
- sequester Na^+ and K^+ ions from the extracellular space;
- isolate neurons from each other;
- metabolize extracellular neurotransmitters, such as serotonin, gamma aminobutyric acid (GABA), and glutamate;
- form glial scar tissue in an attempt to repair damage to the CNS; and
- form a framework along which developing neurons migrate to their destination during embryogenesis.

Oligodendroglia are small cells that possess only a few processes and their cytoplasm is devoid of GFAP. They are

Neuroglia	Origin	Location	Function
Protoplasmic astrocyte	Neural tube	CNS, gray matter	Support and isolate neurons; sequester Na$^+$ ions; metabolize extracellular neurotransmitters; repair damage to CNS by forming glial scar tissue; surround unmyelinated axons; in the embryo they establish pathways along which neurons migrate
Fibrous astrocyte	Neural tube	CNS, white matter	Same as protoplasmic astrocyte
Oligodendroglia	Neural tube	CNS, mostly white matter	In white matter they form myelin sheaths around axons of the CNS; in gray matter they surround neurons
Microglia	Bone marrow	CNS	Phagocytose damaged nerve tissue in the CNS
Ependymal cells	Neural tube	Lining ventricles of the brain and central canal of spinal cord	Promotes movement of cerebrospinal fluid; forms simple cuboidal epithelium of the choroid plexus; in third ventricle differentiates to form tanycytes
Schwann cells	Neural crest	Peripheral nervous system only	Myelinate axons and surround unmyelinated axons of the PNS; function during degeneration and regeneration of axons

Table 3.3 ● Properties of neuroglia.

present in gray matter, where they abut neurons and are sometimes referred to as **satellite oligodendrocytes**. They are most numerous in white matter, where they form myelin sheaths around axons. Each oligodendroglion may myelinate a single internode of as many as 30 axons.

Microglia are the smallest of the neuroglia and, unlike the others, they are derived from monocytes that, as they leave the bloodstream and enter the substance of the CNS, differentiate into small macrophages. Microglia function in the phagocytosis of damaged tissues and participate in inflammatory and degenerative reactions.

Ependymal cells form the simple cuboidal to simple columnar epithelial lining of the ventricles of the brain and the central canal of the spinal cord. These cells possess cilia in some regions of the spinal canal and ventricles facilitating the circulation of cerebrospinal fluid (CSF). Ependymal cells in certain regions of the ventricles become modified and participate in the formation of the choroid plexus, the structures that are responsible for the elaboration of the CSF. Some of the ependymal cells of the third ventricle are modified and are known as **tanycytes**. These modified ependymal cells possess long processes that approximate capillaries and certain neurosecretory cells of the hypothalamus. It is speculated that they may transport CSF to these cells.

Schwann cells are present only in the PNS. They are derived from neural crest cells that migrate during development to the sites of axon formation and elongation. These cells envelop the forming axons, isolating them from the surrounding environment. Schwann cells invest all unmyelinated axons as well as forming the myelin sheath of all myelinated axons of the PNS. Unlike oligodendroglia, a Schwann cell is capable of myelinating only a single internode of a single axon. Schwann cells form their own basal lamina and extracellular matrix, hence they are capable of synthesizing type IV collagen, the glycoproteins fibronectin and laminin, as well as various proteoglycans. Schwann cells also function during degeneration and regeneration of axons.

Myelin

Myelin is formed from the layers of oligondendroglia and Schwann cell plasmalemma wrapped around axons of certain neurons

Each axon is served by a large number of oligodendroglia or neuroglia, since a single one of these cells is capable of myelinating only a short segment of an axon. These short, myelin-wrapped segments are known as **internodes** (200–1,000 μm in length), and the unmyelinated regions of the axon located between adjacent internodes are known as **nodes of Ranvier** (Fig. 3.9). As described above, oligodendroglia myelinate in the CNS

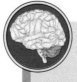

Note that the clinical case at the beginning of the chapter refers to a sudden appearance of sensory loss and motor disturbances.

1 Is a tumor usually responsible for bilateral paralysis of the leg?

2 Is a single CNS lesion usually responsible for a relapsing and remitting course of events?

3 Does a single lesion usually affect both sensory and motor functions?

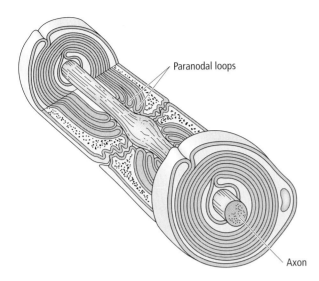

Figure 3.9 ● Longitudinal section of a nerve fiber at the node of Ranvier. Note that as the two Schwann cell membranes approach each other they form cytoplasm-filled regions known as paranodal loops.

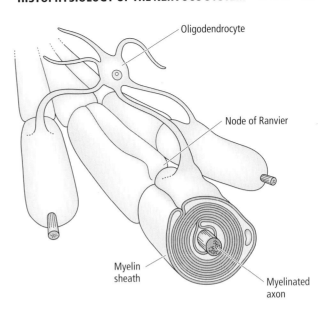

Figure 3.10 ● Myelination is very similar in the central nervous system where a single oligodendrocyte is capable of myelinating a single internode of numerous axons.

only and Schwann cells myelinate in the PNS only. Moreover, a single oligodendroglion is able to myelinate a single internode of as many as 30 different axons (Fig. 3.10), whereas a single Schwann cell is capable of myelinating only one internode of one axon.

Although the mechanism of myelination is not understood, it is believed that the process is similar whether it occurs in the peripheral or the central nervous system, therefore, only Schwann cell myelination will be discussed here. As the axon reaches 1 μm in diameter, Schwann cells proliferate, forming a continuous chain of cells along the length of the axon. As they envelop the axon, they begin to layer their membranes (as many as 50 or more layers) in a spiral fashion around the axon (Fig. 3.11). As the developing myelin sheath becomes more tightly wound, the cytoplasm of the wrapped region retracts into the Schwann cell body, and the cytoplasmic aspects of the apposing cell membranes approximate each other. Moreover, the extracytoplasmic aspects of the cell membranes also approach one another.

Viewed with the electron microscope the myelin sheath presents the appearance of concentric, wider, electron-dense lines alternating with concentric, narrower, less electron-dense lines. The wider lines (3 nm in width) represent the apposition of the cytoplasmic surfaces of the Schwann cell plasmalemma, and are called **major dense lines**. The narrower lines represent the apposition of the outer surfaces of the Schwann cell plasmalemma, and are known as **intraperiod lines**. Although these lines *appear* to be concentric, they are actually spiral lines. The outer surfaces of the Schwann cell plasmalemma do not contact each other, necessitating a change of terminology to **intraperiod gap**. This intraperiod gap is believed to be a conduit so that small molecules can reach the axon. The beginning of the internal aspect (closest to the axolemma) of the intraperiod gap is known as the

internal mesaxon, whereas the distal aspect of the intraperiod gap (at the external surface of the myelin sheath) is referred to as the **external mesaxon**.

At the edges of the Schwann cell, in the region of the node of Ranvier, bubbles of cytoplasm remain that separate the major dense line. Additionally, some of the cytoplasm may remain in the region of the internode, forming oblique arrays of bubbles of cytoplasm. When whole mounts of teased myelinated nerve fibers are viewed with the light microscope these areas appear as clear slanted lines in the myelin sheaths and are known as **clefts (incisures) of Schmidt–Lantermann**.

The process of myelination occurs over a period of several years and, as such, some axons are myelinated much sooner than others. Motor nerves are the first to be myelinated whereas sensory nerves are not myelinated until several months after birth. Certain regions of the CNS do not become completely myelinated until several years after birth.

Myelin is composed of approximately 70–80% lipids and the remainder consists of proteins and water. The preponderant lipid constituent is cholesterol, followed by phospholipids and glycosphingolipids. There are several proteins whose roles in the structural integrity of the myelin sheath are beginning to be understood (Table 3.4). P_0 and P_2 are present mostly in PNS myelin, P_1 is located in both PNS and CNS myelin, and **proteolipid protein** (PLP) is the major structural protein that is present only in CNS myelin. All of these proteins are transmembrane proteins and are believed to play a role in the compaction of the major dense line, since their cytoplasmic aspects are composed of highly charged amino acids that attract their counterparts on the other side of the membrane. Another protein, **myelin-associated glycoprotein** (MAG), has globular subunits that extend into the extracellular space (into the intraperiod gap) of the myelin sheaths of both the CNS and PNS. Here they contact MAGs from the

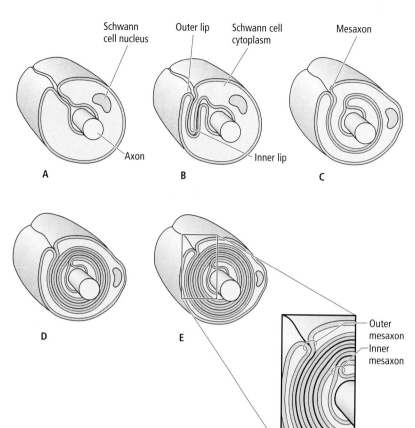

Figure 3.11 ● Myelin formation and structure in the peripheral nervous system. (A) The axon is surrounded by a Schwann cell. (B) The Schwann cell begins to rotate around the axon. (C) As rotation progresses, the mesaxon is being formed. (D) Continued rotation of the Schwann cell squeezes the cytoplasm out of the myelin sheath. (E) Higher magnification, displaying the inner and outer mesaxons as well as the major dense lines and intraperiod lines.

Protein	Location	Function
P_0	Mostly in PNS	Compaction of major dense line
P_1	Mostly in PNS	Compaction of major dense line
P_2	Both PNS and CNS	Compaction of major dense line
PLP (proteolipid protein)	CNS only	Compaction of major dense line
MAG (myelin-associated glycoprotein)	Both PNS and CNS	Compaction of intraperiod gap

CNS, central nervous system; PNS, peripheral nervous system.

Table 3.4 ● Proteins of myelin.

other side, thus establishing adhesive forces that hold the external aspects of the Schwann cell plasmalemma in close proximity. The cytoplasmic aspects of this transmembrane protein are associated with the cytoskeletal components spectrin and actin, thus reinforcing the rigorous architecture of the myelin sheath.

GENERATION AND CONDUCTION OF NERVE IMPULSES

Nerve fibers transmit information along their membranes, which become depolarized subsequent to suitable stimulation. Modulation of the transmembrane **resting potential**,

due to the actions of voltage-gated ion channels, results in the transmission of an electrical signal along the dendrites, soma, and/or axon either as an **action potential** or as a **postsynaptic potential**.

Resting potential, Nernst equation, and Goldman equation

The resting potential is the voltage difference between the cytoplasmic and extracellular sides of the plasmalemma; it can be calculated using the Nernst or Goldman equations

The **resting potential** is the voltage difference existing between the two sides (cytoplasmic and extracellular) of the semipermeable membrane of any cell. This voltage difference is present only in the *immediate vicinity* of the membrane, since deeper in the cytoplasm and farther out in the extracellular space the electric charges are neutral. Neurons possess constant permeability K⁺ ion channels that establish a specific charge difference (**potential difference**) between the two sides of the membrane, so that its cytoplasmic aspect appears negative with respect to its extracellular aspect. In order to understand the establishment of a resting potential one must realize that there are two factors operating on this semipermeable membrane, the concentration gradient and the electrical gradient.

Since the intracellular concentration of K⁺ is greater than the extracellular concentration, potassium is being driven by a concentration gradient from the cell into the extracellular space. Potassium ions travel through ion channels that are not gated and are known as **K⁺ leak channels**. Because only K⁺ ions are permitted through these channels an electrical imbalance is established (more positive ions are present on the extracellular aspect of the membrane than on the intracellular aspect). It should be understood that a K⁺ ion may travel in either direction through the same K⁺ leak channel. At the point where the concentration gradient's "desire" to push potassium out of the cell and the electrical imbalance's "desire" to return potassium into the cell *equal each other*, the net flow of K⁺ ions becomes zero. This does not mean that there is no flow of K⁺ ions across the membrane, it simply means that the same number of K⁺ ions flow into the cell as out of the cell. The establishment of this equilibrium potential (modified for K⁺ ions) is described by the **Nernst equation**:

$$V_m = RT/ZF(\ln[K^+]_{out}/[K^+]_{in})$$

where V_m is the membrane potential in volts; R is the gas constant; T is the temperature in °K; F is Faraday's constant; Z is the ion valence; and $(\ln[K^+]_{out}/[K^+]_{in})$ is the natural logarithm of the ratio of the cytoplasmic to extracellular concentration of K⁺ ions.

The Nernst equation can be applied for all ions, and is solved for the most common ions in Table 3.5. However, the Nernst equation assumes that only the particular ion in question is permitted to traverse the cell membrane. However, this is not a true situation as ion channels of the plasma membrane, particularly of the neuron's membrane, are open simultaneously, thus permitting several ions to cross the plasmalemma. This state of affairs is better described by the Goldman equation.

The **Goldman equation** describes the membrane potential as a function of the relative permeability of the cell membrane to more than a single species of ions. Since the neuron membrane is influenced by at least three ions, Na⁺, K⁺, and Cl⁻, all three are considered in the Goldman equation:

$$V = RT/F \log\{(P_K \cdot [K^+]_{out} + P_{Na} \cdot [Na^+]_{out} + P_{Cl} \cdot [Cl^-]_{in})/$$
$$(P_K \cdot [K^+]_{in} + P_{Na} \cdot [Na^+]_{in} + P_{Cl} \cdot [Cl^-]_{out})\}$$

As is evident the Goldman equation is very similar to the Nernst equation, but it predicts the membrane potential from the concentration of several ions and the permeability of the membrane to those ions. It is interesting to note that the two equations would be identical if the permeability of two of the three ions were zero. Therefore, the Goldman equation is the Nernst equation expanded for multiple ions and consequently it calculates a more realistic resting membrane potential for neurons.

The resting potential of a general neuron plasma membrane is approximately **–71 mV** when the ion concentrations inside and outside the cell equal the values listed in Table 3.5. The chloride ion concentration does not have much of an effect on the resting potential, indicating that it is the K⁺ gradient that has the greatest role in establishing the resting potential. The following mental exercise should help in clarifying this statement. If we assume that originally the potential difference across the membrane is zero but the intracellular concentration of K⁺ is greater than on the outside, K⁺ will follow its concentration gradient and leave the cell via the K⁺ leak channels. As these positive ions leave the cell, the inside of the membrane will become more negative, the outside of the membrane will become more positive, and this electrical imbalance will begin to drive K⁺ back into the cell. At the same time the concentration gradient will continue to drive K⁺ out of the cell and there will come a point where the electric force and the concentration gradient force will equal each other. It is at that point that the same number

Ion	Cytoplasmic concentration (mmol/L)	Extracytoplasmic concentration (mmol/L)	Nernst equilibrium potential (mV)
Na⁺	12	120	+58
K⁺	5	125	−80
Ca²⁺	10^{-4}	1–2	+178
Cl⁻	5–15	110	−80
Organic ions that cannot leave cell	130	1–2	na

na, not applicable.

Table 3.5 ● Ion concentration and Nernst equilibrium potential in mammalian neurons.

of K⁺ ions will leave the cell as enter the cell and, therefore, the net flow of K⁺ equals zero, thus establishing the resting membrane potential. Simultaneously, Cl⁻ ions will be unable to enter the cell because the negative charges oppose their inward movement, thus preventing Cl⁻ ions from having much of an influence on the resting membrane potential. A further point to consider in this mental exercise is the number of ions that have to be involved in the establishment of the membrane potential. Since there are a far greater number of ions inside the cell than just those in the immediate vicinity (that is within 1–2 nm) of the cell membrane, the actual number of K⁺ ions that have to leave the cell per unit area of membrane is miniscule when compared to the concentration of K⁺ inside the cell.

A final point of interest is the effect of the Na⁺/K⁺ pump on the resting membrane potential. It should be recalled that this pump uses energy to move three Na⁺ ions out of the cell into the extracellular space in exchange for two K⁺ ions that it brings into the cell from the extracellular space. If the Na⁺/K⁺ pump is inactivated the membrane resting potential will become somewhat less negative and if the pump remains inactive for a longer period of time (a number of minutes), the resting membrane potential becomes disturbed. However, some time before that happens, cations, especially Na⁺, slowly enter the cell and the intracellular Na⁺ concentration becomes greater. As the concentration of Na⁺ increases, the ion concentration inside the cell will also increase, driving water into the cell. Thus, the major function of the Na⁺/K⁺ pump in the cell is the maintenance of the cell's osmotic balance.

When the resting potential is disturbed at a particular point, voltage-gated ion channels open and the passage of specific ions through the membrane generates a small, localized electric current. If the current is the result of the inward movement of cations (i.e., Na⁺), the resting potential is decreased to such an extent that the polarity of the membrane is reversed (depolarization). This local current is very small and its ability to evoke an **action potential** diminishes:

- as a function of its distance from the **initial segment** of the axon; and
- as a function of the time elapsed between the initiation of the current and its arrival at the initial segment.

If the current is the result of the inward movement of anions through a voltage-gated channel (i.e., Cl⁻) the resting potential is increased (**hyperpolarization**), leading to an increased resistance to depolarization (that is resistance to the formation of an action potential).

Action potentials

An action potential is the change in resting membrane potential when enough Na⁺ ions enter the cytoplasm to reach a threshold level great enough to cause excitation

Action potentials last only a few milliseconds and occur due to the influx of Na⁺ ions into the neuron through voltage-gated Na⁺ ion channels. These channels exist in one of three configurations: closed, open, or refractory. When

the resting potential reaches a threshold level (about −55 mV), the Na⁺ ion channel opens instantaneously (within 10 μs) and remains open, permitting a rapid influx of Na⁺ ions. As the number of Na⁺ ions increases at the *cytoplasmic aspect* of the membrane, the accumulation of positive charges internally (at the interface of the cytoplasm and the plasmalemma) becomes greater than externally (at the interface of the external aspect of the plasmalemma and the extracellular space). Thus the inner aspect appears "more" positive than the external aspect and the membrane is said to have become depolarized (about +40 mV).

At this point we must revise our initial image of the voltage-gated sodium channel. Instead of assuming a single gate on the channel we must envision two gates. The first is the **activation gate** (at the extracellular aspect of the membrane) whereas the second is the **inactivation gate** (at the cytoplasmic aspect of the cell membrane), and both gates must be open for Na⁺ ions to pass through the ion channel. At resting potential the activation gate is closed, the inactivation gate is open, and Na⁺ ions cannot pass through. When the threshold level (−55 mV) is reached the activation gate opens, the inactivation gate remains open, and Na⁺ ions enter the cell through the ion channel. As the positive charge on the internal aspect builds up and the membrane is depolarized (+40 mV), the inactivation gate slowly closes, and Na⁺ ions can no longer pass through the Na⁺ ion channel. For 1–2 ms thereafter the inactivation gate remains closed and the Na⁺ ion channel *cannot* respond to alteration in the resting potential. Thus, the Na⁺ ion *channel is inactivated*; it cannot be opened, and the axon is said to be in the **absolute refractory period**. Once the cell membrane is repolarized the activation gate shuts, the inactivation gate slowly opens, and, although Na⁺ ions still cannot pass through the Na⁺ ion channel, the Na⁺ ion channel once again can respond to alterations in the resting potential.

In response to the sodium influx-induced depolarization of the membrane, voltage-gated K⁺ ion channels slowly open and remain open for a longer period of time than do Na⁺ ion channels. It should be noted that voltage-gate K⁺ channels are different from K⁺-leak channels. They open only during depolarization, whereas K⁺-leak channels are always open. The increased positive charge (due to the influx of Na⁺ ions) on the internal aspect of the membrane drives K⁺ ions out to the external aspect of the cell membrane. This efflux of K⁺ ions is so intense that it hyperpolarizes the membrane, making the initiation of a second depolarization more arduous, until the resting membrane potential is re-established. This period of time is known as the **relative refractory period** and contributes to the total refractory period.

Propagation of an action potential

The advancement of an action potential (i.e., its constant regeneration) in a single direction, along the length of a membrane such as the axolemma, is called propagation of the action potential

An action potential is a local event involving a short segment of an axon and it lasts merely a few milliseconds. In order to utilize action potentials for the transmission of information they must be able to advance along the axon in a single direction, until they reach the axon terminal.

The following points recap the previous discussion of events occurring at a voltage-gated Na$^+$ ion channel:

1   The influx of Na$^+$ ions reversed the polarity of the membrane at that particular point.
2   The positive ions flowed away from the original site of entry, dispersing both toward the soma and toward the axon terminal.
3   As the positive charges reached the neighboring Na$^+$ ion channel (located closer to the axon terminal), the resting membrane potential was disrupted, that is the internal aspect of the axon membrane became more positive due to the presence of excess Na$^+$ ions.
4   Once the threshold level was reached the Na$^+$ ion channel opened permitting the entry of more Na$^+$ ions, resulting in the depolarization of the membrane at the new point and a new action potential was generated.
5   In this fashion the action potential is constantly regenerated (and **propagated**) at sequential Na$^+$ ion channels until the wave of depolarization reaches the axon terminal.
6   Remembering the discussion concerning the refractory period, it should be clear that those Na$^+$ ions that entered at the Na$^+$ ion channel and dispersed toward the soma encountered Na$^+$ ion channels that were still inactivated, and their inactivation gates could not be opened.
7   Since the inactivation gate remained closed Na$^+$ ions could not pass through the Na$^+$ ion channel and the membrane could not be depolarized at the old point.
8   Therefore, the action potential in a normal *in vivo* situation can travel only in a single direction, away from the soma toward the axon terminal.

The conduction velocity of an action potential is directly dependent on the diameter of the axon. The conduction velocity is further increased due to axon myelination (Fig. 3.12). As indicated above, in an unmyelinated axon the propagation of the action potential is dependent on the sequential activation of successive Na$^+$ ion channels. In a myelinated axon voltage-gated Na$^+$ ion channels are much farther apart, located only at the nodes of Ranvier, requiring that the generation of action potentials occurs only at the nodes. Hence, the current must "jump" from node to node (**saltatory conduction**), a much faster process than that occurring in unmyelinated axons.

Postsynaptic potentials

The release of neurotransmitters at the synaptic cleft results in the formation of small, local currents at the postsynaptic membrane, known as postsynaptic potentials

Small local currents, initiated by the release of chemical messengers from synaptic vesicles are spread throughout the cell body of the neuron, and are known as **postsynaptic potentials** (PSPs). As mentioned earlier, the ability of these postsynaptic potentials to evoke an action potential diminishes as a function of:

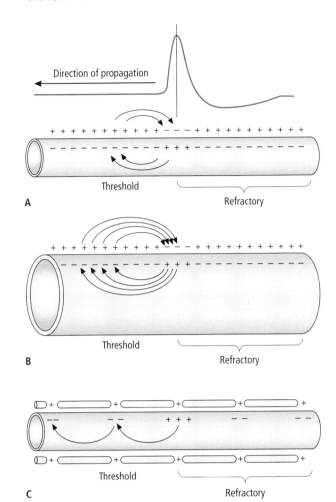

Figure 3.12 ● Propagation of the action potential depicted in three axons: (A, B) unmyelinated axons of different diameters, and (C) a myelinated axon. (A) Because the axon of smaller diameter offers greater axoplasmic resistance, a given localized current can hypopolarize the membrane to a shorter distance than an axon of larger diameter (indicated by the curved arrows) (B). Therefore, the propagation of action potentials occurs much faster in an axon of larger diameter than one of smaller diameter. (C) Myelinated axons offer less resistance than either of the two examples above, since the local current can only leave at the nodes of Ranvier. Therefore, the propagation of the action potential is saltatory, jumping from node to node, and the impulse travels much faster along a myelinated axon than along a nonmyelinated one.

• their distance from the initial segment of the axon; and
• the amount of time that has elapsed from the time the depolarization occurred at the **initial segment** of the axon.

The reason for this is that the dendrites and soma have relatively few voltage-gated channels—a specific requirement for the formation and propagation of action potentials. An increase in the number of postsynaptic potentials (e.g., by the rapid release of multiple quanta of chemical messengers from a single axon terminal or from many axon terminals on the same neuron), however, results in their summation. Hence, hundreds of nearly simultaneous, small postsynaptic potentials may be necessary to achieve the threshold required for the formation of an action potential when those currents arrive at the initial segment of the axon.

Generally, **inhibitory synapses** are closer to the initial segment of the axon than are excitatory synapses. Since inhibitory synapses function to hyperpolarize the postsyn-aptic membrane, they tend to diminish the flow of currents formed at the excitatory potential making it more difficult to reach threshold levels at the initial segment of the axon. This sequence of events is referred to as the **summation of IPSPs and EPSPs** (inhibitory postsynaptic potentials and excitatory postsynaptic potentials).

CLINICAL CONSIDERATIONS

Leigh's syndrome (subacute encephalomyelopathy), a childhood disease, is due to mutations in the mitochondrial DNA as well as mutations in chromosome 9 (*surfeit-1* gene) of neurons located in the basal ganglia. Children afflicted with this disease initially lose their verbal abilities and muscular coordination, and later may exhibit dementia, seizures, and optic atrophy; many die due to respiratory failure.

Tay–Sachs disease is an inherited lysosomal storage disease where specific neurons are unable to synthesize the enzyme hexosaminidase A. These defective lysosomes are unable to digest sphingolipids, which continue to accumulate and impede the normal functioning of the cell, leading to cell death. This autosomal recessive trait is especially prominent in families of Eastern European Jewish descent. Its symptoms—hyperacusis, irritability, hypotonia, reduced motor skills, blindness with red spots in the macula, and seizures—appear before the first year of life and result in the death of the child between the second and fourth year of age.

Multiple sclerosis is characterized by progressive demyelination of the white matter in the brain and spinal cord. This condition, believed to be an autoimmune disease, usually appears in the young adult and is distinguished by periods of deterioration followed by periods of remission that may continue for decades. As the disease progresses the periods of remission become shorter and the disability becomes greater due, among other things, to the decreased velocity of impulse propagation in the affected axons. Any one of the demyelination episodes may lead to death within a short period of time.

Neuroglial tumors account for approximately half of intracranial tumors. They range in severity from the relatively mild oligodendroglioma to the highly malignant, and fatal, **glioblastoma**. The latter disease originates from very rapidly proliferating astrocyte-derived neoplastic cells that invade the cerebrum.

SYNONYMS AND EPONYMS
OF NERVOUS SYSTEM HISTOPATHOLOGY

Name of structure or term	Synonym(s)/ eponym(s)
Axon terminal	Bouton terminaux
Cell body	Perikaryon; soma
Clefts of Schmidt–Lantermann	Incisures of Schmidt–Lantermann
Gap junction	Nexus
Neurofilaments	Intermediate filaments
Rough endoplasmic reticulum	Nissl bodies
Unipolar neuron	Pseudounipolar neuron

FOLLOW-UP TO CLINICAL CASE

The patient underwent an MRI examination of the brain and CSF examination that confirm he has **multiple sclerosis** (MS). MS is a neurologic disease that can vary widely in symptomatology, since it can cause lesions in any part of the CNS. However, it only affects the white matter. More specifically, prototypical MS causes demyelination of axons in the CNS by death or injury to oligodendrocytes. In most cases there is relative preservation of the axons. The understanding of the pathophysiology is incomplete, but it is clear that there is an immunologic attack causing loss of or dysfunction of oligodendrocytes. However, it is not a typical autoimmune condition since most of the medications used for autoimmune diseases such as rheumatoid arthritis do not work (or do not work well).

The diagnosis can be confirmed by MRI of the appropriate area of the CNS. The patient in the case study had multiple demyelinating plaques in the cerebellum and brain, including the corpus callosum (which is characteristic). The lesions of MS are often periventricular in location. There are often lesions seen that are clinically "silent." Using CSF and serum electrophoresis, synthesis of antibodies within the CNS and not the serum is often demonstrated. This is pathologic.

One definition for MS is that it causes multiple lesions in the CNS in space and time. Multiple focal white matter plaques of demyelination, easily seen by MRI, are present in different parts of the brain, brainstem, and/or spinal cord at different times. Peripheral nerve myelin is not affected at all since it is produced differently. The most common syndrome is a relapsing/remitting course. Over the course of many years symptoms occur in episodes lasting typically weeks or months, and then symptoms spontaneously impróve. Over the course of years, after a number of relapses, this can lead to disability.

Common symptoms of relapses include, but are certainly not limited to, focal numbness/tingling or weakness, gait ataxia, visual loss (optic neuritis), slurred speech, paraplegia and sensory disturbance up to a thoracic dermatome level, and ocular motility problems (producing double vision). One characteristic of MS is that heat or a rise in body temperature can temporarily bring about symptoms typical of that particular patient's MS. This is not due to any new lesions happening within the CNS. A rise in temperature actually reduces the efficiency of conduction along axons. The effects are not seen in people with normal CNS function because there is a large reserve capacity for conduction, but this is not so in the old plaques of demyelination in patients with MS. It is common for MS patients to complain of symptoms surfacing temporarily with fevers, hot baths or showers, prolonged exertion, or sunbathing.

QUESTIONS TO PONDER

1. Why is the neuron cell body so rich in organelles?

2. What is the functional difference between a node and an internode?

3. Why are results obtained by the use of the Goldman equation a more accurate prediction of resting membrane potential than the results obtained by the use of the Nernst equation?

4. Although action potentials can travel in both directions along an axon *in vitro*, why is it that they travel only in the anterograde direction *in vivo*?

5. Why are the locations of inhibitory synapses and excitatory synapses important?

CHAPTER 4

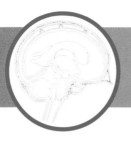
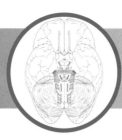
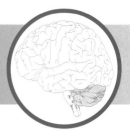

Neurotransmitter Substances

CLINICAL CASE

A 60-year-old man presents to your office with imbalance and a few falls. He has had some severe bumps and bruises from the falls, which prompted him to come in to see the doctor. Symptoms seemed to begin about 6 months previously, and are slowly getting worse. Also noted is a tremor that primarily involves the right hand, and is most prominent when at rest and when walking. In fact, the patient barely notices it but it is very bothersome to his wife. His movements, according to his wife, seem very slow and stiff.

The patient does not make good eye contact when being spoken to, and gaze is directed downward. Facial expression is limited, and there seems to be a paucity of spontaneous movements. All movements, including walking, speaking, reaching, etc., are very slow but performed accurately. There is a tremor, most prominent in the right hand, which is most noticeable at rest and goes away when reaching for objects. It is also enhanced when walking, and writing is poor. Walking is slow with short, shuffling steps.

Cells of the nervous system communicate with each other at synapses either via electrical signals or by the release of relatively small messenger molecules. The morphology and physiology of electrical and chemical synapses were presented in Chapter 3, whereas the current chapter discusses the most common and significant of the neurotransmitter substances (of which there are more than 100) (Table 4.1). These messenger molecules may be classified into two major types, those that bind directly to **ion channels (ligand-gated receptors)** and those that bind to **G-protein-coupled receptors**. The neurotransmitter substances that bind specifically to ligand-gated ion channels cause those channels to open directly, thus the target neuron responds immediately, resulting in an **ionotropic effect** (Fig. 4.1). Those neurotransmitter substances that bind to G-protein-coupled receptors exert an indirect effect on ion channels. Since the G-proteins act as intermediaries, the effect on the target neuron is slower than in the previous instance. Thus, these neurotransmitter substances are frequently known as **neuromodulators**, and they are said to exert a **metabotropic effect** (Fig. 4.2).

In order for a substance to be considered a neurotransmitter (or neuromodulator) it must possess five basic characteristics: (i) they must be synthesized by presynaptic neurons; (ii) they have to reside within the synaptic terminals (enclosed in synaptic vesicles); (iii) they are released from the presynaptic terminals by way of a calcium-dependent mechanism; (iv) they have to bind to specific receptors on the postsynaptic membrane; and (v) they must be inactivated in the synaptic cleft. Each neuron has at least one, but usually a number of neurotransmitter substances—**co-transmitters**—in its presynaptic terminal (frequently a classic neurotransmitter as well as neuropeptides). These co-transmitters may be

Table 4.1 ● Properties of the principal neurotransmitters (organized in alphabetically)

Neurotransmitter	Major function	Precursor	Enzyme	Location in nervous system	Additional pertinent information
Acetylcholine	Excitatory/inhibitory	Acetyl CoA and choline	Choline acetyl-transferase	Myoneural junction; autonomic nervous system; striatum	Removed by the enzyme acetylcholinesterase; cholinergic neurons degenerate in Alzheimer's disease
Adenosine triphosphate (ATP)	Excitatory	ADP	Oxidative phosphorylation; glycolysis	Motoneurons of the spinal cord; autonomic ganglia	Also co-released with numerous neurotransmitters
Beta-endorphin	Inhibitory	Amino acids	Protein synthesis	Hypothalamus; nucleus solitarius?	Least numerous of the opioid neurotransmitter-containing cells; function in pain suppression
Dopamine	Excitatory	Tyrosine (L-DOPA)	Tyrosine hydroxylase	Neurons of the substantia nigra, arcuate nucleus, and tegmentum	Associated with Parkinsonism; inhibition of prolactin release; schizophrenia
Dynorphin	Inhibitory	Amino acids	Protein systhesis	Hypothalamus; amygdala; limbic system	More numerous than beta-endorphin-containing cells; function in pain suppression
Enkephalins	Inhibitory	Amino acids	Protein synthesis	Raphe nuclei; striatum; limbic system; cerebral cortex	More numerous than beta-endorphin- and enkephalin-containing cells; function in pain suppression
Epinephrine	Excitatory	Norepinephrine	Phenylethanolamine-N-methyltransferase	Rostral medulla	Not commonly present in the CNS
Gamma aminobutyric acid (GABA)	Inhibitory	Glutamate	Glutamic acid decarboxylase	Mostly local circuit interneurons	Decreased GABA synthesis in vitamin B_6 deficiency
Glutamate	Excitatory	Glutamine	Glutaminase	Most excitatory neurons of the CNS	Glutamate–glutamine cycle; excitotoxicity
Glycine	Inhibitory	Serine	Serine hydroxymethyl-transferase	Neurons of the spinal cord	Activity blocked by strychnine
Nitric oxide (NO)	Inhibitory	L-arginine	Nitric oxide synthase	Cerebellum; hippocampus; olfactory bulb	Smooth muscle relaxant, thus strong vasodilator
Norepinephrine (noradrenaline)	Excitatory	Tyrosine (dopamine)	Dopamine beta-hydroxylase	Postganglionic sympathetic neurons; locus ceruleus	Associated with mood and mood disorders (mania, depression, anxiety, and panic)
Serotonin (5-hydroxytryptamine)	Excitatory	Tryptophan	Tryptophan-5-hydroxylase	Pineal body; raphe nuclei of midbrain, pons, and medulla	Associated with sleep modulation; arousal, cognitive behaviors
Somatostatin	Inhibitory	Amino acids	Protein synthesis	Amygdala, small spinal ganglion cells, and hypothalamus	Also known as somatotropin release-inhibiting factor
Substance P	Excitatory	Amino acids	Protein synthesis	Dorsal root and trigeminal ganglia (C and Aδ fibers)	Composed of 11 amino acids; associated with transmission of pain

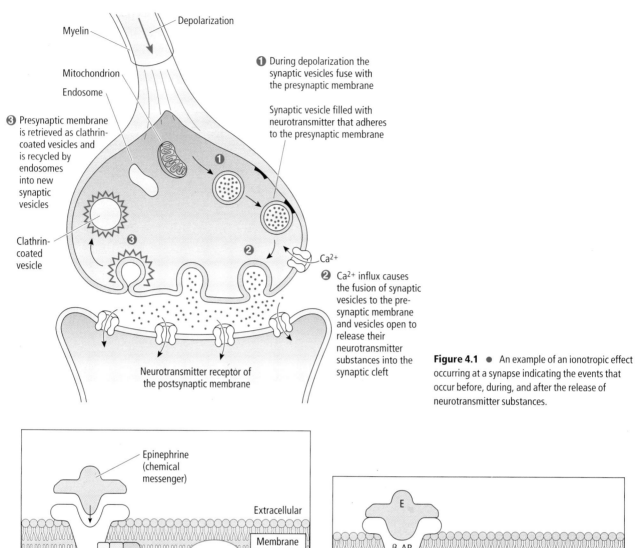

Figure 4.1 ● An example of an ionotropic effect occurring at a synapse indicating the events that occur before, during, and after the release of neurotransmitter substances.

Myelin

Depolarization

Mitochondrion

Endosome

1 During depolarization the synaptic vesicles fuse with the presynaptic membrane

Synaptic vesicle filled with neurotransmitter that adheres to the presynaptic membrane

3 Presynaptic membrane is retrieved as clathrin-coated vesicles and is recycled by endosomes into new synaptic vesicles

Clathrin-coated vesicle

2 Ca²⁺ influx causes the fusion of synaptic vesicles to the pre-synaptic membrane and vesicles open to release their neurotransmitter substances into the synaptic cleft

Ca²⁺

Neurotransmitter receptor of the postsynaptic membrane

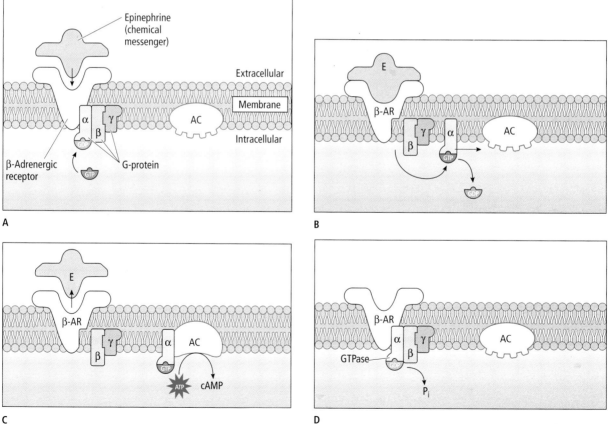

A

Epinephrine (chemical messenger)

Extracellular

Membrane

AC

Intracellular

β-Adrenergic receptor

G-protein

GTP

B

E

β-AR

γ

β

α

AC

GTP

GDP

C

E

β-AR

γ

β

α

AC

GTP

ATP → cAMP

D

β-AR

α

γ

β

AC

GTPase

GDP

Pᵢ

Figure 4.2 ● A diagram of G-protein action during a metobotropic event. (A) Binding of epinephrine (E) to its beta-adrenergic receptor (β-AR) activates the replacement of GDP by GTP on the alpha-subunit of the G-protein. (B, C) The alpha-subunit dissociates from the G-protein and activates adenylate cyclase (AC) to convert ATP to cAMP, and epinephrine dissociates from its beta-adrenergic receptor. (D) GTPase cleaves an inorganic phosphate molecule from GTP, converting it into GDP and the alpha-subunit rejoins its G-protein.

released individually or together, and they are usually housed in different synaptic vesicles. It is interesting to note that the "classic" neurotransmitters (e.g., acetylcholine and monoamines) are stored in small, electron-lucent synaptic vesicles, whereas neuropeptides are stored in somewhat larger, dense-cored secretory granules.

CLASSIFICATION OF NEUROTRANSMITTER SUBSTANCES

Neurotransmitter substances may be classified into four different groups: biogenic amines, neuropeptides, small molecule neurotransmitters, and other ligands.

Biogenic amines

Biogenic amines are derived from amino acids and exert a metabotropic effect

Biogenic amines, amino acid derivatives, bind to G-protein-coupled receptors and activate the second messenger system within the target neuron, which in turn will open ion channels. Biogenic amines include dopamine, norepinephrine, and epinephrine (all considered under the heading **catecholamines**), and histamine and serotonin. Upon release from the presynaptic terminal, biogenic amines are endocytosed by the nerve terminals and glial cells, and are digested by the enzymes **cathecol *O*-methyltranferase** and **monoamine oxidase** (MAO). In this fashion, each release of these neurotransmitters is responsible for only a limited number of depolarizations/hyperpolarizations. **Monoamine oxidase inhibitors** (MAOIs) are drugs that act within the presynaptic neuron to inactivate catecholamines and indoleamines. They also act to increase the concentration of other neurotransmitters such as serotonin, dopamine, and norepinephrine, and, by some unknown mechanism, relieve depression.

Catecholamines

The three major catecholamines, dopamine, norepinephrine, and epinephrine, have similar characteristics. They are all derivatives of the amino acid **tyrosine**, they have a **catechol** component, and the enzyme **tyrosine hydroxylase** participates in the conversion of tyrosine to **dihydroxyphenylalanine (L-DOPA)** (Fig. 4.3).

Dopamine

Dopamine is an excitatory neurotransmitter present in neurons of various regions of the central nervous system (CNS). They include the neurons of the arcuate nucleus, a group of nerve cell bodies that project to the infundibulum of the hypophysis, the neurons of the ventral tegmentum whose axons project to the limbic system, and the neurons of the substantia nigra whose axons project to the striatum.

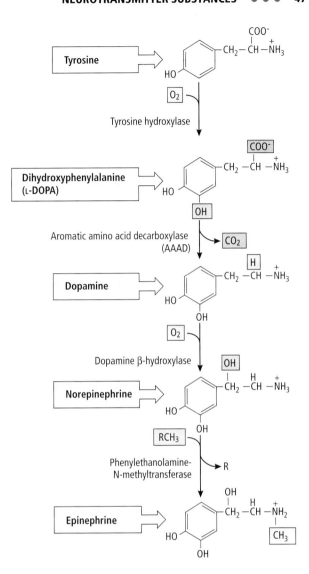

Figure 4.3 ● Synthesis of catecolamines from tyrosine.

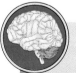

Note that the clinical case at the beginning of the chapter refers to a patient with imbalance and tremors.

1 What region of the brain should be suspected when a patient exhibits movement disorders?

2 What condition should a physician suspect when the symptoms include tremors of the hand at rest but not during the process of reaching for something?

3 What condition should a physician suspect when the patient's actions are slowed and his facial expressions are limited?

Norepinephrine

Norepinephrine (noradrenaline), an excitatory neurotransmitter located in postganglionic sympathetic neurons, is derived from dopamine. The conversion occurs in the presynaptic terminals of adrenergic neurons and is facilitated by the enzyme **dopamine β-hydroxylase**. An additional site where norepinephrine is the neurotransmitter is the **locus ceruleus**. Neurons of the locus ceruleus project to the reticular formation as well as to various other regions of the CNS.

Higher than normal levels of norepinephrine in the CNS have been associated with mania, whereas lower than normal levels have been associated with depression. Additionally, panic disorders have also been associated with abnormal levels of norepinephrine in the CNS.

Epinephrine

Epinephrine (adrenaline) is an excitatory neurotransmitter derived from norepinephrine. The conversion is catalyzed by the enzyme **phenylethanolamine-*N*-methyltransferase**. Very few neurons of the CNS use epinephrine as a neurotransmitter substance, and those that do are restricted to the rostral medulla oblongata.

Serotonin

Serotonin is a derivative of tryptophan, an amino acid that is converted into 5-hydroxytryptophan by the rate-limiting enzyme **tryptophan-5-hydroxylase**. Decarboxylation of 5-hydroxytryptophan results in the formation of 5-hydroxytryptamine, serotonin, which is an excitatory neurotransmitter (Fig. 4.4). Neurons that use serotonin as

their neurotransmitter substance are known as serotonergic neurons, and they are present in the pons, medulla, raphe nuclei of the midbrain, and pineal body. These neurons function in arousal and sleep modulation as well as in regulating certain higher cognitive functions. Moreover these neurons may exert modulatory effects on cathecolamine levels.

Histamine

Histamine is an inflammatory pharmacologic agent released by mast cells and basophils. It is responsible for causing capillaries to become leaky and also for contraction of bronchiolar smooth muscles. In the nervous system it is located mostly in the hypophysis and the median eminence of the hypothalamus. It appears that histamine may affect emotion, memory, and learning, through H1 receptors.

Neuropeptides

Neuropeptides are small polypeptides cleaved from their larger propeptides on the RER immediately after synthesis, then packaged in the Golgi apparatus, and transferred to the presynaptic terminal

Initially, many of the **neuropeptides** were known as hormones in the digestive and respiratory systems, but subsequently they were observed to function also as neurotransmitters in the nervous system. Neuropeptides are small polypeptides, cleaved, post-translationally before they reach the Golgi apparatus, from larger **propeptide molecules** synthesized on the rough endoplasmic reticulum (RER) in the soma. The cleaved neuropeptides are packaged into secretory vesicles in the *trans*-Golgi network and transferred, via the rapid anterograde transport, to the presynaptic terminal. Often, a presynaptic terminal may possess and release a number of different neuropeptides simultaneously, but once released, instead of being recycled, they are destroyed by peptidases. Thus, a single release of a quantum of neuropeptides cannot elicit multiple responses from the postsynaptic cell. Depending on the specific neuropeptides and/or their receptors, these small peptides may be excitatory or inhibitory neurotransmitters or neuromodulators. Although there are numerous neuropeptides, only the most common ones will be detailed in this textbook, namely somatostatin, substance P, and the opioid neuropeptides, endorphins, enkephalins, and dynorphins.

Somatostatin

Somatostatin (also known as **somatotropin release-inhibiting factor**) was first observed in the digestive tract as one of the paracrine hormones manufactured and released by one of the **diffuse neuroendocrine system (DNES) cells**. It was noted to function in inhibiting the release of other paracrine and endocrine hormones manufactured by nearby DNES cells. Somatostatin, in the CNS, is an inhibitory neurotransmitter and is localized in the hypothalamus, amygdala, and the small spinal ganglion cells.

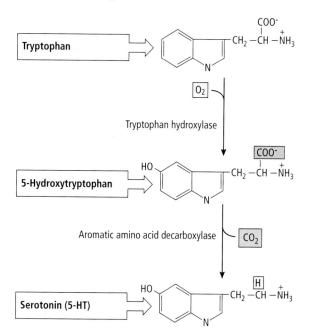

Figure 4.4 ● Synthesis of serotonin from tryptophan.

Substance P

Substance P is a small polypeptide, composed of 11 amino acids, that was first discovered in the digestive system as a product of the DNES cells. Subsequently, it was observed in the spinal cord, hippocampus, and the neocortex, as well as in the unipolar neurons of the trigeminal ganglia and dorsal root ganglia. Substance P is an excitatory neuropeptide that is one of the most important neurotransmitters in nociception.

Opioid neuropeptides

The **opioid neuropeptides** constitute a major subgroup of neuropeptides, composed of at least 20 neurotransmitter substances. Although they may be subdivided into three categories—enkephalins, endorphins, and dynorphins—they have three major characteristics in common in that they are mostly inhibitory, they bind to opium receptors of the postsynaptic membrane, and they serve as substance P agonists, inducing analgesia.

Enkephalins

Enkephalins are of two types, methionine enkephalins (met-enkephalins) and leucine enkephalins (leu-enkephalins). **Met-enkephalins** are derived from **proenkephalin** and **pro-opiomelanocortin** (POMC), a large propeptide precursor that is cleaved to form the following: beta endorphins, adrenocorticotropic hormone (ACTH), beta lipoprotein, and melanocyte-stimulating hormone (Fig. 4.5). **Leu-enkephalin** is a derivative of the propeptides **prodynorphin** and **proenkephalin**. Enkephalins are the neurotransmitter substances used by many interneurons as well as at synapses in the dorsal horn of the spinal cord. Enkephalins are also used as neurotransmitters in the limbic system, the cerebral cortex, in the striatum, and in the raphe nuclei of the brainstem.

Endorphins

The most common form of the endorphins are **beta endorphins**, also POMC derivatives. They are present in the hypothalamus where they exert an analgesic effect. As with most other opioid neuropeptides, beta endorphins are inhibitory neurotransmitter substances.

Dynorphin

Dynorphin is an inhibitory neurotransmitter substance derived from the propeptide **prodynorphin**. This neurotransmitter substance is inhibitory, and functions in pain suppression. Dynorphin is localized in the amygdala, limbic system, and in the hypothalamus.

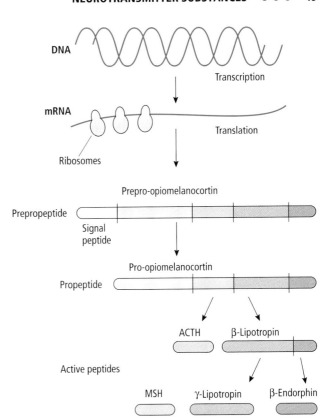

Figure 4.5 ● Synthesis of enkephalins from prepro-opiomelanocortin. ACTH, adrenocorticotropic hormone; MSH, melanocyte-stimulating hormone.

Small molecule neurotransmitters

Small molecule neurotransmitters are low molecular weight substances that are synthesized in the presynaptic terminals

Small molecule neurotransmitters, such as acetylcholine, glycine, glutamate, and gamma aminobutyric acid (GABA), are low weight substances that are usually synthesized in the presynaptic terminals. The enzymes required for their synthesis are translated in the soma and reach the presynaptic terminals via anterograde axonal transport.

Acetylcholine

Acetylcholine is the neurotransmitter at myoneural junctions, presynaptic and postsynaptic terminals of the parasympathetic nervous system, and presynaptic terminals of the sympathetic nervous system, as well as in various regions of the CNS

Acetylcholine, a neurotransmitter substance localized both in the central and peripheral nervous systems, is synthesized in the presynaptic terminal from acetyl coenzyme A (CoA) and choline by **choline acetyltransferase**, the rate-limiting enzyme of its synthesis (Fig. 4.6). Acetylcholine, as with many other neurotransmitters, has the ability to bind to both

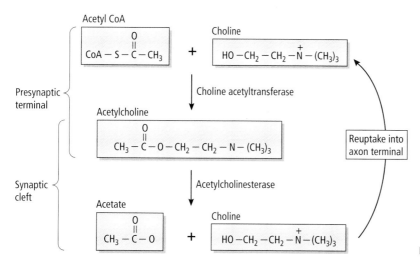

Figure 4.6 ● Acetylcholine synthesis and degradation.

ionotropic receptors and **metabotropic receptors**. In skeletal muscle it is an **excitatory neurotransmitter substance**, binding directly to ligand-gated sodium (nicotinic receptors) as well as to potassium ion channels and causing them to open. In cardiac muscle it is an **inhibitory neurotransmitter substance**, binding to G-protein-linked receptors (muscarinic receptors) that facilitate the opening of potassium ion channels.

Acetylcholine is also present in the autonomic nervous system, specifically at the preganglionic sympathetic, preganglionic parasympathetic, and postganglionic parasympathetic synapses, as well as in localized areas of the CNS such as the projection neurons of the tegmentum, interneurons of the striatum, projection neurons of the forebrain, and motoneurons of the brainstem and spinal cord.

The enzyme **acetylcholinesterase** is present in the synaptic cleft at the postsynaptic membrane. This enzyne cleaves the released acetylcholine into its two component molecules, choline and acetyl CoA, preventing multiple depolarizations from the release of a single quantum of acetylcholine. The cleaved moieties, acetyl CoA and choline, are transported, individually, into the presynaptic terminal where they are reassembled into acetylcholine and stored in synaptic vesicles.

Glycine

Glycine, one of the most common inhibitory neurotransmitters of the spinal cord, is synthesized by the enzyme **serine hydroxymethyl transferase** from the amino acid serine (Fig. 4.7A). Usually, glycine binds to ligand-gated chloride channels. Subsequent to its release into the synaptic cleft, glycine is recaptured by glycine-specific, membrane-bound carrier proteins (transport proteins) ferried into the presynaptic terminal and is transported into synaptic vesicles for future use.

Glutamate

Glutamate is present in almost every region of the brain as well as in the spinal cord at presynaptic terminals of the central processes of Aδ and C fibers of the dorsal root ganglion

Glutamate, probably the most common excitatory neurotransmitter, is synthesized in the presynaptic terminal from glutamine, catalyzed by the enzyme **glutaminase**. Once glutamate is released into the synaptic cleft within the CNS, it must be quickly removed, or it will cause the postsynaptic neuron to undergo repeated excitations, resulting in neuronal degeneration and subsequent death. This process, known as **excitotoxicity**, results from repeated stimulation of the postsynaptic membrane receptors that open Ca^{2+} channels. The increased influx of Ca^{2+} into the soma results in free radical formation and damage to the neuron and its membranes.

To prevent excitotoxicity, the free glutamate in the vicinity of the synapse is endocytosed by the presynaptic terminal as well as by local **glia cells**. The glutamate endocytosed by the presynaptic terminal is converted, by the enzyme **glutamine synthetase**, to glutamine, which then is converted to form glutamate. The same reaction occurs within the glia cells; however, these cells release the newly formed glutamine into the vicinity of the presynaptic terminal that endocytoses the glutamine and, as before, converts it into glutamate (Fig. 4.8). This entire sequence is known as the **glutamine–glutamate cycle**.

Gamma aminobutyric acid

Approximately 30% of the neurons of the CNS use **gamma aminobutyric acid (GABA)** as an inhibitory neurotransmitter substance. GABA is derived from glucose by way of glutamate, whose conversion to GABA is catalyzed by the enzyme **glutamic acid decarboxylase**, utilizing **pyridoxal phosphate**

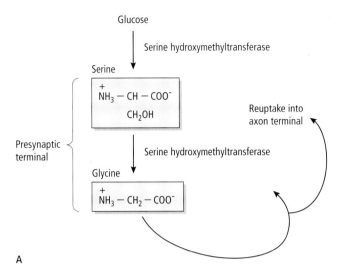

A

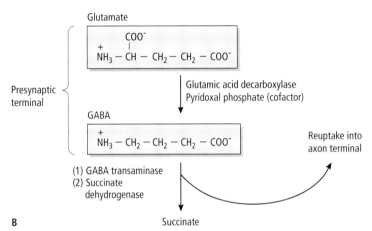

B

Figure 4.7 ● (A) Synthesis of glycine from glucose. (B) Synthesis of gamma aminobutyric acid (GABA) from glutamate.

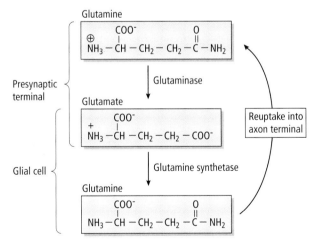

Figure 4.8 ● Glutamine–glutamate cycle.

presynaptic terminals by using GABA-specific membrane-bound protein transporters.

GABA is present in local circuit interneurons and Purkinje cells of the cerebellum. Depending on the receptor, the binding of GABA either opens chloride or potassium ion channels or closes calcium ion channels.

Other neurotransmitters

Although there is a plethora of other neurotransmitter and neuromodulator substances, many of them are sufficiently rare in the nervous system that they will not be addressed in this textbook. Only adenosine triphosphate and nitric oxide will be discussed.

Adenosine triphosphate

Adenosine triphosphate (ATP) is a high energy phosphate molecule that is customarily associated with energy storage in cells. Not much is understood concerning its functions as a neurotransmitter substance, but it is known to be co-released with other neurotransmitters and it has an excitatory effect. It

(a vitamin B_6 derivative) as a cofactor (Fig. 4.7B). Once GABA is released from the presynaptic terminal, the free neurotransmitter molecules (those not bound to postsynaptic receptors) are rapidly reabsorbed by neuroglia and the

is present in autonomic postganglionic neurons as well as in motoneurons of the spinal cord.

Nitric oxide

Nitric oxide (NO) is a gas, derived from the amino acid L-**arginine** by the action of the enzyme **nitric oxide synthase**.

It is a very reactive molecule and, therefore, has a very short half-life. This inhibitory neurotransmitter is unusual not only because it is a gas but also due to the fact that it does not bind to membrane receptors. It may function in memory formation since it is located in the hippocampal formation. Additionally, NO is also present in the olfactory system, the cerebellum, striatum, cerebral cortex, and the hypothalamus.

CLINICAL CONSIDERATIONS

Parkinsonism
Parkinsonism is a neurologic disorder characterized by progressive deterioration with time. The chief symptoms are rigidity of movement, increased tremors and trembling, being slow in initiating movement, muscle stiffness, stooping gait, and difficulties in maintaining balance. This disease is the result of the degeneration and death of dopaminergic neurons in the **substantia nigra**, which causes a decrease in the availability of the neurotransmitter substance **dopamine**. The reason for the degeneration of the dopaminergic neurons is not understood. It is interesting to note that excess levels of dopamine in the ventral tegmentum has been associated with schizophrenia.

Eaton–Lambert syndrome and myasthenia gravis
Eaton–Lambert syndrome is an autoimmune disorder affecting mostly men older than 50 years of age, many of whom are long-time smokers who are also suffering from small cell lung carcinoma. The symptoms of this syndrome include weakness of the axial and limb muscles. Additional symptoms include xerostomia (dry mouth), impaired accommodation of the eyes, impotence, and the inability to elicit deep tendon reflexes. Since some of these symptoms also appear in **myasthenia gravis**, the two conditions resemble one another. However, in the Eaton–Lambert syndrome the ocular and bulbar muscles are rarely affected, whereas ocular paresis is normally present in myasthenia.

The two diseases affect different regions of the myoneural junction. In the Eaton–Lambert syndrome, the autoimmune response is against the calcium ion channels of the presynaptic membrane, interfering with the flow of calcium ions into the presynaptic terminal. The diminished number of calcium ions prevents the adherence of the normal number of synaptic vesicles to the presynaptic membrane, decreasing the release of acetylcholine with each stimulus, and resulting in a weak muscle contraction.

In myasthenia gravis, the autoimmune reaction is against the acetylcholine receptors of the postsynaptic membrane. Therefore, even though the release of acetylcholine from the presynaptic membrane is normal, the reduced number of normal acetylcholine receptors of the postsynaptic membrane results in weak muscle contraction. The muscles of the head, and especially of the eye, are the first ones to be affected, but as the disease progresses the respiratory muscles also become involved and the patient dies of respiratory insufficiency.

Apha latrotoxin (black widow spider venom)
Alpha latrotoxin, the venom of the black widow spider, is inserted into the presynaptic membrane of the myoneural junction, where it acts as an ungated, nonselective ion channel, permitting the entry of Na^+, K^+, and Ca^{2+} into the presynaptic terminal. The altered intracellular univalent cation concentration results in constant depolarization of the presynaptic terminal. Moreover, the elevated Ca^{2+} levels facilitate synaptic vesicle docking and the release of copious amount of acetylcholine into the synaptic cleft. The continuous release of acetylcholine initially results in muscle rigidity and then in paralysis of the affected muscles.

Huntington's disease
Huntington's disease is a genetic disorder resulting in degeneration of GABAergic neurons in the caudate nucleus and putamen. The reduction in GABA results in increased release of dopamine and a corresponding decrease in acetylcholine release in the striatum, causing an imbalance in the ratio of these two neurotransmitter substances. It is this imbalance that is responsible for the symptoms of Huntington's disease, whose early signs include the incapacity to form new memory, the inability to make decisions, memory loss, depression, irritability, and mood swings. As the disease progresses, the patient becomes emotionally disturbed, loses cognitive faculties, and will display uncontrolled, erratic movements (Huntington's chorea).

FOLLOW-UP TO CLINICAL CASE

The diagnosis is **Parkinson's disease**, which is very common and usually easy to diagnose. It is a purely clinical diagnosis. All testing is either normal or unrevealing.

This patient was given levodopa three times a day. His symptoms improved dramatically within a half hour of when he took his first dose. He noted that symptoms were bad in the mornings before he took his morning dose of medicine. The patient and his wife both stated that he seemed "normal" with the medicine.

Parkinson's disease is the most common of the class of diseases known as movement disorders. Movement disorders are caused by pathology somewhere within the basal ganglia. In the case of Parkinson's disease, there is a degeneration of neurons in the midbrain's substantia nigra, which is composed of pigmented cells. Dopamine is the neurotransmitter released by these neurons, to communicate with other components of the basal ganglia. In Parkinson's disease there is a relative lack of dopamine in the basal ganglia due to the degeneration of neurons that synthesize it. Levodopa is a precursor to dopamine. It is taken up by the remaining substantia nigra neurons, is converted to dopamine, and the relative deficiency of dopamine in the basal ganglia is temporarily corrected. Dopamine cannot be used as a medicine since it will not cross the blood–brain barrier and get into the brain.

Medications that contain levodopa are very effective treatments for the symptoms of Parkinson's disease. They relieve symptoms very quickly, but the effects typically wear off in a few hours. Dopamine agonists are used in Parkinson's disease, and anticholinergic medicines are also sometimes used. However, none of these medicines alters the underlying pathology of the disease. They only reduce symptoms.

QUESTIONS TO PONDER

1. What is the difference between ionotropic and metabotropic effects?

2. What are the five basic characteristics of neurotransmitter substances?

3. Biogenic amines are one type of neurotransmitters. How are they defined?

4. Neuropeptides are neurotransmitters. What are their major characteristics?

5. Why is acetylcholine sometimes an excitatory and sometimes an inhibitory neurotransmitter substance?

CHAPTER 5

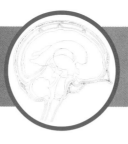
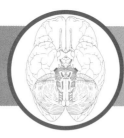
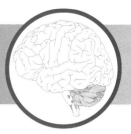

Spinal Cord

CLINICAL CASE

A 45-year-old white female complains of back pain, and weakness and numbness of both legs. The back pain started about a month ago and the other symptoms began 1 week ago as slight imbalance, tingling feet, and "funny" sensations around her abdomen. This has rapidly progressed to the point where she can no longer walk by herself, she burned her leg in the bathtub because she could not feel that the water was too hot, and today she had an episode of urinary incontinence. Sensation seems reduced or altered from her toes all the way up to her chest. The weakness and numbness are in both legs but worse on the left. The arms are normal. Her back pain is in the middle of her back, over the spine, as opposed to the much more common lower back pain.

Exam shows moderate to severe weakness in both legs, which is worse on the right. Arm strength is normal. Pinprick sensation and touch are reduced bilaterally in the legs and abdomen, up to a fairly distinct level at the nipple line. Percussion of the back shows tenderness over the spine in the upper thoracic region. Reflexes at the knees and ankles are pathologically brisk, and Babinski responses are present bilaterally. Reflexes in the arms are normal. The patient cannot walk without assistance.

The **spinal cord**, the grayish-white oblong cylindrical continuation of the medulla oblongata of the brain, begins at the **foramen magnum** of the skull and extends within the vertebral canal to terminate as the cone-shaped **conus medullaris**. In the adult the caudal tip of the conus medullaris is located between vertebral levels **L1** and **L2**. Thus, the adult spinal cord is approximately 45 cm in length with an average diameter of 1–1.5 cm and an average weight of about 30 g.

The spinal cord is a soft, gelatinous substance that is protected from injury by being encased in the bony spinal column. Additional protection is provided by the **meninges**, composed of the three concentric sheaths: the dura matter, arachnoid, and pia mater. There is only a potential space between the outermost dura and the arachnoid, known as the subdural space, but the subarachnoid space, located between the arachnoid and pia, is filled with cerebrospinal fluid (CSF). The meninges surround the entire spinal cord and, in turn, are enveloped by epidural fat and a venous plexus.

Along its length, the lateral aspect of the spinal cord is affixed by about 21 pairs of **denticulate ligaments** (triangular extensions of the pia) to the dura mater. The spinal cord is a two-way conduit to and from the brain. It functions as a *central relay station*, receiving incoming information from the body and the brain, and as a *central processing station*, conveying outgoing information to the body and the brain.

MORPHOLOGY OF THE SPINAL CORD

General structure of the spinal cord

The spinal cord is a cylindrical structure whose circumference varies; in the adult it is shorter than the length of the vertebral canal

The circumference of the spinal cord varies along its length. It presents two regions of thickening—the **cervical enlargement** (C3 to T2) and the **lumbar enlargement** (L1 to S3)—the origins of the spinal nerves destined for the upper and lower limbs, respectively. Each spinal nerve emanates from the spinal cord as dorsal and ventral rootlets, which eventually join within the intervertebral foramen to form that particular spinal nerve.

The spinal cord equals the length of the vertebral canal only until the end of the first trimester of prenatal life. Thereafter the trunk elongates much faster, so that by the time of birth the conus medullaris is only at the level of the third lumbar vertebra and in the adult it extends only as far as the caudal aspect of the first lumbar vertebra. Therefore, lower levels of the spinal cord segments are displaced rostrally in relation to their corresponding vertebral levels (Table 5.1). Because of this differential growth, the subarachnoid space caudal to the conus medullaris, known as the **lumbar cistern**, is devoid of spinal cord (Fig. 5.1).

As the dorsal and ventral rootlets of the lumbar and sacral segments elongate, they descend various distances and form

a loose conglomeration of nerve fibers within the lumbar cistern. Since these fibers resemble a horse's tail, they are known as the **cauda equina**. Moreover, the pial covering of the spinal cord continues beyond the conus medullaris as a thin, non-

Table 5.1 ● Relationship of the spinal segment to the adult vertebral column.

Spinal cord level	Spinous process of vertebrae
C6	C5
T5	T4
T10	T8
L3	T11
L5	T12
S1,2	L1
S4	L2

Note that the clinical case at the beginning of the chapter refers to a rapidly progressing deterioration of sensory and motor functions.

1 Why does the acute onset and rapid progression mandate immediate action?

2 What region of the central nervous system is responsible for the innervation of the upper extremity?

3 Why is the lesion suspected to be in the spinal cord and not in the brain?

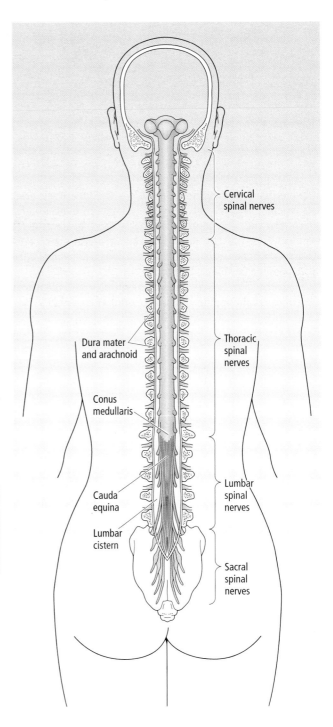

Figure 5.1 ● The spinal cord in a human. Note that the spinal processes of the vertebrae have been removed and that the dura mater and the arachnoid have been opened up so that the spinal cord may be viewed in its entire length. It should be evident that the spinal cord ends at L1,2, and the spinal nerves continue as the cauda equina within the lumbar cistern. It is the lumbar cistern that is accessed during a lumbar puncture to withdraw cerebrospinal fluid for laboratory examination.

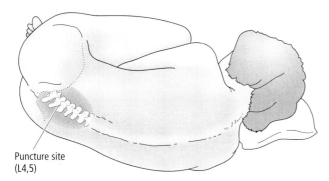

Figure 5.2 ● The preferred method of performing a lumbar puncture is to have the patient assume the lateral decubitus position with the needle piercing the intervertebral space between L4 and L5.

Puncture site
(L4,5)

nervous filament, the **filum terminale**, to the 2nd sacral vertebra where it is covered by the continuation of the dura and arachnoid and is anchored into the 1st coccygeal vertebral segment. The CSF, by filling the **subarachnoid space**, surrounds, suspends, and thus further protects, the spinal cord from possible mechanical injury.

Since the spinal cord of the adult occupies only the upper two-thirds of the spinal column, the **lumbar cistern** is a CSF-filled chamber that is accessible for spinal taps, avoiding damage to the spinal cord (Fig. 5.2). The CSF-filled **central canal** of the spinal cord is continuous rostrally with the fourth ventricle of the brain and extends along the entire length of the cord, terminating within the filum terminale in the young adult and just rostral to the conus medullaris by the fourth decade of life. Frequently the central canal is partially occluded by ependymal cells.

External morphology of the spinal cord

The spinal cord is a bilaterally symmetric structure; it has a ventral median fissure and a dorsal median sulcus along its entire length

The spinal cord possesses a bilateral symmetry, and the ordered presence of the anterior median fissure and the posterior median sulcus

aid in the recognition of this symmetry. The **ventral (anterior) median fissure** is about 3 mm deep and extends along the entire anterior (ventral) length of the spinal cord. The **dorsal (posterior) median sulcus** is not as deep as its anterior counterpart, but it also occupies the entire posterior (dorsal) length of the spinal cord. It is interesting to note that a glial septum, the **dorsal (posterior) median septum**, is continuous with the deep aspect of the posterior median sulcus, and assists in separating the spinal cord into the right and left halves (Fig. 5.3).

Approximately 2 mm on either side of the dorsal median sulcus is the **dorsolateral (posterolateral) sulcus**, distinguished by the presence of the **dorsal rootlets of the spinal nerves** as they penetrate the substance of the spinal cord, that extends the entire length of the spinal cord. The **dorsointermediate sulcus**, located between the posterior median and posterolateral sulci, is present only at the cervical and upper thoracic levels. The **ventral rootlets of the spinal nerves** emerge at the **ventrolateral (anterolateral) sulcus**, between the posterolateral sulcus and the anterior median fissure.

Segmentation of the spinal cord and the roots of the spinal nerves

The segmental design of the spinal cord is evident due to the regular arrangement of the spinal nerves

The segmental design of the spinal cord is displayed by the presence of 31 pairs of spinal nerves and their associated dorsal root ganglia. Each spinal nerve emanates from the spinal cord as a number of **sensory** and **motor rootlets**, leaving the spinal cord's dorsal and ventral surfaces, respectively. Each rootlet is composed of processes of a large number of neurons.

The ventral rootlets, usually no more than eight in number, are seen to join to form a single **ventral root**, housing the axons of motor (and in certain regions, sympathetic) neurons. The dorsal rootlets, also no more than eight in number, join and enter the slight swelling, known as the **dorsal root ganglion** housing the unipolar nerve cell bodies. These dorsal rootlets thus contain the **central processes** of these unipolar

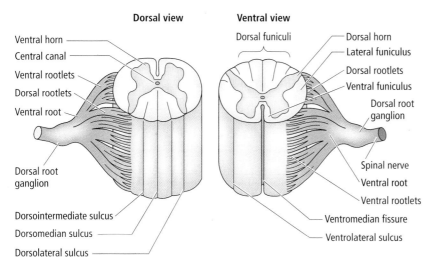

Dorsal view   Ventral view

Ventral horn
Central canal
Ventral rootlets
Dorsal rootlets
Ventral root

Dorsal funiculi

Dorsal horn
Lateral funiculus
Dorsal rootlets
Ventral funiculus
Dorsal root ganglion

Dorsal root ganglion

Spinal nerve
Ventral root
Ventral rootlets

Dorsointermediate sulcus
Dorsomedian sulcus
Dorsolateral sulcus

Ventromedian fissure
Ventrolateral sulcus

Figure 5.3 ● Dorsal and ventral views of the spinal cord, depicting the gray matter as well as the fissures and funiculi of the white matter. Observe also that the dorsal and ventral roots join to form the spinal nerve.

cells. The **peripheral processes** of the unipolar cells, which bring sensory information from sensory receptors distributed throughout the body, leave the dorsal root ganglion to join the ventral root of the same segment to form the mixed **spinal nerve**, which thus contains both sensory and motor fibers.

Each spinal nerve leaves the vertebral column via its **intervertebral foramen** and is named accordingly. The first eight spinal nerves, C1–C8, exit the vertebral canal *above* the correspondingly numbered cervical vertebrae, whereas all subsequent spinal nerves (T1–T12, L1–L5, S1–S5, and Co1) exit *below* the correspondingly named vertebrae (Fig. 5.4). Hence there are 31 pairs of spinal nerves emerging from the spinal cord. The region of the spinal cord associated with a particular pair of spinal nerves is called a **spinal segment**.

Spinal nerves are only a few millimeters in length. They give rise to a slender recurrent meningeal branch and then branch into two components, a smaller **dorsal primary ramus** and a larger **ventral primary ramus**. Every ventral primary ramus receives a **gray ramus communicans** from its corresponding sympathetic chain ganglion. Additionally, each ventral primary ramus from T1 through L2,3 also provides a **white ramus communicans** to its corresponding sympathetic chain ganglion (Fig. 5.5). These connecting branches carry postganglionic and preganglionic **sympathetic fibers** from and to the sympathetic chain ganglia, respectively. White rami communicantes have myelinated fibers, whereas gray rami communicantes house nonmyelinated fibers. Additionally, ventral primary rami S1–S3 also provide spinal preganglionic **parasympathetic fibers** that pass directly to their site of destination.

Sensory innervation of the skin is determined by its developmental origin, and the strip of skin for which a particular spinal nerve is responsible is referred to as a **dermatome**. Along the length of the trunk, each dermatome forms an ordered series of bands, whereas along the limbs the ordering is not as evident. These bands overlap each other, since the sensory nerves of one dermatome are also responsible for innervating regions of adjacent dermatomes (Fig. 5.6). It is interesting to note that the overlap is greater for light touch than for pain. Clinicians should remember the distribution of certain dermatomes (Table 5.2). Additionally, all of the muscle cells that are innervated by the fibers of a particular spinal nerve are referred to as a **myotome**. Furthermore, a **sclerotome** is defined as the ligaments and bones that receive their innervation from the fibers of the same spinal nerve.

Modalities of the spinal nerves

Spinal nerves possess functional components known as modalities: the general somatic afferent, general visceral afferent, general somatic efferent, and general visceral efferent components

Neurons are classified by function into three categories: sensory (afferent), intercalated (connecting), and motor (efferent). The afferent and efferent components are further categorized into more specific divisions, namely somatic and visceral. Thus, a typical spinal nerve has four functional components,

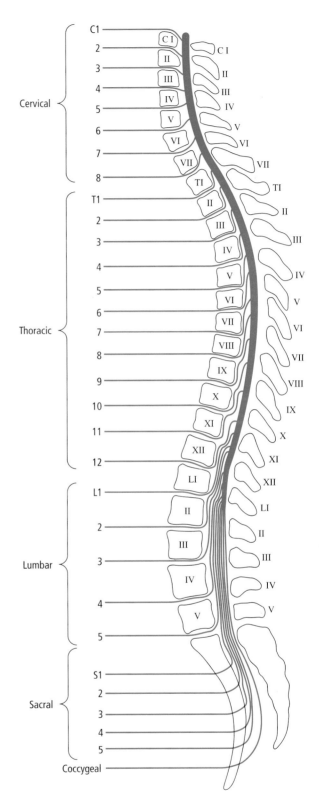

Figure 5.4 • The spinal cord and the relationship between the numbered spinal nerves and the bodies of the associated vertebrae.

known as **modalities**: the general somatic afferent (GSA), general visceral afferent (GVA), general somatic efferent (GSE), and general visceral efferent (GVE) components. Cell bodies of the afferent fibers of a spinal nerve reside in the

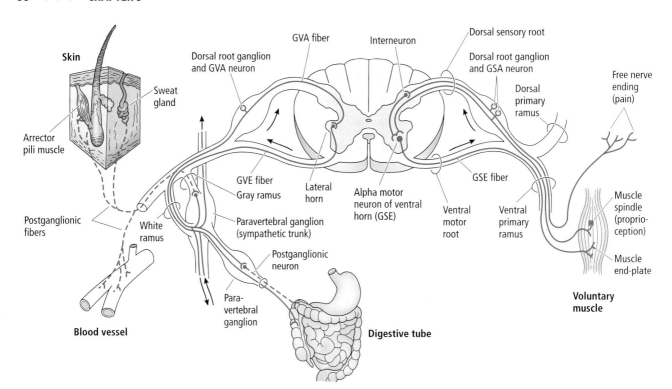

Figure 5.5 ● A typical spinal nerve. The right side depicts the somatic nervous system, while the left side depicts the sympathetic nervous system. The preganglionic fibers are shown as solid lines and the postganglionic fibers are displayed as dashed lines. Note that the left side of the figure shows that the preganglionic sympathetic cell body is in the lateral horn of the thoracic and upper lumbar spinal cord levels (T1 to L1,2). The preganglionic fiber travels along the ventral rootlets, enters the spinal nerve, travels for a very short distance, and then leaves the spinal nerve via the white ramus communicans, which is the connection to the sympathetic chain ganglion. Once in the ganglion, there are three possibilities: (i) it may synapse with the postganglionic cell body located there; (ii) it may travel up or down the sympathetic trunk until it reaches another ganglion and synapse there with a postganglionic sympathethic cell body; or (iii) it may leave the sympathetic trunk altogether and travel to a collateral sympathetic ganglion and synapse there with a postganglionic sympathetic nerve cell body. The text describes the fate of the postganglionic fiber.

Table 5.2 ● List of clinically important dermatomes.

Spinal nerve	Distribution
C2	Occiputum of the head
C3–C5	Neck
C5	Shoulder
C6	Thumb
C7,8	Elbow
C8	Pinkie
T4,5	Nipple
T10	Umbilicus
L1,2	Groin
L3,4	Skin over patella
L5	Big toe
L5–S2	Heel
S1	Little toe
S3	Anus

dorsal root ganglia, whereas the cell bodies of the efferent fibers are located within the gray matter of the spinal cord.

Visceral efferent neurons belong to the autonomic nervous system and they may be part of its sympathetic or parasympathetic component. The cell bodies of the pregan-glionic sympathetic visceral efferent fibers are located in the lateral gray column of the T1 through L2,3 levels of the spinal cord. The cell bodies of the preganglionic parasympathetic visceral efferent fibers are located in the lateral gray column of sacral spinal levels 2–4. The cell bodies of visceral afferent neurons are located in the dorsal root ganglia. Their peripheral processes bring information from the viscera, using white rami communicantes to enter the spinal nerve. The central process of the visceral afferent neuron uses the dorsal rootlets to enter the substance of the spinal cord. Once there it will either complete a reflex path by synapsing with sympathetic or somatic efferent neurons, usually by way of an interneuron, or will synapse with other neurons in the spinal cord or brainstem to deliver the information to higher centers.

General somatic afferent is sensory information, such as touch, pressure, pain, temperature, and proprioception, that is perceived in the body and is transmitted to the spinal cord. **General visceral afferent** is sensory information that is perceived in the viscera—the organs, glands, and membranes—that is transmitted to the spinal cord. The **general somatic efferent** fibers provide motor innervation to skeletal muscles of somatic origin. The **general visceral efferent** fibers provide motor innervation to the glands, cardiac muscle, and smooth muscle.

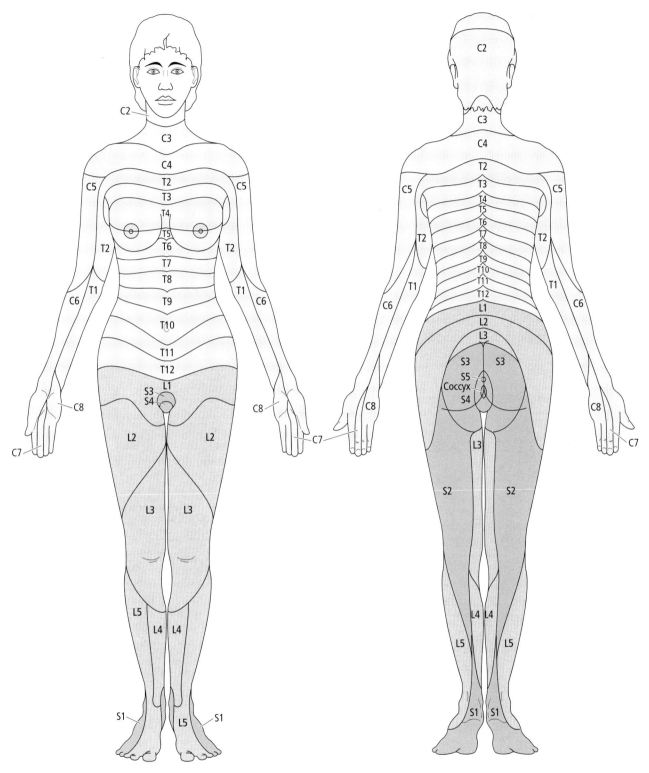

Figure 5.6 ● The sensory supply of the skin is established in bands, known as dermatomes, that represent the distribution of spinal nerves responsible for innervating that particular region. Note that there are overlaps between regions that are not indicated in these diagrams and also that there is no exact agreement among authorities concerning the precise distribution of the nerve supply (e.g., some authors state T4 as the spinal nerve responsible for the nipples, whereas others believe it to be spinal nerve T5).

Fiber type	Myelin sheath	Conduction velocity (m/s)	Fiber diameter (μM)	Function
Afferent				
Ia (Aα)	Yes	70–120	12–22	Primary sensory from muscle spindles
Ib (Aα)	Yes	70–120	10–20	Sensory fibers of Golgi tendon organs
II (Aβ)	Yes	30–70	6–12	Secondary sensory terminals of muscle spindles
III (Aδ)	Thin	10–30	1–6	Nociceptive; touch; pressure
IV (C)	No	0.5–2	>1.5	Nociceptive in muscle; temperature?
Efferent				
Aα	Yes	70–120	12–22	Motor to skeletal muscle fibers (extrafusal)
Aγ	Yes	10–45	2–10	Fusimotor to intrafusal fibers of muscle spindles
Sympathetic	Thin	3–15	3	Preganglionic to soma in ganglion
Sympathetic	No	0.5–2	>1.5	Postganglionic to glands and smooth and cardiac muscles

Table 5.3 ● Classification of afferent and efferent nerve fibers.

Classification of the fiber components of the spinal nerves

Nerve fibers are classified according to their modalities, whether they are afferent or efferent, and based on their conduction velocities

The nerve fibers constituting the spinal nerve are subdivided into two categories, afferent (sensory) and efferent (motor). All afferent fibers enter the spinal cord via the dorsal rootlets and all efferent fibers leave the spinal cord via the ventral rootlets. **Afferent fibers** are classified according to their peak conduction velocities. Unfortunately there are two classifications commonly in use, one using Roman numerals I–IV and a second using the letters A, B, and C, but they are easily reconciled, as evident in Table 5.3. **Efferent fibers** are also classified as A, B, and C fibers as well as by a different system utilizing the Greek letters alpha (α) and gamma (γ). Furthermore, they are also classified according to their modality, into GSE and GVE fibers.

INTERNAL MORPHOLOGY OF THE SPINAL CORD

The spinal cord is composed of gray matter surrounded by white matter

The spinal cord is composed of a column of gray matter surrounded by a sheath of white matter. **Gray matter** is composed of neurons, their processes, and neuroglia. It is the large number of nerve cell bodies that is responsible for the grayish appearance of the gray matter. **White matter** is composed of myelinated and unmyelinated processes of neurons, neuroglia, and blood vessels, and it is the white coloration of the myelin that gives white matter its name.

Inspection of cross-sections of the spinal cord displays a bilateral symmetry. The gray matter is arranged in the shape of a butterfly and the appearance of this image, as well as the ratio of white matter to gray matter, vary with level of the segment being examined.

The cross-sectional area of gray matter is largest in the mid to low cervical and mid to lower lumbar levels, which are the regions of the spinal cord responsible for the neural supply of the upper and lower limbs, respectively. The region of the spinal cord that displays the least area of gray matter is at the thoracic level. The cross-sectional area of the white matter is greatest at the cervical level and smallest at the sacral level of the spinal cord, since the total number of ascending and descending nerve fibers increase in a rostral direction. Because of these characteristics the segmental level of a cross-section of the spinal cord can easily be distinguished.

It is interesting to note that generally speaking the processes of the neurons run *parallel* to the longitudinal axis of the spinal cord in white matter, but *perpendicular* to the longitudinal axis of the spinal cord in gray matter.

Gray matter

Gray matter, composed of neurons, their processes, and neuroglia, is subdivided into the ventral, dorsal, and lateral columns

During examination of a cross-section of the gray matter it becomes evident that the two "wings" of the butterfly-shaped gray matter are connected to each other by a narrow strip of gray matter, known as the **gray commissure**, the center of which is occupied by the **central canal**. Viewed in three dimensions, the lateral aspect of the gray matter is concave and displays a **ventral (anterior) gray column** and a **dorsal (posterior) gray column**, as well as a small projection, the **lateral (intermediolateral) gray column**, which appears only between spinal

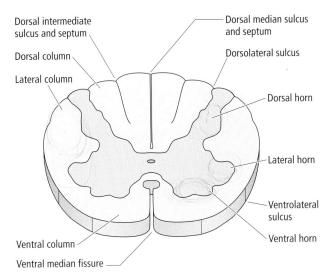

Figure 5.7 ● Cross-section of the spinal cord showing its major landmarks. Observe that the various regions of the white matter are described on the left side and the regions of the gray matter on the right side of the diagram.

cord levels T1 and L2,3 (Fig. 5.7). The lateral gray column represents the location of the cell bodies of the preganglionic sympathetic neurons. It should be noted that these three columns are also referred to as the anterior (ventral), posterior (dorsal), and lateral horns when the spinal cord is examined in cross-sections, and therefore these terms are frequently used interchangeably. Although the gray matter is completely surrounded by white matter, the dorsal horn approaches the limit of the spinal cord and is separated from the dorsolateral sulcus by a small bundle of nerve fibers, known as the **dorsolateral tract** (of Lissauer). The narrow region of the dorsal horn in contact with the dorsolateral tract is subdivided into two regions, the outer **dorsomarginal nucleus** and the somewhat deeper situated **substantia gelatinosa**.

Reticular formation and central canal

The central canal of the spinal cord, lined by ependymal cells, is surrounded by gray matter, the substantia gelatinosa centralis, and the gray commissure

The interface between the gray matter and white matter is usually well defined, but at cervical levels the base of the anterior gray column forms network-like interdigitations with the adjoining white matter. This interwoven structure, known as the **reticular formation**, is similar to other regions present in the brain and caudal spinal cord levels and thus is part of the **reticular system**, discussed later in this book (see Chapter 14). The central canal of the spinal cord contains CSF and is lined by ciliated cuboidal to columnar epithelium composed of **ependymal cells**. In some regions the canal may be partially or completely occluded by clusters of ependymal cells. Immediately surrounding the ependymal cells is the **substantia gelatinosa centralis**, a layer of neuroglia interspersed with occasional nerve cell bodies and fine nerve fibers. The remainder of gray matter surrounding the sub-

stantia gelatinosa centralis is referred to as the **gray commissure**. The white matter surrounding the gray commissure is called the **anterior** and **posterior white commissure**.

Neuronal architecture

Processes of neurons are intertwined within the gray matter of the spinal cord; these form a complex web known as the neuropil

Much of the gray matter is composed of an intricate network of neuronal processes. These may be the central processes of unipolar neurons, the initial segments of motoneurons (somatic and autonomic), axons that are crossing over from one side of the spinal cord to the other, as well as the highly complex and not well understood **neuropil**. The latter is composed of nerve fibers whose extent is limited to the gray matter. Neurons of the spinal cord gray matter are **multipolar** and are collected in various sized clusters, which, for the sake of convenience, are described as belonging to the dorsal gray column, lateral gray column, or ventral gray column.

The gray matter of the spinal cord can be organized into nine layers plus the region surrounding the central canal, named Rexed laminae I–X, after the Swedish neuroanatomist who mapped out their distribution. These laminae are numbered in a dorsoventral direction, and generally correspond to the nerve cell clusters in the three columns (Fig. 5.8; Table 5.4).

Neuronal groups of the dorsal gray column

The nuclei of the dorsal gray column are sensory in nature and are arranged in four groups: the dorsomarginal nucleus, substantia gelatinosa, nucleus proprius, and nucleus dorsalis

The nuclei of the dorsal gray column function in the reception and processing of sensory input from the central processes of

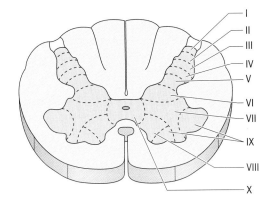

Figure 5.8 ● Cross-section of the spinal cord displaying the divisions of the gray matter into nine regions, referred to as Rexed laminae, as well as a tenth region, around the central canal of the spinal cord, known as the gray commissure (central gray, periependymal gray). These divisions are based on the cellular composition of the gray matter and they bear some relationship to the nuclei of the spinal cord (see Table 5.4).

Column	Neuronal group	Extent	Rexed lamina
Dorsal gray	Dorsomarginal nucleus	C1–S5	I
Dorsal gray	Substantia gelatinosa (of Rolando)	C1–S5	II
Dorsal gray	Nucleus proprius	C1–S5	III and IV (and V?)
Dorsal gray	Nucleus dorsalis (Clarke's column)	C8–L3	VII
Dorsal gray		C1–S5	VI
Lateral gray	Lateral nucleus	T1–L2 (or L3)	VII
Lateral gray	Sacral parasympathetic nucleus (of Onufrowicz)	S2–S4	VII
Ventral gray		C1–S5	VIII
Ventral gray	Medial group	C1–S5 (?except L5 and S1)	IX
Ventral gray	Central group	C1–C6 and L2–S2	IX
Ventral gray	Central group: phrenic nucleus	C3–C6	IX
Ventral gray	Central group: accessory nucleus	C1–C6	IX
Ventral gray	Central group: lumbosacral group	L2–S2	IX
Ventral gray	Lateral group	C4–T1 and L2–S3	IX
Pericentral canal	Gray commissure	C1–S5	X
Pericentral canal	Substantia gelatinosa centralis	C1–S5	X

Table 5.4 ● Neuronal groups of the spinal cord gray matter and their relationship to Rexed laminae.

the unipolar neurons whose cell bodies are located in the dorsal root ganglia. These nerve cells are subdivided into four groups: the dorsomarginal nucleus, substantia gelatinosa, nucleus proprius, and nucleus dorsalis.

The **dorsomarginal nucleus (Rexed lamina I)** extends the entire length of the spinal cord, capping the dorsal horn, and receives afferent fibers carrying pain, temperature, and light touch sensations. It also contributes fibers for the lateral and ventral spinothalamic tracts. It contacts the dorsolateral tract of Lissauer of the white matter.

The **substantia gelatinosa** of Rolando **(Rexed lamina II)** extends the entire length of the spinal cord. It is densely packed with Golgi type II neurons, known as **gelatinosa cells**, that possess highly branched, unmyelinated axons. These cells receive sensory input from the central fibers of unipolar neurons of the dorsal root ganglia, delivering pain, temperature, and light touch information. Descending fibers from higher centers (such as the cerebral cortex) form excitatory and inhibitory synapses with the gelatinosa cells, thus modifying the arriving pain and temperature sensations.

The **nucleus proprius (Rexed laminae III and IV)** extends the entire length of the spinal cord. It is composed of densely clustered large nerve cell bodies, located just ventral to the substantia gelatinosa, and receives the central processes of the majority of the unipolar neurons of the dorsal root ganglia. The nucleus proprius receives pain, light touch, and temperature sensations and provides input to the lateral and ventral spinothalamic tracts.

The **nucleus dorsalis**, also known as **Clarke's column (Rexed lamina VII)** extends from C8 to L3. It is located at the base of the dorsal gray column and houses relatively large cell bodies that receive synapses from proprioceptive fibers, which bring information from Golgi tendon organs and

muscle spindles. Some of the axons of these large nerve cell bodies travel in the dorsal spinocerebellar tracts.

Neuronal groups of the lateral gray column

The **lateral nucleus (Rexed lamina VII)** is composed of the relatively small multipolar cell bodies of preganglionic sympathetic neurons. They are present only between T1 and L2,3, and they send their axons into the ventral root of the spinal cord to enter the sympathetic trunk via the white rami communicantes.

A similar nucleus, the sacral parasympathetic nucleus, is located at sacral levels 2–4. These preganglionic neurons of the sacral outflow of the parasympathetic nervous system are also considered to belong to Rexed lamina VII.

Neuronal groups of the ventral gray column

Neurons of the ventral gray column include motoneurons and interneurons, and are subdivided into three groups: medial, central, and lateral

The nuclei of the ventral gray column are large and small multipolar motoneurons whose axons leave the spinal cord via the ventral rootlets. The large motoneurons give rise to **alpha efferents** that supply skeletal muscles with motor innervation, whereas the smaller motoneurons supply **gamma efferents** to intrafusal muscle fibers of muscle spindles, still others are **interneurons**. These nerve cells are subdivided into three major groups, medial, central, and lateral.

The **medial group (Rexed lamina IX)** extends almost the entire length of the spinal cord (with the possible exceptions

Funiculi	Sulci/fissures	Sulci/fissures	Spinal cord levels
Dorsal funiculus	Dorsal median sulcus	Dorsolateral sulcus	All cord levels
Fasciculus gracilis	Dorsal median sulcus	Dorsointermediate sulcus	All cord levels
Fasciculus cuneatus	Dorsointermediate sulcus	Dorsolateral sulcus	C1–T6
Lateral funiculus	Dorsolateral sulcus	Ventrolateral sulcus	All cord levels
Ventral funiculus	Ventrolateral sulcus	Ventral median fissure	All cord levels
Ventral white commissure	Central canal	Ventral median fissure	All cord levels

Table 5.5 ● Subdivisions of the spinal cord white matter.

of L5 and S1). Between T1 and L4 it is subdivided into two components, the dorsomedial and ventromedial groups. The motoneurons of the medial group provide innervation for the skeletal muscles of the abdomen, the intercostal muscles, and the muscles of the neck.

The **central group (Rexed lamina IX)** is the smallest of the three groups and its distribution is not very extensive. The central group is present only in the cervical and lumbosacral segments of the spinal cord. Two regions of the cervical aspect of the central group have special names, the phrenic nucleus and the accessory nucleus. The **phrenic nucleus** (extending from C3 to C6) is responsible for the innervation of the diaphragm and the **accessory nucleus** (extending from C1 to C6) is responsible for innervation of the sternocleido-mastoid and trapezius muscles. Cells of the accessory nucleus provide fibers for the spinal root of cranial nerve XI (the spinal accessory nerve). The lumbosacral aspect of the central group (L2 to S2) is known as the **lumbosacral group** and its function is not known.

The **lateral group (Rexed lamina IX)** is present only in the regions of the spinal cord responsible for the motor innervation of the upper and lower extremities (C4 to T1 and L2 to S3).

Neuronal groups of the gray commissure

The gray matter that surrounds the central canal of the spinal cord is known as the **gray commissure (periependymal gray)** and the **substantia gelatinosa centralis** (both **Rexed lamina X**). The gray commissure is subdivided into a posterior gray commissure and an anterior gray commissure by the central canal. The gray commissures and the substantia gelatinosa centralis extend the entire length of the spinal cord and are believed to be associated with the autonomic nervous system.

White matter

White matter is also bilaterally symmetric and is composed of myelinated and unmyelinated fibers; it is subdivided into three major columns: the dorsal, lateral, and ventral funiculi

The **white matter** of the spinal cord is also bilaterally symmetric. It surrounds the gray matter and is composed mostly of myelinated and unmyelinated nerve fibers. It has two main functions:

1 To bring information into the central nervous system (CNS) and transmit it to higher levels.
2 To transmit information from the higher levels to the spinal cord and to muscles and glands.

Based on the presence of sulci and fissures, the white matter is subdivided into three major columns: the dorsal, lateral, and ventral funiculi (Table 5.5). The **dorsal funiculus** is bounded by the dorsal median and dorsolateral sulci; hence, it is between the dorsal midline and the dorsal nerve rootlets. The **lateral funiculus** is between the dorsolateral and ventro-lateral sulci; hence it is between the dorsal and ventral rootlets. The **ventral funiculus** is between the ventrolateral sulcus and the ventral median fissure, that is the ventral rootlets and the ventral midline. The cervical and upper thoracic aspects of the dorsal funiculus (C1 to T6) is further subdivided by the dorsal intermediate sulcus and septum into a medial **fasciculus gracilis** and a lateral **fasciculus cuneatus**. Moreover, the ventral funiculus houses the **ventral white commissure,** the region of decussation for the spino-thalamic tracts.

Within the funiculi, the nerve fibers that have similar destinations are arranged in bundles known as **tracts (fasciculi)**. Some of these fiber bundles, especially in the dorsal funiculus, are clearly defined into well recognizable tracts that are separated from each other by glial sheaths, whereas most tracts appear to have overlapping boundaries. Tracts are classified into three categories, **ascending**, **descending**, and **intersegmental**. Ascending tracts transmit sensory information to higher centers, whereas descending tracts relay motor information originating at higher centers. The intersegmental tracts convey information between spinal cord segments, thus orchestrating intersegmental spinal reflexes. Although these tracts will be discussed in detail in later chapters of this book, the positions of these tracts are indicated in the transverse section of the spinal cord in Fig. 5.9 and Table 5.6.

VASCULAR SUPPLY OF THE SPINAL CORD

The spinal cord receives its blood supply from two pairs of longitudinally arranged vessels, the anterior and posterior spinal arteries as well as from small, segmental radicular arteries

The **anterior spinal arteries**, direct branches of the verte-bral arteries, join with each other to form a single median vessel, the **anterior spinal artery**, which occupies

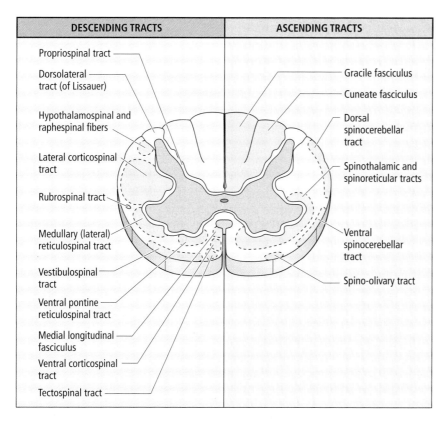

Figure 5.9 ● The white matter of the spinal cord is organized into fiber bundles known as tracts or fasciculi. These tracts have relatively well-defined boundaries and are subdivided into three major groups: descending, ascending, and intersegmental. The descending fibers tracts convey motor information from higher centers, ascending tracts carry sensory information to higher centers, and intersegmental tracts (not illustrated here) transmit information between spinal cord segments and are therefore restricted to the spinal cord.

Funiculi	Ascending tracts	Descending tracts	Intersegmental
Dorsal	Fasciculus gracilis Fasciculus cuneatus		Dorsal intersegmental
Lateral	Dorsal spinocerebellar Ventral spinocerebellar Lateral spinothalamic Spinotectal Posterolateral (of Lissauer) Spinoreticular Spino-olivary	Lateral corticospinal Rubrospinal Lateral (medullary) reticulospinal Descending autonomic fibers Olivospinal	Lateral intersegmental
Ventral	Ventral spinothalamic	Ventral corticospinal Vestibulospinal Tectospinal Reticulospinal	Anterior intersegmental

Table 5.6 ● Tracts of the spinal cord white matter.

and follows the ventral median fissure of the spinal cord. This vessel extends from within the cranial cavity throughout the entire length of the spinal cord and provides small branches that penetrate and supply the white and gray matter of the spinal cord. The anterior spinal artery may be quite small in the thoracic region (Fig. 5.10).

The **posterior spinal arteries** also arise from the vertebral arteries directly or frequently indirectly by way of the inferior cerebellar branch of the vertebral artery. Each posterior spinal artery bifurcates to form two longitudinal vessels that extend from within the cranial cavity throughout the entire length of the spinal cord, sandwiching the dorsal rootlets

between them. These three vessels provide small branches that penetrate and serve the white and gray matter of the spinal cord.

The 32 pairs of **radicular arteries** are small vessels that arise from arteries in the immediate vicinity of the spinal column. Each radicular artery enters the intervertebral foramen where it bifurcates, forming an **anterior** and a **posterior radicular artery**, which follow the ventral and dorsal roots, respectively, to gain entrance into the vertebral canal. The anterior and posterior radicular arteries anastomose with branches of the anterior and posterior spinal arteries on the surface of the spinal cord, and arborize to supply the white

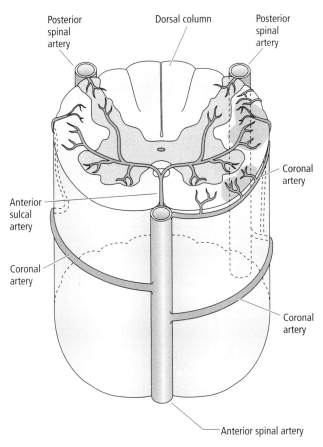

Figure 5.10 ● The vascular supply of the spinal cord. Note that there are two posterior spinal arteries but only a single anterior spinal artery. These three vessels, the coronal arteries, and branches of the anterior spinal artery vascularize the anterolateral aspect of the spinal cord, whereas the deep anterior aspect is vascularized by branches of the anterior sulcal artery. Much of the posterior aspect of the spinal cord is vascularized by branches of the posterior spinal arteries.

and gray matter of the spinal cord. It should be stressed that the radicular arteries are extremely important for the vascularization of the spinal cord, because, with the exception of the cervical region, the anterior and posterior spinal arteries by themselves are unable to provide an adequate vascular supply to the spinal cord. Therefore, an injury to the spinal nerve damages not only the afferent and efferent fibers of a particular spinal cord level, but may also damage the segmental white and gray matter by producing ischemic conditions due to the reduction in blood supply from the radicular artery serving that region. It should be noted that the **great ventral radicular artery** (artery of Adamkiewicz) is the largest, albeit inconsistent, of the radicular arteries (Fig. 5.11). It usually arises on the left-hand side and serves much of the inferior half of the spinal cord, entering the vertebral canal between L2 and L3, and contributes to the formation of the inferior aspect of the ventral spinal artery.

Several longitudinally arranged tortuous veins of the pia mater are responsible for the venous drainage of the spinal cord. These are the **ventral** and **dorsal spinal veins** that communicate with the segmentally arranged radicular veins. The

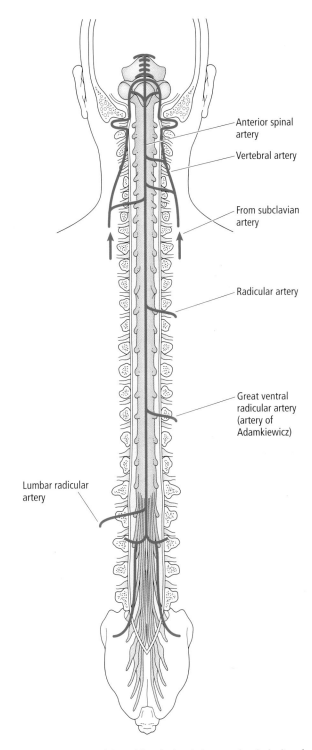

Figure 5.11 ● Ventral view of the spinal cord, drawn so that the bodies of all the vertebrae have been removed and the anterior spinal artery is displayed. Note that although there are 32 pairs of radicular arteries, only a few are displayed in this image and, to limit confusion, their anterior and posterior branches are not displayed. It should be noted that the anterior branches join the anterior spinal artery whereas their posterior branches join the posterior spinal arteries.

radicular veins follow the paths of their companion radicular arteries to leave the vertebral canal via the intervertebral foramina. Along the way they also communicate with the **epidural venous network** embedded in the epidural fat of the vertebral canal. The epidural venous network delivers its blood into the cavernous sinus of the cranial cavity. Cranially, the ventral and dorsal spinal veins drain into the veins and venous sinuses of the cranial cavity.

CLINICAL CONSIDERATIONS

Syringomyelia
Syringomyelia is a spinal cord disorder marked by the loss of the sense of temperature and pain at levels involving several consecutive spinal cord segments. Frequently, the other senses, such as touch and pressure, are unaffected and then a **dissociated anesthesia** is said to be present. A number of conditions may cause this disorder, including the presence of a cleft within the spinal cord as well as an anomalous increase in the size of the central canal of the spinal cord.

Spinal shock
Spinal shock occurs infrequently and is characterized by complete anesthesia and paralysis, including the absence of all reflexes, somatic or autonomic, involving the body segments caudal to the site of damage. This condition may be permanent if the spinal cord is transected or of temporary duration if the spinal cord receives a sudden, but transient, injury, such as an unusually high dose of spinal anesthesia.

Tabes dorsalis
Tabes dorsalis is a late stage effect of syphilis, arising about 10–20 years after the disease was contracted. The condition is characterized by infection of the dorsal column and dorsal roots causing sudden, sharp, shooting pain in the lower extremities. Occasionally, the condition is accompanied by ulceration of the feet, violent stomach cramps, and deterioration of the joints.

Brown-Séquard's syndrome
Brown-Séquard's syndrome is the result of unilateral spinal cord lesions characterized by contralateral pain and temperature loss and ipsilateral weakness and loss of proprioception.

Ependymomas
Ependymomas are tumors involving usually the caudal end of the spinal cord and the filum terminale. The unchecked cell division of the ependymal cells results in the presence of small to medium-sized growth in the affected area. These cells produce large quantities of proteins that elevate the protein levels in the CSF with a consequent reduction in the ability of the arachnoid granulations to deliver CSF into the lacunae lateralis/superior sagittal sinus. Therefore, the patient begins to suffer from hydrocephalus with headaches, and MRI examinations display the presence of enlarged cerebral ventricles.

Spina bifida
Spina bifida is a prenatally acquired developmental defect of incomplete fusion of one or more vertebral arches along with the incomplete fusion of the lips of the neural tube. It is a relatively frequent anomaly, whose incidence is about 1–2% of all births. The subtypes of spina bifida depend on the severity of the lack of fusion. The most common ones are spina bifida anterior, spina bifida cystica, and spina bifida occulta. **Spina bifida anterior** occurs along the ventral surface of the vertebral column. This incomplete closure of the vertebrae is often accompanied by anomalous development of the thoracic and abdominal viscera. **Spina bifida cystica** (also known as **spina bifida aperta**) is a more serious defect involving herniation of the spinal cord (myelocele) and/or of the meninges (meningocele) through the congenital defect in the vertebral column. The meningocele and myelocele may protrude far enough to reach the skin and may even rupture the skin with subsequent leakage of CSF and the possibility of bacterial infection resulting in meningitis. **Spina bifida occulta** is the most common of the spina bifida cases, being present in about 5% of the population. This is the mildest form of spina bifida and may not even be symptomatic. In cases like this the patient may even be unaware of the defect until for other reasons radiographs or MRI are taken of the region of the defect. Then it appears as an osseous defect without the accompanying herniation of the spinal cord or of the meninges. Frequently, the site of the defect is apparent on the overlying skin by the presence of a tuft of hair and/or of a dimple over the region of the osseous lesion.

SYNONYMS AND EPONYMS
OF THE SPINAL CORD

Name of structure or term	Synonym(s)/ eponym(s)
Afferent fibers	Sensory fibers
Anterior gray column	Ventral gray column
Anterior median fissure	Ventral median fissure
Anterolateral sulcus	Ventrolateral sulcus
Dorsolateral tract	Dorsolateral tract of Lissauer
Efferent fibers	Motor fibers
Gray commissure	Periependymal gray
Great ventral radicular artery	Artery of Adamkiewicz
Intermediolateral gray column	Lateral gray column
Lateral reticulospinal tract	Medullary reticulospinal tract
Posterior gray column	Dorsal gray column
Posterior median septum	Dorsal median septum
Posterior median sulcus	Dorsal median sulcus
Posterolateral sulcus	Dorsolateral sulcus
Substantia gelatinosa	Substantia gelatinosa of Rolando

FOLLOW-UP TO CLINICAL CASE

This patient has an **acute myelopathy**, meaning spinal cord pathology, which in this case seems to be in the upper thoracic region. This is located at T4 or above, but not below. The sensory level makes that very clear. The location of the back pain is also consistent. The brisk reflexes and Babinski response (a pathologic reflex of dorsiflexion of the big toe with a scratch on the lateral bottom of the foot) point to a CNS cause, as opposed to a peripheral nervous system cause. Bilateral weakness in the legs, and not the arms, also makes a thoracic cord pathology most likely. A lesion in the brain that causes leg weakness rarely leaves the arm or face unaffected, and is almost always unilateral (although there are exceptions).

This case represents a neurologic emergency. She should be admitted to the hospital without delay. The cause is not immediately clear, but the acute onset and rapid progression mandate immediate action. Work-up would include imaging of the thoracic spine, preferably with MRI. This would almost certainly reveal the pathology; probably in this case a mass of some sort. The mass would have to be rapidly growing and the rapid deterioration and back tenderness indicates that the mass is most likely extra-axial (outside the cord). This could either be intradural or extradural. These types of masses can cause vascular compromise as well as physical compression of the cord.

Some causes of extra-axial masses include metastatic tumors (lung, breast, prostate, etc.), primary tumors (meningiomas, fibromas, etc.), epidural abscess, vascular malformations, or hemorrhage. Compression from vertebral fracture or intervertebral disc herniation can look similar. Treatment for any of these is surgical removal of the offending mass.

QUESTIONS TO PONDER

1. Why does the spinal cord have cervical and lumbar enlargements instead of having a uniform diameter throughout its length?

2. Why is the spinal nerve so important if it is only a couple of millimeters in length?

3. What is the significance of fasciculi (tracts) in the white matter of the spinal cord?

4. Why are the small radicular arteries important for the vascularization of the spinal cord?

5. What is the significance of the lumbar cistern?

CHAPTER 6

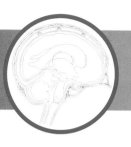
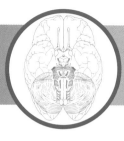
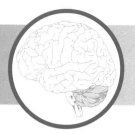

Gross Anatomy of the Brain

CLINICAL CASE

A 28-year-old man was struck in the back of the head by a steel beam while at work. He apparently lost consciousness for approximately 30 minutes. He was hospitalized since he was still confused and disoriented throughout his stay in the emergency room. By the next day he was felt to be back to normal except for a headache and was discharged. The patient had no memory of the event, and he had no memory of an important conversation he had had with his boss 5 minutes before the head trauma. He also had no memory of being in the emergency room and no memories of events subsequent to the injury until the next day. He also noted, besides persistent headache, that he was somewhat forgetful since the injury. Neurologic examination was unremarkable.

The brain, a bilaterally symmetric, soft, gelatinous structure surrounded by its meninges and enclosed in its bony cranium, is continuous with the spinal cord at the foramen magnum at the base of the skull. At birth the brain weighs less than 400 g, but by the beginning of the second year of life it has more than doubled in weight to 900 g. The adult brain weighs between 1,250 and 1,450 g, and demonstrates a gender differential, since brains of males generally weigh more than those of females. This statement, however, should be tempered by the evidence that, in adults, the ratio of brain to body weight is greater in females than in males and that the increase in weight is due more to the proliferation of neuroglia than to the mitotic activity of neurons. An additional point of interest is that there does not appear to be a relationship between brain weight and intelligence.

As detailed in Chapter 2, it is evident during embryogenesis that the brain is subdivided into five continuous regions, from rostral to caudal: the telencephalon, diencephalon, mesencephalon, metencephalon, and myelencephalon. As the brain grows in size and complexity, these regions fold upon and over one another, so that in the adult the evidence of these subdivisions is no longer clearly apparent.

The present chapter will not discuss the functional aspects of the brain; instead its basic morphology and architecture

Note that the clinical case at the beginning of the chapter refers to a patient who loses consciousness subsequent to head trauma.

1 Why is it important to do a CT scan or MRI in the case of a head injury that involves loss of consciousness?

2 What happened to the patient's brain as his head was struck by the steel beam?

3 Most tissues swell when they are exposed to blunt trauma. Does that happen to the brain?

are detailed to provide an anatomical framework of reference for the chapters that follow, and many of the major topics introduced in this chapter are discussed in further detail in specific chapters in this textbook. Much of this terminology should be memorized so that when, in later chapters, functional connections among regions of the brain are discussed the student has a visual image of the location of the various structures and the pathways the connections take.

If the adult brain is viewed in three dimensions, only three regions are clearly visible, and these are the **cerebrum**, **cerebellum**, and part of the **brainstem**.

CEREBRUM

The cerebrum, observed from above, hides the remainder of the brain from view, and is composed of two large, oval, cerebral hemispheres

The **cerebral hemispheres** are narrower posteriorly, at the **occipital pole**, than anteriorly, at the **frontal pole**. They are large, oval struc-

tures that superficially resemble the surface of a shelled walnut (Fig. 6.1). The midline **longitudinal cerebral fissure**, occupied in life by the falx cerebri, incompletely separates the two cerebral hemispheres from one another. The floor of the cerebral fissure is formed by the **corpus callosum**, a large myelinated fiber tract that forms an anatomical and functional connection between the right and left hemispheres.

The surface few millimeters of the cerebral hemisphere are composed of a highly folded collection of gray matter, known as the **cerebral cortex**. This folding increases the surface area and presents elevations, **gyri**, and depressions, **sulci**. Deep to the cortex is a central core of **white matter** that forms the bulk of the cerebrum and represents fiber tracts, supported by neuroglia, ferrying information destined for the cortex and cortical responses to other regions of the central nervous system (CNS). Buried within the mass of white matter are collections of neuron cell bodies, some of which are lumped together under the rubric of **basal ganglia**, even though, technically, they are *nuclei*. Large collections of gray matter are

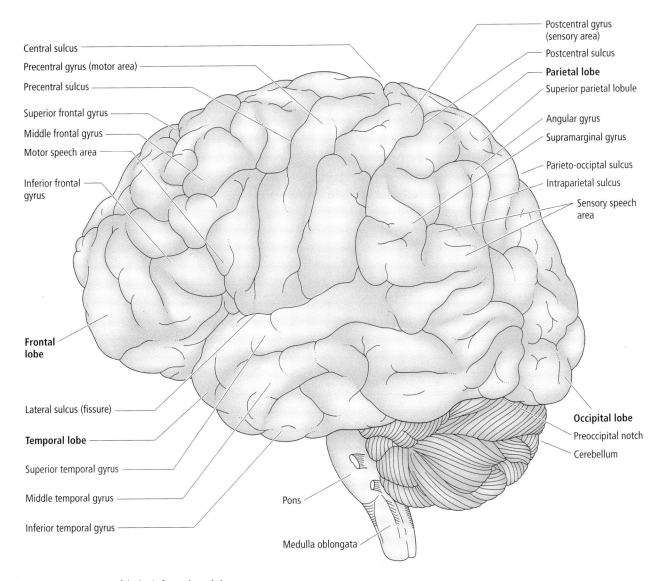

Central sulcus
Precentral gyrus (motor area)
Precentral sulcus
Superior frontal gyrus
Middle frontal gyrus
Motor speech area
Inferior frontal gyrus
Frontal lobe
Lateral sulcus (fissure)
Temporal lobe
Superior temporal gyrus
Middle temporal gyrus
Inferior temporal gyrus

Postcentral gyrus (sensory area)
Postcentral sulcus
Parietal lobe
Superior parietal lobule
Angular gyrus
Supramarginal gyrus
Parieto-occiptal sulcus
Intraparietal sulcus
Sensory speech area
Occipital lobe
Preoccipital notch
Cerebellum
Pons
Medulla oblongata

Figure 6.1 ● Diagram of the brain from a lateral view.

also present in the diencephalons, namely, the epithalamus, thalamus, hypothalamus, and subthalamus.

The **cerebrum** is a hollow structure and the cavities within the cerebral hemispheres are called the **right** and **left lateral ventricles**, which communicate with the third ventricle via the **interventricular foramen** (foramen of Monro) (Fig. 6.2A). The two lateral ventricles are separated from one another by two closely adjoined non-nervous membranes, each known as a **septum pellucidum**. Ependymal cells line each lateral ventricle, and protruding into each ventricle is a choroid plexus that functions in the manufacture of cerebrospinal fluid.

Lobes of the cerebral hemispheres

The five lobes of the cerebral hemispheres are the frontal, parietal, temporal, and occipital lobes, and the insula

Each cerebral hemisphere is subdivided into five lobes: the frontal, parietal, temporal, and occipital lobes, and the insula (Table 6.1). Additionally, the cortical constituents of the limbic system are also considered to be a region of the cerebral hemisphere and some consider it to be the sixth lobe, the **limbic lobe**.

Viewed from the side, each cerebral hemisphere resembles the shape of a boxing glove, where the thumb is the **temporal lobe** and is separated from the **parietal lobe** by the **lateral fissure** (fissure of Sylvius) (Fig. 6.1). The floor of the lateral fissure is formed by the **insula** (island of Reil) that

is hidden by the **frontal**, **parietal**, and **temporal opercula** (L., "lids"), regions of the same named lobes. Although the geographic distributions of many of the sulci and gyri are relatively inconsistent, some regularly occupy specific locations, are recognizable in most brains, and are named. The sulci are generally smaller and shallower than the fissures, and one of these, the **central sulcus** (central sulcus of Rolando), separates the frontal lobe from the parietal lobe. The division between the parietal and occipital lobes is not readily evident when viewed from the lateral aspect because it is defined as the imaginary line between the **preoccipital notch** and the **parieto-occipital notch**. However, it is clearly delimited on the medial aspect of the cerebral hemisphere, where the boundary between these two structures is the **parieto-occipital sulcus** and its continuation, the **calcarine fissure** (Fig. 6.3).

Frontal lobe

The frontal lobe extends from the frontal pole to the central sulcus

On its *lateral aspect*, the **frontal lobe** extends from the frontal pole to the central sulcus, constituting the anterior one-third of the cerebral cortex. Its posteriormost gyrus, the **precentral gyrus**, consists of the primary motor area and is bordered anteriorly by the **precentral sulcus** and posteriorly by the

Table 6.1 ● Lobes of the cerebral hemispheres.

Lobe	Surface	Major gyri	Function/comment
Frontal	Lateral	Precentral gyrus	Primary motor area
		Inferior frontal gyrus	Broca's area in dominant hemisphere; functions in speech production
	Medial	Anterior paracentral lobule	Continuation of precentral gyrus
	Inferior	Gyrus rectus and orbital gyri	Olfactory bulb and tract in the olfactory sulcus
Parietal	Lateral	Postcentral gyrus	Primary somesthetic area
		Superior parietal lobule	Association area involved in somatosensory function
		Inferior parietal lobule	
		Supramarginal gyrus	Integrates auditory, visual, and somatosensory information
		Angular gyrus	Receives visual input
	Medial	Posterior paracentral lobule precuneus	Continuation of the postcentral gyrus
Temporal	Lateral	Superior temporal gyrus	Wernicke's area in dominant hemisphere; ability to read,
		Middle and inferior temporal gyri	understand, and speak the written word
	Superior	Transverse temporal gyri (of Heschl)	Primary auditory cortex
	Inferior	Fusiform gyrus	Borders the parahippocampal gyrus of the limbic lobe
Occipital	Lateral	Superior and inferior occipital gyri	Separated from each other by the lateral occipital sulcus
	Medial	Cuneate gyrus (cuneus)	Separated from each other by the calcarine fissure; striate cortex
		Lingual gyrus	(primary visual cortex) is on the banks of this fissure
Insula	Lateral	Short and long gyri	Forms the floor of the lateral sulcus; associated with taste
Limbic	Medial	Cingulate gyrus	Above the body of the corpus callosum and continues as the isthmus
		Parahippocampal gyrus	Anterior continuation of isthmus; ends in the uncus
		Hippocampal formation	Composed of hippocampus, subiculum, and dentate gyrus
		Subcallosal, parolfactory, and preterminal gyri	Collectively known as the subcallosal area

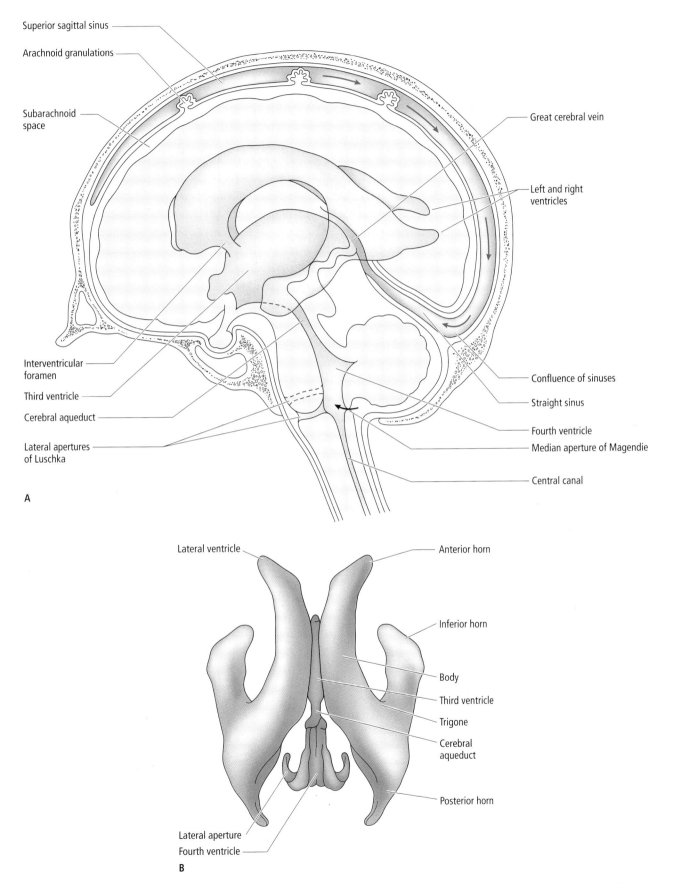

Superior sagittal sinus

Arachnoid granulations

Subarachnoid space

Great cerebral vein

Left and right ventricles

Interventricular foramen

Third ventricle

Cerebral aqueduct

Lateral apertures of Luschka

Confluence of sinuses

Straight sinus

Fourth ventricle

Median aperture of Magendie

Central canal

A

Lateral ventricle

Anterior horn

Inferior horn

Body

Third ventricle

Trigone

Cerebral aqueduct

Posterior horn

Lateral aperture

Fourth ventricle

B

Figure 6.2 ● (A) Diagram of the ventricles of the brain and central canal of the spinal cord *in situ*. (B) A three-dimensional representation of the ventricles of the brain.

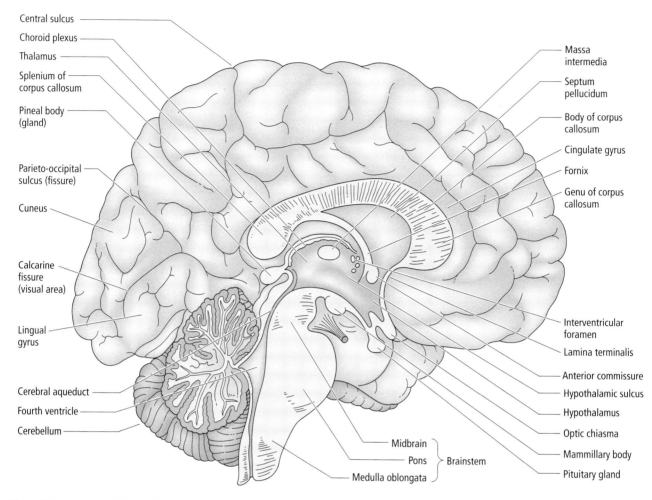

Figure 6.3 ● Diagram of the medial view of a sagittal section of the brain.

central sulcus. The region of the frontal lobe located anterior to the precentral sulcus is subdivided into the **superior, middle**, and **inferior frontal gyri**. This subdivision is due to the presence, though inconsistent, of two longitudinally disposed sulci, the superior and inferior frontal sulci. The inferior frontal gyrus is demarcated by extensions of the lateral fissure into three subregions: the pars triangularis, pars opercularis, and pars orbitalis. In the dominant hemisphere, a region of the inferior frontal gyrus is known as **Broca's area**, which functions in the production of speech.

On its *inferior aspect*, the frontal lobe presents the longitudinally disposed **olfactory sulcus**. Medial to this sulcus is the **gyrus rectus** (also known as the **straight gyrus**), and lateral to it are the **orbital gyri**. The olfactory sulcus is partly occupied by the **olfactory bulb** and **olfactory tract** (Figs 6.4, 6.5). At its posterior extent, the olfactory tract bifurcates to form the lateral and medial olfactory striae. The intervening area between the two striae is triangular in shape and is known as the **olfactory trigone** and it abuts the **anterior perforated substance**.

On its *medial aspect*, the frontal lobe is bordered by the arched **cingulate sulcus**, which forms the boundary of the superior aspect of the cingulate gyrus. The quadrangular-shaped

cortical tissue anterior to the central sulcus is a continuation of the precentral gyrus and is known as the **anterior paracentral lobule**.

Parietal lobe

The parietal lobe extends from the central sulcus to the parieto-occipital sulcus

The **parietal lobe** is interposed between the frontal and occipital lobes and is situated above the temporal lobe. On its *lateral aspect*, its anteriormost gyrus, the **postcentral gyrus**, is the primary somesthetic area to which primary somatosensory information is channeled from the contralateral half of the body. The remainder of the parietal lobe, separated from the postcentral gyrus by the **postcentral sulcus**, is subdivided by the inconsistent intraparietal sulcus, into the **superior** and **inferior parietal lobules**. The former is an association area involved in somatosensory function, whereas the latter is separated into the **supramarginal gyrus**, which integrates auditory, visual, and somatosensory information, and the **angular gyrus**, which receives visual input.

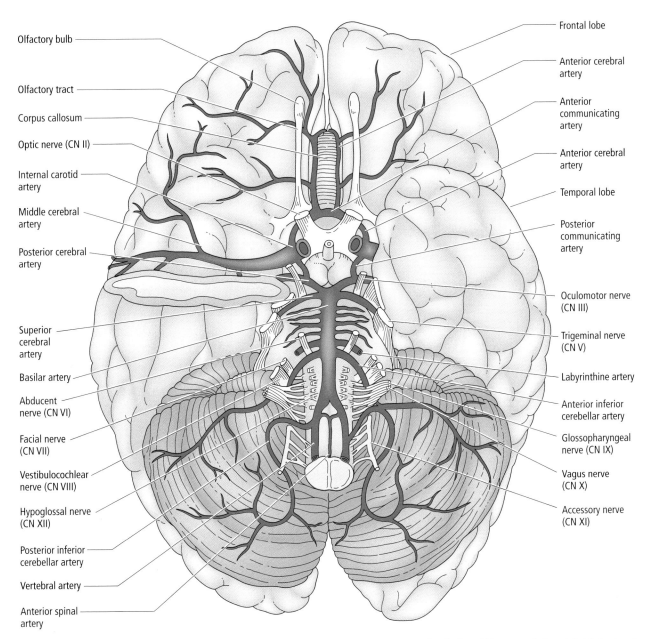

Olfactory bulb

Olfactory tract

Corpus callosum

Optic nerve (CN II)

Internal carotid
artery

Middle cerebral
artery

Posterior cerebral
artery

Superior
cerebral
artery

Basilar artery

Abducent
nerve (CN VI)

Facial nerve
(CN VII)

Vestibulocochlear
nerve (CN VIII)

Hypoglossal nerve
(CN XII)

Posterior inferior
cerebellar artery

Vertebral artery

Anterior spinal
artery

Frontal lobe

Anterior cerebral
artery

Anterior
communicating
artery

Anterior cerebral
artery

Temporal lobe

Posterior
communicating
artery

Oculomotor nerve
(CN III)

Trigeminal nerve
(CN V)

Labyrinthine artery

Anterior inferior
cerebellar artery

Glossopharyngeal
nerve (CN IX)

Vagus nerve
(CN X)

Accessory nerve
(CN XI)

Figure 6.4 ● Diagram of the base of the brain displaying the cranial nerves and the arterial supply. Note that the frontal lobes are pulled apart slightly to show the corpus callosum and the anterior cerebral arteries; also the right temporal lobe is sectioned to demonstrate the middle cerebral artery.

On its *medial aspect*, the parietal lobe is separated from the occipital lobe by the parieto-occipital sulcus and its inferior continuation, the calcarine fissure. This region of the parietal lobe is subdivided into two major structures, the anteriorly positioned **posterior paracentral lobule** (a continuation of the postcentral gyrus) and the posteriorly situated **precuneus**.

Temporal lobe

The temporal lobe, the "thumb of the boxing glove," is situated inferiorly to the lateral fissure and anterior to the parieto-occipital sulcus

The **temporal lobe** is separated from the frontal and parietal lobes by the lateral fissure and from the occipital lobe by an imaginary plane that passes through the parieto-occipital sulcus. The anteriormost aspect of the temporal lobe is known as the **temporal pole**. On its *lateral aspect*, the temporal lobe exhibits three parallel gyri, the **superior**, **middle**, and **inferior temporal gyri**, separated from each other by the inconsistently present superior and middle temporal sulci. The superior temporal gyrus of the dominant hemisphere contains **Wernicke's area**, which is responsible for the individual's ability to speak and understand the spoken and written word.

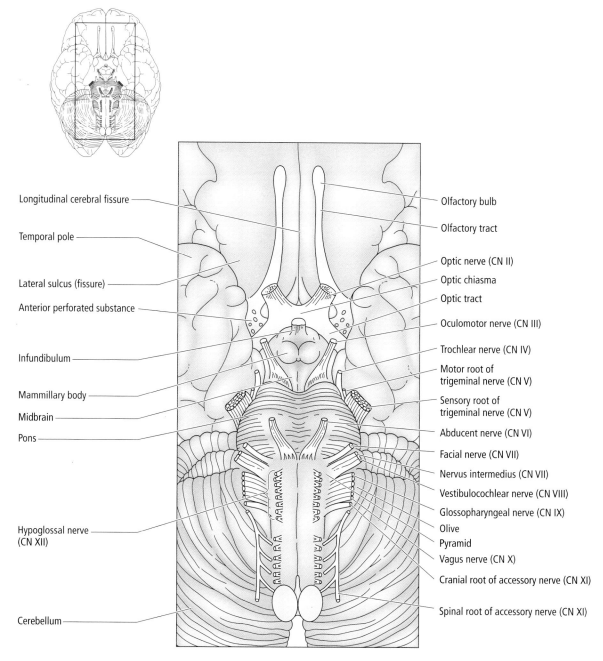

Figure 6.5 ● Diagram of the base of the brain displaying the location of the cranial nerves.

Hidden within the lateral fissure is the *superior aspect* of the temporal lobe whose surface is marked by the obliquely running **transverse temporal gyri** (of Heschl), the primary auditory cortex.

The *inferior aspect* of the temporal lobe is grooved by the **inferior temporal sulcus** that is interposed between the inferior temporal gyrus and the **lateral occipitotemporal gyrus (fusiform gyrus)**. The **collateral sulcus** separates the fusiform gyrus from the **parahippocampal gyrus** of the limbic lobe.

Occipital lobe

The occipital lobe extends from the parieto-occipital sulcus to the occipital pole

The **occipital lobe** extends from the occipital pole to the parieto-occipital sulcus. On its *lateral aspect*, the occipital lobe presents the **superior** and **inferior occipital gyri**, separated from each other by the horizontally running **lateral occipital sulcus**.

On its *medial aspect*, the occipital lobe is subdivided into the superiorly located **cuneate gyrus (cuneus)** and the inferiorly positioned **lingual gyrus**, separated from each other by the **calcarine fissure**. The cortical tissue on each bank of this fissure is known collectively as the **striate cortex (calcarine cortex)**, and forms the **primary visual cortex**.

Insula

The insula forms the floor of the lateral sulcus

In order to view the **insula** the frontal, temporal, and parietal opercula have to be pulled apart, since this lobe is submerged within and forms the floor of the lateral sulcus. It is completely circumscribed by the **circular sulcus**. The lateral surface of the insula is subdivided into several short and long gyri, the most prominent of which is located posteriorly. The insula is believed to be associated with taste, and perhaps other visceral functions.

Limbic lobe

The limbic lobe is a hemispherical region on the medial aspect of the cerebral cortex that surrounds the corpus callosum and the diencephalon

The **limbic lobe** is a complex region and includes the cingulate gyrus, parahippocampal gyrus, hippocampal formation, subcallosal gyrus, parolfactory gyrus, and the preterminal gyrus.

The following description is a view of the *medial aspect* of the hemisected brain and the various regions of the corpus callosum are obvious landmarks. Therefore, the corpus callosum will now be described, even though it is not a part of the limbic lobe. The anterior extent of the corpus callosum, known as the **genu**, bends inferiorly and turns posteriorly, where it forms a slender connection, the **rostrum**, with the anterior commissure. The posterior extent of the corpus callosum is bulbous in shape, and is known as the **splenium** (see Fig. 6.3).

The **cingulate gyrus** is located above the corpus callosum and is separated from it by the **callossal sulcus**. As the cingulate gyrus continues posteriorly, it follows the curvature of the corpus callosum and dips beneath the splenium to continue anteriorly as the **isthmus** of the cingulate gyrus. The anterior continuation of the isthmus is the **parahippocampal gyrus** whose anteriormost extent is known as the **uncus**. Above the parahippocampal gyrus is the **hippocampal sulcus**, which separates the parahippocampal gyrus from the **hippocampal formation** (composed of the hippocampus, subiculum, and dentate gyrus).

Just beneath the rostrum of the corpus callosum is the **subcallosal gyrus**. The connection between the anterior commissure and the optic chiasma is the lamina terminalis and the cortical tissue anterior to the lamina terminalis is the **parolfactory gyrus** and **preterminal gyrus**. The subcallosal, parolfactory, and preterminal gyri are referred to as the **subcallosal area**.

Brodmann's classification of the cerebral cortex

The best accepted system of functional regionalization of the cerebral cortex was developed by the neuroanatomist, K. Brodmann, who in the late nineteenth and early twentieth centuries mapped the cortex into 47 unique areas, each associated with specific morphological characteristics. Although later investigators refined and expanded his map into more than 200 areas and assigned functional characteristics to them, Brodmann's original classification is still widely used. The major areas, their location, and function are presented in Table 6.2.

Histology of the cerebral cortex

The histological organization of the cerebral cortex permits its subdivision into three regions: the archicortex, mesocortex, and neocortex

The cerebral cortex is well endowed with neurons, neuroglia, nerve fibers, and a rich vascular supply. The

Area number	Area name	Location
1, 2, and 3	Primary somatosensory cortex	Parietal lobe
4	Primary motor cortex	Frontal lobe
5 and 7	Somatosensory association cortex	Parietal lobe
6	Supplementary motor area and premotor cortex	Frontal lobe
8	Frontal eye field	Frontal lobe
9–12 and 46–47	Prefrontal cortex	Frontal lobe
17	Primary visual cortex	Occipital lobe
18 and 19	Visual association cortex	Occipital lobe
22	Wernicke's speech area (dominant hemisphere)	Temporal lobe (and perhaps into the parietal lobe also)
	Auditory association cortex	
41 and 42	Primary auditory cortex	Temporal lobe
44 and 45	Broca's speech area (dominant hemisphere)	Frontal lobe

Table 6.2 ● Selected Brodmann's areas.

Name	Numeral	Components
Molecular layer	I	Afferent fibers from the thalamus or from the cerebral cortex
External granular layer	II	Stellate neurons
External pyramidal layer	III	Small pyramidal cells
Internal granular layer	IV	Fusiform neurons
Internal pyramidal layer	V	Larger pyramidal cells
Fusiform layer	VI	Fusiform neurons

Table 6.3 ● Layers of the neocortex.

arrangement of the three types of neurons that populate the cortex—pyramidal cells, stellate neurons, and fusiform neurons—permit the classification of the cortex into three types: the archicortex (allocortex), mesocortex (juxtallocortex), and neocortex (isocortex).

The **archicortex**, phylogenetically the oldest region, is composed of only three layers and is located in the limbic system. The **mesocortex**, phylogenetically younger, is composed of three to six layers, and is located predominantly in the insula and cingulate gyrus. The **neocortex**, phylogenetically the youngest region of the cerebral cortex, is composed of six layers and comprises the bulk of the cerebral cortex.

Although the cerebral cortex is arranged in layers, superimposed upon this cytoarchitecture is a functional organization of **cell columns**. Each cell column is less than 0.1 mm in diameter, is perpendicular to the superficial surface of the cortex, passes through each of the six cortical layers, and is composed of neurons with similar functions. All neurons of a single column respond to like stimuli from the same region of the body.

The organization of the six layers of the neocortex is known as its cytoarchitecture, where each layer has a name and an associated Roman numeral (Table 6.3).

White matter of the cerebral hemispheres

There are three categories of fiber components in the cerebral hemispheres: commissural, projection, and association fibers

The central core of white matter that forms the substance of the cerebrum is composed of myelinated nerve fibers of varied sizes and their supporting neuroglia. These fibers may be classified into the following three categories: commissural, projection, and association fibers.

Commissural fibers

Commissural fibers are bundles of axons that connect the right and left cerebral hemispheres

Commissural fibers (transverse fibers) interconnect the right and left cerebral hemispheres. There are four bundles of commissural fibers, the corpus callosum, anterior commissure, posterior commissure, and hippocampal commissure (see Fig. 6.3).

The largest group of the commissural fibers, the **corpus callosum**, is comprised of four regions: the anteriormost **rostrum**, the curved **genu**, the relatively flattened **body**, and its posteriormost region, the **splenium**. The corpus callosum connects the **neocortex** of the right hemisphere with that of the left.

The **anterior commissure** connects the right and left amygdalas, the olfactory bulbs, and several cortical regions of the two temporal lobes.

The **posterior commissure** connects the right and left pretectal region and related cell groups of the mesencephalon.

The **hippocampal commissure (commissure of the fornix)** joins the right and left hippocampi to one another.

Projection fibers

Projection fibers are restricted to a single hemisphere and connect the cerebral hemispheres with lower levels

Projection fibers are restricted to a single hemisphere and connect the cerebral cortex with lower levels, namely the corpus striatum, diencephalon, brainstem, and spinal cord. The majority of these fibers are axons of pyramidal cells and fusiform neurons. These fibers are component parts of the **internal capsule**, which is subdivided into the anterior limb, genu, posterior limb, retrolentiform, and sublentiform regions. The projection fibers may be subdivided into corticopetal and corticofugal fibers.

Corticopetal fibers are *afferent fibers* that bring information from the thalamus to the cerebral cortex. They consist of **thalamocortical fibers**.

Corticofugal fibers are *efferent fibers* that transmit information from the cerebral cortex to lower centers of the brain and spinal cord. They consist of the corticobulbar, corticopontine, corticospinal, and corticothalamic fibers.

Association fibers

Association fibers connect regions of a hemisphere to other regions of the same hemisphere

Association fibers, also known as **arcuate fibers**, are restricted to a single hemisphere and are subdivided into two major categories, short arcuate fibers and long arcuate fibers.

Fiber group	Extends from	Extends to
Uncinate fasciculus	Anterior temporal lobe and uncus	Motor speech area and orbital gyri of frontal lobe
Cingulum	Medial cortex below rostrum	Parahippocampal gyrus and parts of temporal lobe
Superior longitudinal fasciculus	Anterior frontal lobe	Occipital, parietal, and temporal lobes
Inferior longitudinal fasciculus	Posterior region of the parietal and temporal lobes	Anterior region of the occipital lobe
Fronto-occipital fasciculus	Ventrolateral regions of the frontal lobe	Temporal and occipital lobes

Table 6.4 ● Extent of the long arcuate fiber groups.

They are the axons of pyramidal cells and fusiform neurons. **Short arcuate fibers**, which connect adjacent gyri, do not usually reach the subcortical white matter of the cerebral cortex; most of them are confined to the cortical gray matter. The **long arcuate fibers**, which connect nonadjacent gyri, consist of the following fiber tracts (Table 6.4): the uncinate fasciculus, cingulum, superior longitudinal fasciculus, inferior longitudinal fasciculus, and fronto-occipital fasciculus.

Basal ganglia

The basal ganglia consist of some deep cerebral nuclei and brainstem nuclei that, when damaged, produce movement disorders

The **basal ganglia**, called ganglia even though they are nuclei, are large collections of cell bodies that are embedded deep in the white matter of the brain (Fig. 6.6). These soma include those deep nuclei of the brain and brainstem which, when damaged, produce *movement disorders*. Thus the basal ganglia are composed of the caudate nucleus, lenticular nucleus (putamen and globus pallidus), subthalamic nucleus of the ventral thalamus, and the substantia nigra of the mesencephalon (the caudate nucleus and the putamen together are referred to as the striatum). These nuclei have numerous connections with various regions of the CNS; some receive input and are categorized as input nuclei, some project to other regions and are referred to as output nuclei, whereas some receive input, project to other regions of the CNS, and have local interconnections and these are known as intrinsic nuclei.

DIENCEPHALON

The diencephalon is that portion of the prosencephalon that surrounds the third ventricle

The **diencephalon**, interposed between the cerebrum and the midbrain, has four regions: the epithalamus, thalamus (Gr., "bed, bedroom"), hypothalamus, and subthalamus. The right and left halves of the diencephalon are separated from one another by a narrow slit-like space, the ependymal-lined **third ventricle**. Rostrally, the interventricular foramina (of Monro) leads from the lateral ventricles into the third ventricle, whereas caudally, the third ventricle is connected to the **fourth ventricle** by the **cerebral aqueduct (of Sylvius)**.

The **epithalamus**, composed of the **pineal body**, **stria medullaris**, and **habenular trigone**, constitutes the dorsal surface of the diencephalon. The right and left thalami compose the bulk of the diencephalon and form the superior aspect of the lateral walls of the third ventricle. The two thalami, structures composed of numerous nuclei, are connected to each other by a bridge of gray matter, the **interthalamic adhesion (massa intermedia)**. Some of the nuclei of the thalamus form distinctive bulges on its surface, namely the **pulvinar** (L., "cushion") and the **medial** and **lateral geniculate bodies**. The boundary between the thalamus and the **hypothalamus** is marked by a groove, the **hypothalamic sulcus**, located along the lateral walls of the third ventricle. Structures associated with the hypothalamus are the **pituitary gland** and its **infundibulum**, the **tuber cinereum**, and the two **mammillary bodies**. The subthalamic nuclei and fiber tract form the **subthalamus**.

CEREBELLUM

The cerebellum is located below the occipital lobe of the cerebral hemispheres. It is connected to the brainstem via the superior, middle, and inferior cerebellar peduncles

The **cerebellum** is located in the posterior aspect of the brain, just below the occipital lobes of the cerebrum (Figs 6.7–6.8). It is separated from the cerebrum via a horizontal dural reflection, the tentorium cerebelli. The cerebellum is connected to the midbrain, pons, and medulla of the brainstem via three pairs of fiber bundles, the **superior, middle**, and **inferior cerebellar peduncles**, respectively. Viewing the cerebellum, it can be seen that it is composed of the right and left **cerebellar hemispheres** and the narrow, intervening **vermis**. The vermis is also subdivided into a superior and an inferior portion, where the superior portion is visible between the two hemispheres, while its inferior portion is buried between the two hemispheres.

The surface of the cerebellum has horizontal elevations, known as **folia**, and indentations between the folia, known as **sulci**. Some of these sulci are deeper than others and they are said to subdivide each hemisphere into three lobes, the

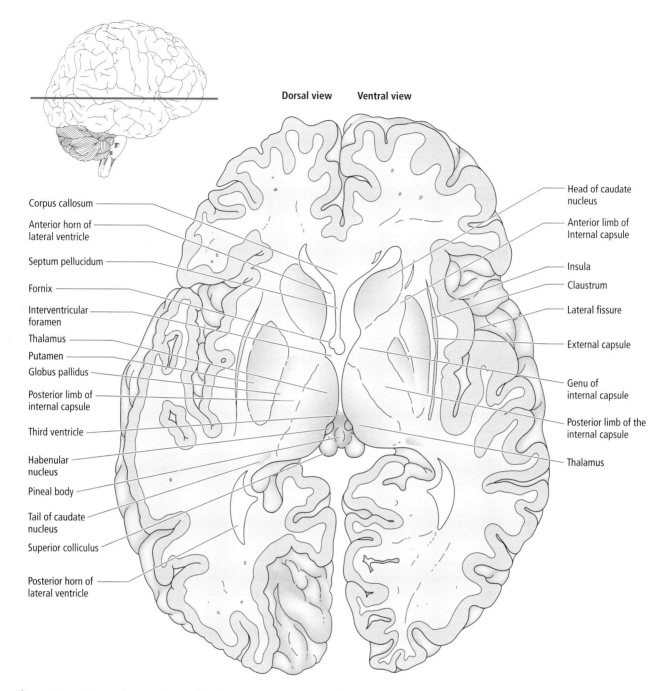

Dorsal view   **Ventral view**

Corpus callosum

Anterior horn of
lateral ventricle

Septum pellucidum

Fornix

Interventricular
foramen

Thalamus

Putamen

Globus pallidus

Posterior limb of
internal capsule

Third ventricle

Habenular
nucleus

Pineal body

Tail of caudate
nucleus

Superior colliculus

Posterior horn of
lateral ventricle

Head of caudate
nucleus

Anterior limb of
Internal capsule

Insula

Claustrum

Lateral fissure

External capsule

Genu of
internal capsule

Posterior limb of the
internal capsule

Thalamus

Figure 6.6 ● Diagram of a coronal section of the brain displaying the basal ganglia.

small **anterior lobe**, the much larger **posterior lobe**, and the inferiorly positioned **flocculonodular lobe** (formed from the **nodule** of the vermis and the **flocculus** of each cerebellar hemisphere). The anterior lobe is separated from the posterior lobe by the **primary fissure**, and the **posterolateral fissure** separates the flocculonodular lobe from the posterior lobe (Figs 6.7–6.9).

Similar to the cerebrum, the cerebellum has an outer rim of gray matter, the **cortex**, an inner core of nerve fibers, the **medullary white matter**, and the **deep cerebellar nuclei**, located within the white matter. The cortex and white matter

are easily distinguished from each other in a midsagittal section of the cerebellum, where the white matter arborizes, forming the core of what appears to be a tree-like architecture, known as the **arbor vitae**.

Histologically, the cerebellar cortex is a three-layered structure, the outermost **molecular layer**, the middle **Purkinje layer**, and the innermost **granular layer**. The granular layer is well defined due to the presence of nucleic acids in the nuclei of its numerous, small cells. The Purkinje layer, composed of a single layer of large Purkinje cell perikaryons, is also easily recognizable. The molecular layer is

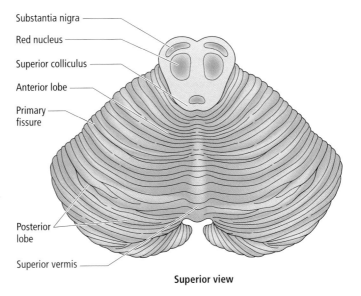

Substantia nigra

Red nucleus

Superior colliculus

Anterior lobe

Primary fissure

Posterior lobe

Superior vermis

Superior view

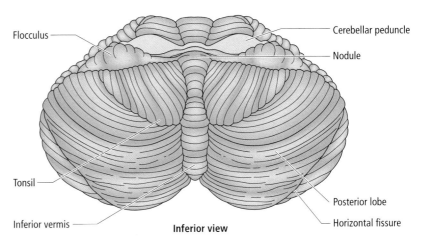

Flocculus

Cerebellar peduncle

Nodule

Tonsil

Inferior vermis

Inferior view

Posterior lobe

Horizontal fissure

Figure 6.7 ● Superior and inferior views of the cerebellum.

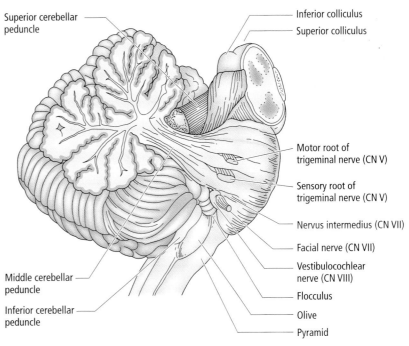

Superior cerebellar peduncle

Inferior colliculus

Superior colliculus

Motor root of trigeminal nerve (CN V)

Sensory root of trigeminal nerve (CN V)

Nervus intermedius (CN VII)

Facial nerve (CN VII)

Vestibulocochlear nerve (CN VIII)

Flocculus

Olive

Pyramid

Middle cerebellar peduncle

Inferior cerebellar peduncle

Figure 6.8 ● Diagram of a lateral view of the cerebellum and medulla.

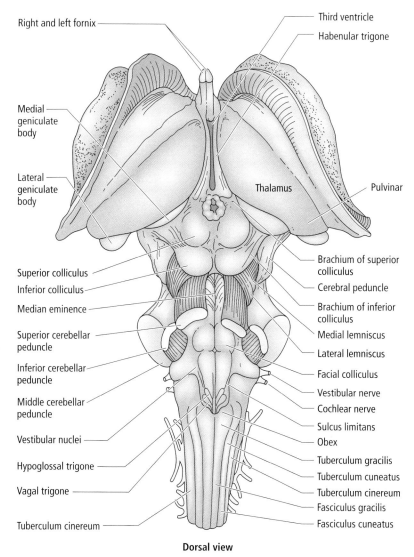

Right and left fornix
Third ventricle
Habenular trigone
Medial geniculate body
Lateral geniculate body
Thalamus
Pulvinar
Superior colliculus
Inferior colliculus
Median eminence
Superior cerebellar peduncle
Inferior cerebellar peduncle
Middle cerebellar peduncle
Vestibular nuclei
Hypoglossal trigone
Vagal trigone
Tuberculum cinereum
Brachium of superior colliculus
Cerebral peduncle
Brachium of inferior colliculus
Medial lemniscus
Lateral lemniscus
Facial colliculus
Vestibular nerve
Cochlear nerve
Sulcus limitans
Obex
Tuberculum gracilis
Tuberculum cuneatus
Tuberculum cinereum
Fasciculus gracilis
Fasciculus cuneatus

Dorsal view

Figure 6.9 ● Diagram of the dorsal view of the brainstem.

rich in axons and dendrites as well as capillaries that penetrate deep into this layer.

Four pairs of nuclei are located within the substance of the cerebellar white matter. These are the **fastigial**, **dentate**, **emboliform**, and **globose nuclei**. The connections between the cortical regions and the deep nuclei of the cerebellum permit the subdivision of the cerebellum into three zones—the **vermal**, **paravermal**, and **hemispheric**—where each zone is composed of deep cerebellar nuclei, white matter, and cortex.

BRAINSTEM

The brainstem is composed of the mesencephalon, metencephalon, and myelencephalon

The **brainstem**, the oldest part of the CNS, is composed of the **mesencephalon**, **metencephalon**, and **myelencephalon** (although some authors also include the diencephalon) (Figs 6.9, 6.10). Since these are embryologic terms, one may also state that the brainstem is composed of the mesencephalon, pons, cerebellum, and medulla oblongata. As parts of it have been overgrown by the cerebrum and the cerebellum, its dorsal aspect is mostly hidden from view in the whole brain, whereas its ventral and lateral aspects are visible. Removal of the cerebral and cerebellar hemispheres exposes the brainstem in its entirety and it is usually examined in that fashion as well as by hemisecting the entire brain.

Mesencephalon

The mesencephalon is that region of the brainstem that surrounds the cerebral aqueduct (of Sylvius)

The **mesencephalon (midbrain)** is a relatively narrow band of the brainstem surrounding the cerebral aqueduct, extending from the diencephalon to the pons. The dorsal aspect of the midbrain is known as the **tectum** (L., "roof") and incorporates the paired **superior** and **inferior colliculi** (also known as the **corpora quadrigemina**). These structures are associated with the **lateral** and **medial geniculate bodies**, respectively, and they are all associated with

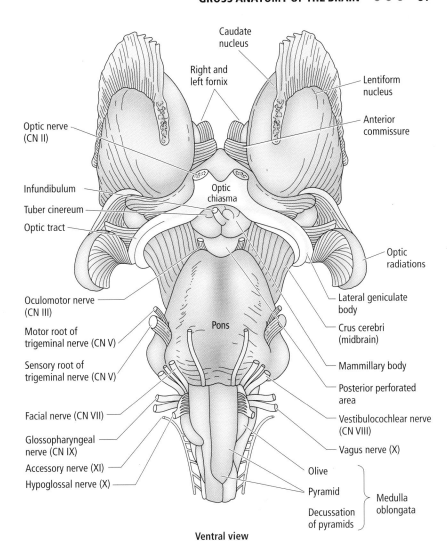

Caudate
nucleus

Right and
left fornix

Lentiform
nucleus

Optic nerve
(CN II)

Anterior
commissure

Infundibulum

Tuber cinereum

Optic chiasma

Optic tract

Optic
radiations

Oculomotor nerve
(CN III)

Lateral geniculate
body

Motor root of
trigeminal nerve (CN V)

Pons

Crus cerebri
(midbrain)

Sensory root of
trigeminal nerve (CN V)

Mammillary body

Posterior perforated
area

Facial nerve (CN VII)

Vestibulocochlear nerve
(CN VIII)

Glossopharyngeal
nerve (CN IX)

Vagus nerve (X)

Accessory nerve (XI)

Olive

Hypoglossal nerve (X)

Pyramid

Medulla
oblongata

Decussation
of pyramids

Figure 6.10 ● Diagram of the ventral view of the brainstem.

Ventral view

visual and auditory functions. The **trochlear nerve (CN IV)** exits the dorsal aspect of the mesencephalon just below the inferior colliculus. All other cranial nerves exit the ventral aspect of the brainstem. The region of the mesencephalon below the cerebral aqueduct is known as the **midbrain (mesencephalic) tegmentum** (L., "cover"). The cerebral hemispheres are connected to the brainstem by two large fiber tracts, the **cerebral peduncles**, and the depression between the peduncles is known as the interpeduncular fossa, the site of origin of the **oculomotor nerve (CN III)**.

Metencephalon

The metencephalon is located below the cerebellum; its ventral bulge, the pons, is clearly visible

The cerebellum overlies and hides the dorsal aspect of the brainstem, but its ventral aspect, the **pons**, is clearly evident. Rostrally, the **superior pontine sulcus** acts as the boundary between the **metencephalon** and the midbrain and the **inferior pontine sulcus** as the boundary between the metencephalon and the myelencephalon. Part of the floor of the fourth ventricle is formed by the dorsal aspect of the pons,

and is known as the **pontine tegmentum**, the structure that houses the nuclei of the trigeminal, abducent, facial, and vestibulocochlear nerves. Cranial nerves VI, VII, and VIII leave the brainstem at the inferior pontine sulcus, whereas the trigeminal nerve exits the brainstem through the middle cerebellar peduncle.

Myelencephalon

The myelencephalon, the caudal-most portion of the brainstem, houses the fourth ventricle

The caudal-most portion of the brainstem, the **myelencephalon**, also known as the **medulla oblongata**, extends from the inferior pontine sulcus to the spinal cord. The boundary between them is the region where the lateral walls of the fourth ventricle converge in a V shape at the midline **obex** (at the level of the foramen magnum).

The ventral surface of the myelencephalon displays the **anterior midline fissure**, bordered on each side by the **pyramids** and crossed by the pyramidal decussations, connecting the right and left pyramids to each other. The **olives** are olivepit-shaped swellings lateral to each pyramid.

The hypoglossal nerve is evident as a number of thin filaments on each side of the brainstem, arising from the **anterior lateral sulcus** between the pyramids and olives. The glossopharyngeal, vagus, and accessory nerves arise from the groove dorsal to the olives.

The dorsal surface of the myelencephalon presents the posterior median fissure, which is interposed between the right and left **tuberculum gracilis**, swellings formed by the nucleus gracilis. Just lateral to the tuberculum gracilis is another swelling, the **tuberculum cuneatus**, a bulge formed by the underlying nucleus cuneatus. The caudal continuation of the tuberculum gracilis is the **fasciculus gracilis**, and the continuation of the tuberculum cuneatus is the **fasciculus cuneatus**. Just lateral to the tuberculum cuneatus is another

swelling, the **tuberculum cinereum**, formed by the **descending tract of the trigeminal nerve**.

CLINICAL CONSIDERATIONS

As indicated at the beginning of this chapter, most of the major topics discussed here are presented in detail in subsequent chapters. Therefore the pertinent clinical considerations are presented in the chapters dealing with the specific topics.

SYNONYMS AND EPONYMS OF THE BRAIN

Name of structure or term	Synonym(s)/ eponym(s)
Archicortex	Allocortex
Central sulcus	Central sulcus of Rolando
Commissural fibers	Transverse fibers
Cuneate gyrus	Cuneus
Hippocampal commissure	Commissure of the fornix
Interthalamic adhesion	Massa intermedia
Interventricular foramen	Foramen of Monro
Lateral fissure	Fissure of Sylvius
Lateral occipitotemporal gyrus	Fusiform gyrus
Mesocortex	Juxtallocortex
Myelencephalon	Medulla oblongata
Neocortex	Isocortex
	Neopallium
	Homogenetic cortex
Striate cortex	Calcarine cortex
Superior and inferior colliculi	Corpora quadrigemina
Transverse temporal gyri	Transverse temporal gyri of Heschl

FOLLOW-UP TO CLINICAL CASE

A review of the head CT that was performed in the emergency room revealed the extent of the patient's injuries. There were modest contusions of the bilateral anterior and orbital regions of the frontal lobes and the left anterior temporal lobe. Contusions are brain "bruises." The patient had a **concussion**, meaning any alteration of consciousness resulting from head trauma. Persistent headache and memory difficulties are often characteristics of "postconcussion syndrome," which can also include dizziness, poor balance, poor concentration, and other vague symptoms.

There are several ways in which head trauma can cause brain injury. As in the above case, contusion can result. The locations of these are often predictable. *Coup* and *contrecoup* are terms used to define the location of contusion related to the site of head trauma. A *coup* injury refers to a contusion that occurs to the part of the brain that directly underlies the site of head trauma. A *contrecoup* injury refers to a contusion that occurs in parts of the brain directly opposite the site of head trauma. The patient above suffered *contrecoup* contusions. The anterior and orbital regions of the frontal lobes and the anterior temporal lobes are the most common locations of contusions. The skull is somewhat rigid and is the first to have

contact with the object of injury. There is a very sudden acceleration or deceleration of the skull. The brain within is somewhat mobile. As the skull accelerates or decelerates, the brain crashes into the skull at certain points. The damage occurs mostly to those parts of the brain surface that are most angular and also in close proximity to the bones of the skull.

There are other locations and mechanisms of injury that are often more important, especially in cases where disability or death occur from head trauma. There is also a rotational component to brain movement inside the skull at the moment of impact. This causes shearing stresses, especially to the upper brainstem region, which can damage the reticular system, which maintains consciousness and awareness. This is probably the mechanism by which head injury causes loss or alteration of consciousness. Damage to the corpus callosum is also often demonstrated pathologically, secondary to its rotational momentum against the rigid falx. Diffuse axonal injury refers to diffuse damage to white matter, specifically to axons, which has been demonstrated pathologically. This is also thought to be due to shearing or stretching injury to the long and thin axons due to sudden and severe rotational and angular stresses.

QUESTIONS TO PONDER

1. How are the categories of the three fiber components of the cerebral white matter classified?

2. Why is it inaccurate to call the basal ganglia, "ganglia?"

3. What are peduncles?

4. Describe the reason why the trochlear nerve is an unusual cranial nerve.

CHAPTER 7

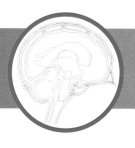
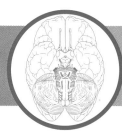
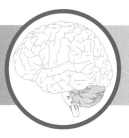

Meninges and Cerebrospinal Fluid

CLINICAL CASE

A 23-year-old male comes to the emergency room complaining of 2 days of fever, headache, stiff neck, and general ill feeling. Symptoms have been getting worse over the course of these 2 days. He notes pain on movement of his eyes and sensitivity to light. His roommate who accompanies him noted he has been somewhat lethargic. Before the onset of the present symptoms he had been quite well. He had had no seizure.

Upon examination in the ER, he appeared ill and lethargic but easily arousable. He had a fever of 38.5°C. Blood pressure, heart rate, and respirations were normal. With the patient supine the neck was passively flexed. The neck was abnormally stiff (i.e., it did not flex to the normal degree). At the same time as the neck was flexed, his knees flexed slightly. When eye movement was tested, the patient noted his eyes hurt when they moved. Strength, sensation, reflexes, and all other parts of the neurologic and general exams were normal or unremarkable.

The central nervous system (CNS) is enclosed in the bony cranium and vertebral column. Separating the brain and spinal cord from the calcified tissue are three more or less concentric membranes, the outermost, dense, irregular collagenous connective tissue, the **dura mater**, also known as the **pachymeninx**, the middle spiderweb-like **arachnoid**, and the very flimsy, innermost **pia mater**. The arachnoid and pia mater, together, are also known by the term **leptomeninges** and are separated from one another by the subarachnoid space. The dura mater forms reflections upon itself, some of which contain **dural venous sinuses**. The meninges surrounding the brain and spinal cord are compared in Table 7.1.

Cerebrospinal fluid (CSF), a clear fluid, manufactured by the **choroid plexuses** of the ventricles of the brain, circulates in the subarachnoid space, the ventricles of the brain, and the central canal of the spinal cord. It is delivered into the lacunae lateralis, and from there into the vascular supply by structures, derived from both the pia mater and arachnoid, known as **arachnoid granulations**. The four ventricles of the brain are fluid-filled, ependymal-lined cavities that are continuous with each other as well as with the central canal of the spinal cord. These spaces are the remnants of the lumen of the embryonic neural tube.

Skull (bone)	Vertebra (bone)
Periosteal layer of dura mater	Periosteum
Epidural space (potential space)	Epidural space (a real space that contains the venous plexus in a connective tissue surrounded by fat)
Meningeal layer of dura mater	Dura mater (meningeal layer only)
Subdural space (potential space)	Subdural space (potential space)
Arachnoid	Arachnoid
Subarachnoid space (real space; contains CSF)	Subarachnoid space (real space; contains CSF and cauda equina; expands into the lumbar cistern caudal to L2)
Pia mater	Pia mater (forms denticulate ligaments and filum terminale)
Subpial extracellular matrix	Subpial extracellular matrix
Astrocyte end-feet	Astrocyte end-feet
Brain tissue	Spinal cord tissue
CSF, cerebrospinal fluid.	

Table 7.1 ● Comparison of the layers of meninges around the brain and spinal cord.

CRANIAL MENINGES

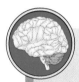

Note that the clinical case at the beginning of the chapter refers to a patient suffering with increasing severity of fever, headache, and stiff neck.

1 What should the physician suspect when the symptoms include fever accompanied by light sensitivity?

2 Why is a stiff neck an important clue in this case?

3 Should the fever be treated with antibiotics? Why or why not?

Cranial dura mater

The cranial dura mater is composed of an outer periosteal dura mater and an inner meningeal dura mater

Although the **dura mater** surrounding the brain is continuous with the dura mater surrounding the spinal cord at the level of the foramen magnum, it is customary to discuss the two separately. The cranial dura mater has two layers (Fig. 7.1), an outer **periosteal dura mater** that is attached to the internal table of the diploë and acts as a true periosteum, and an internal **meningeal dura mater** that is in intimate contact with the arachnoid. The periosteal and meningeal layers of the dura mater are tightly attached to each other throughout much of their extent; however, in certain regions the two layers are separated from each other to form venous channels, known as sinuses.

The periosteal dura mater is a coarse type of connective tissue composed of dense irregular collagenous connective tissue interlaced with some elastic fibers. It is a very tough, mostly inelastic tissue that is tightly attached to the surrounding bony vault of the skull. It is especially firmly attached at the sutures and to the floor of the cranial cavity. At the foram-ina of the skull the periosteal dura mater forms a connective tissue sheath around the cranial nerves as they leave the skull and this dural layer is quickly replaced by the epineurium, derived from the extracranial connective tissue. At the rim of the foramen magnum the periosteal dura becomes continuous with the periosteum of the vertebral canal.

The meningeal layer of the dura is also composed of dense irregular collagenous connective tissue. Its innermost aspect is lined by a single layer of flattened **fibroblasts** that form an **epithelioid sheath** that is in direct contact with, and separates the **arachnoid** from, the collagenous connective tissue component of the meningeal dura.

Vascular and nerve supply of the dura mater

The periosteal layer of the dura mater has a very rich vascular supply, whereas the meningeal layer of the dura mater has no vascular supply

The periosteal layer of the dura mater is richly supplied by blood vessels, whereas the meningeal layer has no vascular supply. The blood vessels of the periosteal layer include the **middle meningeal** and **accessory meningeal arteries** of the middle cranial fossa, as well as the **meningeal branches of the anterior** and **posterior ethmoidal arteries** and **meningeal branches of the internal carotid artery** of the anterior cranial fossa. **Meningeal branches of the vertebral, occipital, middle meningeal**, and **ascending pharyngeal arteries** serve the periosteal dura of the posterior cranial fossa. Most of these vessels enter the cranial fossa via foramina and canals of the skull, such as the jugular and mastoid foramina and the hypoglossal canal. Blood is drained from the dura by meningeal veins that empty their blood (indirectly through venous lacunae) into several of the sinuses as well as into nearby **emissary veins** and **diploic veins**.

The dura mater possesses a very rich **sensory nerve** supply, derived mostly from **cranial nerve V (trigeminal nerve)** but also from the first three cervical spinal nerves that serve the dura mater of the posterior cranial fossa. Sympathetic

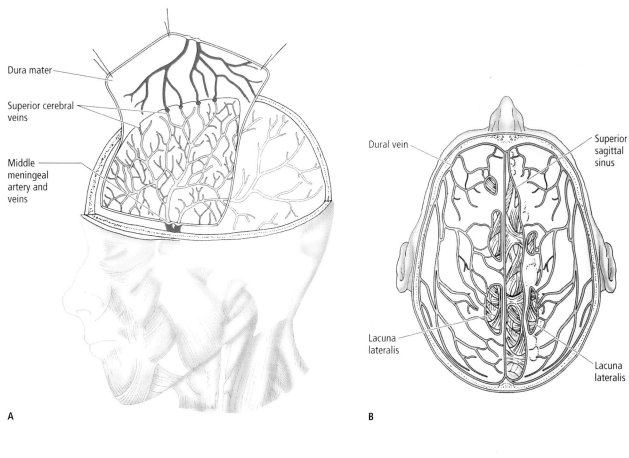

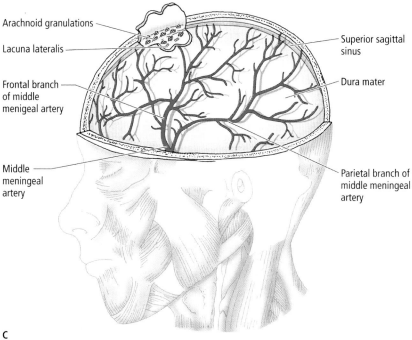

Figure 7.1 ● Three views of the dura mater. (A) The periosteal layer of the dura is reflected to demonstrate the branches of the middle meningeal artery and the tributaries of the middle meningeal vein. (B) The dura is opened to display the superior sagittal sinus and several lacunae lateralis. (C) The dura is reflected to display the arachnoid granulations in a lacuna lateralis.

fibers also reach the dura mater, arising from the vertebral and carotid plexuses, to serve the dural blood vessels.

Reflections of the meningeal layer of the dura mater

The meningeal layer of the dura mater is reflected upon itself to form dural folds

The meningeal layer of the dura mater is responsible for the formation of several folds that serve to separate parts of the brain from one another (Figs 7.2, 7.3). These folds are reflections of the meningeal layer of the dura upon itself and are known as the **falx cerebri, tentorium cerebelli**, and **falx cerebelli**. Additionally, the meningeal layer of the dura also forms a diaphragm over the hypophyseal fossa, known as the **diaphragma sella**, as well as a roof over the trigeminal ganglion, thus forming a shallow compartment known as the **cavum trigeminale (Meckel's cave)**.

Falx cerebri

The falx cerebri is a sickle-shaped fold of the meningeal layer of the dura mater

The **falx cerebri** is located in the midline **longitudinal cerebral fissure**, which separates the right and left cerebral hemisphere from one another. Its narrow anterior aspect is attached to the **crista galli** and its broader, posterior aspect is attached to the superior surface of the **tentorium cerebelli**, extending posteriorly as far as the internal occipital protuberance. The superior, convex surface of the falx cerebri is attached to the periosteal layer of the dura, leaving only a narrow, endothelially lined channel, the **superior sagittal sinus**. This sinus is the largest dural venous sinus, which begins just behind the crista galli, at the **foramen cecum**, and terminates posteriorly at the **confluence of sinuses**. The inferior surface of the falx cerebri is a free, concave-shaped

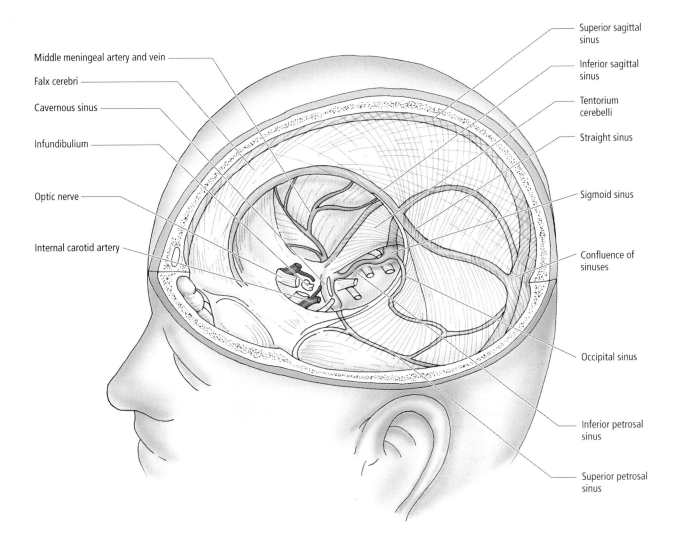

Figure 7.2 ● Diagram of the dura and dural folds containing the venous sinuses.

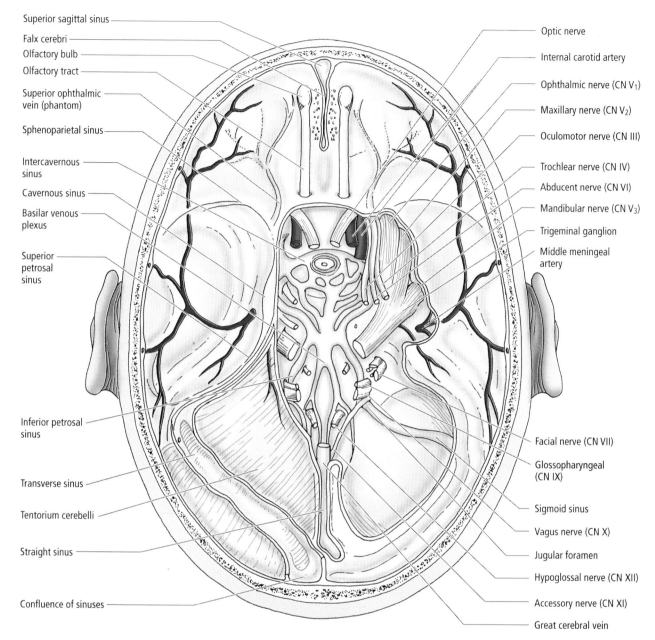

Superior sagittal sinus
Falx cerebri
Olfactory bulb
Olfactory tract
Superior ophthalmic vein (phantom)
Sphenoparietal sinus
Intercavernous sinus
Cavernous sinus
Basilar venous plexus
Superior petrosal sinus
Inferior petrosal sinus
Transverse sinus
Tentorium cerebelli
Straight sinus
Confluence of sinuses

Optic nerve
Internal carotid artery
Ophthalmic nerve (CN V₁)
Maxillary nerve (CN V₂)
Oculomotor nerve (CN III)
Trochlear nerve (CN IV)
Abducent nerve (CN VI)
Mandibular nerve (CN V₃)
Trigeminal ganglion
Middle meningeal artery
Facial nerve (CN VII)
Glossopharyngeal (CN IX)
Sigmoid sinus
Vagus nerve (CN X)
Jugular foramen
Hypoglossal nerve (CN XII)
Accessory nerve (CN XI)
Great cerebral vein

Figure 7.3 ● Diagram of the dura and dural reflections housing the venous sinuses. Note that on the right-hand side the tentorium cerebelli was incised to display the trigeminal ganglion, the three divisions of the trigeminal nerve, and the contents of the cavernous sinus.

edge, which contains the **inferior sagittal sinus**. At the junction where the falx cerebri joins and fuses with the tentorium cerebelli is another endothelially lined space, the **straight sinus**, that receives blood from the inferior sagittal sinus and the **great cerebral vein**. Blood from the straight sinus also enters the confluence of sinuses.

Tentorium cerebelli

The tentorium cerebelli separates the occipital lobe of the cerebral hemispheres from the cerebellum

The **tentorium cerebelli**, a horizontal reflection of the meningeal layer of the dura mater, is interposed between the cerebellum and the occipital lobes of the cerebrum. Its anterior sharp concave margin is free, cradling the midbrain. The lateral borders of the tentorium cerebelli extend much farther anteriorly than does its midline (where it is joined by the falx cerebri). The superior surface of the central region is convex, being highest along the length of the **straight sinus**. The **transverse sinuses**, endothelially lined vascular spaces, sit in the lateral aspect of the tentorium cerebelli, where this dural reflection is attached to the lips of the **grooves** for the left and right **transverse sinuses of the occipital bone**.

Anteriorly, the lateral aspect of the tentorium is attached to the superior surface of the **petrous** portion of the **temporal bone** and forms endothelially lined spaces, the right and left **superior petrosal sinuses**, and continues anteriorly to attach to the **posterior clinoid processes of the sphenoid bone**. The free, medial edge of the tentorium cerebelli crosses over the lateral edge and attaches to the **anterior clinoid processes** of the sphenoid bone. Because of the separate attachments of the free and attached aspects of the tentorium cerebelli, an oval opening is created in the dura mater. This opening, known as the **tentorial incisure**, surrounds the midbrain and permits the ascent of the **posterior cerebral arteries** to reach the **cerebral hemispheres**.

Falx cerebelli

The **falx cerebelli**, a relatively small reflection of the meningeal layer of the dura folded upon itself, is interposed between the right and left cerebellar hemispheres. The posterior border of the falx cerebelli meets the periosteal layer of the dura mater on the internal aspect of the occipital bone, where it is attached along the entire length of the **internal occipital crest**, and forms the endothelially lined **occipital sinuses**.

Diaphragma sella

The **diaphragma sella** is a thin reflection of the meningeal layer of the dura mater. Its lateral aspect is attached to the **clinoid processes**, whereas its central aspect is open, thus forming an incomplete roof over the hypophyseal fossa that is penetrated by the **infundibulum of the hypophysis**. The anterior and posterior edges of the diaphragma sella house the **anterior** and **posterior intercavernous sinuses**.

Cavum trigeminale (Meckel's cave)

The **cavum trigeminale (Meckel's cave)** is a narrow, slit-like region interposed between the periosteal and meningeal layers of the dura mater positioned on the **trigeminal impression** of the petrous portion of the **temporal bone**. It is occupied by the **trigeminal ganglion** as well as by the sensory and motor roots of the trigeminal nerve.

Cranial arachnoid

The cranial arachnoid is a fine, spiderweb-like, nonvascular membrane that is interposed between the meningeal layer of the dura mater and the pia mater

There is a potential space between the meningeal layer of the cranial dura mater and the **cranial arachnoid** (Figs 7.4, 7.5), known as the **subdural space**, that, according to some neuroanatomists, is occupied by an extremely thin film of fluid. The subarachnoid space may become blood-filled in a case of hemorrhage due to a cerebrovascular accident, although according to some neuroanatomists and histologists the subarachnoid space is not involved; instead an **intradural space** is created. Similar to the dura mater, the

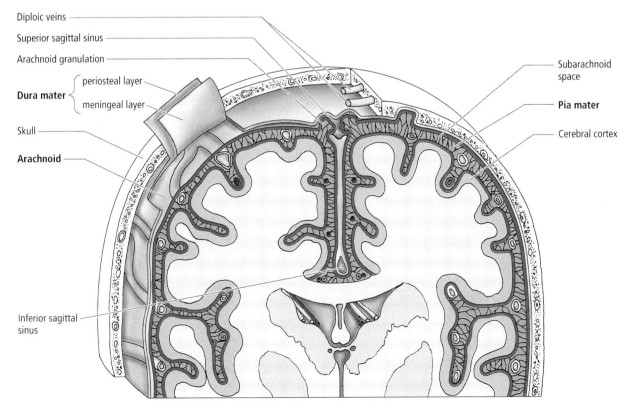

Diploic veins
Superior sagittal sinus
Arachnoid granulation
Dura mater { periosteal layer
meningeal layer
Skull
Arachnoid
Inferior sagittal sinus

Subarachnoid space
Pia mater
Cerebral cortex

Figure 7.4 ● Diagram of a frontal section of the skull and brain to display the three meninges: the dura mater, arachnoid, and pia mater.

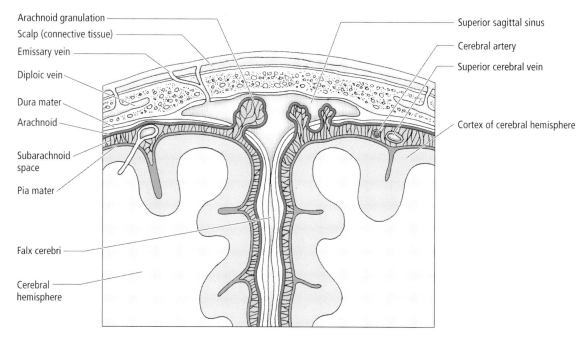

Figure 7.5 ● Diagram of the superior sagittal sinus housing arachnoid granulations.

arachnoid's surface is composed of a single layer of flattened **fibroblasts** that form an **epithelioid sheath**, from which trabeculae, known as **arachnoid trabeculae**, extend toward and attach to the external surface of the pia mater. These trabeculae are formed from highly attenuated fibroblasts that surround some collagen fibers. The space between the epithelioid sheath and the pia mater, known as the **subarachnoid space**, is occupied by **cerebrospinal fluid** and is traversed by numerous arachnoid trabeculae. Blood vessels from the vascular meninges perforate the arachnoid to reach the pia mater; however, each vessel is completely surrounded by arachnoid fibroblasts and, therefore, the vessels never actually enter the subarachnoid space. It should be recalled that the **blood–brain barrier**, established by the endothelial cells of the blood vessels, prevents large molecules from leaving the bloodstream.

Arachnoid cisternae

The arachnoid resembles the dura mater in that it does not follow closely the contours of the brain; therefore, over the sulci, the subarachnoid space is much deeper than over the gyri. Moreover, in certain areas of the brain the arachnoid completely diverges from the pia mater, forming expanded subarachnoid spaces known as **subarachnoid cisterns**. As the CSF percolates through the subarachnoid spaces it also enters the subarachnoid cisterns, filling them. The major subarachnoid cisterns are the cisterna magna (cisterna cerebellomedullaris), pontine cistern, and interpeduncular and chiasmatic cisterns (cisterna basalis), as well as the superior cistern (cistern of the great cerebral vein).

The **cisterna magna**, the largest of the subarachnoid cisterns, is formed between the caudal aspect of the cerebellum and the dorsal surface of the medulla oblongata as the arachnoid stretches across these two structures rather than following the contour of the brain. It is the cisterna magna that communicates with the fourth ventricle of the brain via the medial **foramen of Magendie**, through which the CSF formed by the choroid plexuses of the ventricles of the brain enters the subarachnoid space. The **pontine cistern** is a much smaller space than the cisterna magna. It is located along the ventral surface of the pons and communicates with the subarachnoid space of the spinal cord caudally, and with the pontine cistern rostrally. The **basilar artery** traverses the pontine cistern. The **interpeduncular cistern** is located between the right and left cerebral peduncles and receives CSF by way of the two **lateral foramina of Luschka**, from the fourth ventricle. The interpeduncular cistern is continuous with the **chiasmatic cistern** and, frequently, the two are considered to be a single cistern, the **cisterna basalis**, even though the **optic chiasma** is interjected between them. The pontine cistern is traversed by the **posterior** and **middle cerebral arteries** as well as by the **cerebral arterial circle**, whereas the **anterior cerebral artery** traverses the chiasmatic cistern. The **superior cistern (cistern of the great cerebral vein)** is located in the vicinity of the superior aspect of the cerebellum, the corpora quadrigemina, and the pineal body. As its alternate name implies, the great cerebral vein traverses the superior cistern.

Arachnoid granulations

Arachnoid granulations function in transporting CSF manufactured by the choroid plexuses of the ventricles of the brain into the vascular system

Arachnoid granulations (also known as **arachnoid villi**) are small, but visible with the unaided eye, mushroom-shaped

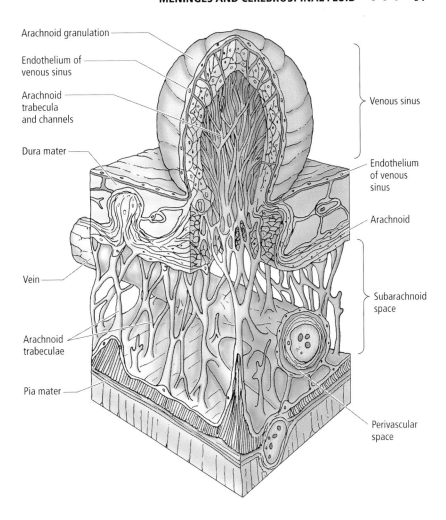

Arachnoid granulation

Endothelium of venous sinus

Arachnoid trabecula and channels

Dura mater

Vein

Arachnoid trabeculae

Pia mater

Venous sinus

Endothelium of venous sinus

Arachnoid

Subarachnoid space

Perivascular space

Figure 7.6 ● Schematic diagram of an arachnoid granulation protruding into the superior sagittal sinus.

evaginations of the arachnoid protruding into the lumen of the dural sinuses (Fig. 7.6). Most of the arachnoid granulations are associated with **lacunae lateralis**, diverticula of the **superior sagittal sinus**, although some jut into the lumen of the sinus. The core of an arachnoid granulation, composed of arachnoid trabeculae, is continuous with the subarachnoid space and is surrounded by the epithelioid layer of the arachnoid and of the dura, forming a membrane that is two cell layers thick. As the arachnoid granulation evaginates into the lacuna lateralis it is invested by some cellular and collagenous elements of the meningeal dura mater, which in turn is surrounded by the endothelial lining of the blood vessel. CSF from the subarachnoid space enters into the core of the arachnoid granulation and from there penetrates, probably by osmosis, the epithelioid layers of the arachnoid granulation and the endothelial lining to escape into the lacuna lateralis. Therefore, the function of the arachnoid granulations is transporting CSF manufactured by the choroid plexuses of the ventricles of the brain into the vascular system. It is important to note that although the arachnoid granulations protrude into the venous sinuses, they are always separated from the blood by the endothelial lining of the dural sinus/lacuna lateralis.

Cranial pia mater

Cranial pia mater is a vascular tissue that closely invests the contours of the brain

The **cranial pia mater** is composed of a single layer (or occasionally two layers) of attenuated **fibroblasts** that form a transparent **epithelioid membrane**, which closely invests the contours of the brain. The pia mater, unlike the arachnoid or the dura mater, follows the gyri and the sulci, maintaining an uninterrupted contact with the surface of the brain. Since the pia mater is vascular it has numerous blood vessels associated with it; however, because this layer is so thin, the vessels are in part surrounded by cells derived from the arachnoid trabeculae and, in part, by cells of the pia mater. Deep to the epithelioid sheath is a thin, discontinuous layer of collagen and elastic fibers. The end-feet of the astrocytes form a protective layer that underlies this subpial extracellular matrix, separating it from the neural tissue. In addition to separating the subarachnoid space from the brain tissue, the pia mater also serves to degrade neurotransmitter substances and to prevent material in the subarachnoid space from entering the nervous tissue, as evidenced by the inability of erythrocytes to cross the pia mater in cases of subarachnoid hemorrhages.

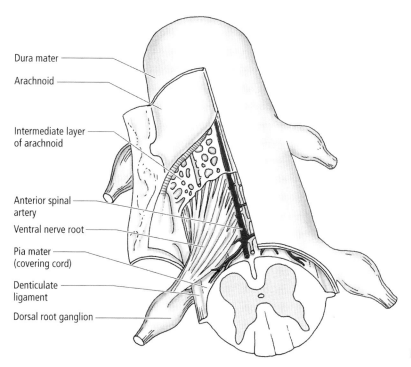

Dura mater

Arachnoid

Intermediate layer
of arachnoid

Anterior spinal
artery

Ventral nerve root

Pia mater
(covering cord)

Denticulate
ligament

Dorsal root ganglion

Figure 7.7 ● Schematic diagram of the spinal meninges.

SPINAL MENINGES (Fig. 7.7)

Spinal dura mater

Spinal dura mater, unlike cranial dura mater, is composed only of a meningeal layer

The **dura mater** of the spinal cord differs from that of the cranial cavity because it is composed only of the meningeal layer. The periosteal layer is the true **periosteum** of the vertebral canal and is separated from the meningeal layer by a loose connective tissue and fat-filled **epidural space**. A plexus of veins is embedded in the connective tissue and fat layer. At the level of the second lumbar vertebra the spinal cord ends in the conical-shaped **conus medullaris**, but the dura mater continues as a cylindrical sheath until it narrows into a cone-shaped structure at the second sacral vertebra. It then continues as a very narrow cylindrical sheath, which becomes anchored into the periosteum of the first and second coccygeal vertebra.

Spinal arachnoid

The **spinal arachnoid** is seamlessly continuous with the cranial arachnoid at the foramen magnum. It closely adheres to the spinal dura mater and there is a potential subdural space between the two layers. The narrow subarachnoid space is filled with CSF that percolates through and around the arachnoid trabeculae. At the level of the conus medullaris the subarachnoid space becomes much larger, is referred to as the **lumbar cistern**, and is filled with the dorsal and ventral

rootlets of the spinal nerves, collectively referred to as the **cauda equina**. These nerve rootlets extend to the lumbar, sacral, and coccygeal intervertebral foramina through which they exit to form their respective spinal nerves. As the rootlets of the spinal nerves leave the vertebral canal, they are surrounded by a thin arachnoid sheath to be replaced by the proper connective tissue layers (endoneurium, perineurium, and epineurium) as they enter the realm of the peripheral nervous system.

Spinal pia mater

The spinal pia mater is continuous with the cranial pia mater at the foramen magnum and the two are essentially identical to each other

The **spinal pia mater** very closely invests the spinal cord and at the level of the conus medullaris it is gathered into a very thin, non-nervous filament, the **filum terminale**, that extends for about 20 cm from the tip of the conus medullaris to become attached to the periosteum of the first coccygeal vertebra. Narrow, triangular, fibrous extensions of the pia mater extend laterally through the arachnoid to attach to the meningeal layer of the dura mater, helping to anchor the spinal cord along its entire length. These triangular extensions of the pia resemble shark's teeth and, therefore, are known as **denticulate ligaments**. There are 21 pairs of denticulate ligaments, positioned in such a fashion that they are situated about half way between successive spinal nerves. The first pair is located at the level of the foramen magnum and the last pair is situated caudal to the 12th thoracic vertebra.

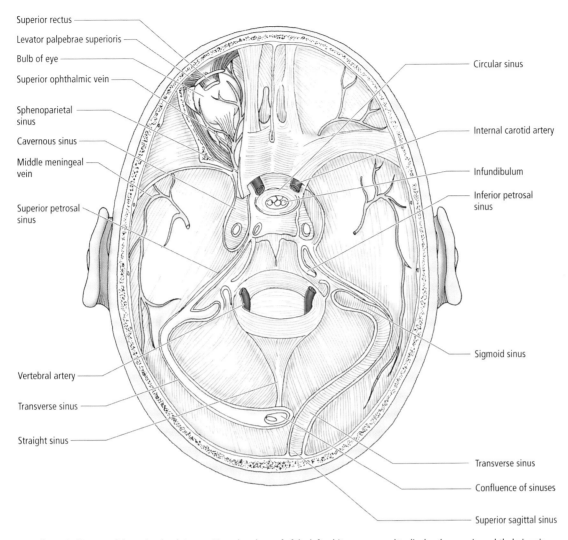

Superior rectus

Levator palpebrae superioris

Bulb of eye

Superior ophthalmic vein

Sphenoparietal sinus

Cavernous sinus

Middle meningeal vein

Superior petrosal sinus

Vertebral artery

Transverse sinus

Straight sinus

Circular sinus

Internal carotid artery

Infundibulum

Inferior petrosal sinus

Sigmoid sinus

Transverse sinus

Confluence of sinuses

Superior sagittal sinus

Figure 7.8 ● Schematic diagram of the major dural sinuses. Note that the roof of the left orbit was removed to display the superior ophthalmic vein.

VENOUS SINUSES OF THE CRANIAL DURA MATER

Venous sinuses of the cranial dura mater are endothelially lined vascular spaces formed in reflections of the meningeal layer of the cranial dura mater

The **venous sinuses** of the dura mater, formed within reflections of the meningeal dura, are endothelially lined venous channels that are devoid of valves (Fig. 7.8). These sinuses collect blood from the brain and from emissary veins and also receive CSF from the subarachnoid spaces. They empty their contents into the superior jugular bulb of the **internal jugular vein** as that bulb sits in the jugular foramen. Based on their location and draining patterns the dural venous sinuses are grouped into two major categories, the **anterior inferior** and **posterior superior groups**.

Anterior inferior group

The **anterior inferior group** of dural sinuses include the cavernous, anterior and posterior intercavernous, spheno-

parietal, and superior and inferior petrosal sinuses and the basilar plexus.

Cavernous sinus

The cavernous sinuses, located on either side of the body of the sphenoid, are associated with the internal carotid artery as well as with a number of cranial nerves

The two, rather large **cavernous sinuses** (Fig. 7.9), located on either side of the body of the sphenoid just inferior to the hypophyseal fossa, are connected to each other by the very small **anterior** and **posterior intercavernous sinuses**, thus forming the **circular sinus**, encircling the infundibulum of the pituitary gland. The lumen of each cavernous sinus is criss-crossed by a spongy network of endothelially covered filamentous structures that reduce the luminal size and reduce the velocity of blood flow. The cavernous sinus receives its blood from a number of sources, including the **pterygoid plexus of veins** (via the emissary veins), the

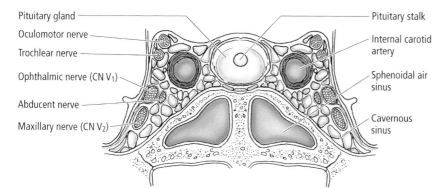

Figure 7.9 ● Diagram of the cavernous sinuses and their contents.

angular vein (via the inferior and superior ophthalmic veins), as well as the **middle** and **inferior cerebral veins**. There are numerous interrelationships of the cavernous sinus with the venous channels on the outside of the skull, which presents many possible pathways for the entry of infectious agents with a possibility of **meningitis**. The **superior** and **inferior petrosal sinuses** drain blood from the cavernous sinus into the transverse sinus and into the superior bulb of the internal jugular vein, respectively.

The cavernous sinus is associated with the internal carotid artery as well as a number of cranial nerves, four of which are embedded in its wall and one other that passes through the lumen of the sinus. Embedded in the lateral wall of the cavernous sinus are the **ophthalmic** and **maxillary divisions of the trigeminal nerve** and the **oculomotor** and **trochlear nerves**. The **internal carotid artery** and its associated **carotid sympathetic plexus** of fibers, as well as the **abducent nerve**, pass through the lumen of the cavernous sinus. It should be stressed, however, that the vessel and nerves travel in a sheath of endothelial cells that isolate them from the bloodstream.

Sphenoparietal sinus

The **sphenoparietal sinus** is a very small sinus that is located on the inferior aspect of the edge of the lesser wing of the sphenoid bone. It receives blood from several tiny meningeal veins and from the anterior temporal diploic vein, and drains into the cavernous sinus.

Superior petrosal sinus

The **superior petrosal sinus** is located in a shallow groove on the superior aspect of the petrous portion of the temporal bone. It receives blood via small veins from the tympanic cavity, as well as from the cerebellar and inferior cerebral veins and drains into the transverse sinus just prior to its joining the sigmoid sinus.

Inferior petrosal sinus

The **inferior petrosal sinus**, located in the shallow groove formed between the petrous temporal and occipital bones, receives blood from the cavernous and superior petrosal

sinuses, the veins of the pons, medulla, and cerebellum, and from the labyrinthine veins. The inferior petrosal sinus drains into the superior bulb of the internal jugular vein.

Basilar plexus

The **basilar plexus**, a group of slender venous channels located in the meningeal dura mater on the basilar portion of the occipital bone, acts as a venous connection between the right and left inferior petrosal sinuses. It drains into the anterior vertebral plexus of veins.

Posterior superior group

The **posterior superior group** of dural sinuses includes the superior sagittal, inferior sagittal, straight, transverse, sigmoid, petrosquamous, and occipital sinuses as well as the confluence of sinuses (see Figs 7.1–7.3, 7.9, 7.10).

Superior sagittal sinus

The superior sagittal sinus begins at the foramen cecum and ends in the transverse sinus of the right hand side

The **superior sagittal sinus**, located in the superior, convex aspect of the falx cerebri, begins at the **foramen cecum**, where blood from the **emissary vein of the foramen cecum** enters it and, usually, ends in the **transverse sinus** of the right side. Along its length the superior sagittal sinus grooves the internal aspects of the frontal bone, the suture line between the two parietal bones, and the squamous portion of the occipital bone, forming the **groove for the superior sagittal sinus**. This sinus receives blood from many of the cerebral veins, from the superior cerebellar veins, and the emissary veins traversing the parietal foramina. Additionally, **lacunae lateralis**, endothelially lined spaces housing arachnoid granulations, drain their blood mixed with CSF into the superior sagittal sinus.

Inferior sagittal sinus

The **inferior sagittal sinus** is much smaller, narrower, and shorter than the superior sagittal sinus. It is located in the concave, inferior aspect of the **falx cerebri** occupying a little more than its posterior half. Occasional veins from the medial aspect of the cerebral hemispheres and small veins of the falx cerebri deliver their blood into the inferior sagittal sinus, which, in turn, drains into the straight sinus.

Straight sinus

The **straight sinus** occupies the interface between the tentorium cerebelli and the falx cerebri and is formed by the junction of the great cerebral vein with the inferior sagittal sinus. It receives blood from those two structures as well as from some of the cerebellar veins and drains, usually, into the left transverse sinus.

Transverse sinuses

The paired **transverse sinuses** begin at the internal occipital protuberance of the occipital bone and are located in the lateral aspect of the tentorium cerebelli. They are responsible for the formation of the grooves for the transverse sinuses. The right transverse sinus is usually larger and is the continuation of the superior sagittal sinus, whereas the left transverse sinus is the continuation of the straight sinus, although, occasionally the reverse occurs. Each transverse sinus ends in, and delivers its blood to, the sigmoid sinus; whereas each receives blood from the inferior cerebellar vein, the diploic veins from the temporal and occipital regions, the veins from the cerebral hemispheres, and from the petrosquamous and superior petrosal sinuses.

Sigmoid, petrosquamous, and occipital sinuses and the confluence of sinuses

Each **sigmoid sinus**—a continuation of each transverse sinus—follows an S-shaped curve as it grooves the temporal and occipital bones to terminate in the posterior aspect of the superior bulb of the internal jugular vein in the jugular foramen. The **petrosquamous sinus**, when present, is located in the meningeal reflection of the dura along the intersection of the petrous and squamous portions of the temporal bone. It receives blood from a diploic vein in its vicinity and drains into the transverse sinus. The smallest of the sinuses is the **occipital sinus** located in the posterior margin of the falx cerebelli. It delivers its blood into the transverse sinus or, with equal frequency, into the **confluence of sinuses** located just lateral to the internal occipital protuberance. The confluence of sinuses receives blood from the superior sagittal, straight, and occipital sinuses. Blood flow in the confluence of sinuses is somewhat turbulent and pressures are established in such a fashion that, usually, blood arriving from the straight sinus is shunted into the left transverse sinus, whereas blood from the superior sagittal sinus reaches the right transverse sinus.

CEREBROSPINAL FLUID

Cerebrospinal fluid is manufactured by the choroid plexuses of the ventricles of the brain

Although the choroid plexuses located in every ventricle of the brain manufacture **cerebrospinal fluid**, the majority of this fluid is formed in the two lateral ventricles. The average rate of CSF production is approximately 14–35 mL per hour for a total daily production of less than 800 mL. However, only about 150 mL of CSF occupies the ventricles, central canal of the spinal cord, perivascular space, and the subarachnoid space and its dilated cisterna at any one time because there is a constant drainage of CSF into the superior sagittal sinus by the numerous arachnoid granulations. CSF, a clear fluid with a low density, is rich in sodium, potassium, and chloride ions but has almost no protein and only occasional lymphocytes and a few desquamated epithelioid cells (Table 7.2). CSF forms a protective cushion for the brain and spinal cord and is also a recipient of the brain metabolites, which then reach the systemic circulation as the CSF is returned to the bloodstream.

The **blood–CSF barrier**, composed of zonulae occludentes —tight junctions formed by the fusion of cell membranes of contiguous cells of the simple cuboidal epithelium of the choroid plexus—maintains the chemical stability of the CSF. These tight junctions prevent paracellular movement of substances, thus requiring them to take the transcellular route via facilitated and active transports across the epithelium of the choroid plexus, resulting in differences in the composition of CSF and plasma.

VENTRICLES OF THE BRAIN

The four ventricles of the brain—the two lateral ventricles, the third ventricle, and the fourth ventricle—are lined by ependymal cells that isolate CSF from the brain tissues

Although the ventricles of the brain have been described previously (see Chapter 6), they are addressed here for completeness of discussion of the CSF. The four ventricles and the central canal of the spinal cord are the remnants of the lumen of the embryonic neural tube.

The largest ventricles, the paired **lateral ventricles**, are horseshoe-shaped cavities separated from one another by

Table 7.2 ● Composition of cerebrospinal fluid.

Constituent	Amount
White blood cells	0–5 cells/mL
Protein	Almost none
Glucose	2.1–4.0 mmol/L
Na^+	135–150 mmol/L
K^+	2.8–3.2 mmol/L
Cl^-	115–130 mmol/L
Ca^{2+}	1.0–1.4 mmol/L
Mg^{2+}	0.8–1.3 mmol/L
pH	7.3

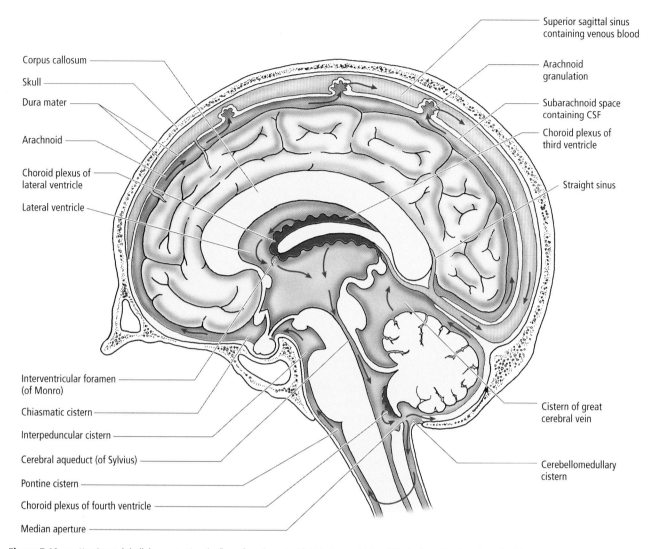

Corpus callosum

Skull

Dura mater

Arachnoid

Choroid plexus of
lateral ventricle

Lateral ventricle

Interventricular foramen
(of Monro)

Chiasmatic cistern

Interpeduncular cistern

Cerebral aqueduct (of Sylvius)

Pontine cistern

Choroid plexus of fourth ventricle

Median aperture

Superior sagittal sinus
containing venous blood

Arachnoid
granulation

Subarachnoid space
containing CSF

Choroid plexus of
third ventricle

Straight sinus

Cistern of great
cerebral vein

Cerebellomedullary
cistern

Figure 7.10 ● Hemisected skull demonstrating the flow of cerebrospinal fluid in the ventricles of the brain and in the subarachnoid spaces.

the **septum pellucidum**, and are located in the right and left cerebral hemispheres. Each lateral ventricle possesses a body and four horns, the anterior, posterior, lateral, and inferior horns. The **anterior horn** hollows out the frontal lobe; the **inferior lobe** is the cavity of the temporal lobe, whereas the occipital lobe houses the variable-sized **posterior lobe** of the cerebral hemisphere. The **body** of each lateral ventricle is located mostly in the parietal lobe. The body and the inferior horn contain a relatively extensive **choroid plexus** that is responsible for the manufacture of most of the CSF. The two lateral ventricles communicate with the third ventricle via the right and left **interventricular foramina (of Monro)** (Fig. 7.10).

The **third ventricle** is the quadrilateral, slit-like, vertically positioned space whose walls are formed by the right and left thalami. It is interrupted by a mass of gray matter, the **massa intermedia**, that forms a bridge between the two thalami. The roof of the third ventricle is formed by the tela choroidea, whereas its floor is formed by the hypothalamus, whose separation from the thalamus is indicated on the wall of the third ventricle by the **hypothalamic sulcus**. The third ventricle has several outpocketings: the preoptic, infundibular, mammillary, and pineal recesses. It is drained by the **cerebral aqueduct (of Sylvius)** that conveys CSF into the fourth ventricle.

The **fourth ventricle** is an irregularly shaped space in the hindbrain, extending from the cerebral aqueduct (of Sylvius) posteriorly to the **obex** anteriorly. It is continuous with the central canal of the spinal cord. The lateral aspect of the fourth ventricle has two openings, the right and left **foramina of Luschka** and the single, median **foramen of Magendie**, all three foramina draining the CSF from the fourth ventricle into the **subarachnoid space**. Specifically, the foramina of Luschka lead to the **interpeducular cistern**, whereas the foramen of Magendie delivers the CSF into the **cerebellomedullary cistern**.

CLINICAL CONSIDERATIONS

Meningitis

Meningitis, a bacterial or viral inflammation of the meninges, is an exceptionally dangerous condition affecting about two or three people per 100,000 in the USA annually (the incidence in neonates is lower, about five in 1,000,000). The symptoms in neonates and babies include fever, lethargy, respiratory distress, poor feeding, vomiting, irritability, an unusual high-pitched cry when held and quiet when placed down in a stationary position, and occasionally bulging at the fontanelle. In children and adults the symptoms are different and include high fever and chills, severe headache, painful and stiff neck, nausea and/or vomiting, and in later stages, sleepiness, confusion, and difficulty in waking up. Meningitis has a high degree of morbidity and mortality, especially if not diagnosed properly.

Meningiomas

Meningiomas are benign, encapsulated tumors composed of fusiform cells originating in the leptomeninges, specifically the arachnoid. Usually these tumors occur in adults and reach a fairly large size, on average 3 cm, before being diagnosed. Approximately 20% of all brain tumors and 10% of all spinal cord tumors are meningiomas, but, depending on their location, most can be treated with relative ease with good prognosis. The symptoms include headaches, seizures, weakness, and possibly paralysis or impairment of some brain functions due to pressure being applied to specific areas of the brain by the tumor. Diagnosis requires either radiographic or MRI techniques.

Blood–brain barrier

The integrity of the blood–brain barrier prevents many substances, including some neurotransmitters and drugs, from penetrating it. In order to permit the delivery of certain drugs through the blood–brain barrier, procedures were developed such as perfusion with a hypertonic solution, **mannitol**. This temporarily disables the fasciae occludentes of the capillary endothelial cells, allowing the delivery of certain therapeutic drugs.

Hydrocephalus

The constant production of CSF by the choroid plexus must be mirrored by its constant resorption by the arachnoid villi. If too little CSF is resorbed or if there is a blockage of CSF flow within the ventricular system of the brain, the result will be swelling of the brain tissue, a condition known as **hydrocephalus** (G., "water head"). This situation results in an increased head size in the neonate and fetus, and impaired muscular, cognitive, or other mental functions in the adult, possibly resulting in death if left untreated.

SYNONYMS AND EPONYMS OF THE CRANIAL MENINGES

Name of structure or term	Synonym(s)/eponym(s)
Arachnoid granulations	Arachnoid villi
Cavum trigeminale	Meckel's cave
Chiasmatic cistern	Cisterna basalis
Cisterna magna	Cisterna cerebellomedullaris
Superior cistern	Cistern of the great cerebral vein

FOLLOW-UP TO CLINICAL CASE

The immediate concern for any ER physician should be the possibility of meningitis (infection of the meninges) or possibly even encephalitis (infection within the brain itself). These are two examples of neurologic emergencies, and require careful evaluation. Both of these conditions could result in death, depending on the particular infectious organism involved (among other things).

Work-up did reveal that this patient had **acute meningitis**. Because the initial presentation was so suggestive of meningitis, he should have been started immediately on appropriate antibiotics. Any acute infectious illness can be accompanied by dangerously low blood pressure (i.e., sepsis) or other abnormalities of vital signs. A head CT was performed to look particularly for bleeding or a mass lesion. This was normal (as it almost always is in cases of meningitis). A lumbar puncture was performed to look at the CSF. This showed elevated protein (80 mg/L), elevated white blood cells (210 cells/mm^3), and no red blood cells. The white cells were mostly lymphocytes. Staining for bacteria, fungi, and parasites was negative. CSF cultures were negative (although these are not known until a few days after the CSF is drawn).

After several days, the patient fully recovered. This case represents aseptic meningitis since no organism was identified. Most cases of aseptic meningitis are assumed to be viral. This is actually a fairly common infection, and very mild cases are certainly missed since patients may not even go to the doctor for it. Viral meningitis is usually a self-limiting infection and is often mild. However, bacterial meningitis is very serious and often results in death or permanent disability. Both viral and bacterial infections are acute, but other organisms cause subacute or chronic meningitis such as tuberculosis or fungi.

QUESTIONS TO PONDER

1. How is the cranial dura mater different from the spinal dura mater?

2. How does the vascular supply of the cranial periosteal layer of the dura mater differ from that of the meningeal layer?

3. It is well known that the brain itself does not "feel" pain, yet patients with epidural or subdural hematomas may experience severe pain.

4. How does cerebrospinal fluid located in the ventricles of the brain reach the subarachnoid cisterns?

5. How does the cerebrospinal fluid leave the subarachnoid space and where does it go?

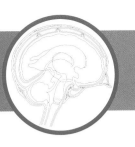
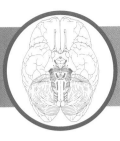
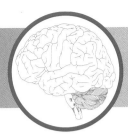

CHAPTER 8

Vascular Supply of the Central Nervous System

CLINICAL CASE

VASCULAR SUPPLY OF THE SPINAL CORD

ARTERIAL SUPPLY OF THE BRAIN

VENOUS DRAINAGE OF THE BRAIN

CLINICAL CONSIDERATIONS

SYNONYMS AND EPONYMS

FOLLOW-UP TO CLINICAL CASE

QUESTIONS TO PONDER

CLINICAL CASE

A 68-year-old woman presents to the emergency room with a sudden onset of right arm and leg weakness and altered speech. The right side of her face is noted by the family to be "droopy" and they say she is speaking "gibberish." This began very suddenly about 3 hours before presenting to the ER. The symptoms have been about the same since the onset. The history cannot be obtained from the patient herself since her speech is not intelligible.

The exam shows the patient to be alert and attentive. She can speak words but they are contextually inaccurate and she cannot form understandable sentences or even phrases. She cannot speak the names of simple objects that are presented to her, and she cannot follow direction appropriately. The right side of her face and her right arm are very weak, while the right leg is only mildly weak. The rest of the neurologic exam is unremarkable.

The average brain weighs only about 1,250–1,450 g but receives about 750 mL of blood per minute, almost 20% of the total blood volume, indicating its need for a large supply of oxygen and nutrients, especially glucose. In order to provide the brain with such a high volume of blood, two pairs of major arteries—the right and left **vertebral arteries** and the right and left **internal carotid arteries**—deliver all of their blood almost exclusively to the brain. These four vessels form an anastomotic network, the **cerebral arterial circle** (of Willis), a very effective system that is designed to ensure an uninterrupted blood supply to the brain. The brain's requirement for a constant blood flow is evidenced by the fact that interruption of the blood supply for 10–15 seconds results in losing consciousness and after 5 minutes without blood flow to the brain irreversible brain damage occurs. With the notable exceptions of the basilar artery and the anterior communicating artery, all other arteries of the brain are paired.

Before discussing the blood supply of the brain, it should be noted that although the description that follows implies very specifically established vascular patterns, there are numerous variations even in larger vessels. The vertebral arteries serve the occipital lobes of the cerebral hemispheres, brainstem, parts of the thalamus, as well as the cerebellum, whereas the internal carotid artery supplies blood to the remainder of the brain. One tends to think of larger vessels as having thick walls, but those of the brain are thin walled. Furthermore, since the arteries of the brain travel in the subarachnoid space, if there is a hemorrhage the blood accumulates in that space. Finally, it should be realized that there is only a limited amount of collateral circulation in the brain, even though the cerebral arterial circle forms anastomotic connections between the right and left sides of the brain.

Although the vascular supply of the spinal cord has been covered in Chapter 5, it will be repeated here for two reasons:

so that the reader does not have to refer back and so that the reader can appreciate the vascular supply of the entire central nervous system (CNS).

VASCULAR SUPPLY OF THE SPINAL CORD

The spinal cord receives its blood supply from two pairs of longitudinally arranged vessels, the anterior and posterior spinal arteries as well as from small, segmental radicular arteries

The **anterior spinal arteries**, direct branches of the vertebral arteries, join with each other to form a single median vessel, the anterior spinal artery, which occupies and follows the ventral median fissure of the spinal cord (Fig. 8.1). This vessel extends from within the cranial cavity throughout the entire length of the spinal cord and provides small branches that penetrate and supply the white and gray matter of the spinal cord. Moreover, this vessel also supplies the medulla oblongata. The anterior spinal artery may be quite small in the thoracic region.

The **posterior spinal arteries** also arise from the vertebral arteries directly, or frequently indirectly, by way of the inferior cerebellar branch of the vertebral artery. Each posterior spinal artery bifurcates to form two longitudinal vessels that extend from within the cranial cavity throughout the entire length of the spinal cord, sandwiching the dorsal rootlets between them. These three vessels provide small branches that penetrate and serve the white and gray matter of the spinal cord as well as the medulla oblongata.

The 32 pairs of radicular arteries are small vessels that arise from arteries in the immediate vicinity of the spinal column. Each radicular artery enters the intervertebral foramen where it bifurcates, forming an **anterior** and a **posterior radicular artery**, which follow the ventral and dorsal roots, respectively, to gain entrance into the vertebral canal. The anterior and posterior radicular arteries anastomose with branches of the anterior and posterior spinal arteries on the surface of the spinal cord, and arborize to supply the white and gray matter of the spinal cord. It should be stressed that the radicular arteries are extremely important for the vascularization of the spinal cord, because, with the exception of the cervical region, the anterior and posterior spinal arteries by themselves are unable to provide an adequate vascular supply to the spinal cord. Therefore, an injury to a spinal nerve damages not only the afferent and efferent fibers of a particular spinal cord level, but may also damage the segmental white and gray matter by producing ischemic conditions due to the reduction in blood supply from the radicular artery serving that region. It should be noted that the **great ventral radicular artery** (artery of Adamkiewicz) is the largest, albeit inconsistent, of the radicular arteries. It usually arises on the left-hand side and serves much of the inferior half of the spinal cord, entering the vertebral canal between L2 and L3, and contributes to the formation of the inferior aspect of the ventral spinal artery.

Several longitudinally arranged tortuous veins of the pia mater are responsible for the venous drainage of the spinal

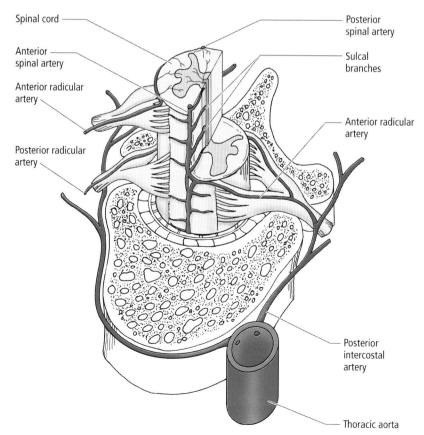

Figure 8.1 ● Arterial supply of the spinal cord.

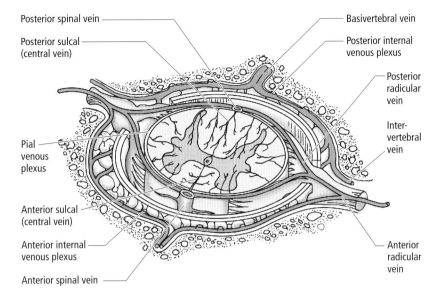

Figure 8.2 ● Venous drainage of the spinal cord.

cord (Fig. 8.2). These are the **ventral** and **dorsal spinal veins** that communicate with the segmentally arranged radicular veins. The **radicular veins** follow the paths of their companion radicular arteries to leave the vertebral canal via the intervertebral foramina. Along the way they also communicate with the **epidural venous network** embedded in the epidural fat of the vertebral canal. The epidural venous network delivers its blood into the cavernous sinus of the cranial cavity. Cranially, the ventral and dorsal spinal veins drain into the inferior cerebellar veins and inferior petrosal sinuses.

ARTERIAL SUPPLY OF THE BRAIN

In order to protect the brain from certain substances carried in the bloodstream, the blood–brain barrier is established by endothelial cells

Blood–brain barrier

The blood–brain barrier prevents certain molecules and macromolecules from entering the substance of the brain by the formation of occluding junctions by the endothelial cells

The basal lamina-lined endothelial cells of the capillaries of the brain and spinal cord form a **blood–brain barrier**. These endothelial cells not only form **fasciae occludentes** with each other, but they have only a limited ability to form **caveolae**, relying instead mostly on **receptor-mediated transport** to transfer material between the capillary lumen and the neural tissue of the CNS. Therefore, most macromolecules injected into the capillary lumen are unable to gain access into the intercellular spaces of the brain and spinal cord. Similarly, most macromolecules injected into the intercellular compartment of the CNS are unable to enter the capillary lumen, unless the endothelial cells possess specific receptors for them. Small, noncharged molecules (e.g., O_2, H_2O, CO_2) and numerous small lipid-soluble materials, including some drugs, can dissolve through the lipid membrane of the endothelial cells and thus are able to penetrate

the blood–brain barrier. Molecules, such as some of the vitamins, amino acids, glucose, and nucleosides, can penetrate the blood–brain barrier via carrier proteins, with or without passive diffusion. Ion channels are also present in the endothelial cell membranes and they are responsible for the transport of ions across the blood–brain barrier.

The end-feet of astrocytes contact and form a sheet around the basal lamina of the capillaries of the CNS. These end-feet are referred to as the **perivascular glia limitans**. These astrocytes function not only in maintaining the neurochemical balance of the intercellular compartment of the CNS by removing excess K^+ ions and neurotransmitters that were released into the intercellular spaces, but also in transferring metabolites from the capillary lumen to neurons in their vicinity.

Internal carotid artery

The internal carotid artery, one of the terminal branches of the common carotid artery, forms numerous branches supplying the brain and also participates in the formation of the cerebral arterial circle

The **internal carotid artery**, a terminal branch of the common carotid artery, ascends in the neck, enters the cranial cavity through the carotid canal of the petrous portion of the temporal bone, and reaches the cavernous sinus from below. It passes through, and subsequently pierces, the roof of the cavernous sinus and enters the cranial cavity where it is flanked by the oculomotor and optic nerves (Fig. 8.3). The internal carotid artery then approximates the anterior perforated substance where it terminates into its various branches. Along this path, from the neck to its termination, the internal carotid artery makes a number of almost 90° turns, thus reducing both the pressure and the velocity of blood it brings to the thin-walled vessels of the brain. Although the internal carotid artery is said to be divided into four regions—the cervical, petrous, cavernous, and cerebral—only the **cavernous** and **cerebral portions** are discussed in this textbook. Readers interested in the

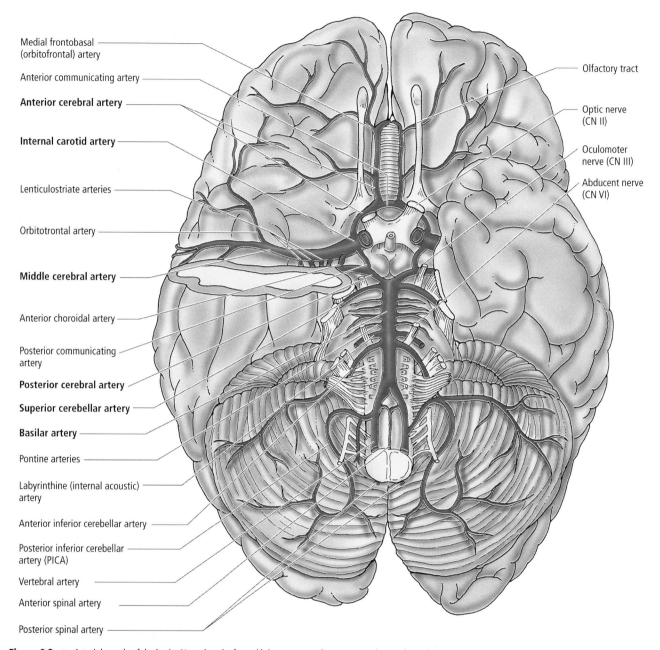

Medial frontobasal
(orbitofrontal) artery

Anterior communicating artery

Anterior cerebral artery

Internal carotid artery

Lenticulostriate arteries

Orbitotrontal artery

Middle cerebral artery

Anterior choroidal artery

Posterior communicating
artery

Posterior cerebral artery

Superior cerebellar artery

Basilar artery

Pontine arteries

Labyrinthine (internal acoustic)
artery

Anterior inferior cerebellar artery

Posterior inferior cerebellar
artery (PICA)

Vertebral artery

Anterior spinal artery

Posterior spinal artery

Olfactory tract

Optic nerve
(CN II)

Oculomoter
nerve (CN III)

Abducent nerve
(CN VI)

Figure 8.3 ● Arterial supply of the brain. Note that the frontal lobes are spread apart somewhat to show the anterior cerebral arteries and that the right temporal lobe is severed to show the path and branches of the middle cerebral artery.

distribution and paths of the cervical and petrous portions are urged to read any major textbook of gross anatomy or head and neck anatomy.

Cavernous portion of the internal carotid artery

Branches of the cavernous portion of the internal carotid artery supply the pituitary gland as well as the dura mater of the anterior cranial fossa

The **cavernous portion** of the internal carotid artery passes through the substance of the cavernous sinus, but is isolated from the blood of the cavernous sinus by being invested with

a simple squamous epithelium. The abducent nerve accompanies the internal carotid artery through the cavernous sinus. While in the sinus the artery describes an S-shaped curve and gives off small branches: the cavernous, superior, and inferior hypophyseal, ganglionic, and anterior meningeal arteries. As their names suggest, these vessels serve the areas of their namesake (Table 8.1).

Cerebral portion of the internal carotid artery

The cerebral portion of the internal carotid artery has the following branches: ophthalmic, anterior choroidal, posterior communicating, anterior cerebral, and middle cerebral arteries

Branch	Major areas served	Additional pertinent information
Cavernous	Walls of the cavernous sinus Walls of the inferior petrosal sinus	Anastomoses with branches of the middle meningeal artery
Superior hypophyseal Inferior hypophyseal	Pars tuberalis and infundibulum Posterior lobe of the pituitary	Forms primary capillary bed Sends some twigs to the anterior lobe
Ganglionic	Trigeminal ganglion	Composed of several small branches
Anterior meningeal	Dura mater of the anterior cranial fossa	Anastomoses with the meningeal branch of the posterior ethmoidal artery

Table 8.1 ● Branches of the cavernous portion of the internal carotid artery.

Branch	Major area served	Additional pertinent information
Anterior choroidal	Choroid plexus of the inferior horn of the lateral ventricle	Also serve the optic tract, lateral geniculate body, optic radiation, hippocampus, posterior limb of the internal capsule, and the tail of the caudate nucleus
Posterior communicating	Connects the internal carotid system with the vertebral arterial system	Anastomoses with the posterior cerebral artery
Central branches	Posterior limb of the internal capsule, medial aspect of the thalamus, and tissue forming the lateral border of the third ventricle	Pierce the region of the base of the cerebrum that is posterolateral to the infundibulum of the pituitary

Table 8.2 ● Regions supplied by the anterior choroidal and posterior communicating arteries.

The **cerebral portion** of the internal carotid artery is quite short (Fig. 8.3). Almost as soon as it pierces the roof of the cavernous sinus it gives rise to its branches, the ophthalmic, anterior choroidal, and posterior communicating arteries, and its two terminal branches, the anterior cerebral and middle cerebral arteries. The ophthalmic artery is not discussed in this textbook.

Anterior choroidal artery

The **anterior choroidal artery** is a rather small, narrow artery that arises from the posterior aspect of the internal carotid and follows the path of the optic tract until it reaches the lateral geniculate body, where it enters the choroid fissure to reach and supply the choroid plexus of the inferior horn of the lateral ventricle (Table 8.2). It gives off numerous branches along the way. These branches serve structures in their vicinity, including the optic tract, lateral geniculate body, optic radiation, hippocampus, posterior limb of the internal capsule, and the tail of the caudate nucleus.

Posterior communicating artery

The **posterior communicating artery** connects the cerebral portion of the internal carotid artery to the posterior cerebral branch of the basilar artery (Table 8.2). The right and left

arteries are not identical, in that one is frequently smaller than the other, and, in fact, one may be entirely absent or doubled. The main function of this vessel is to ensure a viable blood supply to the brain in case the internal carotid or vertebral artery becomes occluded. However, it does also have **central branches**—thin, unsubstantial vessels—that pierce the region of the cerebrum base that is posterolateral to the infundibulum of the pituitary, and serve part of the posterior limb of the internal capsule, the medial aspect of the thalamus, and the tissue forming the lateral border of the third ventricle.

Anterior cerebral artery

The anterior cerebral artery has the following branches: the anterior communicating artery and the central and cortical branches

The **anterior cerebral artery**, one of the two terminal branches of the internal carotid artery, passes between the frontal lobes in the beginning of the longitudinal cerebral fissure, where it lies within a few millimeters of the anterior cerebral artery of the other side (Figs 8.3, 8.4). The two vessels follow the genu and then the superior border of the corpus callosum until they each anastomose with the posterior cerebral artery, a branch of the basilar artery. The branches of the anterior cerebral artery are classified into the anterior communicating artery, the central branches, and the cortical branches (Table 8.3).

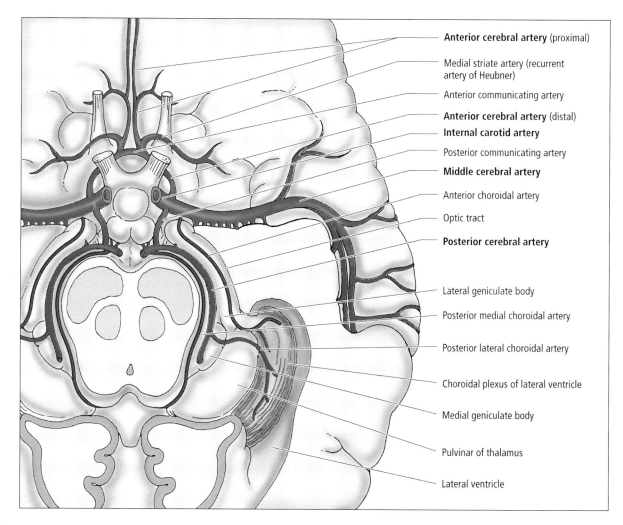

Figure 8.4 ● Region of the arterial cerebral circle displaying the blood supply to the choroidal plexus of the lateral ventricle.

Table 8.3 ● Regions supplied by the anterior cerebral artery and its branches.

Branch	Major area served	Additional pertinent information
Anterior communicating artery	Region of the optic chiasma via its anteromedial branches	Connects the right and left anterior cerebral arteries, forming the anterior boundary of the cerebral arterial circle (of Willis)
Central branches		
Unnamed branches	Septum pellucidum and anterior part of the corpus callosum	Arise just before the origin of the anterior communicating artery
Medial striate artery	Head of caudate nucleus, parts of putamen, globus pallidus, and anterior limb of internal capsule	Also known as the recurrent artery, it arises just after the origin of the anterior communicating artery
Cortical branches		
Orbital branches	Gyrus rectus, medial orbital gyrus, olfactory lobe	Serves area of the frontal lobe that lies on the intracranial roof of the bony orbit
Frontal branches		
Frontopolar artery	Medial surface of the superior frontal gyrus and lateral surface of the superior and middle frontal gyri	Originates at the level of the genu of the corpus callosum
Callosomarginal artery	Corpus callosum, cingulate gyrus, medial aspect of superior frontal gyrus, and precentral and postcentral gyri	Arises at the genu of the corpus callosum and parallels the remainder of the anterior cerebral artery as far posteriorly as the postcentral gyrus
Parietal branches	Medial aspect of precuneate gyrus and neighboring structures	Serve region of the brain as far posteriorly as the parieto-occipital sulcus
Anterior parietal artery		
Posterior parietal artery		

Anterior communicating artery

The **anterior communicating artery** is a very short vessel, no more than 5–6 mm in length, that connects the right and left anterior cerebral arteries to each other, forming the anterior end of the cerebral arterial circle (of Willis). It has two or more small branches, the **anteromedial branches**, which serve the region of the optic chiasma.

Central branches

A number of small, unnamed vessels arise from the initial part of the anterior cerebral artery, just before the origin of the anterior communicating artery; these supply the septum pellucidum as well as the anterior part of the corpus callosum. A larger branch, the **medial striate artery** (also referred to as the recurrent artery), arises just after the origin of the anterior communicating artery. It follows the anterior limb of the internal capsule to supply parts of the following regions of the basal ganglia: the head of the caudate nucleus, part of the putamen, the globus pallidus, and the anterior limb of the internal capsule.

Cortical branches

> The branches of the cortical artery, named by the regions that they serve, are the orbital, frontal, and parietal arteries

The **cortical branches** of the anterior cerebral artery arise from that vessel as it courses along the genu and superior aspect of the corpus callosum. These branches, named by the areas that they serve, are the orbital, frontal, and parietal arteries.

The **orbital branches** distribute to the inferior aspect of the frontal lobes as they lie on the bony roof of the orbit, and serve the gyrus rectus, medial orbital gyrus, and olfactory lobe.

The frontopolar and callosomarginal branches constitute the **frontal branches** of the anterior cerebral artery. The **frontopolar artery** originates at the level of the genu of the corpus callosum and serves the medial surface of the superior frontal gyrus and the region of the lateral surface of the superior and middle frontal gyri. The **callosomarginal artery** branches from the anterior cerebral artery at the genu of the corpus callosum and parallels its parent artery as far posteriorly as the postcentral gyrus. It supplies blood to the corpus callosum, the cingulate gyrus, the medial aspect of the superior frontal gyrus, as well as to the precentral and postcentral gyri.

The remaining portion of the anterior cerebral artery, frequently renamed the **pericallosal artery**, extends as far posteriorly as the parieto-occipital sulcus, and gives rise to the **anterior** and **posterior parietal arteries**. These two vessels and their branches serve the medial aspect of the precuneate gyrus and neighboring structures.

Middle cerebral artery

> The middle cerebral artery has central and cortical branches

The **middle cerebral artery**, the terminal branch and largest branch of the internal carotid artery, enters the lateral fissure

Note that the clinical case at the beginning of the chapter refers to a patient with a sudden onset of unintelligible speech.

1 What should the physician suspect when there is a sudden onset of speech disorder?

2 What lesion of the CNS should be suspected when there is a sudden weakness on one side?

3 Why is the fact that "otherwise the patient is alert and attentive" is not a surprising finding in this case?

(of Sylvius), passes along the free surface of the insula, and gives off several branches that ramify over the dorsal and lateral surfaces of the cerebral cortex (Figs 8.3–8.6). The middle cerebral artery has **central** and **cortical branches**, where the former supply blood to the deeper structures and the latter serve the cortical regions (Table 8.4).

Central branches

There are 10–15 slender vessels, the **striate arteries (lenticulostriate arteries)**, that arise from the middle cerebral artery as it gains entry into the lateral fissure. These vessels pierce the floor of the lateral sulcus to supply structures deep within the white matter of the cerebral cortex, including the corpus striatum, much of the head and body of the caudate nucleus, and large portions of the lenticular nucleus and of the external and internal capsules, passing as deep as the external surface of the thalamus.

Cortical branches

> Branches of the cortical artery are named by the regions that they serve: the orbital, frontal, parietal, and temporal arteries

The **cortical branches** originate from the middle cerebral artery as it courses along the lateral sulcus. These vessels, named according to their location and distribution, are the orbital, frontal, parietal, and temporal branches.

The **orbital branches**, the most prominent of which is the **orbitofrontal artery**, serve the inferior frontal gyrus and the lateral aspect of the orbital surface of the frontal lobe as it lies over the bony roof of the orbit. The **frontal branches** supply the middle frontal and precentral gyri as well as a region of the inferior frontal gyrus. The **anterior** and **posterior parietal branches** serve the postcentral gyrus as well as the caudal aspect of the superior and all of the inferior parietal lobules. Two other branches, the **parietotemporal** and **parietooccipital arteries**, serve the remainder of the parietal lobe, terminating at the parieto-occipital sulcus, thus supplying the angular and supramarginal gyri. The temporal branches consist of three main vessels, the **anterior**, **middle**, and **posterior temporal arteries**. They serve the lateral aspect of the entire temporal lobe as far posteriorly as the occipital gyri.

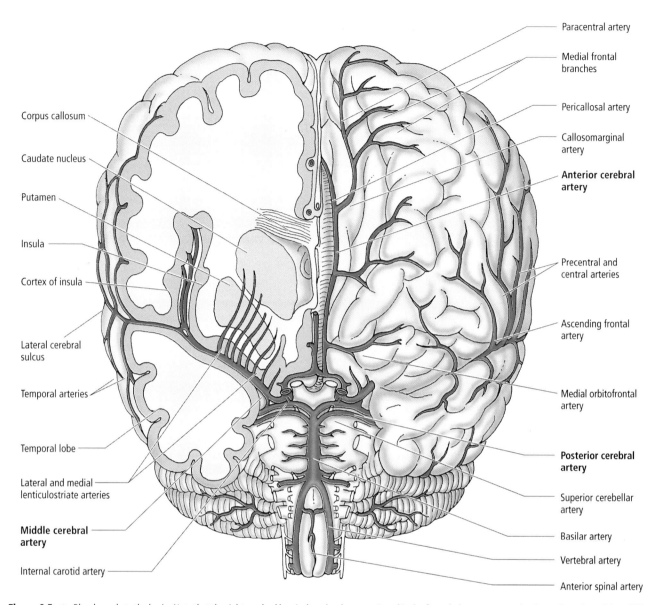

Figure 8.5 ● Blood supply to the brain. Note that the right cerebral hemisphere has been sectioned in the frontal plane to expose the deeper branches of the middle cerebral artery.

Branch	Major area served	Additional pertinent information
Central striate arteries	Corpus striatum, head and body of caudate nucleus, lenticular nucleus, external and internal capsules	These vessels pierce the floor of the lateral sulcus to reach their points of destination located deep within the white matter of the cerebrum
Cortical branches		
Orbital branches	Inferior frontal gyrus, lateral aspect of orbital surface of frontal lobe	Orbitofrontal artery is the most prominent of the orbital branches
Frontal branches	Middle frontal and precentral gyri, part of inferior frontal gyrus	Anterior and posterior parietal branches
Parietal branches	Postcentral gyrus, part of superior and all of inferior parietal lobules, angular and supramarginal gyri	Parietotemporal and parieto-occipital arteries
Temporal branches	Lateral aspect of entire temporal lobe as far posteriorly as occipital gyri	Anterior, middle, and posterior temporal arteries

Table 8.4 ● Regions supplied by the middle cerebral artery and its branches.

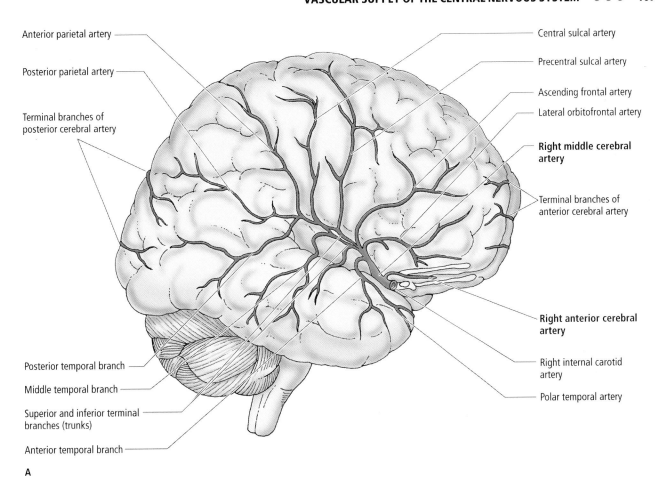

Anterior parietal artery

Posterior parietal artery

Terminal branches of posterior cerebral artery

Posterior temporal branch

Middle temporal branch

Superior and inferior terminal branches (trunks)

Anterior temporal branch

Central sulcal artery

Precentral sulcal artery

Ascending frontal artery

Lateral orbitofrontal artery

Right middle cerebral artery

Terminal branches of anterior cerebral artery

Right anterior cerebral artery

Right internal carotid artery

Polar temporal artery

A

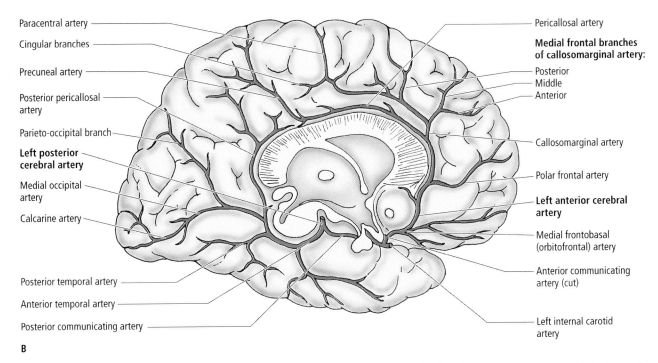

Paracentral artery

Cingular branches

Precuneal artery

Posterior pericallosal artery

Parieto-occipital branch

Left posterior cerebral artery

Medial occipital artery

Calcarine artery

Posterior temporal artery

Anterior temporal artery

Posterior communicating artery

Pericallosal artery

Medial frontal branches of callosomarginal artery:

Posterior

Middle

Anterior

Callosomarginal artery

Polar frontal artery

Left anterior cerebral artery

Medial frontobasal (orbitofrontal) artery

Anterior communicating artery (cut)

Left internal carotid artery

B

Figure 8.6 ● (A) Arterial supply to the lateral aspect of the brain. Note that the temporal lobe is partially reflected to permit a view of the vessels lodged within the lateral fissure (of Sylvius). (B) Arterial supply of the medial aspect of the brain.

Vertebral artery

The right and left vertebral arteries enter the cranial cavity via the foramen magnum and join each other to form the basilar artery

The **vertebral artery**, the largest branch of the subclavian artery, arises from its first part and ascends in the neck, traveling through the **foramina transversaria** of the 6th through 1st (atlas) vertebrae. It describes an S-shaped curve along the posterior arch of the **atlas**, passes through the **foramen magnum** and enters the cranial cavity where it joins its counterpart of the other side to form the **basilar artery**. Only the cranial branches of the vertebral artery are described, and these are the meningeal branches, the posterior inferior cerebellar artery, and the medullary branches (Table 8.5).

Meningeal branches of the vertebral artery

The two or three **meningeal branches** of the vertebral artery serve the falx cerebelli. They ramify between the periosteal and meningeal layers of the dura mater of the cerebellar fossa.

Posterior inferior cerebellar artery

The **posterior inferior cerebellar artery** arises within the cranial cavity from the vertebral artery about 1–2 cm before the formation of the basilar artery (Fig. 8.7). It passes laterally from the vertebral artery, follows the contour of the medulla oblongata to pass between the rootlets of cranial nerves IX and X and divides into a medial and a lateral branch. The **medial branch** supplies the medial aspect of the cerebellar hemispheres, whereas the **lateral branch** serves the inferior aspect of the cerebellum and anastomoses with the anterior inferior cerebellar artery and the superior cerebellar artery. Additional branches of the posterior inferior cerebellar artery supply the choroid plexus of the fourth ventricle as well as the medulla oblongata.

Medullary branches

Several small branches of the cranial portion of the vertebral artery, known as the **medullary branches**, serve the medulla oblongata. It should be noted that this important region is also served by the posterior inferior cerebellar artery (as indicated in the above paragraph), as well as by the anterior and posterior spinal arteries.

Basilar artery

The basilar artery extends from the rostral end of the pyramids to the rostral end of the pons; it has several small branches and three larger ones

The **basilar artery**, formed by the fusion of the right and left vertebral arteries, lies in a shallow groove in the midline of the pons, extending from the rostral end of the pyramids to the rostral end of the pons (Fig. 8.7). It has several small branches, the pontine and labyrinthine arteries, and three larger branches, the anterior inferior cerebellar, superior cerebellar, and posterior cerebral arteries (Table 8.6).

Pontine arteries

The several small **pontine arteries** arise at right angles to the basilar artery and serve the pons and the midbrain, penetrating deep into the substance of these two regions.

Labyrinthine artery

The **labyrinthine (internal auditory) artery** is larger than the pontine arteries and originates somewhat rostral to the anterior inferior cerebellar artery (from which it occasionally arises). It reaches and enters the internal auditory meatus in the company of cranial nerves VII and VIII, and supplies the internal ear.

Anterior inferior cerebellar artery

The **anterior inferior cerebellar artery** arises from the basilar artery just rostral to the pyramids and follows cranial nerve VI for a short distance. It loops around cranial nerves VII and VIII, just before they enter the internal acoustic meatus. Shortly before reaching the cerebellopontine angle, the artery gives rise to small **pontine branches** that pierce the lateral

Branch	Major area served	Additional pertinent information
Meningeal branch	Falx cerebelli	Ramify between periosteal and meningeal layers of the dura
Posterior inferior cerebellar artery		
Medial branch	Medial wall of cerebellum	Additional branches supply choroid plexus of the fourth ventricle
Lateral branch	Inferior aspect of cerebellum	Anastomoses with anterior inferior cerebellar and superior cerebellar arteries of the basilar artery
Medullary branches	Medulla oblongata	Several small branches of the vertebral artery

Table 8.5 ● Regions supplied by the cranial portion of the vertebral artery and its branches.

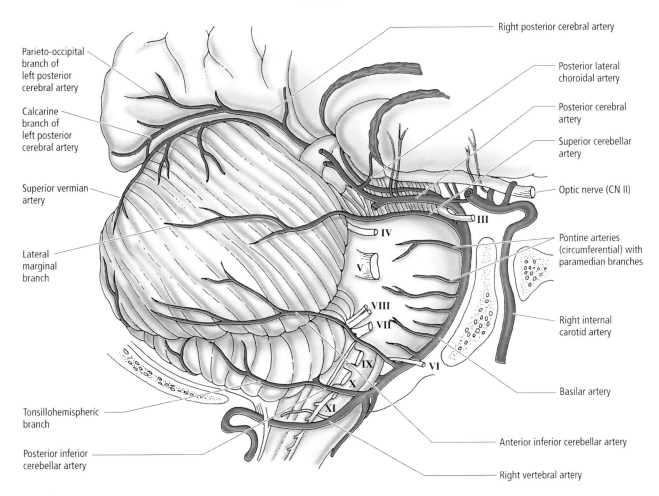

Figure 8.7 ● Arterial supply of the cerebellum.

aspect of the pons. At the cerebellopontine angle the anterior inferior cerebellar artery bifurcates into **medial** and **lateral branches** that serve the anteromedial and anterolateral aspects of the cerebellum, respectively. The branches of the anterior inferior cerebellar artery anastomose with branches of the posterior inferior cerebellar artery and with those of the superior cerebellar artery.

Superior cerebellar artery

The **superior cerebellar artery** originates just caudal to the third cranial nerve. It curves around the cerebral peduncle to gain the superior surface of the cerebellum, which it vascularizes, and as it arborizes its branches provide vascular supply to the pineal body, the midbrain, and the choroid plexus of the third ventricle. Branches of the superior cerebellar artery anastomose with branches of the anterior inferior cerebellar artery.

Posterior cerebral artery

The posterior cerebral artery gives rise to the cortical, central, and posterior choroidal arteries

The right and left **posterior cerebral arteries** are the terminal branches of the basilar artery (Fig. 8.7). Each originates just rostral to the superior cerebellar artery and follows the course of that vessel as they both curve around the cerebral peduncle. It should be noted that the third cranial nerve is located between the posterior cerebral and superior cerebellar arteries. The posterior cerebral artery is connected to the internal carotid artery by the posterior communicating artery, forming the posterior limb of the cerebral arterial circle. Branches of the posterior cerebral artery are the cortical, central, and posterior choroidal arteries.

Cortical branches

The **cortical branches** of the posterior cerebral artery vascularize the medial aspect of the temporal and occipital lobes. They are usually four in number: the anterior and posterior temporal, parieto-occipital, and occipital (calcarine) branches. The **anterior temporal branch** serves the uncus and parahippocampal gyrus; the **posterior temporal branch** vascularizes the lateral and medial occipitotemporal gyri; the **parieto-occipital branch** serves the cuneate and precuneate gyri; and the **occipital (calcarine) branch** follows the calcarine sulcus to serve the lingual and cuneate gyri of the primary visual cortex.

Table 8.6 ● Regions supplied by branches of the basilar artery.

Branch	Major area served	Additional pertinent information
Pontine arteries	Pons and midbrain	Small vessels that arise at right angles from the basilar artery
Labyrinthine (internal auditory) artery	Internal ear	Enters the internal acoustic meatus in company with CN VII and VIII
Anterior inferior cerebellar artery		Its branches anastomose with branches of the posterior inferior cerebellar and superior cerebellar arteries
Pontine	Lateral aspect of pons	
Medial branches	Anteromedial aspect of cerebellum	
Lateral branches	Anterolateral aspect of cerebellum	
Superior cerebellar artery	Superior surface of cerebellum as well as pineal body, midbrain, and choroid plexus of third ventricle	Its branches anastomose with branches of the anterior inferior cerebellar artery
Posterior cerebral artery		It is connected to the internal carotid artery by the posterior communicating artery
Cortical branches		
Anterior temporal	Uncus and parahippocampal gyrus	
Posterior temporal	Lateral and medial occipitotemporal gyri	
Parieto-occipital	Cuneate and precuneate gyri	
Central branches		
Anterior thalamic	Optic tract, mammillary bodies, anterior and ventromedial nuclei of thalamus	
Posterior thalamic	Posterior thalamic nuclei, geniculate bodies	
Mesencephalic	Cerebral peduncles, interpeduncular region, corticospinal tracts, mesencephalic reticular formation, substantia nigra, tegmentum of midbrain	Has a small branch, the circumflex mesencephalic
Posterior choroidal branches		
Lateral choroidal	Choroid plexus of lateral ventricle, lateral geniculate body, pulvinar, dorsomedial nucleus of thalamus	Anastomoses with branches of the medial choroidal
Medial choroidal	Choroid plexus of third ventricle, pineal body, superior and inferior colliculi, dorsal medial nucleus of thalamus	Anastomoses with branches of the lateral choroidal

Central branches

The **central branches** of the posterior cerebral artery are classified into two divisions: the thalamic and mesencephalic (as well as the circumflex mesencephalic) branches.

The **thalamic branches**, supplying regions of the thalamus and hypothalamus, are divided into the anterior and posterior thalamic branches, where the **anterior thalamic branches** serve the optic tract, the mammillary bodies, and the anterior and ventromedial nuclei of the thalamus. The **posterior thalamic branches** vascularize the posterior thalamic nuclei and the geniculate bodies.

The **mesencephalic** and **circumflex mesencephalic branches** serve the cerebral peduncles, the interpeduncular region, the corticospinal tracts, the mesencephalic reticular formation, the substantia nigra, and the tegmentum of the midbrain.

Posterior choroidal arteries

There are at least two **posterior choroidal arteries**—the lateral choroidal and medial choroidal arteries. The **lateral choroidal branches** serve the choroid plexus of the lateral

ventricle as well as the lateral geniculate body, the pulvinar, and the dorsomedial nucleus of the thalamus. The **medial choroidal branches** serve the choroid plexus of the third ventricle as well as the pineal body, the superior and inferior colliculi, the dorsal medial nucleus of the thalamus, and in many cases even vascularize the pulvinar, where they anastomose with the lateral choroidal branches.

Cerebral arterial circle (of Willis)

The cerebral arterial circle (of Willis) is an essential structure in maintaining the normal blood supply to the brain

As described above, the **cerebral arterial circle** connects the branches of the two internal carotid arteries to the branches of the two vertebral arteries, forming a method of shunting blood from one side to the other in case of a blockage in any one of the vessels (Figs 8.8–8.10). The anterior communicating artery forms the anterior connection and the posterior communicating artery forms the posterior connection between the right and left sides. The arteries involved in the circle are: the right internal carotid, right anterior cerebral, anterior communicating, left anterior cerebral, left internal carotid, left posterior communicating, left posterior cerebral, right posterior

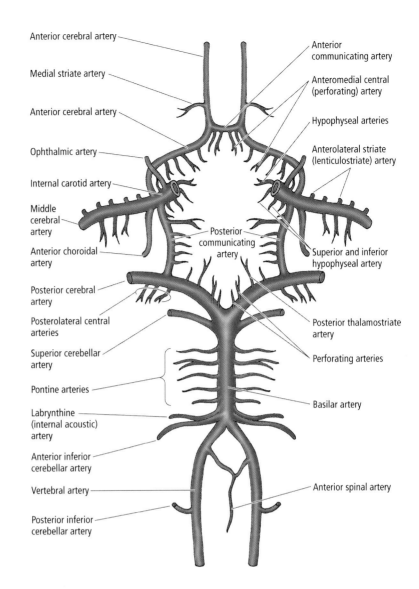

Figure 8.8 ● Diagram of the ventral view of the cerebral arterial circle (of Willis).

Anterior cerebral artery

Medial striate artery

Anterior cerebral artery

Ophthalmic artery

Internal carotid artery

Middle cerebral artery

Anterior choroidal artery

Posterior cerebral artery

Posterolateral central arteries

Superior cerebellar artery

Pontine arteries

Labrynthine (internal acoustic) artery

Anterior inferior cerebellar artery

Vertebral artery

Posterior inferior cerebellar artery

Anterior communicating artery

Anteromedial central (perforating) artery

Hypophyseal arteries

Anterolateral striate (lenticulostriate) artery

Posterior communicating artery

Superior and inferior hypophyseal artery

Posterior thalamostriate artery

Perforating arteries

Basilar artery

Anterior spinal artery

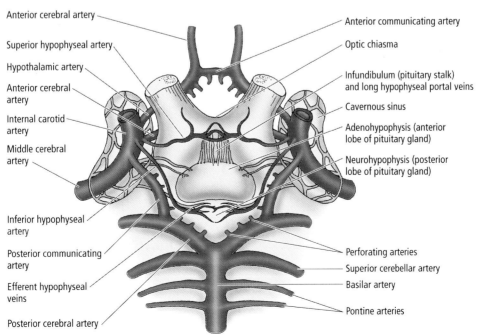

Figure 8.9 ● Close-up diagram of the ventral view of the cerebral arterial circle.

Anterior cerebral artery

Superior hypophyseal artery

Hypothalamic artery

Anterior cerebral artery

Internal carotid artery

Middle cerebral artery

Inferior hypophyseal artery

Posterior communicating artery

Efferent hypophyseal veins

Posterior cerebral artery

Anterior communicating artery

Optic chiasma

Infundibulum (pituitary stalk) and long hypophyseal portal veins

Cavernous sinus

Adenohypophysis (anterior lobe of pituitary gland)

Neurohypophysis (posterior lobe of pituitary gland)

Perforating arteries

Superior cerebellar artery

Basilar artery

Pontine arteries

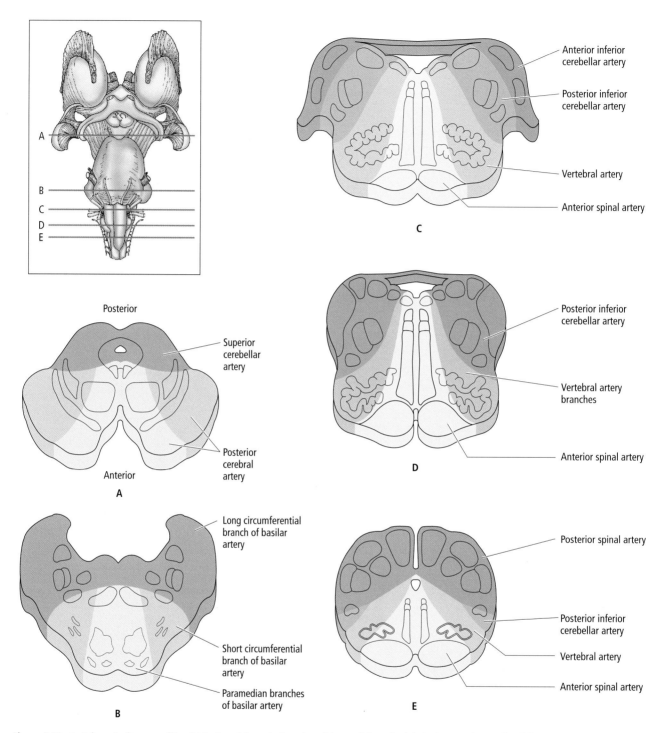

Figure 8.10 ● Schematic diagrams of the distribution of the major branches of the arterial supply of the brainstem, showing five different cross-sections of the brainstem.

cerebral, right posterior communicating, and back to the right internal carotid. The major vessels arising from the anterior, lateral, and posterior aspects of the cerebral arterial circle supply the cerebrum (via the anterior, middle, and posterior cerebral arteries). The arterial circle lies inferior to the hypothalamus and encompasses the mammillary bodies, infundibulum, optic chiasma, and tuber cinereum, among other structures.

VENOUS DRAINAGE OF THE BRAIN

The venous drainage of the brain is accomplished by the cerebral veins, the cerebellar veins, and the veins of the brainstem

Blood from these thin-walled veins reaches the dural venous sinuses via vessels that penetrate both the arachnoid and the meningeal layer of the dura mater. The dural venous sinuses are discussed in Chapter 7.

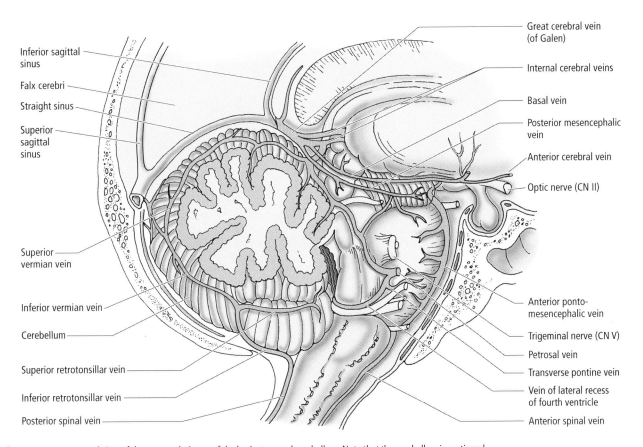

Inferior sagittal sinus

Falx cerebri

Straight sinus

Superior sagittal sinus

Superior vermian vein

Inferior vermian vein

Cerebellum

Superior retrotonsillar vein

Inferior retrotonsillar vein

Posterior spinal vein

Great cerebral vein (of Galen)

Internal cerebral veins

Basal vein

Posterior mesencephalic vein

Anterior cerebral vein

Optic nerve (CN II)

Anterior ponto-mesencephalic vein

Trigeminal nerve (CN V)

Petrosal vein

Transverse pontine vein

Vein of lateral recess of fourth ventricle

Anterior spinal vein

Figure 8.11 ● Lateral view of the venous drainage of the brainstem and cerebellum. Note that the cerebellum is sectioned.

Cerebral veins

The **cerebral veins** are subdivided into two categories: the external veins, which drain the superficial aspect of the cerebrum, and the internal veins, which drain the deep regions of the cerebrum (Figs 8.11–8.13).

External veins

There are three veins in the external vein group, these are the superior, superficial middle, and inferior cerebral veins

There are three **external veins**, the superior, superficial middle, and inferior cerebral veins. The 15 or so **superior cerebral veins** are lodged mostly in the sulci, though they occasionally pass along the surface of the gyri. These vessels drain blood from the medial and superolateral aspects of the cerebrum and empty into the superior sagittal sinus. The **superficial middle cerebral vein** is located within the lateral fissure (of Sylvius) and drains blood from the lateral aspect of the cerebral hemisphere. It delivers its blood into the superior sagittal sinus by way of the **superior anastomotic vein**, into the transverse sinus, via the **inferior anastomotic vein**, and continues posteriorly until it reaches, and empties into, the cavernous sinus. The small **inferior cerebral veins** drain blood from the inferior aspect of the cerebrum and deliver it into the superior

sagittal sinus by way of the superior cerebral veins. The inferior cerebral veins that drain blood from the inferior aspect of the temporal lobe deliver their blood into the cavernous, transverse, sphenoparietal, and superior petrosal sinuses, via the basal and middle cerebral veins.

Internal veins

The internal vein group is composed of the great cerebral vein, its tributaries, and the basal vein

The **internal veins** drain structures deeper within the brain and are composed of the great cerebral vein and their tributaries as well as the basal vein. The **great cerebral vein**, a short vessel formed by the union of the right and left internal cerebral veins, drains into the straight sinus in common with the inferior sagittal sinus. The great cerebral vein receives blood from its tributaries that drain the thalamus, hypothalamus, basal ganglia, and midbrain.

The **thalamostriate vein** receives tributaries that drain the region of the thalamus and corpus striatum, whereas the **choroid vein** follows the choroid plexus of the lateral ventricle and receives tributaries from the fornix, hippocampus, and corpus callosum. At the level of the interventricular foramen (of Monro) the choroid vein joins the thalamostriate vein to form the **internal cerebral vein**, which, shortly after

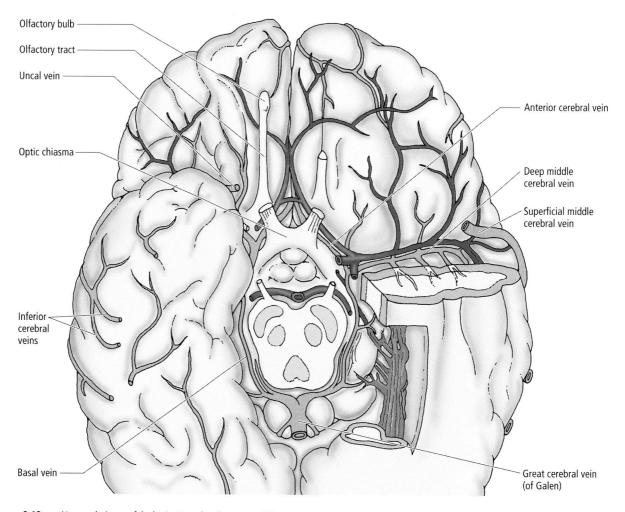

Figure 8.12 ● Venous drainage of the brain. Note that the temporal lobe is sectioned and a window is cut into it to provide a view of the lateral ventricle.

receiving the basal vein, joins its counterpart from the other side to form the **great cerebral vein**.

The **basal vein**, formed by its three tributaries at the anterior perforated substance, the anterior cerebral vein, the deep middle cerebral vein, and the inferior striate veins, receives blood from the parahippocampal gyrus, interpeduncular fossa, midbrain, and lateral ventricle.

Cerebellar veins

The **superior cerebellar veins** drain the superior region of the cerebellum and empty into the straight sinus, the great cerebral vein, and the transverse and superior petrosal sinuses. The **inferior cerebellar veins** drain the inferior aspect of the cerebellum and empty into the occipital, superior petrosal, and transverse sinuses.

Veins of the brainstem

The veins of the brainstem drain the medulla, pons, and midbrain by forming a superficial plexus of veins. These vessels deliver their blood to the vertebral veins, the veins of the spinal cord, and the basilar and inferior petrosal sinuses, as well as into the basal and great cerebral veins.

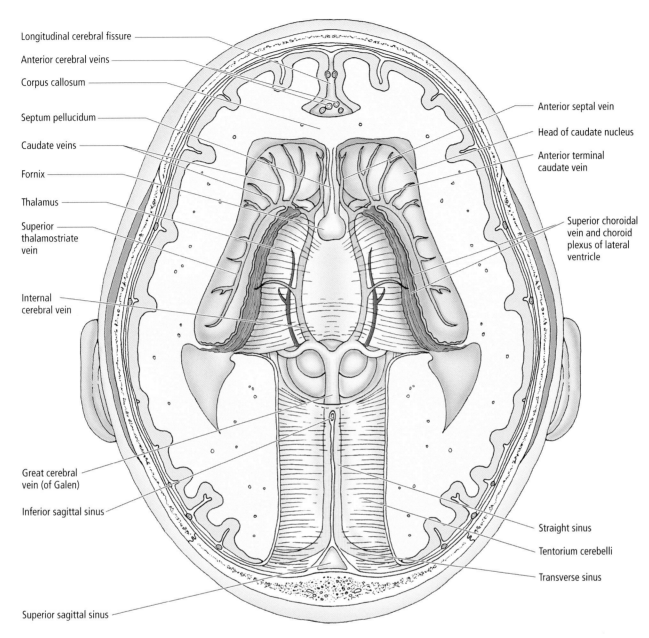

Longitudinal cerebral fissure

Anterior cerebral veins

Corpus callosum

Septum pellucidum

Caudate veins

Fornix

Thalamus

Superior thalamostriate vein

Internal cerebral vein

Great cerebral vein (of Galen)

Inferior sagittal sinus

Superior sagittal sinus

Anterior septal vein

Head of caudate nucleus

Anterior terminal caudate vein

Superior choroidal vein and choroid plexus of lateral ventricle

Straight sinus

Tentorium cerebelli

Transverse sinus

Figure 8.13 ● Diagram of the deep venous drainage of the brain.

CLINICAL CONSIDERATIONS

Aneurysms
Aneurysms are local dilation or ballooning of a vessel due to the weakening of its wall. The most common location for an aneurysm in the brain is the posterior communicating artery as it originates from the internal carotid artery.

Charcot–Bouchard aneurysm
The largest of the slender **striate arteries (lenticulostriate arteries)** is frequently known as the **artery of cerebral hemorrhage** because its aneurysm is the most likely source of strokes in hypertensive patients. This vessel, a branch of the middle cerebral artery, passes between the external capsule and the lentiform nucleus and penetrates as deep as the caudate nucleus.

Ischemia and infarction
The brain receives approximately 750 mL of blood per minute from the right and left internal carotid arteries and from the basilar artery, where each of the three vessels supplies about the same volume of blood flow. This volume translates to about 55 mL of cerebral blood flow per minute per 100 g of brain tissue. **Ischemia** occurs if this blood flow is less than 35 mL/min/100 g of brain tissue, whereas a blood flow of below 15 mL/min/100 g of brain tissue for 5 minutes or longer is considered to be an **infarct** resulting in the death of brain tissue. The infarct may also be due to complete cessation of blood flow because of hemorrhage, thrombosis, embolism, or vasospasm.

Blood–brain barrier
Due to the specificity of the **blood–brain barrier**, certain drugs, antibiotics, and neurotransmitters, such as dopamine, are unable to penetrate the barrier. In order to facilitate the entry of therapeutic substances, a hypertonic solution of **mannitol** is administered which temporarily disables the fasciae occludentes of the capillary endothelial cells. Additionally, it is possible to couple antibodies that have been developed against capillary endothelial cell **transferrin receptors**, to the drugs that need to be administered. The antibody permits the transport of the drug–antibody complex across the blood–brain barrier and into the CNS.

Stroke
A **stroke** (also known as a **cerebrovascular accident**) is a very serious event that results in irreversible damage to a region of the brain whose blood supply has been compromised to such an extent that the involved region can no longer be perfused adequately. The neurons of the region do not receive enough oxygen to sustain them and they die. The severity of the stroke is a function of the region involved and the extent of the damage, therefore the effect may range from minimal damage to death. In the USA, stroke is the third most common cause of death, preceded only by heart disease and cancer. Stroke has numerous risk factors, some of which, such as cigarette smoking and hypertension, can be controlled with relative ease, whereas other factors, such as family history and heart disease, cannot be controlled. There are two types of stroke, ischemic and hemorrhagic stroke. Approximately 85% of all stroke cases are due to **ischemic stroke**, which is the result of embolism of one of the cerebral arteries, vascular disease, or anomalies of the coagulation process. It has been shown that 15–20% of the patients with ischemic stroke die within 30 days of the event. **Hemorrhagic stroke**, which involves bleeding either into the meninges or the brain tissue, has a much higher mortality rate, with 40–80% of patients dying within 30 days.

Lateral medullary syndrome
The **lateral medullary syndrome**, also known as the posterior inferior cerebellar artery (PICA) syndrome, involves occlusion of the branches of the vertebral artery or, less commonly, of the PICA. It is the most commonly occurring brainstem stroke and it has a very good recovery rate. The symptoms of the lateral medullary syndrome include miosis, ptosis, vertigo, dysarthria, and ipsilateral hemiataxia.

Basilar artery thrombosis
Basilar artery thrombosis is a very serious stroke that involves loss of vascular supply to much of the brainstem, resulting in quadriplegia and frequently in death due to respiratory failure.

SYNONYMS AND EPONYMS OF THE VASCULAR SUPPLY OF THE CENTRAL NERVOUS SYSTEM

Name of structure or term	Synonym(s)/ eponym(s)
Cerebral arterial circle	Circle of Willis
Great ventral radicular artery	Artery of Adamkiewicz
Labyrinthine artery	Internal auditory artery
Medial striate artery	Recurrent artery
Occipital branch of the posterior cerebral artery	Calcarine branch of the posterior cerebral artery
Striate arteries	Lenticulostriate arteries

FOLLOW-UP TO CLINICAL CASE

This patient has had a **stroke**. It is in the distribution of the middle cerebral artery (MCA) on the left. The MCA is a common target for stroke; it is sometimes in the full distribution of the MCA, but more commonly only part of it is affected. Some symptoms that are characteristic of MCA territory strokes include hemiparesis and/or hemisensory loss (contralateral), aphasia (usually only if the left MCA is affected), and sometimes hemineglect (contralateral, especially with right MCA stroke). This patient exhibits aphasia and hemiparesis. Some information cannot be ascertained in aphasic patients since they cannot talk about their symptoms.

The two common etiologies of strokes are embolism and cerebral thrombosis. Emboli commonly arise from a cardiac source. A thrombus forms within the heart and a piece or pieces break off, travel downstream, and become lodged within one or more cerebral arteries. A thrombus can also form within a cerebral artery, or one of the arteries leading to the brain (e.g., carotid). The blockage can lead to a reduction of blood flow that, if severe enough and prolonged, leads to infarction.

This patient had an urgent head CT (to rule out hemorrhage). Other testing would include carotid ultrasound or cerebral magnetic resonance angiography (MRA) to look at the appropriate arterial circulation, and echocardiogram. Cardiac thrombus is often prompted by atrial fibrillation, so it would be important to monitor the cardiac rhythm. Treatment for stroke includes intravenous tissue plasminogen activator if it can be started within 3 hours of the stroke onset, intra-arterial thrombolysis if given within 6 hours of onset, carotid endarterectomy if there is severe carotid stenosis from the thrombus (this will only help prevent future strokes), aspirin or similar medications, or heparin.

QUESTIONS TO PONDER

1. What is the significance of the radicular arteries that serve the spinal cord?

2. What is the most significant component of the blood–brain barrier?

3. What is the importance of the posterior communicating artery?

4. What is the significance of the cerebral arterial circle (of Willis)?

5. Where do the veins of the brain drain their blood?

CHAPTER 9

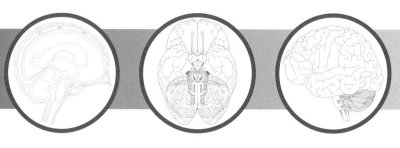

Autonomic Nervous System

CLINICAL CASE

A 55-year-old man presents with generalized weakness and fatigue. This had been ongoing for the past year. He also notes a dry mouth and dry, irritated eyes. He admits to impotence. There is some mild constipation. He has been a heavy smoker since he was 15 years old.

On examination there is mild to moderate weakness noted in the proximal muscles of the arms and legs. He has difficulty rising from a chair without the help of his arms. There is no sensory abnormality and his reflexes are normal. His blood pressure when supine is 150/90 and his heart rate is 80. When standing the blood pressure is 118/76 and the heart rate is 78.

The cells constituting the **autonomic nervous system**, located in both the central and peripheral nervous systems, innervate smooth muscles, cardiac muscles, and glands. They perform their functions below the conscious levels. Functionally, there are three components to the autonomic nervous system, namely **sympathetic**, **parasympathetic**, and **enteric**. Although it is usually treated as a motor system—the **general visceral efferent** (GVE) system—the autonomic nervous system does possess **afferent components**. As a generalization it may be stated that the sympathetic nervous system functions in "fight or flight," the parasympathetic nervous system functions in "digest and rest," whereas the enteric nervous system functions in "overseeing the digestive process."

It is important to note from the outset that there are major differences in the neuronal arrangement of the somatic motor nervous system and the motor limb of the autonomic nervous system (Figs 9.1, 9.2). In the **somatic nervous system** the cell body of the lower motoneuron is located in the **ventral horn** of the spinal cord. The axon of that neuron leaves the spinal cord via the ventral rootlets and passes directly to the muscle fibers it is destined to innervate. Thus, only a single neuron is required to relay the signal for muscle contraction. In the autonomic nervous system two neurons are required to effect a contraction of smooth muscle or cardiac muscle, or to elicit secretion from the cell of a gland. The nerve cell body of the first neuron is in the **central nervous system** (CNS), whereas the nerve cell body of the second neuron is in a **ganglion** in the peripheral nervous system. Because the second nerve cell body resides in an autonomic ganglion, that nerve cell is referred to as the **postganglionic neuron (postsynaptic neuron)**, whereas the first neuron in this two neuron chain, is known as the **preganglionic neuron (presynaptic neuron)**.

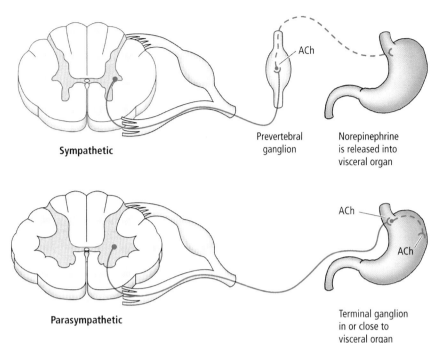

Figure 9.1 ● Schematic diagram demonstrating the difference between the sympathetic nervous system (above) as it arises from spinal cord levels T1 to L1,2 and the spinal component of the parasympathetic nervous system (below) as it originates from the sacral spinal cord. ACh, acetylcholine.

The axon of the preganglionic neuron, the **preganglionic fiber**, is myelinated and it synapses with the postganglionic neuron's soma. The axon of the postganglionic neuron, the **postganglionic fiber**, is not myelinated.

It should be realized that somatic sensory ganglia do not have synapses, whereas synapses do occur in autonomic ganglia. As a generalization, it may be stated that the length of preganglionic and postganglionic fibers differ in that in the sympathetic nervous system the preganglionic fibers are short and the postganglionic fibers are long. In the parasympathetic nervous system the opposite is usually true, in that the preganglionic parasympathetic fibers are long and the postganglionic parasympathetic fibers are usually short.

The **neurotransmitter substance** at the parasympathetic preganglionic and postganglionic and sympathetic preganglionic synapse is **acetylcholine**, whereas at the sympathetic postganglionic synapse it is **norepinephrine (noradrenaline)**. The only exception to this rule is that the postganglionic sympathetic fibers serving the **eccrine sweat glands** release acetylcholine. In addition to the primary neurotransmitter, **co-transmitters** are also usually released.

The fibers of the **sensory** (or afferent) **limb** of the sympathetic and parasympathetic nervous systems travel with blood vessels, cranial nerves, and visceral motor fibers. They frequently *pass through but do not synapse* in the autonomic ganglia. Instead their cell bodies (unipolar/pseudounipolar) are located in the **sensory ganglia** of the cranial and spinal nerves.

SYMPATHETIC NERVOUS SYSTEM

The soma of the preganglionic neurons of the **sympathetic nervous system** are located in the **lateral cell column** of spinal cord levels T1 to L2,3 (Fig. 9.2). Since the axons of these neurons exit the vertebral canal in the ventral root of the spinal nerve at the levels of their origin, the sympathetic nervous system is also known as the **thoracolumbar outflow**. The cell bodies of the postganglionic sympathetic neurons reside in the **sympathetic chain ganglia (paravertebral ganglia** located on either side of the vertebral column), the **pelvic ganglia**, the **preaortic ganglia**, and the small **renal ganglia** (Fig. 9.3). Some of the functions of the sympathetic nervous system are given in Table 9.1.

Preganglionic fibers and paravertebral ganglia of the sympathetic nervous system

Preganglionic fibers of the sympathetic nervous system arise from nerve cell bodies located in the lateral horn of spinal cord levels T1 to L2,3

Preganglionic fibers (preganglionic efferent axons) enter the spinal nerve via the ventral rootlets; they subsequently leave the spinal

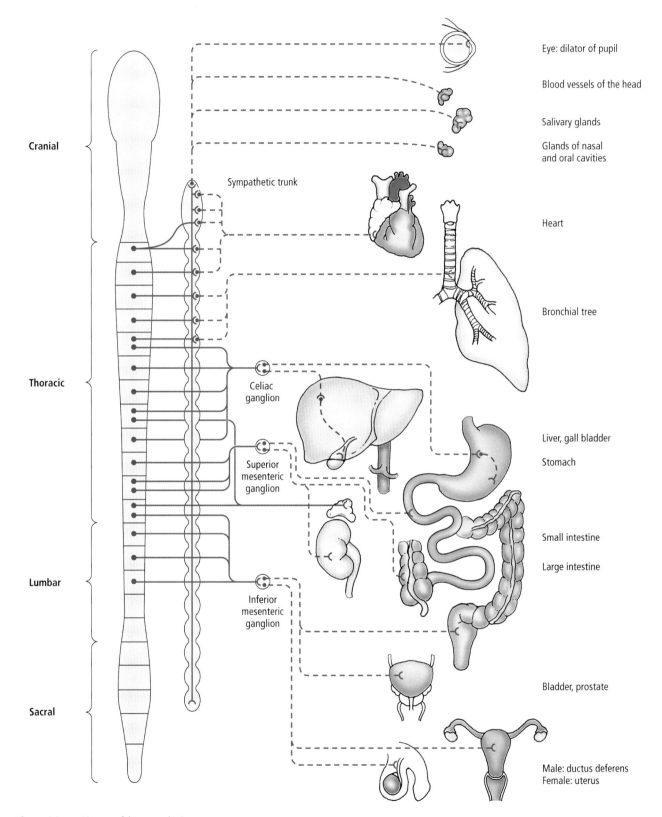

Figure 9.2 ● Diagram of the sympathetic nervous system.

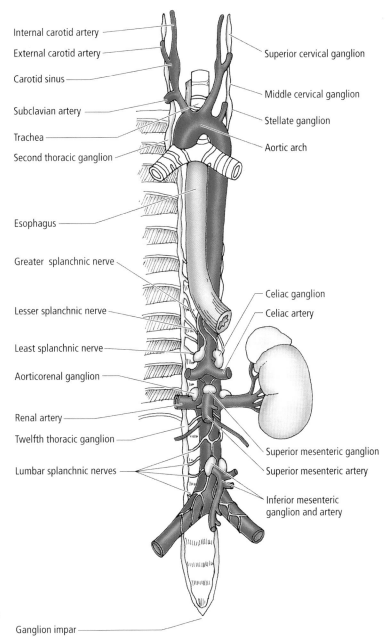

Figure 9.3 ● Diagram of the right and left sympathetic chain ganglia. Observe that the two sides fuse inferiorly to form the single ganglion impar.

Labels on figure:
Internal carotid artery
External carotid artery
Carotid sinus
Subclavian artery
Trachea
Second thoracic ganglion
Esophagus
Greater splanchnic nerve
Lesser splanchnic nerve
Least splanchnic nerve
Aorticorenal ganglion
Renal artery
Twelfth thoracic ganglion
Lumbar splanchnic nerves
Ganglion impar

Superior cervical ganglion
Middle cervical ganglion
Stellate ganglion
Aortic arch
Celiac ganglion
Celiac artery
Superior mesenteric ganglion
Superior mesenteric artery
Inferior mesenteric ganglion and artery

Organ/structure innervated	Function
Eccrine sweat glands of skin	Release of sweat
Arrector pili muscle	Contraction
Blood vessels of skeletal muscle	Dilation
Blood vessels of skin/mucous membranes	Vasoconstriction
Blood vessels of abdominal viscera	Vasoconstriction
Coronary arteries	No effect
Sinoatrial node of heart	Accelerates heart beat
Ventricular myocardium	Increases force of contraction
Alimentary canal	Reduces peristalsis; contraction of sphincters
Iris	Dilates pupils
Levator palpebrae superioris	Contraction of smooth muscles opens upper eyelids
Ductus deferens	Increases peristaltic movements carrying spermatozoa
Bronchial smooth muscle	Relaxation of smooth muscle causes easier breathing
Suprarenal medulla	Releases epinephrine

Table 9.1 ● Functions of the sympathetic nervous system.

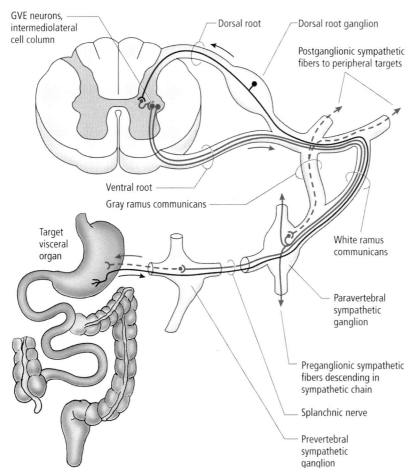

Figure 9.4 ● Diagram of the sympathetic nervous system. Solid red lines represent preganglionic sympathetic fibers and dashed red lines represent postganglionic sympathetic fibers. GVE, general visceral efferent.

nerve via 14 pairs of small branches, known as **white rami communicantes** (white because the axons are myelinated) to reach one of the **sympathetic chain ganglia**. Once preganglionic sympathetic fibers have entered the chain ganglion they have one of three options (Figs 9.4, 9.5):

1 To form synapses with postganglionic, sympathetic soma in the chain ganglion at the level of entry.
2 To proceed superiorly or inferiorly in the sympathetic chain and synapse in a ganglion above or below the point of entry. This may be as far superiorly as the cervical level or as far inferiorly as the sacral level.
3 To pass through the chain ganglion without synapsing in any of the paravertebral ganglia, joining with other preganglionic fibers to form the greater, lesser, or least splanchnic nerves to synapse in one of the prevertebral sympathetic chain ganglia, specifically the pelvic, renal, or preaortic ganglia.

The paravertebral ganglia in the neck fuse to form three ganglia, the largest of which is the **superior cervical ganglion**, the smaller **middle cervical ganglion**, and the smallest **inferior cervical ganglion**. Quite often the inferior cervical ganglion fuses with the first thoracic sympathetic chain ganglion to form the enlarged **stellate ganglion**. The caudal-most ganglia of the right and left paravertebral chains fuse with each other in the coccygeal region, thus forming the unpaired **ganglion impar**.

Distribution of the postganglionic fibers of the sympathetic nervous system

Postganglionic sympathetic fibers may re-enter spinal nerves, may travel with cranial nerves, may travel wrapped around arteries, or may proceed directly to specific organs

The **postganglionic fibers** (axons of the postganglionic soma) arise from the sympathetic chain ganglia and are distributed as branches to the spinal nerves or cranial nerves, or they may travel wrapped around arteries, or they may proceed directly to specific organs or to autonomic plexuses (Fig. 9.4).

1 Branches to **spinal nerves** re-enter the spinal nerve through connections known as **gray rami communicantes** (gray because the postganglionic axons are unmyelinated). Unlike white rami communicantes, there

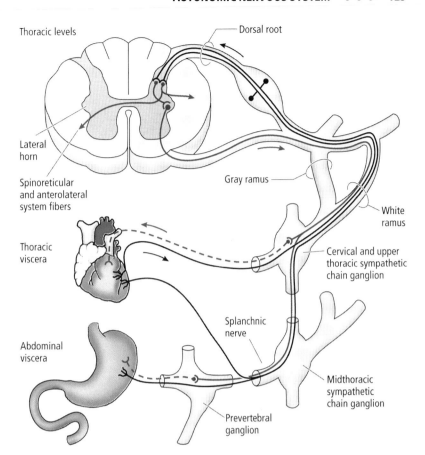

Thoracic levels

Dorsal root

Lateral horn

Spinoreticular and anterolateral system fibers

Gray ramus

White ramus

Thoracic viscera

Cervical and upper thoracic sympathetic chain ganglion

Splanchnic nerve

Abdominal viscera

Midthoracic sympathetic chain ganglion

Prevertebral ganglion

Figure 9.5 ● Diagram demonstrating the difference between the synapse occurring in a sympathetic chain ganglion and that occurring in a prevertebral ganglion. Solid red lines indicate preganglionic sympathetic fibers. Dashed red lines indicate postganglionic sympathetic fibers.

are 31 pairs of gray rami communicantes, one for each spinal nerve. The postganglionic sympathetic fibers are distributed with the cutaneous branches of the spinal nerves, reaching the sweat glands, arrector pili muscles, and smooth muscles of peripheral blood vessels.

2 Branches to **cranial nerves** may reach the cranial nerves directly, namely, the glossopharyngeal (CN IX), vagus (CN X), and hypoglossal (CN XII) nerves or they may follow blood vessels until they are in the vicinity of the cranial nerve that they use to reach their final destination.

3 Branches **wrapped around arteries** travel with these vessels, such as the internal and external carotid arteries and the vertebral artery. There are numerous other arteries that possess postganglionic sympathetic fibers in their tunicae adventitia and they are discussed below.

4 Branches proceeding directly to **specific organs** may travel on arteries, in nerves, or through plexuses, but they travel on their own, at least for a while. These include postganglionic sympathetic fibers destined for the eyes and the heart.

5 Branches that proceed to **autonomic plexuses** possess either postganglionic or preganglionic fibers, depending on the plexus. Those that serve the heart, lungs, and pelvis are probably postganglionic, whereas those that are destined for the abdominal plexuses are preganglionic sympathetic fibers destined for the postganglionic soma in the walls of the organ to be innervated. The **greater**,

lesser, and **least splanchnic nerves** are the major nerve fibers that contain preganglionic sympathetic axons destined for the **abdominal plexuses**.

Topographic distribution of the sympathetic nervous system

The sympathetic nervous system may be subdivided into two categories: (i) those associated with the chain ganglia; and (ii) a collection of autonomic plexuses whose postganglionic fibers are distributed to the abdominal and pelvic viscera. The chain ganglia, although a single entity, may be viewed as being composed of five discrete regions that correspond to the head, neck, thorax, abdominolumbar region, and pelvis.

Cephalic region of the sympathetic nervous system

The cephalic region of the sympathetic nervous system is composed only of postganglionic sympathetic fibers whose cell bodies are located in the superior cervical ganglia

The cephalic region of the sympathetic nervous system has no ganglia of its own, instead it is composed only of **postganglionic sympathetic fibers** whose cell bodies are located in the **superior cervical ganglia**. These fibers are primarily associated with the tunica adventitia of blood vessels passing from the neck into the head, are named according to their vessel of association or by their location, or by the localized region that they serve.

Internal carotid nerves

> The internal carotid nerves are composed of postganglionic sympathetic fibers derived from the superior cervical ganglion

The **internal carotid nerves** travel with the internal carotid arteries as two separate plexuses, the internal carotid plexus and the cavernous plexus.

The **internal carotid plexus** travels on the lateral aspect of the artery and has the following branches:

- Branches **communicating with cranial nerve V** (trigeminal nerve) and **cranial nerve VI** (abducent nerve).
- The **deep petrosal nerve**: this pierces the cartilage of the foramen lacerum and accompanies the greater petrosal nerve as the two nerves enter the pterygoid canal to form the **nerve of the pterygoid canal (vidian canal)**. This nerve proceeds to the pterygopalatine ganglion in the same named fossa. Some branches derived from the greater petrosal nerve synapse in the pterygopalatine ganglion, but none of the branches derived from the deep petrosal nerve synapse (since they are postganglionic sympathetic fibers), instead they become distributed by branches of the maxillary division of the trigeminal nerve to the glands and blood vessels of the pharynx, palate, and nasal cavity.
- The **caroticotympanic nerves**: these are small fibers that are destined to serve regions of the middle ear.

The **cavernous plexus** travels on the medial aspect of the artery and has the following branches:

- Branches communicating with **cranial nerve IV** (trochlear nerve) and **cranial nerve V₁** (ophthalmic division of the trigeminal nerve).
- Branches destined for the **dilator pupillae muscle** of the iris. These travel with the long ciliary nerve as well as with the short ciliary nerves (without synapsing in the ciliary ganglion) to pierce the orb and synapse on the muscle fibers.
- Branches serving the vessels of the pituitary gland, brain, meninges, and orbit.

External carotid nerves

> The external carotid nerves travel with the external carotid artery and its branches in the head

The **external carotid nerves**, composed of postganglionic sympathetic fibers derived from the superior cervical ganglion, travel with the external carotid artery and its branches in the head. These include the following:

- Nerve fibers that follow the facial artery: these travel to and serve the submandibular gland and, using the lingual nerve, reach and serve the sublingual gland.
- Nerve fibers that travel on branches of the facial and superficial temporal arteries, serving them as well as arrector pili muscles and sweat glands of the facial region.
- The **small deep petrosal nerve**: this leaves the middle meningeal artery to pass through (without synapsing in) the otic ganglion. It joins the auriculotemporal nerve and serves the parotid gland.

Cervical region of the sympathetic nervous system

The cervical region of the sympathetic trunk is composed of the **superior, middle**, and **inferior sympathetic cervical ganglia** as well as the **sympathetic cord** that connects them to each other. None of these receive white rami communicantes because the preganglionic fibers enter the chain ganglia at thoracic levels T1–T5, and proceed superiorly in the cord to reach and synapse on postganglionic soma residing in one of the three ganglia. Postganglionic fibers leave the ganglia gathered in nerves of various caliber that join the arteries, cervical spinal nerves, and cranial nerves. Branches are derived from each cervical ganglion and are detailed below.

Superior cervical ganglion

> The superior cervical ganglion is the largest sympathetic ganglion in the neck

The **superior cervical ganglion**, the largest of the three ganglia, is located deep to the carotid sheath, at the level of the atlas. It has numerous branches, some of which (internal and external carotid nerves) were detailed in the section above (see p. 124). The additional branches are those that travel with the cranial nerves and cervical spinal nerves, the pharyngeal branches, the intercarotid plexus, and the superior cardiac nerves:

- Branches traveling with **cranial nerves IX, X**, and **XII**.
- Branches traveling with the first four **cervical nerves**.
- The four to six **pharyngeal branches** that form the pharyngeal plexus in unison with cranial nerves IX and X.
- The **intercarotid plexus** that proceeds to the carotid sinus and carotid body to innervate the smooth muscle of the regional blood vessels.
- The **superior cardiac nerves** of the right and left side: these join the cardiac plexus and innervate the cardiac muscle of the heart. They function in concert with the middle and inferior cardiac nerves to accelerate the rate of heart beat.

Middle cervical ganglion

> The middle cervical ganglion is the smallest of the three sympathetic ganglia in the neck

The smallest of the ganglia, the **middle cervical ganglion**, has an inconstant location and is occasionally absent. The branches arising from the middle cervical ganglion are those that join the cervical spinal nerves, the middle cervical nerve, and the thyroid nerves:

- Gray rami communicantes to the fifth and sixth **cervical nerves** that are distributed with the branches of these cervical nerves.
- The **middle cardiac nerve**, also known as the **great cardiac nerve**: this communicates with the superior cardiac nerve to join the cardiac plexus. It functions, in concert with the superior and inferior cardiac nerves, to accelerate the rate of the heart beat.
- The **thyroid nerves**: these travel on the tunica adventitia of the inferior thyroid artery to reach and supply the thyroid gland.
- The region of the **sympathetic cord** connecting the middle and inferior cervical ganglia. This is usually split into an anterior and a posterior portion; the anterior portion passes around the subclavian artery, forming a loop—the **ansa subclavia**.

Inferior cervical ganglion

> The inferior cervical ganglion often fuses with the first thoracic sympathetic ganglion, forming the stellate ganglion

The **inferior cervical ganglion** is located at the level of the transverse process of the 7th cervical vertebra. The branches arising from the inferior cervical ganglion are the ones that join the cervical spinal nerves, the inferior cardiac nerves, and the vertebral nerve:

- Gray rami communicantes to **cervical spinal nerves 6–8**: these are distributed with the branches of these cervical nerves.
- **Inferior cardiac nerves**: these join the cardiac plexus and function, in concert with the superior and middle cardiac nerves, to accelerate the rate of heart beat.
- **Vertebral nerve**: this travels on the tunica adventitia of the vertebral artery and serves it as well as its intracranial branches with vasomotor function.

The inferior cervical and first thoracic ganglia frequently fuse to form the **stellate ganglion**. This fused ganglion fulfills all the functions of the inferior cervical ganglion and also gives rise to the gray rami communicantes of spinal nerves T1 and T2.

Thoracic region of the sympathetic nervous system

> The thoracic region of the sympathetic nervous system is the only region with white rami communicantes

Theoretically, there are 12 **thoracic sympathetic ganglia** connected to each other by short segments of the sym-

pathetic cord, but fusion of occasional ganglia with each other reduces their number to approximately 10. **White rami communicantes** are connections between the thoracic spinal nerves and the thoracic chain ganglia. They carry **preganglionic sympathetic fibers** from the lateral column of the spinal cord, which enter each thoracic sympathetic ganglion to synapse with **postganglionic sympathetic soma** residing in a sympathetic ganglion at any level of the chain ganglia or in a sympathetic ganglion located elsewhere in the body.

Branches arising from the thoracic sympathetic ganglia are the gray rami communicantes, the visceral branches, and the splanchnic nerves.

Gray rami communicantes

The **gray rami communicantes** arise from each thoracic ganglion to unite with their associated thoracic spinal nerve, carrying postganglionic sympathetic fibers that will be distributed with the branches of the spinal nerve.

Visceral branches

> Visceral branches of the sympathetic nervous system are distributed to specific organs

The **visceral branches** are composed of postganglionic sympathetic fibers that are distributed to plexuses on or in the vicinity of the heart, esophagus, lungs, and aorta:

- **Cardiac branches** arise from the first through fifth thoracic ganglia and are destined for the cardiac plexus. They mix with fibers from the superior, middle, and inferior cardiac nerves. They also function in accelerating the rate of the heart beat.
- **Esophageal branches** arise from many of the thoracic ganglia and serve to modify the function of the enteric nervous system.
- Fibers destined for the **pulmonary plexus** arise from the second through fourth thoracic ganglia and enter the hilum of the lung. They serve the blood vessels of the lung as well as the bronchial musculature.
- The **aortic plexus** is served by fibers arising from the fifth to tenth (or eleventh) thoracic ganglia. These fibers distribute with the branches of the aorta and probably function to modulate the enteric nervous system.

Splanchnic nerves

> Splanchnic nerves are preganglionic fibers destined for the celiac ganglion, the medulla of the suprarenal gland, the aorticorenal ganglia, and the renal plexus

The **splanchnic nerves** are composed of mostly myelinated preganglionic sympathetic fibers (as well as large myelinated visceral afferent fibers bringing information from the viscera), because they have not synapsed in the chain ganglia;

instead they passed through the ganglia on their way to the **preaortic ganglia**. There are three splanchnic nerves: the greater, lesser, and least splanchnic nerves.

1 The **greater splanchnic nerves**, formed into a single trunk from preganglionic sympathetic fibers that pass through the fifth to ninth thoracic ganglia, penetrate the crus of the diaphragm to synapse in the **celiac ganglion** (and **splanchnic ganglion**, if present). Some fibers continue through the celiac ganglion without synapsing, and continue to the **suprarenal gland medulla** and synapse there on **chromaffin cells**.

It is interesting to note that the chromaffin cells of the suprarenal medulla, as well as the neurons of sympathetic ganglia, are derived from neural crest cells. Thus chromaffin cells act as modified postganglionic sympathetic neurons and release their secretory product, **epinephrine** and **norepinephrine**, into the capillary beds of the suprarenal medulla. Approximately 85% of the chromaffin cells release epinephrine and 15% release norepinephrine.

2 The **lesser splanchnic nerve**, formed into a single trunk from preganglionic sympathetic fibers that pass through the tenth and eleventh thoracic ganglia, penetrates the crus of the diaphragm and synapses in the **aorticorenal ganglion**.

3 The **least splanchnic nerve**, formed from preganglionic sympathetic fibers that pass through the twelfth thoracic ganglion, passes through the diaphragm and synapses in the **renal plexus**.

Abdominolumbar region of the sympathetic nervous system

The abdominolumbar portion of the sympathetic nervous system is composed of two to six ganglia and the intervening trunk

The **abdominolumbar sympathetic trunk** is highly variable in that there are two to six ganglia, with an average of four ganglia, connected to one another by cords of varying lengths. The right and left sympathetic trunks in the abdominal cavity are almost hidden by the inferior vena cava and the abdominal aorta, respectively. Branches of the abdominolumbar trunk are composed of gray rami communicantes, lumbar splanchnic nerves, and branches of the celiac ganglion:

- **Gray rami communicantes** in the lumbar area are somewhat longer than those of the thoracic region. They join the spinal nerves to be distributed with them to innervate the smooth muscle of blood vessels as well as the glands and arrector pili of the skin.
- **Lumbar splanchninc nerves**, preganglionic sympathetic fibers that are located caudal to the least splanchnic nerve, synapse in the **inferior mesenteric ganglion**.
- Branches of the **celiac ganglion** are postganglionic sympathetic fibers that follow the aorta and its branches and form a large plexus of nerve fibers, the **celiac plexus**.

PARASYMPATHETIC NERVOUS SYSTEM

Topographic distribution of the parasympathetic nervous system

The preganglionic cell bodies of the **parasympathetic nervous system** are located in cranial nerves as well as in the lateral horn of the sacral spinal cord. Therefore, the parasympathetic nervous system is also referred to as the **craniosacral outflow**. Some of the functions of the parasympathetic nervous system are given in Table 9.2.

Organ/structure innervated	Function
Iris	Constricts pupils (miosis)
Ciliary muscles	Contracts to relax suspensory ligaments of the lens (near vision)
Lacrimal glands	Facilitates flow of tears
Salivary glands	Facilitates flow of serous secretion
Sinoatrial node of heart	Decreases rate of heart beat
Blood vessels	Usually has little effect
Bronchial smooth muscle	Bronchoconstriction
Glands of conducting portion of respiratory system	Facilitates secretion
Peristalsis of alimentary canal	Stimulates peristalsis
Sphincter muscles	Relaxes sphincter muscles (inhibitory function)
Intrinsic glands of the alimentary canal	Facilitates secretion
Pancreas	Facilitates secretion
Gall bladder	Facilitates release of bile
Penis and clitoris	Stimulates erection

Table 9.2 ● Functions of the parasympatheric nervous system.

Cranial portion of the parasympathetic nervous system

The cranial portion of the parasympathetic nervous system is associated with four cranial nerves: the oculomotor, facial, glossopharyngeal, and vagus nerves

The preganglionic parasympathetic fibers of the cranial portion of the parasympathetic nervous system travel with four cranial nerves, the oculomotor, facial, glossopharyngeal, and vagus nerves (Figs 9.6, 9.7).

Oculomotor nerve (CN III)

The **Edinger–Westphal nucleus** houses **preganglionic parasympathetic soma** whose axons travel in the branches of cranial nerve III. When these preganglionic fibers reach the orbit they synapse with postganglionic parasympathetic soma in the **ciliary ganglion** (the parasympathetic ganglion of the oculomotor nerve). The postganglionic parasympathetic fibers, known as the **short ciliary nerves**, exit the ciliary ganglion, pierce the orb (eyeball) to innervate the **sphincter pupillae muscle**, which constricts the pupils. They also innervate the muscles of the **ciliary body**, which function in accommodating the lens of the eye when focusing on nearby objects.

Facial nerve (CN VII)

The **lacrimal** and **superior salivatory nuclei** of the brainstem house the **preganglionic parasympathetic soma** associated with cranial nerve VII.

Preganglionic parasympathetic fibers from the **lacrimal nucleus** reach the **pterygopalatine ganglion** (a parasympathetic ganglion of the facial nerve) where they synapse with postganglionic parasympathetic soma. Postganglionic parasympathetic fibers leave the ganglion and serve the **lacrimal gland**, eliciting the production of tears, as well as **glands in the nasal mucosa**, eliciting the production of mucus.

Preganglionic parasympathetic fibers from the **superior salivatory nucleus** proceed to the **submandibular ganglion** where they synapse with postganglionic parasympathetic soma. Postganglionic parasympathetic fibers leave the ganglion to innervate the submandibular and sublingual glands, eliciting the flow of saliva.

Glossopharyngeal nerve (CN IX)

The **inferior salivatory nucleus** (nucleus of the glossopharyngeal nerve) of the brainstem houses the **preganglionic parasympathetic cell bodies** associated with cranial nerve IX. Preganglionic parasympathetic fibers from this nucleus reach the **otic ganglion** to synapse with postganglionic parasympathetic soma. Their postganglionic parasympathetic fibers leave the ganglion to innervate the parotid gland as well as minor salivary glands in the oral mucosa, eliciting the flow of saliva.

Vagus nerve (CN X)

The nucleus ambiguus and the dorsal motor nucleus of the **vagus nerve** house the **preganglionic parasympathetic soma** associated with cranial nerve X.

Preganglionic parasympathetic nerve fibers from the **nucleus ambiguus** synapse with postganglionic parasympathetic soma located in the **cardiac ganglia** distributed around the great vessels of the heart. Postganglionic parasympathetic axons leave the ganglia and innervate the **sinoatrial (SA) node**. Additionally these fibers also serve occasional atrial and ventricular cardiac muscle fibers. The parasympathetic nervous system decreases the rate of the heart beat.

Preganglionic parasympathetic nerve fibers from the **dorsal motor nucleus of the vagus** synapse with the following soma:

- Postganglionic parasympathetic soma located in ganglia surrounding the **bronchial passages**. Postganglionic parasympathetic fibers derived from these ganglia serve to elicit bronchioconstriction.
- Postganglionic parasympathetic soma located in the vicinity of the **pancreas**. Postganglionic parasympathetic fibers derived from these ganglia serve to elicit the release of pancreatic enzymes and buffer.
- Postganglionic parasympathetic soma along the **gastrointestinal tract** extending from the esophagus to the end of the transverse colon. These postganglionic parasympathetic cell bodies are housed in **Meissner's submucosal** and **Auerbach's myenteric plexus (ganglia)** located within the wall of the alimentary canal. Moreover, many of the preganglionic parasympathetic axons synapse with the intrinsic soma of the enteric nervous system. Parasympathetic activity facilitates the digestive process and relaxes sphincter muscles.

Sacral portion of the parasympathetic nervous system

The preganglionic cell bodies of the sacral portion of the parasympathetic nervous system are housed in the lateral cell column of sacral spinal cord levels 2 through 4

The **lateral cell column** of the second to fourth segments of the sacral spinal cord houses the preganglionic parasympathetic cell bodies composing the **sacral division** of the parasympathetic nervous system. Their preganglionic axons join their corresponding spinal nerves and travel to the **pelvic plexus** and to scattered small **ganglia** in the vicinity of the pelvic organs, where they synapse with the enteric nervous system and with postganglionic cell bodies of the parasympathetic ganglia. Postganglionic parasympathetic fibers from the pelvic plexus and the additional small ganglia serve the urinary bladder, penis, prostate, and seminal vesicles in the male as well as the bladder, uterus, clitoris, and vagina in the female.

The **bladder**, **prostate**, and **seminal vesicles** receive their motor innervation from the small ganglia in their vicinity, except for the **sphincter muscle** controlling the **bladder**, which is **inhibited** by the parasympathetic nervous system.

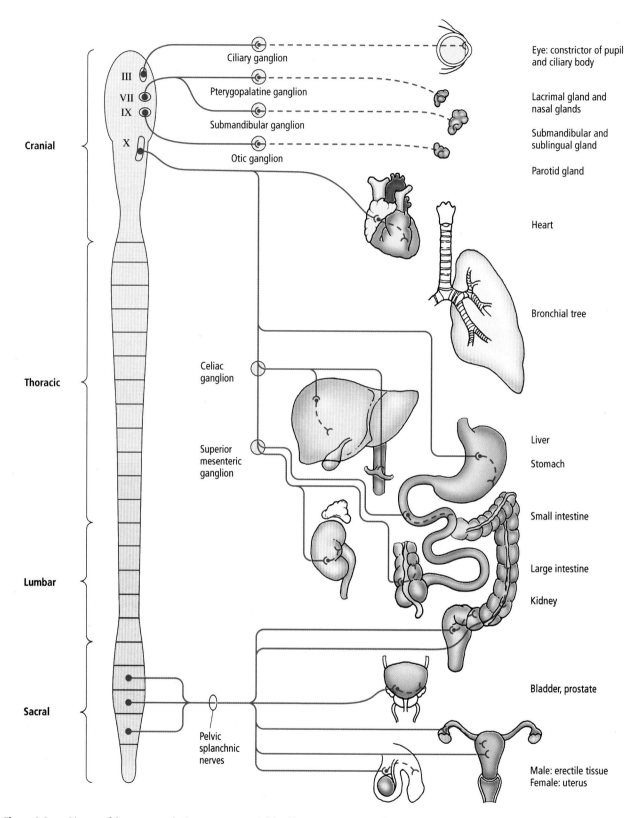

Figure 9.6 ● Diagram of the parasympathetic nervous system. Solid red lines represent preganglionic parasympathetic fibers and dashed red lines represent postganglionic parasympathetic fibers.

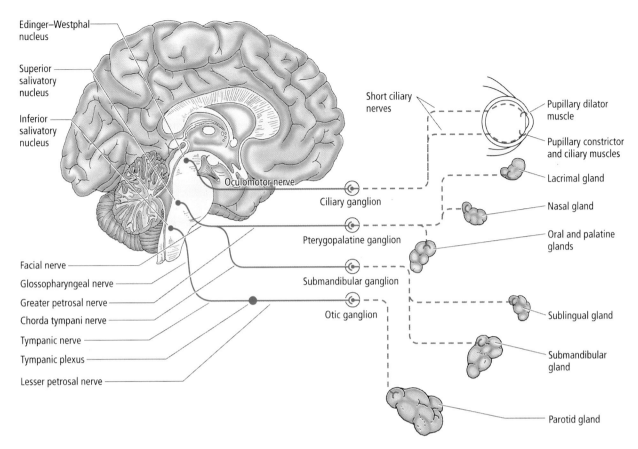

Figure 9.7 ● Schematic diagram of the parasympathetic innervation of the head. Solid red lines represent preganglionic parasympathetic fibers and dashed red lines represent postganglionic parasympathetic fibers.

The **uterus** and **vagina** receive *inhibitory* postganglionic parasympathetic fibers via the **uterovaginal plexus**. Although in the pregnant female the same fibers are believed to have excitatory roles.

The **external genitalia** of the male and the **clitoris** of the female receive postganglionic parasympathetic fibers from the **pelvic plexus** via the **pudendal nerve**; these fibers are responsible for dilation of the cavernous blood sinuses resulting in the erection of the penis and clitoris.

ENTERIC NERVOUS SYSTEM

The intrinsic components of the enteric nervous system are located completely within the wall of the alimentary canal and their neurons are distributed in two sets of ganglia

Meissner's submucosal plexus and Auerbach's myenteric plexus house the intrinsic components of the enteric nervous system. The neurons and neuroglial cells of the enteric nervous system originate from neural crest cells.

Meissner's submucosal plexus is located in the submucosa at its interface with the inner circular layer of the muscularis externa. Generally speaking, Meissner's submucosal plexus is responsible for peristalsis and global, rather than local, actions. **Auerbach's myenteric plexus** is located between the inner circular and outer longitudinal layers of the muscularis externa. Generally speaking, Auerbach's plexus is responsible for localized phenomena and for movement of, and glandular secretions from, the mucosa.

The two sets of **plexuses** interact with the sympathetic and parasympathetic nervous systems as well as with each other and function together to ensure that the alimentary canal performs its functions properly.

The **extrinsic components** of the enteric nervous system are the sympathetic and parasympathetic fibers that modulate the functioning of the intrinsic components. The extrinsic components are necessary but not essential for normal functioning of the digestive tract. Parasympathetic innervation facilitates digestion by increasing peristalsis and relaxing sphincters. Vigorous activity from the sympathetic innervation slows down peristalsis and increases sphincter muscle tonus.

The **intrinsic components** of the enteric nervous system regulate much of the digestive processes by innervating the smooth muscles, glands, as well as the **diffuse neuroendocrine system (DNES) cells** residing in the epithelial lining of the alimentary canal. There are at least 20 different types of DNES cells and each releases a specific paracrine hormone (although many of these hormones also enter the bloodstream to remote target cells). These hormones act in concert to regulate much of the digestive process. A select list of these cells, their hormones, and their function is presented in Table 9.3.

Table 9.3 ● Selected hormones secreted by the diffuse neuroendocrine system (DNES) cells of the alimentary canal.

Paracrine hormone	DNES cell	Site of secretion	Function
Cholecystokinin (CCK)	I	Small intestine	Stimulates contraction of gall bladder (with release of bile) and facilitates the release of pancreatic enzymes
Gastric inhibitory peptide (GIP)	K	Small intestine	Inhibits secretion of gastric HCl
Gastrin	G	Pylorus and duodenum	Stimulates gastric secretion of HCl and pepsinogen
Glicentin	GL	Stomach through colon	Stimulates hepatic glycogenolysis
Glucagon	A	Stomach and duodenum	Stimulates hepatic glycogenolysis
Motilin	Mo	Small intestine	Increases gut motility
Neurotensin	N	Small intestine	Inhibits gut motility; stimulates blood flow to the ileum
Secretin	S	Small intestine	Stimulates bicarbonate secretion by the pancreas and biliary tract
Serotonin and substance P	EC	Stomach through colon	Increase gut motility
Somatostatin	D	Pylorus and duodenum	Inhibits nearby DNES cells
Vasoactive intestinal peptide (VIP)	VIP	Stomach through colon	Increases gut motility; stimulates intestinal ion and water secretion

HCl, hydrochloric acid.

NEUROTRANSMITTERS AND RECEPTORS OF THE AUTONOMIC NERVOUS SYSTEM

Because the two primary neurotransmitters are acetylcholine and norepinephrine, it is customary to speak of **cholinergic** and **adrenergic** divisions of the autonomic nervous system. Preganglionic and postganglionic parasympathetic neurons, preganglionic sympathetic neurons, and those postglanglionic sympathetic neurons that innervate eccrine sweat glands are all cholinergic. All other postganglionic sympathetic neurons are adrenergic.

Autonomic receptors

Autonomic receptors are classified as **cholinergic** or **adrenergic** (noradrenergic), based on their ability to bind and to be activated by acetylcholine or norepinephrine, respectively. Subtypes of both cholinergic and adrenergic receptors have been identified. Additionally, other types of receptors are also present.

Cholinergic receptors

Muscarinic and nicotinic receptors are the two types of cholinergic receptors

There are two types of **cholinergic receptors**, namely, muscarinic receptors and nicotinic receptors. The former are also activated by muscarine, a toxin derived from toadstools, and the latter are also activated by nicotine. It is important to note that nicotine will not activate muscarinic receptors and muscarine will not activate nicotinic receptors, but both types will be activated by acetylcholine.

Muscarinic receptors are located in the membranes of cells synapsing with postganglionic parasympathetic fibers and in the membranes of eccrine sweat glands (innervated by postganglionic sympathetic fibers).

Nicotinic receptors are located in the membranes of postganglionic sympathetic and postganglionic parasympathetic soma where they synapse with their preganglionic counterparts. They are also located in the sarcolemma of the myoneural junctions of skeletal muscle cells.

Adrenergic receptors

Adrenergic receptors are of two major types: alpha adrenergic and beta adrenergic

There are two types of adrenergic receptors, alpha adrenergic receptors and beta adrenergic receptors, each with its own subtypes.

Alpha adrenergic receptors are more easily activated by epinephrine than by norepinephrine and are least activated by isoproterenol. Alpha receptors are located in the plasma membranes of vascular smooth muscle cells, dilatator pupillae muscle cells, and soma of enteric neurons controlling sphincter muscle contraction.

Beta adrenergic receptors are more responsive to isoproterenol than to epinephrine and are least activated by norepinephrine. Beta receptors are located in the plasma membranes of cardiac muscle cells, bronchiolar smooth muscle cells, and soma of enteric neurons that facilitate peristaltic activity of the alimentary canal.

Additional receptors

There are **additional receptors**, especially in the enteric nervous system, that are neither cholinergic nor adrenergic. These respond to various other neurotransmitter substances, such as somatostatin, substance P, adenosine, vasoactive intestinal peptide, etc., many of which are detailed in Chapter 4.

PELVIC AUTONOMIC FUNCTIONS

The somatic and autonomic nervous systems interact with each other to perform numerous functions, among them those that control urination, defecation, and erection and ejaculation.

Urine retention and urination

Urine retention and urination require the interaction of the sympathetic, parasympathetic, and somatic motor nervous systems and are controlled by the cerebral cortex and pons

The process of retaining urine in, and evacuating urine from, the urinary bladder is a learned function that requires the interactions of the sympathetic, parasympathetic, and somatic motor nervous systems and is controlled by the cerebral cortex and pons. As the urinary bladder distends, nociceptors and stretch receptors in its wall transmit the information to the dorsal horn of the spinal cord. These afferent nerves are **unipolar (pseudounipolar) neurons** whose cell bodies are located in the dorsal root ganglia. If the volume of urine in the bladder is low, the skeletal muscles of the **external sphincter** undergo reflex contraction in response to stimulation by axons of somatic motoneurons whose cell bodies are located in the **Onuf nucleus** (ventral horn of spinal cord levels S2–S4). Cell bodies of the motor neurons in the Onuf nucleus are activated by projections from the pons and cerebral cortex (Fig. 9.8). Concurrently, the smooth muscle cells of the **internal sphincter** also undergo **reflex contraction** and the **detrusor muscles**, smooth muscles located in the wall of the urinary bladder, undergo **reflex relaxation**, due to the activities of preganglionic sympathetic innervation from the intermediate cell column at spinal cord levels T12 to S2.

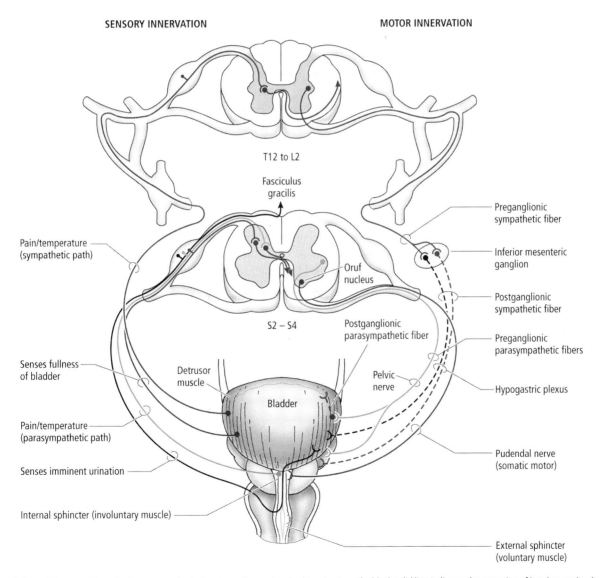

SENSORY INNERVATION   MOTOR INNERVATION

Figure 9.8 ● Diagram of the spinal sensory and spinal motor pathways involved in urination. The black solid line indicates the sensation of imminent urination and the black dashed line indicates the inhibition of relaxation of the urinary bladder permitting postganglionic sympathetic fibers to cause contraction of the detrusor muscles, thus causing emptying of the bladder.

The process of **urination** is facilitated by the micturition centers located in the cerebral cortex and the pons. As the bladder distends and the urine volume reaches a threshold level, sensory information reaches the **ventral posterolateral (VPL) nucleus of the thalamus** traveling via the medial lemniscal pathway, the dorsal column, and the anterolateral column. The information is transmitted by tertiary neurons from the thalamus to the **postcentral sulcus** and the individual becomes conscious of the need to urinate. When the individual is ready to void the retentive reflexes described above become inhibited, thus the internal and external sphincters relax. Additionally, projections from the pons activate the preganglionic parasympathetic neurons in the lateral horn of spinal cord levels S2–S4, whose post-ganglioic counterparts stimulate the detrusor muscles of the bladder to undergo contraction, thus emptying the urinary bladder.

Defecation

The sigmoid colon distends as the feces continues to accumulate in its lumen causing the urge to defecate

As feces accumulate, the sigmoid colon distends and the individual becomes conscious of the need to **defecate**, but the feces are retained in the colon by the two sphincter muscles, the **internal smooth muscle sphincter** and the **external skeletal muscle sphincter**. The former is supplied by **postganglionic sympathetic fibers** from the hypogastric plexus as well as by postganglionic parasympathetic fibers located in Auerbach's plexus (whose preganglionic fibers arise from the sacral spinal cord). The external sphincter is supplied by the somatic nervous system, namely the **inferior rectal nerve**. Thus, when the sigmoid colon becomes distended, the internal sphincter muscle relaxes (due to the parasympathetic nerve supply) and at the same time the external sphincter muscle contracts, preventing the feces from exiting the bowel. While the individual is asleep, this contraction of the external sphincter muscle is a reflex response. When the individual is awake, the contraction of the external sphincter is a voluntary response. When the individual is ready to defecate, the voluntary relaxation of the external sphincter, the peristaltic action of the sigmoid colon, and the intra-abdominal pressure created by contraction of the anterior abdominal wall musculature cooperate in expelling the feces from the sigmoid colon and the rectum through the anus.

Erection and ejaculation

Erection of the penis and of the clitoris is an autonomic function initiated by tactile or psychogenic stimulation and mediated by parasympathetic innervation derived from sacral spinal cord levels. The parasympathetic fibers are responsible for engorgement of the spongy tissue of the penis and clitoris as well as of the vascular channels of the labia minora, and cause the release of secretions from the vaginal glands, lubricating the vagina. Preganglionic sympathetic fibers from spinal cord levels T10 to L2 synapse on postganglionic sympathetic nerve cell bodies housed in the inferior mesenteric ganglion. **Postganglionic sympathetic fibers** from that ganglion are responsible in females for rhythmic contractions of the vagina and uterus, and in males for the release of secretions from the prostate gland and seminal vesicles as well as for **ejaculation**.

CLINICAL CONSIDERATIONS

Congenital megacolon
Congenital megacolon, also known as Hirschsprung's disease, is an excessive enlargement of the distal part of the colon due to the lack of, or a marked reduction in, the neuronal population in Auerbach's myenteric plexus. Due to the absence of these neurons a region of the colon becomes constricted, the muscles cannot relax, and feces accumulate in the region of the colon proximal to the constriction. With the accumulation of feces the proximal region enlarges, resulting in megacolon.

Horner's syndrome
Horner's syndrome is a condition resulting from damage to the cervical sympathetic trunk, sympathetic fibers of the carotid plexus, or any region of the spinal cord or brainstem involving the sympathetic pathways. The syndrome is characterized by the following conditions on the affected side: constriction of the pupil (miosis), lack of the ability to sweat (anhydrosis), recession of the orb within the orbit (enophthalmos), and drooping of the upper eyelid (ptosis). It is interesting to note that cancer of the apex of the lung may involve the cervical sympathetic trunk, thus precipitating Horner's syndrome.

Shy–Drager syndrome
Shy–Drager syndrome patients suffer from orthostatic hypertension and faint frequently because the autonomic nervous system neurons responsible for adjusting blood pressure during postural changes have either degenerated or died. These postural changes can involve the patient standing up from a reclining (or even from a sitting) position.

SYNONYMS AND EPONYMS
OF THE AUTONOMIC NERVOUS SYSTEM

Name of structure or term	Synonym(s)/eponym(s)
Auerbach's myenteric plexus	Auerbach's plexus
Meissner's submucosal plexus	Meissner's plexus
Middle cardiac nerve	Great cardiac nerve
Nerve of the pterygoid canal	Nerve of the vidian canal
Postganglionic neuron	Postsynaptic neuron
Preganglionic neuron	Presynaptic neuron

FOLLOW-UP TO CLINICAL CASE

Serologic testing confirmed that this patient had **Lambert–Eaton myasthenic syndrome**. This is an autoimmune condition.

Acetylcholine is released at presynaptic peripheral nerve terminals in response to an action potential. The action potential at the presynaptic terminal opens voltage-gated calcium channels, leading to an influx of calcium, which leads to acetylcholine release. This acetylcholine diffuses across the synapse to reach receptors on the target organ. This is most apparent at the neuromuscular junction, where an action potential along the muscle membrane is induced by the released acetylcholine from the presynaptic nerve terminal. It occurs for both autonomic nerves as well as nerves supplying skeletal muscle, and the effects are seen at both nicotinic and muscarinic receptors.

In Lambert–Eaton syndrome antibodies to the voltage-gated calcium channels are produced. This reduces calcium influx at the presynaptic terminal in response to an action potential, and acetylcholine release is therefore impaired. This produces both skeletal muscle weakness and autonomic dysfunction. Common autonomic symptoms include dry mouth, dry eyes, impotence, heart rate irregularities, constipation, and orthostatic hypotension (can cause dizziness). Both parasympathetic and sympathetic function can be affected. Most often, however, it is the muscle weakness and fatigue that causes the most disability.

Lambert–Eaton syndrome is a paraneoplastic disorder, meaning it is often associated with cancer. Small cell lung cancer is the one most often associated. The immune system is induced by an as yet undetermined mechanism to produce antibodies to the voltage-gated calcium channel. Therefore, a cancer work-up should be undertaken in all patients with this syndrome. In particular, this patient needs, at the least, a chest X-ray and/or chest CT since he has been a heavy smoker.

Autonomic dysfunction can occur with many other conditions affecting acetylcholine release or metabolism. A major culprit is medication with anticholinergic effects (there are many). Botulism, which also reduces acetylcholine release at the presynaptic terminal, causes autonomic dysfunction as well as weakness.

QUESTIONS TO PONDER

1. Why are there only 14 pairs of white rami communicantes, whereas there are 32 or 31 pairs of gray rami communicantes?

2. Why is it that preganglionic sympathetic fibers are usually short, whereas preganglionic parasympathetic fibers are usually long?

3. Why can the same neurotransmitter (acetylcholine) be used in both preganglionic sympathetic and parasympathetic synapses, but not at postganglionic synapses?

4. Why is it that the short ciliary nerves have both sympathetic post-ganglionic and parasympathetic postganglionic fibers, whereas the long ciliary nerves have only postganglionic sympathetic fibers?

5. Why is the contraction of the external skeletal muscle sphincter, which controls the emptying of the colon, sometimes a voluntary response and sometimes a reflex response?

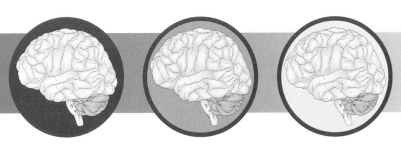

PART 2

Integrative Components of the Nervous System

CHAPTER 10

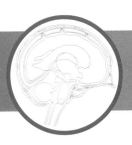 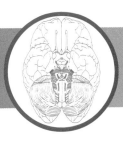 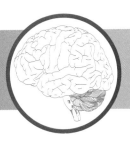

Ascending Sensory Pathways

CLINICAL CASE

A 60-year-old woman complains of falls, imbalance, and numbness and tingling in her hands and legs. There is also some incoordination of hand use and she has difficulty manipulating small items such as buttons. She is unable to play the piano now since she cannot position her fingers correctly on the piano keys. She thinks the strength in her arms and legs is adequate. Symptoms started with very slight tingling sensations, which she noticed about 5 years ago. The falls and difficulty walking have been present for about 2 months. Higher order cognitive functions are intact according to her husband. Her vision is normal.

On examination, the patient shows normal mental status. Strength seems essentially normal throughout. Sensation, particularly to vibration and joint position, is severely diminished in the distal upper and lower limbs (arms, legs, hands, and feet). Tendon reflexes are normal in the arms, but somewhat brisk in the legs at the knees and ankles. Gait is moderately ataxic and she has to reach out for support by touching the walls of the hallway at times. Fine movements of the fingers are performed poorly, even though finger and wrist strength seems normal.

A variety of **sensory receptors** scattered throughout the body can become activated by exteroceptive, interoceptive, or proprioceptive input. Exteroceptive input relays sensory information about the body's interaction with the external environment. Interoceptive input relays information about the body's internal state, whereas proprioceptive input conveys information about position sense from the body and its component parts. Each receptor is specialized to detect mechanical, chemical, nociceptive (L. nocere, "to injure," "painful"), or thermal stimuli. Activation of a sensory receptor is converted into nerve impulses and this sensory input is then conveyed via the fibers of the cranial or spinal nerves to their respective relay nuclei in the central nervous system (CNS). The sensory information is then further processed as it

progresses, via the **ascending sensory systems (pathways)**, to the cerebral cortex or to the cerebellum. Sensory information is also relayed to other parts of the CNS where it may function to elicit a reflex response, or may be integrated into pattern-generating circuitry.

The ascending sensory pathways are classified according to the functional components (modalities) they carry as well as by their anatomical localization. The two functional categories are the **general somatic afferent (GSA) system**, which transmits sensory information such as touch, pressure, vibration, pain, temperature, stretch, and position sense from **somatic** structures; and the **general visceral afferent (GVA) system**, which transmits sensory information such as pressure, pain, and other visceral sensation from **visceral** structures.

Anatomical system	Anatomical tracts	Functional component(s)
Anterolateral (ALS)	Spinothalamic* Spinoreticular Spinomesencephalic Spinotectal Spinohypothalamic	Pain, temperature, nondiscriminative (crude) touch, pressure, and some proprioceptive sensation
Dorsal column–medial lemniscal (DCML)*	Fasciculus gracilis Fasciculus cuneatus	Discriminative (fine) touch, vibratory sense, position sense
Somatosensory to the cerebellum	Anterior spinocerebellar Posterior spinocerebellar Rostral spinocerebellar Cuneocerebellar	Primarily proprioceptive information (also some pain and pressure information)

*Indicates conscious level.

Table 10.1 ● A general description of the anatomical and functional aspects of the ascending sensory pathways.

Anatomically, the ascending sensory systems consist of three distinct pathways: the anterolateral system (ALS), the dorsal column–medial lemniscal (DCML) pathway, and the somatosensory pathways to the cerebellum.

The **anterolateral system**, which includes the **spinothalamic**, **spinoreticular**, **spinomesencephalic**, **spinotectal**, and **spinohypothalamic tracts**, relays predominantly pain and temperature sensation, as well as nondiscriminative (crude or poorly localized) touch, pressure, and some proprioceptive sensation (Table 10.1).

The **dorsal column–medial lemniscal pathway** (which includes the **fasciculus gracilis**, **fasciculus cuneatus**, and **medial lemniscus**) relays discriminative (fine) tactile sense, vibratory sense, and position sense (Table 10.1).

The **somatosensory pathways to the cerebellum**, which include the **anterior**, **posterior**, and **rostral spinocerebellar**, as well as the **cuneocerebellar tracts**, relay primarily proprioceptive (but also some pain and pressure) information (Table 10.1).

The ascending sensory pathways are the main avenues by which information concerning the body's interaction with the external environment, its internal condition, and the position and movement of its parts, reach the brain. One similarity shared by all three ascending sensory pathways from the body (not including the head or face) is that the first order neuron cell bodies reside in the **dorsal root ganglia**. It is interesting to note that **conscious perception** of sensory information from external stimuli is mediated by the **spinothalamic** and **DCML pathways** to the ventral posterior lateral nucleus of the **thalamus**, whereas sensations that do *not* reach consciousness are mediated by the **spinoreticular**, **spinomesencephalic**, **spinotectal**, **spinohypothalamic**, and the **anterior**, **posterior**, and **rostral spinocerebellar**, and **cuneocerebellar tracts**. These tracts terminate in the reticular formation, mesencephalon, hypothalamus and cerebellum, respectively.

Sensory input may ultimately elicit a reflex or other motor response because of the functional integration of the ascending (somatosensory) pathways, the cerebellum, and the somatosensory cortex, as well as the motor cortex and descending (motor) pathways. Furthermore, descending projections from the **somatosensory cortex**, as well as from the **raphe nucleus magnus** and the **dorsolateral pontine reticular formation** to the **somatosensory relay nuclei** of the brainstem and spinal cord, modulate the transmission of incoming sensory impulses to higher brain centers.

This chapter includes a description of the sensory receptors and the ascending sensory pathways from the body, whereas the ascending sensory pathways from the head, transmitted mostly by the trigeminal system, are described in Chapter 15.

SENSORY RECEPTORS

Although sensory receptors vary, they generally all function in a similar fashion

Although sensory receptors vary according to their morphology, the velocity of conduction, and the modality to which they respond, as well as to their location in the body, they generally all function in a similar fashion. The stimulus to which a specific receptor responds causes an alteration in the ionic permeability of the nerve endings, generating a **receptor potential** that results in the formation of **action potentials**. This transformation of the stimulus into an electrical signal is referred to as **sensory transduction**.

Some receptors that respond quickly and maximally at the onset of the stimulus, but stop responding even if the stimulus continues, are known as **rapidly adapting (phasic) receptors**. These are essential in responding to changes but they ignore ongoing processes, such as when one wears a wristwatch and ignores the continuous pressure on the skin of the wrist. However, there are other receptors, **slowly adapting (tonic) receptors**, that continue to respond as long as the stimulus is present.

Sensory receptors are classified according to the **source of the stimulus** or according to the **modality** to which they respond. It is important to note that, in general, receptors do not transmit only one specific sensation.

Classification according to stimulus source

Receptors that are classified according to the source of the stimulus are placed in one of the following three categories: exteroceptors, proprioceptors, or interoceptors.

Exteroceptors are close to the body surface and are specialized to detect sensory information from the external environment

1 **Exteroceptors** are close to the body surface and are specialized to detect sensory information from the external environment (such as visual, olfactory, gustatory, auditory, and tactile stimuli). Receptors in this class are sensitive to touch (light stimulation of the skin surface), pressure (stimulation of receptors in the deep layers of the skin, or deeper parts of the body), temperature, pain, and vibration. Exteroceptors are further classified as teloreceptors or contact receptors:

    * **teloreceptors** (G. tele, "distant"), include receptors that respond to distant stimuli (such as light or sound), and do not require direct physical contact with the stimulus in order to be stimulated;
    * **contact receptors**, which transmit tactile, pressure, pain, or thermal stimuli, require direct contact of the stimulus with the body.

Proprioceptors transmit sensory information from muscles, tendons, and joints about the position of a body part, such as a limb in space

2 **Proprioceptors** transmit sensory information from muscles, tendons, and joints about the position of a body part, such as a limb in space. There is a *static* position sense relating to a stationary position and a *kinesthetic* sense (G. kinesis, "movement"), relating to the movement of a body part. The receptors of the vestibular system located in the inner ear, relaying sensory information about the movement and orientation of the head, are also classified as proprioceptors.

Interoceptors detect sensory information concerning the status of the body's internal environment

3 **Interoceptors** detect sensory information concerning the status of the body's internal environment, such as stretch, blood pressure, pH, oxygen or carbon dioxide concentration, and osmolarity.

Classification according to modality

Receptors are further classified into the following three categories according to the modality to which they respond: nociceptors, thermoreceptors, and mechanoreceptors (Table 10.2).

Nociceptors

Nociceptors are rapidly adapting receptors that are sensitive to noxious or painful stimuli

Nociceptors are rapidly adapting receptors that are sensitive to noxious or painful stimuli. They are located at the peripheral terminations of lightly myelinated free nerve endings of **type Aδ fibers**, or unmyelinated **type C fibers**, transmitting pain. Nociceptors are further classified into three types.

1 **Mechanosensitive nociceptors** (of Aδ fibers), which are sensitive to intense mechanical stimulation (such as pinching with pliers) or injury to tissues.
2 **Temperature-sensitive (thermosensitive) nociceptors** (of Aδ fibers), which are sensitive to intense heat and cold.
3 **Polymodal nociceptors** (of C fibers), which are sensitive to noxious stimuli that are mechanical, thermal, or chemical in nature. Although most nociceptors are sensitive to one particular type of painful stimulus, some may respond to two or more types.

Nociception is the reception of noxious sensory information elicited by tissue injury, which is transmitted to the CNS by nociceptors. **Pain** is the perception of discomfort or an agonizing sensation of variable magnitude, evoked by the stimulation of sensory nerve endings.

Thermoreceptors

Thermoreceptors are sensitive to warmth or cold

Thermoreceptors are sensitive to warmth or cold. These slowly adapting receptors are further classified into three types.

1 **Cold receptors**, which consist of free nerve endings of lightly myelinated Aδ fibers.
2 **Warmth receptors**, which consist of the free nerve endings of unmyelinated C fibers that respond to *increases* in temperature.
3 **Temperature-sensitive nociceptors** that are sensitive to excessive heat or cold.

Mechanoreceptors

Mechanoreceptors are activated following physical deformation of the skin, muscles, tendons, ligaments, and joint capsules in which they reside

Mechanoreceptors, which comprise both exteroceptors and proprioceptors, are activated following physical deformation due to touch, pressure, stretch, or vibration of the skin, muscles, tendons, ligaments, and joint capsules, in which they reside. A mechanoreceptor may be classified as **nonencapsulated** or **encapsulated** depending on whether a structural device encloses its peripheral nerve ending component.

Table 10.2 ● Sensory receptors.

Sensory receptors	Mediate/ respond to	Endings	Location	Associated with	Pathways	Rate of adaptation
Nociceptors						
Pain Temperature	Tissue damage Extreme temperature	Branching free nerve (Aδ, C) endings (unmyelinated nonencapsulated)	Epidermis, dermis, cornea, muscle, joint capsules	Aδ (group III) myelinated fibers, C (group IV) unmyelinated fibers	Anterolateral system	Slow
Mechanoreceptors						
Free nerve endings	Touch, pressure	Nonencapsulated	Epidermis, dermis, cornea, dental pulp, muscle, tendons, ligaments, joint capsules, bones, mucous membranes	Aδ, C fibers	Anterolateral system	Slow
Merkel's tactile discs	Discriminative touch, superficial pressure	Nonencapsulated	Basal epidermis	Aβ (group II) myelinated fibers	DCML pathway	Slow
Meissner's corpuscles	Two-point discriminative (fine) touch	Encapsulated	Papillae of dermis of hairless skin	Aβ (group II) myelinated fibers	DCML pathway	Rapid
Pacinian corpuscles	Deep pressure and vibratory sensation	Encapsulated	Dermis, hypodermis, interosseous membranes, ligaments, external genitalia, joint capsules, peritoneum, pancreas	Aβ (group II) myelinated fibers	DCML pathway	Rapid
Peritrichial nerve endings	Touch, hair movement (bending)	Nonencapsulated	Around hair follicle	Aβ (group II) myelinated fibers	DCML pathway	Rapid
Ruffini's organs	Pressure on, or stretching of, skin	Encapsulated	Joint capsules, dermis, hypodermis	Aβ (group II) myelinated fibers	DCML pathway	Slow
Muscle and tendon mechanoreceptors						
Nuclear bag fibers	Detects onset of muscle stretch		Skeletal muscle	Aα (group Ia) myelinated fibers	DCML pathway and ascending sensory pathways to the cerebellum	Both slow and rapid
Nuclear chain fibers	Muscle stretch in progress		Skeletal muscle	also secondary afferents, muscle spindle afferents		
Golgi tendon organs	Stretching of tendon		Skeletal muscle	Aα (group Ib) myelinated fibers		Slow

DCML, dorsal column–medial lemniscal.

Nonencapsulated mechanoreceptors

Nonencapsulated mechanoreceptors are slowly adapting and include free nerve endings and tactile receptors

Free nerve endings (Fig. 10.1) are present in the epidermis, dermis, cornea, dental pulp, mucous membranes of the oral and nasal cavities and of the respiratory, gastrointestinal, and urinary tracts, muscles, tendons, ligaments, joint capsules, and bones. The peripheral nerve terminals of the free nerve endings lack Schwann cells and myelin sheaths. They are stimulated by touch, pressure, thermal, or painful stimuli.

Peritrichial nerve endings (Fig. 10.2) are specialized members of this category. They are large-diameter, myelinated, Aβ fibers that coil around a hair follicle below its associated sebaceous gland. This type of receptor is stimulated only when a hair is being bent.

Tactile receptors (Fig. 10.3) consist of disc-shaped, peripheral nerve endings of large-diameter, myelinated, Aβ fibers. Each disc-shaped terminal is associated with a specialized epithelial cell, the Merkel cell, located in the stratum basale of the epidermis. These receptors, frequently referred to as **Merkel's discs** (Fig. 10.4), are present mostly in glabrous (hairless), and occasionally in hairy skin. Merkel's discs

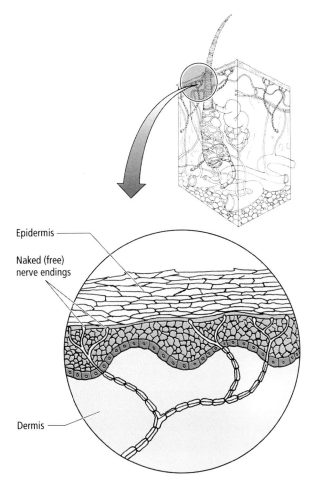

Figure 10.1 ● Free nerve endings in the skin. The free nerve endings terminating in the epidermis lose their myelin sheath. Many free nerve endings have unmyelinated axons.

respond to discriminative touch stimuli that facilitate the distinguishing of texture, shape, and edges of objects.

Encapsulated mechanoreceptors

Encapsulated mechanoreceptors include Meissner's corpuscles, pacinian corpuscles, and Ruffini's end organs.

Meissner's corpuscles are present in the dermal papillae of glabrous skin of the lips, forearm, palm, and sole, and in the connective tissue papillae of the tongue

Meissner's corpuscles (Fig. 10.5) are present in the dermal papillae of glabrous skin of the lips, forearm, palm, and sole, as well as in the connective tissue papillae of the tongue. These corpuscles consist of the peripheral terminals of Aβ fibers, which are encapsulated by a peanut-shaped structural device consisting of a stack of concentric Schwann cells surrounded by a connective tissue capsule. They are rapidly adapting and are sensitive to two-point tactile (fine) discrimination, and are thus of great importance to the visually impaired by permitting them to be able to read Braille.

Pacinian corpuscles are the largest of the mechanoreceptors

Pacinian corpuscles (Fig. 10.6), the largest of the mechanoreceptors, are rapidly adapting and resemble an onion in cross-section. Each Pacinian corpuscle consists of Aβ-fiber terminals encapsulated by layers of modified fibroblasts that are enclosed in a connective tissue capsule. Pacinian corpuscles are located in the dermis, hypodermis, interosseous membranes, ligaments, external genitalia, joint capsules, and peritoneum, as well as in the pancreas. They are more rapidly adapting than Meissner's corpuscles and are believed to respond to pressure and vibratory stimuli, including tickling sensations.

Ruffini's end organs are located in the joint capsules, dermis, and underlying hypodermis of hairy skin

Ruffini's end organs (corpuscles of Ruffini) (Fig. 10.7) are located in joint capsules, the dermis, and the underlying hypodermis of hairy skin. The unmyelinated peripheral terminals of Aβ myelinated fibers are slowly adapting. They intertwine around the core of collagen fibers, which is surrounded by a lamellated cellular capsule. Ruffini's end organs respond to *stretching* of the collagen bundles in the skin or joint capsules and may provide proprioceptive information.

Muscle spindles and **Golgi tendon organs** (GTOs) are also encapsulated mechanoreceptors, but, due to their specialized function, are discussed separately.

Muscle spindles and Golgi tendon organs

Two types of proprioceptors, the neuromuscular (muscle) spindles and the GTOs (neurotendinous spindles), are associated with skeletal muscle only

The mucle spindles and GTOs detect sensory input from the skeletal muscle and transmit it to the spinal cord where it plays an important role in reflex activity and motor control involving the cerebellum. In addition, sensory input from these muscle receptors is also relayed to the cerebral cortex by way of the DCML pathway, which mediates information concerning posture, position sense, as well as movement and orientation of the body and its parts.

Muscle spindles

Structure and function

Skeletal muscle consists of extrafusal and intrafusal fibers

Extrafusal fibers are ordinary skeletal muscle cells constituting the majority of gross muscle, and their stimulation results in muscle contraction. **Muscle spindles**, composed of small bundles of encapsulated **intrafusal fibers**, are dispersed throughout gross muscle. These are *dynamic stretch receptors* that continuously check for changes in muscle length.

Each muscle spindle is composed of two to 12 intrafusal fibers enclosed in a slender capsule, which in turn is

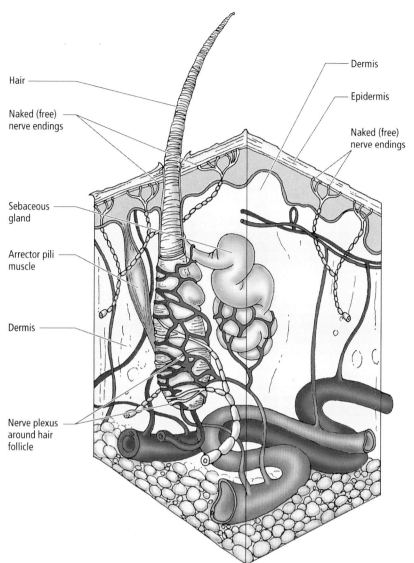

Hair

Naked (free)
nerve endings

Sebaceous
gland

Arrector pili
muscle

Dermis

Nerve plexus
around hair
follicle

Dermis

Epidermis

Naked (free)
nerve endings

Figure 10.2 ● Peritrichial nerve endings. These free
nerve endings spiral around the base of a hair follicle.

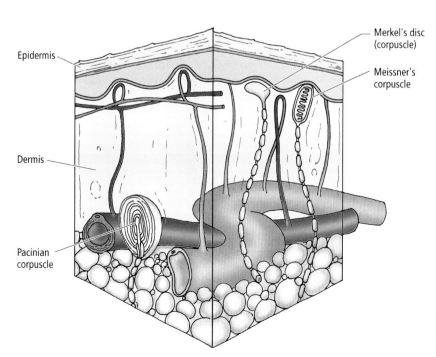

Epidermis

Dermis

Pacinian
corpuscle

Merckel's disc
(corpuscle)

Meissner's
corpuscle

Figure 10.3 ● A section of dermis showing a
Merckel's disc, Meissner's corpuscle, and Pacinian
corpuscle.

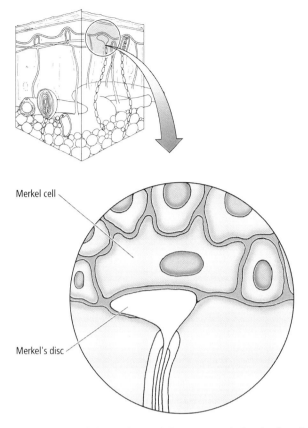

Merkel cell

Merkel's disc

Figure 10.4 ● Merkel's discs (corpuscles) terminate on the basal surface of the epidermis.

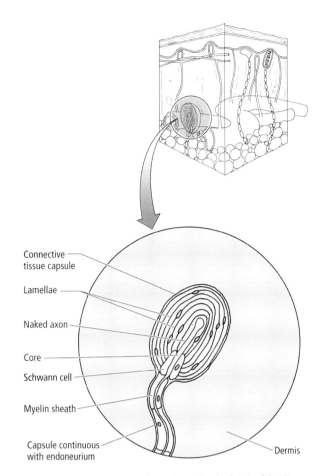

Connective tissue capsule

Lamellae

Naked axon

Core

Schwann cell

Myelin sheath

Capsule continuous with endoneurium

Dermis

Figure 10.6 ● Pacinian corpuscles are located in the dermis of the skin.

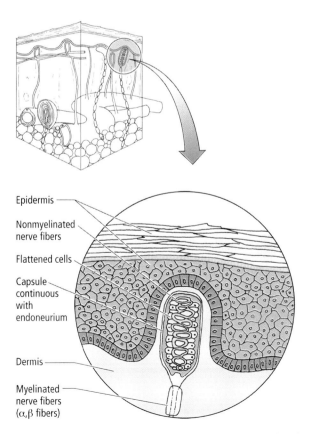

Epidermis

Nonmyelinated nerve fibers

Flattened cells

Capsule continuous with endoneurium

Dermis

Myelinated nerve fibers (α,β fibers)

Figure 10.5 ● Meissner's corpuscles are located in dermal papillae of the skin.

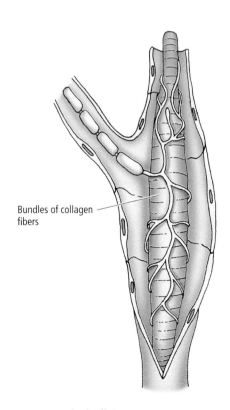

Bundles of collagen fibers

Figure 10.7 ● A corpuscle of Ruffini.

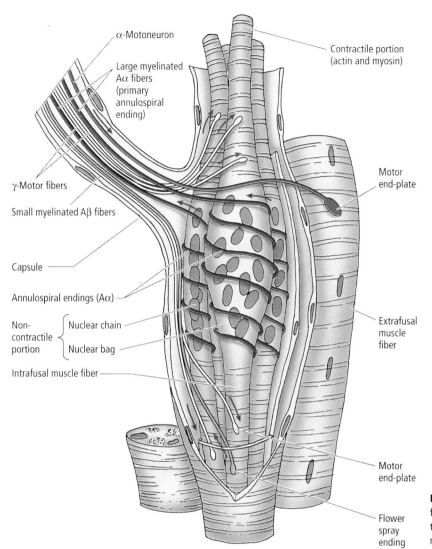

α-Motoneuron

Large myelinated
Aα fibers
(primary
annulospiral
ending)

Contractile portion
(actin and myosin)

Motor
end-plate

γ-Motor fibers

Small myelinated Aβ fibers

Capsule

Annulospiral endings (Aα)

Non-
contractile
portion { Nuclear chain

Nuclear bag

Intrafusal muscle fiber

Extrafusal
muscle
fiber

Motor
end-plate

Flower
spray
ending
(Aβ)

Figure 10.8 ● Right: an extrafusal skeletal muscle fiber. Left: a neuromuscular spindle containing the two types of intrafusal fibers—the nuclear bag fiber with multiple nuclei in the dilated central region and a nuclear chain fiber with a row of nuclei in its central region.

surrounded by an outer fusiform connective tissue capsule whose tapered ends are attached to the connective tissue sheath surrounding the extrafusal muscle fibers (Fig. 10.8). The compartment between the inner and outer capsules contains a glycosaminoglycan-rich viscous fluid.

There are two types of intrafusal fibers based on their morphological characteristics: nuclear bag fibers and nuclear chain fibers. Both nuclear bag and nuclear chain fibers possess a central, noncontractile region housing multiple nuclei, and a skeletal muscle (myofibril-containing) contractile portion at each end of the central region. The **nuclear bag fibers** are larger, and their multiple nuclei are clustered in the "bag-like" dilated central region of the fiber. The **nuclear chain fibers** are smaller and consist of multiple nuclei arranged sequentially, as in a "chain" of pearls, in the central region of the fiber.

Each intrafusal fiber of a muscle spindle receives sensory innervation via the peripheral processes of pseudounipolar sensory neurons whose cell bodies are housed in dorsal root ganglia, or in the sensory ganglia of the cranial nerves (and in the case of the trigeminal nerve, within its mesencephalic nucleus). Since the large-diameter Aα fibers spiral around the noncontractile region of the intrafusal fibers, they are known as **annulospiral** or **primary** endings. These endings become activated at the **beginning of muscle stretch** or **tension**. In addition to the annulospiral endings, the intrafusal fibers, mainly the nuclear chain fibers, also receive smaller diameter, Aβ peripheral processes of pseudounipolar neurons. These nerve fibers terminate on both sides of the annulospiral ending, are referred to as **secondary** or **flower spray endings**, and are activated during the time that the stretch is in progress (Fig. 10.8).

Each intrafusal fiber of a muscle spindle receives sensory innervation via the peripheral processes of pseudounipolar sensory neurons

In addition to sensory innervation, intrafusal fibers also receive motor innervation via gamma motoneurons that innervate the contractile portions of the intrafusal fibers, causing them to contract

In addition to the sensory innervation, intrafusal fibers also receive motor innervation via gamma motoneurons (fusimotor neurons) that innervate the contractile portions of the intrafusal fibers, causing them to undergo contraction. Since the intrafusal fibers are oriented parallel to the longitudinal axis of the extrafusal fibers, when a muscle is *stretched*, the central, noncontractile region of the intrafusal fibers is also stretched, distorting and stimulating the sensory nerve endings coiled around them, causing the nerve endings to fire. However, when the muscle *contracts*, tension on the central noncontractile region of the intrafusal fibers decreases (which reduces the rate of firing of the sensory nerve endings coiled around it).

During voluntary muscle activity simultaneous stimulation of the extrafusal fibers by the alpha motoneurons, and the contractile portions of the intrafusal fibers by the gamma motoneurons, serves to modulate the sensitivity of the intrafusal fibers. That is, the gamma motoneurons cause corresponding contraction of the contractile portions of the intrafusal fibers, which stretch the central noncontractile region of the intrafusal fibers. Thus, the sensitivity of the intrafusal fibers is constantly maintained by continuously readapting to the most current status of muscle length. In this fashion the muscle spindles can detect a change in muscle length (resulting from stretch or contraction) irrespective of muscle length at the onset of muscle activity. It should be noted that even though they contract, the intrafusal fibers, due to their small number and size, do not contribute to any significant extent to the overall contraction of a gross muscle.

Simple stretch reflex

The **simple stretch reflex**, whose mechanism is based on the role of the intrafusal fibers, functions to maintain muscle length caused by external disturbances. As a muscle is stretched, the intrafusal fibers of the muscle spindles are also stretched. This in turn stimulates the sensory afferent annulospiral and flower spray endings to transmit this information to those alpha motoneurons of the CNS (spinal cord, or cranial nerve motor nuclei) that innervate the agonist (stretched) muscle as well as to those motoneurons that innervate the antagonist muscle(s). The degree of stretching is proportional to (or related to) the load placed on the muscle. The larger the load, the more strongly the spindles are depolarized and the more extrafusal muscle fibers are in turn activated. As these alpha motoneurons of the stretched muscle fire, they stimulate the contraction of the required number of extrafusal muscle fibers of the *agonist* muscle. The alpha motoneurons of the *antagonist* muscle(s) are inhibited so the antagonist muscle relaxes. The simple reflex arc involves the firing of only two neurons—an **afferent sensory neuron** and an **efferent motoneuron**—providing dynamic information concerning the changes of the load on the muscle and position of the body region in three-dimensional space.

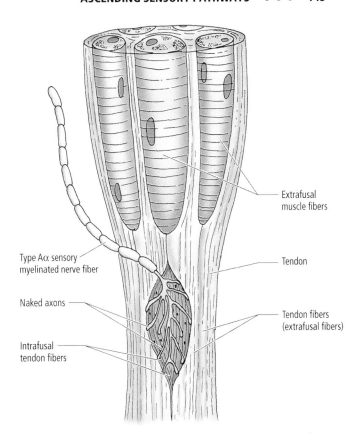

Figure 10.9 ● A Golgi tendon organ (neurotendinous spindle).

Golgi tendon organs

GTOs (neurotendinous spindles) are fusiform-shaped receptors located at sites where muscle fibers insert into tendons

Unlike muscle spindles, which are oriented parallel to the longitudinal axis of the extrafusal muscle fibers, GTOs are *in series*. Furthermore, GTOs do not receive motor innervation as the muscle spindles do. GTOs consist of interlacing **intrafusal** collagen bundles enclosed in a connective tissue capsule (Fig. 10.9). A large-diameter, type Aα sensory fiber, whose cell body is housed in a dorsal root sensory ganglion or a cranial nerve sensory ganglion, passes through the capsule and then branches into numerous delicate terminals that are interposed among the intrafusal collagen bundles. The central processes of these Aα afferent neurons enter the spinal cord via the dorsal roots of the spinal nerves to terminate and establish synaptic contacts with inhibitory interneurons that, in turn, synapse with alpha motoneurons supplying the contracted agonist muscle.

Combined muscle spindle and Golgi tendon organ functions during changes in muscle length

During slight stretching of a relaxed muscle, the muscle spindles are stimulated while the GTOs remain undisturbed and quiescent; with further stretching both the muscle spindles and GTOs are stimulated

During muscle contraction, as the muscle shortens, tension is produced in the tendons anchoring that muscle to bone, compressing the nerve fiber terminals interposed among the inelastic intrafusal collagen fibers. This compression activates the sensory terminals in the GTOs, which transmit this sensory information to the CNS, providing proprioceptive information concerning muscle activity and preventing the placement of excessive forces on the muscle and tendon. In contrast, the noncontractile portions of the muscle spindles are not stretched, and are consequently undisturbed. The contractile regions of the muscle spindles, however, undergo corresponding contraction that enables them to detect a future change in muscle length (resulting from stretch or contraction).

During slight stretching of a relaxed muscle, the muscle spindles are stimulated whereas the GTOs remain undisturbed and quiescent. During further stretching of the muscle, which produces tension on the tendons, both the muscle spindles and the GTOs are stimulated. Thus GTOs monitor and check the amount of tension exerted on the muscle (regardless of whether it is tension generated by muscle stretch or contraction), whereas muscle spindles check muscle fiber length and rate of change of muscle length (during muscle stretch or contraction).

ANTEROLATERAL SYSTEM

The ALS transmits nociceptive, thermal, and nondiscriminatory touch information to higher brain centers, generally by a sequence of three neurons and interneurons

The anterolateral system (ALS) transmits nociceptive, thermal, and nondiscriminatory (crude) touch information to higher brain centers (see Table 10.2), generally by a sequence of three neurons and interneurons (Fig. 10.10). The neuron sequence consists of:

1 A **first order neuron** (pseudounipolar neuron) whose cell body is located in a dorsal root ganglion. It transmits sensory information from peripheral structures to the dorsal (posterior) horn of the spinal cord.
2 A **second order neuron** whose cell body is located within the dorsal horn of the spinal cord, and whose axon usually decussates and ascends:

- in the **direct pathway of the ALS (spinothalamic tract)** to synapse in the contralateral thalamus, and sending some collaterals to the reticular formation;
- in the **indirect pathway of the ALS (spinoreticular tract)** to synapse in the reticular formation, and sending some collaterals to the thalamus; or

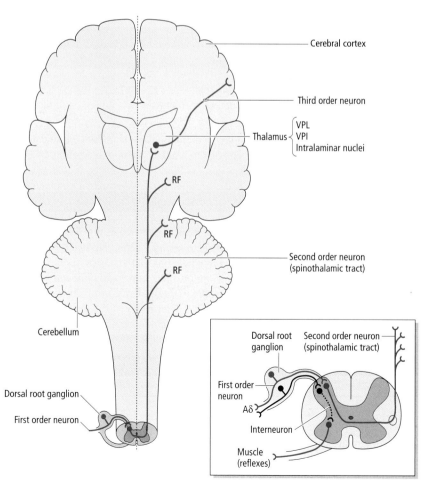

Figure 10.10 ● The direct pathway of the anterolateral system. Note the first order neuron in the dorsal root ganglion, the second order neuron in the dorsal horn of the spinal cord, and the third order neuron in the thalamus. The second order neuron sends collaterals to the reticular formation (RF). VPI, ventral posterior inferior; VPL, ventral posterior lateral.

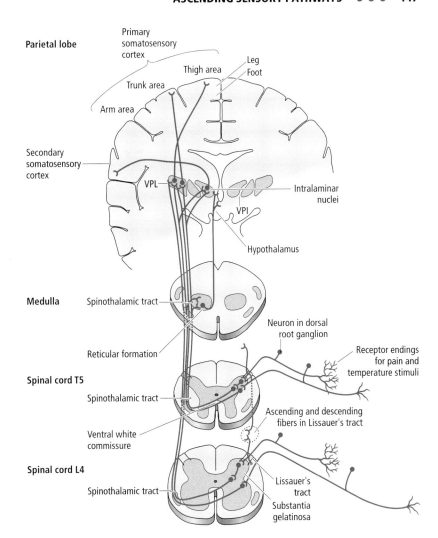

Figure 10.11 ● The ascending sensory pathway that transmits nondiscriminative (crude) touch, pain, and temperature sensations from the body. (Modified from Gilman, S, Winans Newman, S (1992) *Essentials of Clinical Neuroanatomy and Neurophysiology*. FA Davis, Philadelphia; fig. 19.)

- as **spinomesencephalic**, **spinotectal**, or **spinohypo-thalamic fibers** to synapse in several brainstem nuclei.

3 A **third order neuron** whose cell body is located in the thalamus, and whose axon ascends ipsilaterally to terminate in the somatosensory cortex.

In some cases, the first order neuron may synapse with an **interneuron** that resides entirely within the dorsal horn, and whose axon synapses with the second order neuron.

Pain pathways from the body

First order neurons (sensory receptors)

Receptors that transmit nociceptive information consist of high-threshold free nerve endings ramifying near the external surface and internal environment of the organism

Receptors that transmit nociceptive information consist of high-threshold free nerve endings ramifying near the external surface and internal environment of the organism. These are dendritic arborizations of small, pseudounipolar,

first order neurons (Fig. 10.11) whose somata are housed in a dorsal root ganglion. The peripheral processes of these pseudounipolar neurons consist of two main types of fiber (Fig. 10.12):

1 Thinly myelinated **Aδ (fast-conducting) fibers**, which relay sharp, short-term, well-localized pain (such as that resulting from a pinprick). These fibers transmit sensations that do not elicit an affective component associated with the experience.
2 Unmyelinated **C (slow-conducting) fibers**, which relay dull, persistent, poorly localized pain (such as that resulting from excessive stretching of a tendon). These fibers transmit sensations that elicit an affective response.

The central processes of these pseudounipolar neurons enter the spinal cord at the dorsal root entry zone, via the lateral division of the dorsal roots of the spinal nerves, and upon entry collectively form the **dorsolateral fasciculus (tract of Lissauer)**, which is present at all spinal cord levels. These central processes bifurcate into short ascending and descending branches. These branches either ascend or descend one to three spinal cord levels within this tract, to terminate in their

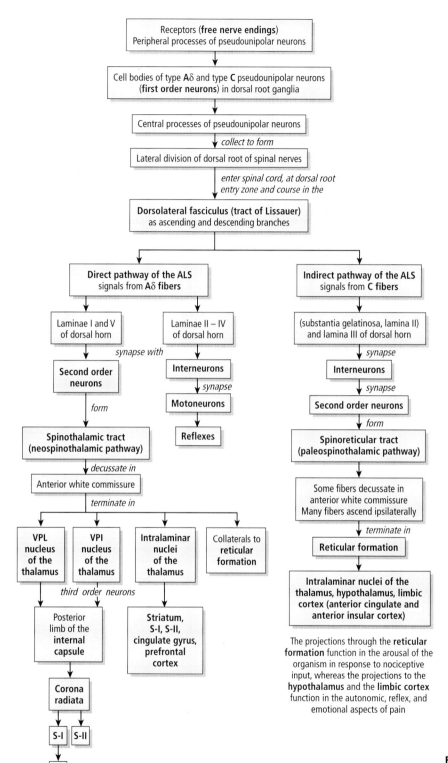

Figure 10.12 ● The spinothalamic (direct) and spinoreticular (indirect) pathways of the anterolateral system (ALS) transmitting nondiscriminative (crude) touch, pain, and temperature sensation from the body. VPI, ventral posterior inferior; VPL, ventral posterior lateral.

target laminae of the dorsal horn, where they synapse with second order neurons (or with interneurons). Therefore, although stimulation of the peripheral endings of fibers carried by one spinal nerve may enter the spinal cord at a specific spinal level, collaterals of the ascending and descending branches spread the signal to neighboring spinal levels above and below the level of entry. These collaterals play an important function in intersegmental reflexes.

Second order neurons

The cell bodies of the second order neurons transmitting nociception reside in the dorsal horn of the spinal cord

The cell bodies of the second order neurons transmitting nociception reside in the dorsal horn of the spinal cord (Fig. 10.12). Recent findings indicate that the axons of these second order neurons course in either the **direct (spinothalamic)** or **indirect (spinoreticular) pathways** of the ALS, or as three sets of fibers (the remaining components of the ALS): the **spinomesencephalic, spinotectal,** or **spinohypothalamic fibers**. Approximately 15% of nociceptive fibers project directly to the thalamus whereas 85% project to the thalamus via a relay in the reticular formation.

Direct pathway of the anterolateral system

The spinothalamic tract transmits not only nociceptive input, but also thermal and nondiscriminative touch input to the contralateral ventral posterior lateral nucleus of the thalamus

Type **Aδ fibers** of first order neurons synapse primarily with **second order neurons** in lamina I (posteromarginal nucleus, or zone) and lamina V (reticular nucleus) of the spinal cord gray matter. However, many first order neurons synapse with spinal cord **interneurons** that are associated with reflex motor activity. The axons of the second order neurons flow across the midline to the contralateral side of the spinal cord in the anterior white commissure, forming the **spinothalamic tract** (Fig. 10.13).

The spinothalamic tract transmits not only nociceptive input, but also thermal and nondiscriminative (crude) touch input to the contralateral ventral posterior lateral nucleus of the thalamus. It also sends some projections to the **ventral posterior inferior**, and the **intralaminar nuclei of the thalamus**. Although the spinothalamic tract ends at the thalamus, as it ascends through the brainstem it also sends collaterals to the reticular formation. Since the spinothalamic tract (direct pathway of the ALS: spinal cord → thalamus) is phylogenetically a newer pathway, it is referred to as the **neospinothalamic pathway**.

Only about 15% of the nociceptive fibers from the spinal cord, ascending in the ALS and carrying nociceptive information, terminate directly in the thalamus via the spinothalamic tract. Although referred to as the "spinothalamic tract," it actually consists of two anatomically distinct tracts: the **lateral**

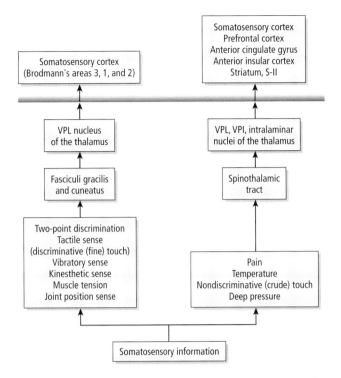

Figure 10.13 ● Somatosensory information to consciousness. VPI, ventral posterior inferior; VPL ventral posterior lateral.

spinothalamic tract (located in the lateral funiculus) and the very small **anterior spinothalamic tract** (located in the anterior funiculus). Earlier studies indicated that the lateral spinothalamic tract transmitted only nociceptive and thermal input, whereas the anterior spinothalamic tract transmitted only nondiscriminative (crude) touch. Recent studies however, support the finding that both the anterior and lateral spinothalamic tracts (as well as the other component fibers of the ALS: spinoreticular, spinomesencephalic, spinotectal, and spinohypothalamic), transmit **nociceptive**, **thermal**, and **nondiscriminative (crude) tactile signals** to higher brain centers.

Indirect pathway of the anterolateral system

Type C fibers of first order neurons terminate on interneurons in laminae II (substantia gelatinosa) and III of the dorsal horn. Axons of these **interneurons** synapse with **second order neurons** in laminae V–VIII. Many of the axons of these second order neurons ascend ipsilaterally, however a small number of axons sweep to the opposite side of the spinal cord in the anterior white commissure. These axons form the more prominent **ipsilateral** and smaller **contralateral spinoreticular tracts**. The spinoreticular tracts transmit **nociceptive**, **thermal**, and **nondiscriminatory (crude) touch** signals from the spinal cord to the thalamus indirectly, by forming multiple synapses in the reticular formation prior to their thalamic projections. Since the spinoreticular tract (indirect pathway of the ALS: spinal cord → reticular formation → thalamus) is phylogenetically an older pathway, it is referred to as the **paleospinothalamic pathway** (Fig. 10.14).

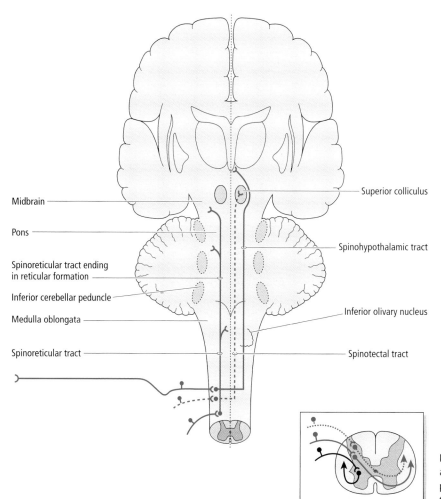

Midbrain

Pons

Spinoreticular tract ending
in reticular formation

Inferior cerebellar peduncle

Medulla oblongata

Spinoreticular tract

Superior colliculus

Spinohypothalamic tract

Inferior olivary nucleus

Spinotectal tract

Figure 10.14 ● Spinotectal, spinoreticular, and spinohypothalamic tracts of the indirect pathway of the anterolateral system. Note that the spinomesencephalic tract is not shown.

The spinoreticular tract is a bilateral (primarily uncrossed) tract that conveys sensory information to the brainstem reticular formation, the region responsible for producing arousal and wakefulness, thus alerting the organism following an injury. Impulses from the reticular formation are then relayed bilaterally to the **intralaminar nuclei of the thalamus**, via reticulothalamic fibers. Since these nuclei lack somatotopic organization, there is only an indistinct localization of sensory signals carried by this pathway. The reticular formation and its continuation into the diencephalon, the intralaminar nuclei of the thalamus, are components of the **reticular-activating system** (RAS). The RAS functions in activating the organism's entire nervous system, so as to elicit responses that will enable it to evade painful stimuli. In addition, there are some second order neurons from the dorsal horn that bypass the reticular formation and relay sensory input from C fibers directly to the intralaminar nuclei of the thalamus.

Other component fibers of the anterolateral system

In addition to the spinothalamic and spinoreticular tracts, the ALS also contains spinomesencephalic, spinotectal, and spinohypothalamic fibers

The **spinomesencephalic fibers** terminate in the periaqueductal gray matter and the midbrain raphe nuclei, both of which are believed to give rise to fibers that modulate nociceptive transmission and are thus collectively referred to as the "descending pain-inhibiting system" (see discussion later). Furthermore, some spinomesencephalic fibers terminate in the parabrachial nucleus, which sends fibers to the amygdala—a component of the limbic system associated with the processing of emotions. Via their connections to the limbic system, the spinomesencephalic fibers play a role in the emotional component of pain.

The **spinotectal fibers** terminate mainly in the deep layers of the superior colliculus. The superior colliculi have the reflex function of turning the upper body, head, and eyes in the direction of a painful stimulus (Fig. 10.14).

The **spinohypothalamic fibers** ascend to the hypothalamus where they synapse with neurons that give rise to the hypothalamospinal tract. This pathway is associated with the autonomic and reflex responses (i.e., endocrine and cardiovascular) to nociception (Fig. 10.14).

Approximately 85% of the nociceptive fibers from the spinal cord ascending in the ALS, terminate in the brainstem reticular formation. From there, the information eventually reaches the thalamus via multiple additional synapses that occur in the brainstem. The reticular formation sends fibers transmitting nociceptive input not only to the thalamus but also to the hypothalamus, which is associated with the autonomic and reflex responses to nociception, and the limbic system, which mediates the emotional component of nociception.

Third order neurons

Cell bodies of third order neurons of the nociception-relaying pathway are housed in: the ventral posterior lateral, the ventral posterior inferior, and the intralaminar thalamic nuclei

The **ventral posterior lateral nucleus** gives rise to fibers that course in the **posterior limb of the internal capsule** and in the **corona radiata** to terminate in the **postcentral gyrus** (primary somatosensory cortex, S-I) of the parietal lobe of the cerebral cortex. Additionally, the ventral posterior lateral nucleus also sends some direct projections to the secondary somatosensory cortex, S-II (Fig. 10.15).

The **ventral posterior inferior nucleus** projects mostly to the **secondary somatosensory cortex** (S-II), although some of its fibers terminate in the **primary somatosensory cortex** (S-I).

The **intralaminar nuclei** send fibers to the **striatum** (the **caudate nucleus** and the **putamen**), the **S-I** and **S-II**, as well as to the **cingulate gyrus** and the **prefrontal cortex**.

It should be noted that most of the nociception-relaying fibers arriving at the **intralaminar nuclei** transmit nociceptive information relayed there from the reticular formation. Multiple synapses have been formed in the reticular formation prior to synapsing in the intralaminar nuclei, and thus, strictly speaking, the intralaminar relay neurons for this pathway are not the third order neurons in the sequence, but they function as if they were third order neurons.

Projections to the somatosensory (somesthetic) cortex

The **primary somatosensory cortex** (S-I) consists of the postcentral gyrus of the parietal lobe, which corresponds to

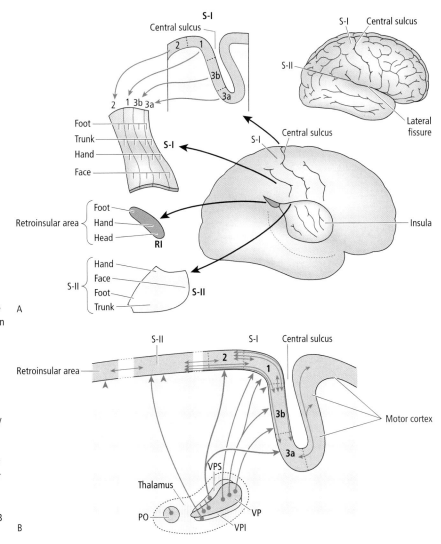

Figure 10.15 ● Primary and secondary somatosensory cortex and retroinsular cortex: three major cortical areas receiving somatosensory information from the thalamus. (A) Counter clockwise from top right: lateral view of the brain; a cross-section of the central sulcus (of Rolando); and the primary somatosensory cortex (postcentral gyrus, S-I) forming the posterior border of the sulcus. Note the components of the primary somatosensory cortex areas 3a, 3b, 1, and 2, and the cortical representation of the foot, trunk, hand, and face. The lateral view of the brain shows the exposed insular cortex, secondary somatosensory cortex (S-II), and retroinsular (RI) cortex. (B) Thalamocortical projections to the primary somatosensory cortex (S-I), secondary somatosensory cortex (S-II), and retroinsular cortex (RI). PO, posterior complex; VP, ventral posterior; VPI, ventral posterior inferior; VPS, ventral posterior superior. (Modified from Burt, AM (1993) *Textbook of Neuroanatomy*. WB Saunders, Philadelphia; figs 10.20, 10.22.)

Brodmann's areas 3a, 3b, 1, 2 (Fig. 10.15A). The **secondary somatosensory cortex** (S-II) consists of Brodmann's area 43, located on the superior bank of the lateral fissure, at the inferior extent of the primary motor and sensory areas.

Axons of the thalamic third order neurons terminate in somatotopically corresponding regions of the primary somatosensory cortex. Regions of the head are represented in the inferior half of the postcentral gyrus near the lateral fissure, whereas those of the upper limb and the trunk are represented in its superior half. The lower limb is represented in the medial surface of the postcentral gyrus, and the perineum in the paracentral lobule. The body areas with the largest cortical area representation are the head and upper limb, reflecting the great discriminative capability that structures in these regions possess (Fig. 10.16).

In summary, nociceptive signals relayed from the spinal cord directly to the ventral posterior lateral, the ventral posterior inferior, and the intralaminar nuclei of the thalamus via the spinothalamic tract (neospinothalamic, direct pathway of the ALS) are transmitted to the somatosensory cortex (both to S-I and S-II). The postcentral gyrus is the site where processing of pain localization, intensity, quality, and sensory integration takes place at the conscious level. The primary somatosensory cortex sends projections to the secondary somatosensory cortex, which is believed to have an important function in the memory of sensory input.

In contrast, nociceptive signals relayed from the spinal cord to the reticular formation via the spinoreticular tracts (paleospinothalamic, indirect pathway of the ALS) are then transmitted to:

- the **intralaminar nuclei of the thalamus** (the cranial extension of the reticular formation into the thalamus), which in turn project to the primary somesthetic cortex;
- the **hypothalamus**; and
- the **limbic system**.

The projections through the reticular formation function in the arousal of the organism in response to nociceptive input, whereas the projections to the hypothalamus and limbic system have an important function in the autonomic, reflex, and emotional (suffering) responses to a painful experience.

Projections to the cingulate and insular cortices

Cerebral imaging studies such as electroencephalography (EEG), functional magnetic resonance imaging (fMRI), magnetoencephalography (MEG), and positron emission tomography (PET) have demonstrated that nociceptive signals are not only processed at the primary and secondary

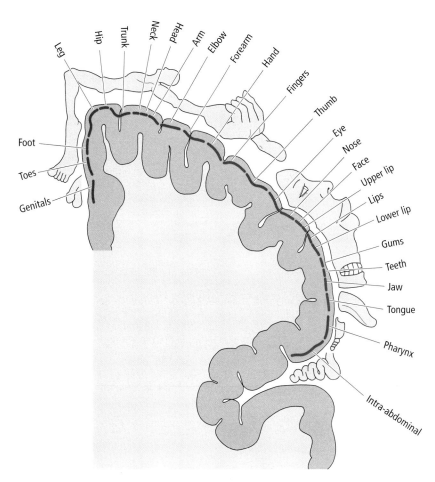

Figure 10.16 ● Coronal section through the primary somatosensory cortex (postcentral gyrus), showing the sensory homunculus. Note that the amount of cerebral cortex representing each body part is proportional to the extent of its motor innervation.

somatosensory cortices, but also in the **anterior cingulate cortex**, **anterior insular cortex**, and even the **supplemental motor area** of the motor cortex. The anterior cingulate and anterior insular cortices are connected with the limbic cortex, which plays a role in the emotional aspect of pain.

Visceral pain

A striking characteristic of the brain is that although it receives and processes nociceptive information, the brain itself has no sensation of pain. During brain surgery, the patient is often awake and has no pain sensation from the brain tissue itself. The structures that have to be anesthetized during brain surgery are the dura mater, the bones of the skull, and the extracranial soft tissues. Moreover, although the internal (visceral) organs themselves have no pain receptors, pain receptors are present embedded in the walls of the arteries serving these organs.

Visceral pain is characterized as diffuse and poorly localized, and is often "referred to" and felt in another somatic structure distant or near the source of visceral pain. Nociceptive signals from the viscera generally follow the same pathway as signals arising from somatic structures. General visceral afferent nociceptive information from visceral structures of the trunk is carried mostly by type **C**, **Aδ**, or **Aβ fibers** (Fig. 10.17). The peripheral terminals of these fibers are associated with Pacinian corpuscles that respond to excessive stretching of the intestinal wall, a lesion in the wall of the gastrointestinal tract, or to smooth muscle spasm. The cell bodies of these sensory (pseudounipolar), **first order neurons** are housed in the dorsal root ganglia, and their central processes carry the information, via the **dorsolateral fasciculus (tract of Lissauer)**, to the dorsal horn and lateral gray matter of the spinal cord. Here, these central processes synapse with second order neurons as well as with neurons associated with reflex activities.

The axons of the **second order neurons** join the **anterolateral system** to relay nociceptive signals from visceral structures to the **reticular formation** and the **thalamus**. Fibers from the reticular formation project to the **intralaminar nuclei of the thalamus**, which in turn project to the **cerebral cortex** and the **hypothalamus**. Recall that the intralaminar nuclei of the thalamus lack somatotopic organization, resulting in only an indistinct localization of sensory signals carried by this pathway.

Visceral pain signals relayed to the primary somatosensory cortex may be associated with referred pain to a somatic structure. In addition to projections to the somatosensory cortex, recent studies indicate that nociceptive signals are also relayed to the **anterior cingulate** and **anterior insular cortices**, two cortical areas implicated in the processing of visceral pain.

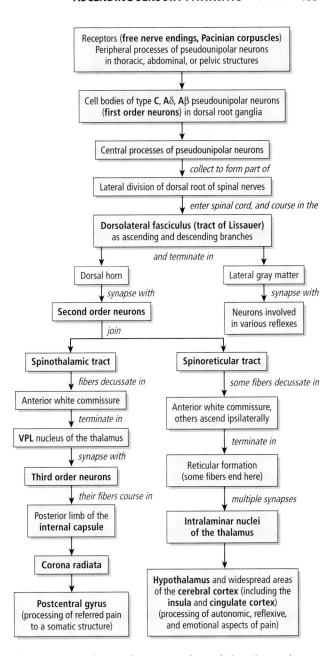

Figure 10.17 ● The ascending sensory pathway relaying pain sensation from the viscera. VPL ventral posterior lateral.

Temperature pathways from the body

Temperature sensory input is transmitted to the CNS via unmyelinated C fibers that are activated by warm stimuli, or by lightly myelinated Aδ fibers that are activated by cold stimuli (see Fig. 10.12; Table 10.2).

All fibers enter the spinal cord at the dorsal root entry zone in the lateral division of the dorsal root of the spinal nerves. These fibers accompany nociceptive fibers and, upon

Table 10.3 ● Ascending sensory pathways to consciousness.

Sensation	Sensory receptor	Location of cell body of first order neuron	Location of cell body of second order neuron (origin of pathway)	Pathway	Decussation
Pain and thermal sense from the body	Aδ and C fiber endings	Dorsal root ganglion	Dorsal horn	Spinothalamic tract of ALS	Anterior white commissure
Nondiscriminative (crude) touch and superficial pressure from the body	Free nerve endings, Merkel's discs, peritrichial nerve endings	Dorsal root ganglion	Dorsal horn	Spinothalamic tract of ALS	Anterior white commissure
Two-point discriminative (fine) touch, vibratory sense, proprioceptive sense from muscles and joints of body	Meissner's corpuscles, Pacinian corpuscles, muscle stretch receptors, Golgi tendon organs	Dorsal root ganglion	Nucleus gracilis, nucleus cuneatus	First order fibers: fasciculi gracilis and cuneatus Second order fibers: medial lemniscus	Medial lemniscal decussation

ALS, anterolateral system; VPI, ventral posterior inferior; VPL, ventral posterior lateral.

entering the spinal cord, join the **dorsolateral fasciculus (tract of Lissauer)**. In the dorsolateral fasciculus, they bifurcate into short *ascending* and *descending* fibers. These fibers ascend or descend respectively, one to three spinal cord levels to synapse in laminae I, II, and III of the dorsal horn gray matter. Temperature input is relayed to **interneurons** which, in turn, transmit the information to **second order neurons** in lamina V.

The axons of the second order neurons, accompanied by nociceptive fibers, decussate in the anterior white commissure to join the contralateral **anterolateral system**. Some of these fibers ascend to terminate in the brainstem **reticular formation**; however, most terminate primarily in the **ventral posterior lateral nucleus of the thalamus**. **Third order neuron** fibers from the thalamus relay thermal sensory information to the **somesthetic cortex**.

TACTILE SENSATION AND PROPRIOCEPTION

Tactile sensation is divisible into nondiscriminative (crude) touch and discriminative (fine) touch

Tactile sensation is divisible into nondiscriminative (crude) touch and discriminative (fine) touch. Crude touch, transmitted via the ALS (discussed above), is sensed following gentle stroking of the skin with a fine cotton strand, but this sensation does not include detailed information about the stimulus. Tactile examination of an object is dependent on discriminative (fine) touch sense, which enables one to detect fine detail regarding the location, size, shape, and texture of an object even when the eyes are closed.

Conscious proprioception may be categorized into static and dynamic proprioception. **Static proprioception (static position sense)** is the awareness of the position of a body part such as a limb, whereas **dynamic proprioception (kinesthetic sense)** is the awareness of movement of a body part, and balance.

Discriminative (fine) touch, **pressure**, **vibratory sense**, as well as **proprioceptive** sensory information are transmitted to higher brain centers, reaching consciousness, by three neurons arranged in sequence (Fig. 10.18; Table 10.3).

1 A **first order neuron** (pseudounipolar neuron) whose cell body is located in a dorsal root ganglion. The neuron transmits sensory information from the periphery to the spinal cord (for reflex activity) and to the **dorsal column nuclei** (the **nucleus gracilis** and the **nucleus cuneatus**).
2 A **second order neuron** whose cell body is located in the **dorsal column nuclei** in the medulla, and whose axon decussates and ascends to terminate in the contralateral **thalamus**.
3 A **third order neuron** whose cell body resides in the **thalamus**, and whose axon ascends ipsilaterally to terminate in the **somatosensory cortex**. The specifics of these pathways are discussed below.

Discriminative (fine) touch and pressure sense from the body

First order neurons (sensory receptors)

The receptors that transmit discriminative (fine) touch, pressure, and conscious proprioception information consist of:

Table 10.3 ● *Continued.*

Location of pathway in spinal cord	Pathway (second order neuron) termination	Location of cell body of third order neuron	Termination of third order neuron	Conscious/ subconscious	Function(s)
Lateral funiculus	VPL, VPI, and intralaminar nuclei of the thalamus	VPL nucleus of the thalamus Intralaminar nuclei	Postcentral gyrus Cingulate gyrus Prefrontal cortex	Conscious	Relays pain and thermal sensation from the body
Anterior funiculus	VPL nucleus of the thalamus	VPL nucleus of the thalamus	Postcentral gyrus	Conscious	Relays nondiscriminative (crude) touch sensation from the body
Posterior funiculus Medulla	VPL nucleus of the thalamus	VPL nucleus of the thalamus	Postcentral gyrus	Conscious	Relays two-point discriminative (fine) touch tactile sensation, vibratory sense, proprioceptive sense from muscles and joints of the body

- **free nerve endings** responding to touch, pressure, and proprioception in the skin, muscles, and joint capsules;
- **tactile (Merkel's) discs** responding to touch and pressure in the skin;
- **peritrichial endings** stimulated by touch of the hair follicles;
- **Meissner's corpuscles** activated by touch of the skin; and
- **Pacinian corpuscles** stimulated by touch, pressure, vibration, and proprioception in the deep layers of the skin, and in visceral structures.

These **first order pseudounipolar neurons**, whose cell bodies are located in the dorsal root ganglia, send peripheral processes to somatic or visceral structures. These peripheral processes are medium-size type **Aβ** and large-size type **Aα** **fibers**. Upon being stimulated, the peripheral processes transmit the sensory information to the spinal cord by way of the central processes of the pseudounipolar neurons, which enter the spinal cord at the dorsal root entry zone via the medial division of the dorsal roots of the spinal nerves. Upon entry into the posterior funiculus of the spinal cord, the afferent fibers bifurcate into long ascending and short descending fibers.

Bifurcating fibers

The long ascending and short descending fibers give rise to collateral branches that may synapse with several distinct cell groups of the dorsal horn interneurons and with ventral horn motoneurons. These fibers collectively form the **dorsal column pathways**, either the **fasciculus gracilis** or the **fasci-**

culus cuneatus, depending on the level of the spinal cord in which they enter.

Below level T6
The central processes that enter the spinal cord below level T6 include the lower thoracic, lumbar, and sacral levels that bring information from the lower limb and lower half of the trunk

The central processes that enter the spinal cord below level T6 include the lower thoracic, lumbar, and sacral levels. They bring information from the lower limb and lower half of the trunk. The central processes enter the ipsilateral **fasciculus gracilis** (L. gracilis, "slender") and ascend to the medulla to terminate in the ipsilateral **nucleus gracilis**. It should be recalled that the fasciculus gracilis is present in the entire length of the spinal cord.

Level T6 and above
The central processes that enter the spinal cord at level T6 and above bring information from the upper thoracic and cervical levels, that is from the upper half of the trunk and upper limb

The central processes that enter the spinal cord at level T6 and above bring information from the upper thoracic and cervical levels, that is from the upper half of the trunk and upper limb. These central processes enter the ipsilateral **fasciculus cuneatus** (L. cuneus, "wedge") and ascend to the medulla to synapse with second order neurons in the ipsilateral **nucleus cuneatus**. It should be noted that the fasciculus cuneatus is present only at the upper six thoracic and at all cervical spinal cord levels.

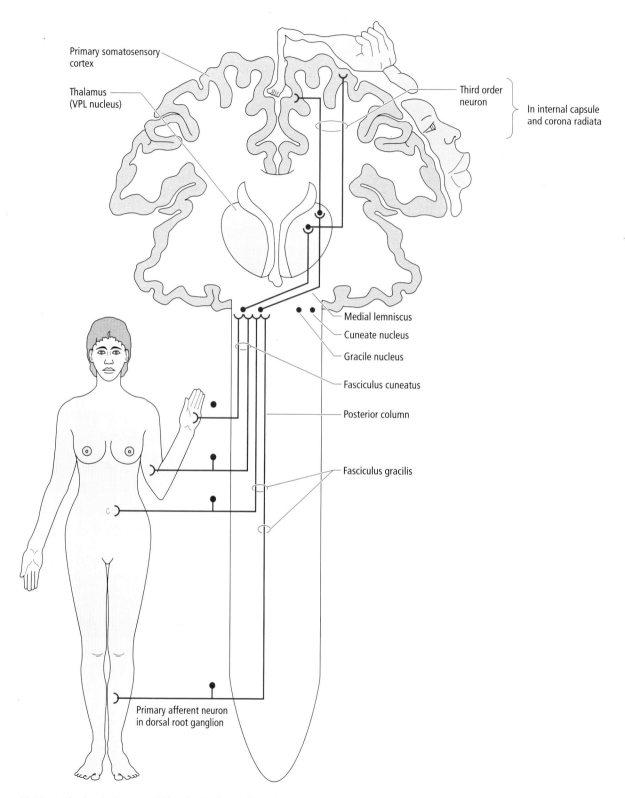

Primary somatosensory cortex

Thalamus (VPL nucleus)

Third order neuron

In internal capsule and corona radiata

Medial lemniscus

Cuneate nucleus

Gracile nucleus

Fasciculus cuneatus

Posterior column

Fasciculus gracilis

Primary afferent neuron in dorsal root ganglion

Figure 10.18 ● The dorsal column–medial lemniscal pathway relaying discriminative (fine) touch and vibratory sense from the body to the somatosensory cortex. VPL, ventral posterior lateral.

Note that the clinical case at the beginning of the chapter refers to a patient who has a sensory disturbance of the distal upper and lower limbs. Symptoms include numbness and tingling of the hands and legs, incoordination in movements of the hands, imbalance, and difficulty walking. Sensation, particularly to vibration and joint position, is severely impaired in the distal limbs.

1 Which ascending sensory pathway(s) is/are affected in this patient?

2 Where are the nerve cell bodies of the affected pathways located?

3 In which part of the spinal cord are the affected ascending pathways located?

4 How extensive is the damage if symptoms are present in both the upper and lower limbs?

As the descending fibers of all of the first order neurons descend to various spinal cord levels within the fasciculus gracilis or the fasciculus cuneatus, they give rise to collateral branches along the way. These collateral branches form synapses with interneurons and alpha motoneurons, thus participating in intersegmental reflexes.

Second order neurons

The first order fibers terminating in the nucleus gracilis and nucleus cuneatus synapse with second order neurons whose cell bodies are housed in these nuclei

The first order fibers terminating in the nucleus gracilis and nucleus cuneatus synapse with second order neurons whose cell bodies are housed in these nuclei. The fibers of the second order neurons form the **internal arcuate fibers** as they curve ventromedially through the reticular formation to the opposite side. These fibers ascend as the **medial lemniscus** (L. lemniscus, "ribbon") in the caudal part of the medulla, cranial to the prominent pyramidal (motor) decussation, to synapse with third order neurons in the **ventral posterior lateral nucleus of the thalamus**.

Third order neurons

The ventral posterior lateral nucleus of the thalamus houses the cell bodies of the third order neurons of the DCML pathway

The ventral posterior lateral nucleus of the thalamus houses the cell bodies of the third order neurons of the DCML pathway. The fibers arising from the thalamus ascend in the **posterior limb of the internal capsule** and the **corona radiata** to terminate in the primary somatosensory cortex of the **postcentral gyrus** (which occupies Brodmann's areas 3a, 3b, 1, and 2, of the parietal cortex).

Projections to the somatosensory cortex

Brodmann's area 3b receives most of the projections arising from the ventral posterior lateral nucleus of the thalamus, and is where initial cortical processing of tactile discrimination input occurs

Brodmann's area 3b receives most of the projections arising from the ventral posterior lateral nucleus of the thalamus, and is the site where the initial cortical processing of tactile discrimination input takes place. Brodmann's area 3b in turn projects to Brodmann's areas 1 and 2. Area 1 is responsible for determining the *texture* and area 2 the *size* and *shape* of objects. In contrast, area 3a is stimulated by signals arising from muscle spindles and is believed to participate in motor functions.

The primary somatosensory cortex projects to the secondary somatosensory cortex, located on the superior border of the lateral fissure. Some third order neuron fibers from the thalamus terminate directly in the secondary somatosensory cortex.

SENSORY PATHWAYS TO THE CEREBELLUM

Most of the proprioceptive information does not reach conscious levels, and instead is transmitted directly to the cerebellum

Only a small portion of the proprioceptive information enters consciousness. Most of the proprioceptive information does not reach conscious levels, and instead is transmitted directly to the cerebellum via the ascending somatosensory cerebellar pathways without projecting to the thalamus or the cerebral cortex. These pathways, which process subconscious proprioception from muscles, tendons, and joints, are two-neuron pathways, consisting of first order and second order neurons. The pathways include (Fig. 10.19; Tables 10.1, 10.4): the dorsal (posterior) spinocerebellar tract, the cuneocerebellar tract, the ventral (anterior) spinocerebellar tract, and the rostral spinocerebellar tract.

Dorsal (posterior) spinocerebellar tract

The primary function of the dorsal spinocerebellar tract is to relay proprioceptive input from the neuromuscular spindles and GTOs of the ipsilateral trunk and lower limb, to the cerebellum

The primary function of the dorsal (posterior) spinocerebellar tract (Fig. 10.19A; Table 10.5) is to relay proprioceptive input from the neuromuscular spindles and GTOs of the ipsilateral trunk and lower limb, to the cerebellum. It should be recalled, however, that it also relays some touch and pressure sensation from the skin of the ipsilateral trunk and lower limb.

First order neurons (pseudounipolar neurons) whose cell bodies are housed in the dorsal root ganglia send their peripheral processes to the skin, muscles, tendons, and joints. Here they perceive proprioceptive information, which is then transmitted to the spinal cord by their central processes. These central processes join the medial division of the dorsal roots of the spinal nerves to synapse in the **nucleus dorsalis**

Table 10.4 ● Ascending sensory pathways (subconscious).

Sensation	Sensory receptor	Location of cell body of first order neuron	Location of cell body of second order neuron	Pathway	Decussation of pathway (ipsilateral/ contralateral)
Pain and thermal sense from the body	Aδ and C fibers	Dorsal root ganglion	Dorsal horn	Spinoreticular	Anterior white commissure
				Spinotectal	
				Spinomesencephalic	
				Spinohypothalamic	
Two-point discriminative (fine) touch, tactile sensation, vibratory sense	Touch and pressure receptors	Dorsal root ganglion	Dorsal horn	Anterior spinocerebellar	Decussates in anterior white commissure and decussates again within cerebellum
Proprioceptive sense from muscles and joints of the body, limb position sense	Muscle stretch receptors, Golgi tendon organs	Dorsal root ganglion	Dorsal horn (Clark's column) C8–L2,3	Posterior spinocerebellar	Ipsilateral
		Dorsal root ganglion	Accessory cuneate nucleus	Cuneocerebellar	Ipsilateral
		Dorsal root ganglion	Dorsal horn	Rostral spinocerebellar	Ipsilateral

Table 10.5 ● Functions of the ascending sensory tracts to the cerebellum (subconscious).

Tract	Location of first order neuron cell body	Location of second order neuron cell body	Termination	Function
Dorsal (posterior) spinocerebellar	Dorsal root ganglion	Dorsal horn (Clark's column) C8–L2,3	Ipsilateral cerebellar vermis	Relays proprioceptive input from the ipsilateral trunk and lower limb Coordination of movements of the lower limb muscles Posture maintenance
Cuneocerebellar	Dorsal root ganglion	Accessory cuneate nucleus	Ipsilateral anterior lobe of the cerebellum	Relays proprioceptive information from the ipsilateral neck and upper limb Movement of head and upper limb
Ventral (anterior) spinocerebellar	Dorsal root ganglion	Dorsal horn	Ipsilateral cerebellar vermis	Relays proprioceptive input from the ipsilateral trunk and lower limb Coordination of movements of lower limb muscles Posture maintenance
Rostral spinocerebellar	Dorsal root ganglion	Dorsal horn	Cerebellum	Relays proprioceptive input primarily from the ipsilateral head and upper limb Movement of head and upper limb

Table 10.4 ● *Continued.*

Location of pathway in spinal cord	Pathway (second order neuron) termination	Location of cell body of third order neuron	Termination of third order neuron	Conscious/ subconscious	Function(s)
Lateral funiculus	Reticular formation	Multiple synapses in brainstem reticular formation; fibers terminate in the intralaminar nuclei of the thalamus	Anterior cingulate cortex, anterior insular cortex	Subconscious	Relays pain and thermal sense from the body; input functions in arousal of the organism in response to pain
	Superior colliculus	–	–	Subconscious	Mediates reflex movement of the head, eyes, and upper trunk in direction of the stimulus
	Periaqueductal gray matter and raphe nucleus magnus	–	–	Subconscious	Involved in pain modulation
	Hypothalamus	–	–	Subconscious	Functions in the autonomic, reflex, and emotional aspects of pain
Lateral funiculus	Cerebellar vermis	–	–	Subconscious	Mediates coordination of muscle activity of the trunk and lower limb
Lateral funiculus	Cerebellar vermis	–	–	Subconscious	Relays proprioceptive information to the cerebellum, and functions in the coordination of movement of the lower limb and posture maintenance
–	Anterior lobe of the cerebellum	–	–	Subconscious	Neck and upper limb equivalent of the dorsal spinocerebellar tract
Lateral funiculus	Cerebellum	–	–	Subconscious	Mediates proprioception from the head and upper limb

(**Clark's column**, lamina VII of spinal cord levels C8 to L2,3) at their level of entry. Sensory information transmitted by spinal nerves entering at the sacral and lower lumbar spinal cord levels (below Clark's column) is relayed to the caudal extent of the nucleus dorsalis (L2,3) by ascending in the fasciculus gracilis.

Clark's column houses the cell bodies of **second order neurons** whose axons form the **dorsal spinocerebellar tract**, which ascends ipsilaterally in the lateral funiculus of the spinal cord. When this tract reaches the brainstem it joins the restiform body (of the inferior cerebellar peduncle), and then passes (as "mossy fibers") into the vermis of the cerebellum. The dorsal spinocerebellar tract relays proprioceptive information directly to the cerebellum where this information is processed; it plays an important role in the coordination of movements of individual lower limb muscles and in the maintenance of posture.

Cuneocerebellar tract

Proprioceptive sensory information from the neck, upper limb, and upper half of the trunk enters at spinal cord segments C2 to T5

Proprioceptive sensory information from the neck, upper limb, and upper half of the trunk enters at spinal cord segments C2 to T5. The central processes of the pseudounipolar first order neurons ascend in the fasciculus cuneatus and terminate in the external (accessory) cuneate nucleus—the nucleus dorsalis of Clark homologue at cervical levels above C8 (Fig. 10.19A; Table 10.5).

The axons of the **second order neurons**, whose cell bodies are housed in the **accessory cuneate nucleus**, form the **cuneocerebellar tract**. This tract is referred to as the neck and upper limb counterpart of the dorsal spinocerebellar tract. Fibers of the cuneocerebellar tract join the restiform body (of the inferior cerebellar peduncle) and then enter the anterior lobe of the cerebellum ipsilaterally. Information carried by the cuneocerebellar tract plays a role in movements of the head and upper limbs.

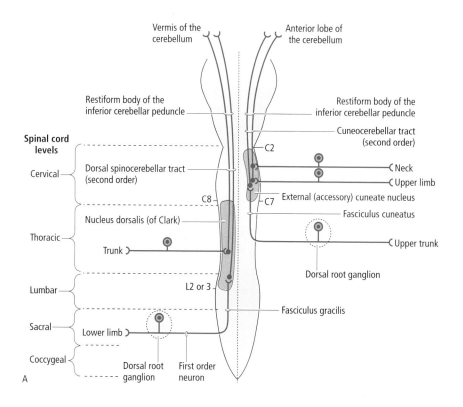

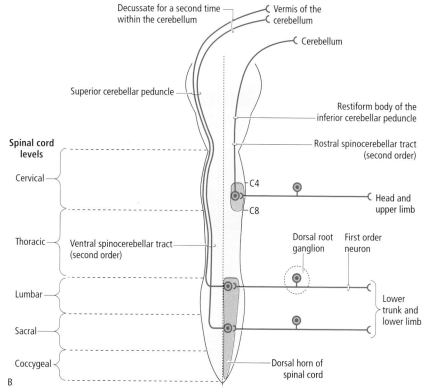

Figure 10.19 ● (A) Two of the ascending sensory pathways to the cerebellum: the dorsal spinocerebellar tract transmitting sensory information from the lower limb and trunk, and the cuneocerebellar tract transmitting sensory information from the neck, upper limb, and upper trunk to the cerebellum. (B) Two of the ascending sensory pathways to the cerebellum: the ventral spinocerebellar tract transmitting sensory information from the lower trunk and lower limb, and the rostral spinocerebellar tract transmitting sensory information from the head and upper limb to the cerebellum.

Ventral (anterior) spinocerebellar tract

The ventral (anterior) spinocerebellar tract relays proprioceptive information from the muscle spindles and GTOs of the trunk and lower limb

The ventral (anterior) spinocerebellar tract relays proprioceptive information from the muscle spindles and GTOs of the trunk and lower limb. It functions in the coordination of movement of the lower limb, and maintenance of posture (Fig. 10.19B; Table 10.5).

First order neurons (pseudounipolar neurons) transmit sensory input to laminae V–VII of the lumbar, sacral, and coccygeal spinal cord levels, where they terminate and synapse with second order neurons.

The axons of these **second order neurons,** known as spinal border cells, form the **ventral (anterior) spinocerebellar tract**, which decussates in the anterior white commissure and ascends in the lateral funiculus of the spinal cord to the medulla. At pontine levels these fibers join the superior cerebellar peduncle to pass as "mossy fibers" into the vermis of the cerebellum. These fibers then decussate again to their actual side of origin within the cerebellum.

Rostral spinocerebellar tract

Proprioceptive information from the head and upper limb is transmitted to C4–C8 spinal cord levels

Proprioceptive information from the head and upper limb is transmitted to C4–C8 spinal cord levels. The central processes of **first order neurons** synapse with second order neurons whose cell bodies reside in lamina VII of the dorsal horn. The fibers of the **second order neurons** form the primarily uncrossed **rostral spinocerebellar tract**, the head and upper limb counterpart of the ventral spinocerebellar tract. These fibers join the restiform body (of the inferior cerebellar peduncle) to enter the cerebellum. Additionally, some fibers pass into the cerebellum via the superior cerebellar peduncle (Fig. 10.19B; Table 10.5). This tract plays a role in movement of the head and upper limb.

CLINICAL CONSIDERATIONS

Lesions involving peripheral nerves

The damage that occurs to a peripheral nerve, and the resulting sensory symptoms, differ depending on whether the damaged nerve carries sensory fibers and which fibers are involved in the lesion

The extent of damage that may occur to a peripheral nerve, and the sensory symptoms that will arise following a lesion, differ depending on whether the damaged nerve carries sensory fibers and which fibers are involved in the lesion. Diminished cutaneous sensation due to damage of the sensory fibers of a particular nerve is usually narrower than the range of distribution of the nerve, due to the overlapping areas of distribution of adjacent nerves.

Dorsal root and spinal nerve lesions

The sensory deficits that arise following a lesion to a dorsal root or to a spinal nerve are usually revealed in a segmental distribution

The sensory deficits that arise following a lesion to a dorsal root or to a spinal nerve are usually revealed in a segmental distribution (Fig. 10.20). Since peripheral nerves branch and extend their innervation into territories of adjacent nerves, a peripheral nerve lesion may include areas supplied by several adjacent spinal cord levels. Due to this innervation overlap, it is difficult to trace the sensory deficit to a single spinal nerve or dorsal root. Dorsal root irritation results in pain and **paresthesia** (G., "abnormal sensations"), such as tingling, itching, or pricking of the skin.

Spinal cord lesions

In order to be able to identify the site of a spinal cord lesion, one has to be familiar with the anatomical arrangement of the various ascending and descending tracts in the spinal cord. In general, the pathways relaying **pain**, **temperature**, and **nondiscriminative (crude) touch** from the body, ascend in the opposite side of origin, in the anterolateral aspect of the spinal cord. Pathways relaying **discriminative (fine) touch** and **proprioceptive** modalities ascend ipsilateral to the side of origin, in the dorsal white columns.

Brown-Séquard syndrome

Although spinal cord injuries are rarely limited to a particular tract, quadrant, or side of the spinal cord, the hemisection of the spinal cord is used for instructive purposes. One such example is the **Brown-Séquard syndrome** (Fig. 10.21).

When the **spinal cord** is **hemisected** (only the right or left half is severed), all of the tracts (both ascending and descending) coursing through the level of the lesion are severed, and the following will be observed.

1 The lower motoneurons ipsilateral to and at the level of the lesion will be damaged, leading to **ipsilateral lower motoneuron paralysis** at the level of the lesion.
2 Since the corticospinal tract (upper motoneurons) will be severed, the individual will exhibit an **ipsilateral loss of motor function** below the level of the lesion, followed by **spastic paralysis** (see Chapter 11).

For **sensory deficits** at or below the level of the lesion, the following will be observed.

1 Since the **anterolateral system** (which includes the spinothalamic, spinoreticular, spinomesencephalic, spinotectal, and spinohypothalamic fibers) has been severed, there will be a contralateral loss of:

    • **pain and temperature sensation** beginning one or two segments below the level of the lesion; and
    • **nondiscriminative (crude) touch sensation** beginning three to four segments below the level of the lesion.

2 Since the **dorsal column pathways** (**fasciculus gracilis** and **fasciculus cuneatus**) have been severed, there will be an ipsilateral loss of the following, below the level of the lesion:

    • **discriminative (fine) touch;**
    • **vibratory sensation;**

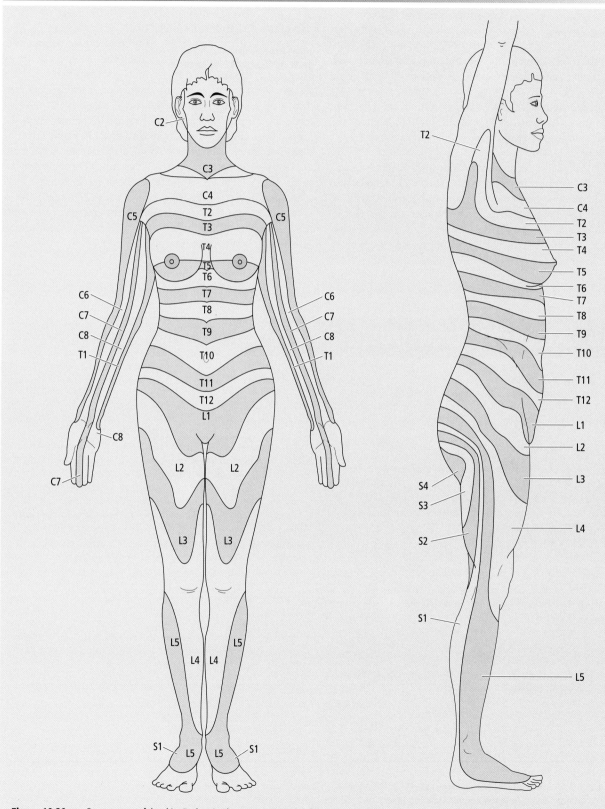

Figure 10.20 ● Dermatomes of the skin. Each striped area represents the skin innervated by a single dorsal root ganglion (on each side).

CLINICAL CONSIDERATIONS (*continued*)

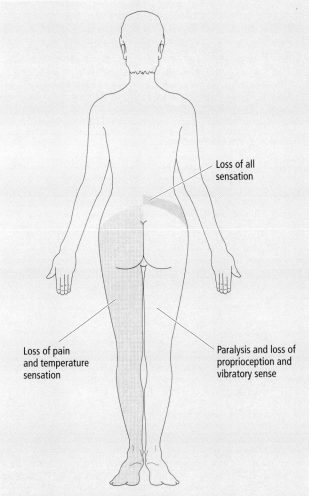

Figure 10.21 ● Brown-Séquard syndrome. The figure shows the deficits resulting following hemisection of the right side of the spinal cord at the level of T12.

Loss of all sensation

Loss of pain and temperature sensation

Paralysis and loss of proprioception and vibratory sense

- **proprioceptive (joint position) sensation:** an individual with this type of lesion will have coordination difficulties (**dorsal column sensory ataxia**); if the lesion involves the sensory innervation of the lower limbs the individual will have difficulty in maintaining his balance when his feet are closely approximated and when his eyes are closed (positive **Romberg sign**);
- **astereognosis (stereoanesthesia)** (G. astereognosis, "inability to know solids"): an individual with astereognosis is unable to identify the shape and form of a known object (such as a fork) following manual examination with the eyes closed, but can identify the object by sight; and
- **two-point discrimination:** the individual is unable to perceive simultaneous stimulation by a blunt instrument at two separate points on the skin as two distinct points of stimulation.

Since crude touch is carried by more than one ascending sensory pathway, ascending on *both* sides of the spinal cord, some touch sensation remains intact in individuals with Brown-Séquard syndrome. Furthermore, if *only* the

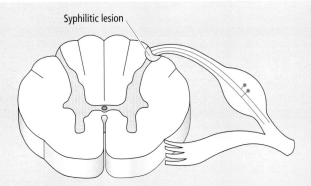

Syphilitic lesion

Figure 10.22 ● Location of a syphilitic lesion on the spinal cord.

dorsal right quadrant of the spinal cord is damaged, pain and temperature sensation will not be affected, whereas there will be a loss of discriminative (fine) touch and proprioceptive sensation, below the level of the lesion on the ipsilateral (right) side of the body.

Tabes dorsalis

Tabes dorsalis, a form of tertiary neurosyphilis, is a rare condition which is manifested during the second decade after an individual becomes infected with the microorganism causing syphilis

Tabes dorsalis, a form of tertiary neurosyphilis, is a rare condition which is manifested during the second decade after an individual becomes infected with the microorganism causing syphilis. This condition is characterized by sensory ataxia (G. ataxia, "without order") resulting from impairment of two-point discrimination, vibratory sense, position sense, and kinesthesis. Individuals with this condition find it necessary to look at their lower limbs during walking. Additionally, they have difficulty standing up straight if their feet are closely approximated when their eyes are closed, or if they are standing in the dark (referred to as **Romberg's sign**). There is also degeneration of the large-diameter, heavily myelinated fibers coursing in the medial division of the dorsal root; thus sensory information from the mechanoreceptors to the ascending sensory pathways is also affected (Fig. 10.22). Additionally, these individuals experience abnormal pain sensations.

Friedreich's ataxia

Friedreich's ataxia is a hereditary disorder that is manifested prior to, or during, puberty

Friedreich's ataxia is a hereditary disorder that is manifested prior to, or during, puberty. In this condition, the **spinocerebellar tracts** as well as the **dorsal column pathways** degenerate and, consequently, produce an increasingly deteriorating ataxia.

Subacute combined degeneration

In subacute combined degeneration both the corticospinal tracts and the dorsal column pathways undergo degeneration

In **subacute combined degeneration**, as a result of vitamin B_{12} deficiency, both the corticospinal tracts and the dorsal column pathways undergo degeneration. The deficits in the affected individual are characterized by muscle weakness as a result of the degeneration of the corticospinal (motor) tracts, and loss of vibratory sense, two-point discrimination, and proprioception as a result of the degeneration of the dorsal column pathways.

CLINICAL CONSIDERATIONS (*continued*)

Syringomyelia

Syringomyelia is a disease in which the central canal of the spinal cord, usually at the lower cervical or upper thoracic spinal cord levels, becomes enlarged

Syringomyelia (G. syrinx, "tube") is a disease in which the central canal of the spinal cord, usually at the lower cervical or upper thoracic spinal cord levels, becomes enlarged (although the enlargement of the central canal may extend cranially and/or caudally) (Fig. 10.23). The enlarging canal stretches and damages the surrounding nerve tissue. The tissue affected first is the anterior white commissure containing crossing fibers, followed by the damage to the anterior horn. This results in:

1 **Loss of pain** and **temperature sensation** from the skin of both shoulders and upper extremities due to the destruction of the second order neuron decussating fibers that relay pain and temperature input. If the lesion involves only the cervical levels of the spinal cord, the anterior surface of the arm and forearm is not affected since it is innervated by T1 and T2.

2 **Weakness** and **atrophy** of the intrinsic muscles of the hands due to the degeneration of the motoneurons in the anterior horn of the spinal cord. If the disease progresses to include additional spinal cord levels and more nerve tissue surrounding the increasingly enlarged space, additional deficits will become apparent.

Vascular problems of the spinal cord

Anterior spinal artery syndrome

Occlusion of the anterior spinal artery, either by a thrombus or by compression, will obstruct blood flow to the ventral two-thirds of the spinal cord, and result in infarction

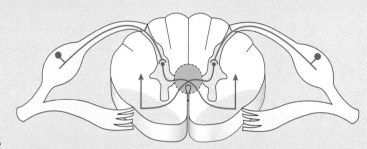

A

Area in which sensations of pain and temperature are lost

B

Figure 10.23 ● Syringomyelia. (A) Damage of decussating fibers of the pain and temperature pathway. (B) Skin area in which there is loss of pain and temperature sensation following the development of syringomyelia.

CLINICAL CONSIDERATIONS (*continued*)

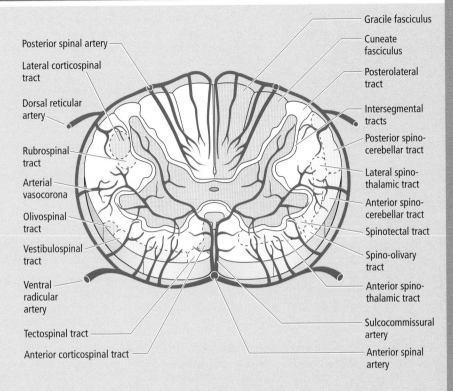

Figure 10.24 ● Cross-section of the spinal cord and its arterial supply.

Labels (clockwise from top): Gracile fasciculus; Cuneate fasciculus; Posterolateral tract; Intersegmental tracts; Posterior spinocerebellar tract; Lateral spinothalamic tract; Anterior spinocerebellar tract; Spinotectal tract; Spino-olivary tract; Anterior spinothalamic tract; Sulcocommissural artery; Anterior spinal artery; Anterior corticospinal tract; Tectospinal tract; Ventral radicular artery; Vestibulospinal tract; Olivospinal tract; Arterial vasocorona; Rubrospinal tract; Dorsal reticular artery; Lateral corticospinal tract; Posterior spinal artery

Occlusion of the anterior spinal artery, either by a thrombus or by compression, will obstruct blood flow to the ventral two-thirds of the spinal cord, and will result in infarction (Fig. 10.24). If the anterior spinal artery is occluded or compressed near the artery's origin in the medulla, structures located in the anterior aspect of the medulla, such as the pyramid and medial lemnisci, will be affected. Damage of the corticospinal fibers in the pyramid above its decussation will result in contralateral hemiparesis. Damage of the medial lemniscus will result in loss of proprioception and vibratory sense from the opposite side of the body.

If occlusion or compression of the anterior spinal artery occurs at spinal levels, it will result in damage of the corticospinal tract fibers and the anterior horns of the spinal cord. This is characterized by motor function deficits ipsilateral to, and below, the level of the lesion. Since the dorsal column pathways are not affected by occlusion of the anterior spinal artery at spinal levels, discriminatory (fine) touch and position sense remain intact.

Posterior spinal artery occlusion or compression

The two posterior spinal arteries supply the dorsal one-third of the spinal cord; if either is occluded or compressed, it results in infarction of the dorsal white columns and the ALS

The two posterior spinal arteries supply the dorsal one-third of the spinal cord (Fig. 10.24). If one or both of the posterior spinal arteries is/are occluded or compressed, it results in infarction of the dorsal white columns and the ALS. If only one of the posterior spinal arteries is occluded, or compressed, it will result in loss of discriminatory (fine) touch and proprioceptive sensation, ipsilaterally, and loss of pain and temperature sensation, contralaterally, below the level of the lesion. If infarction occurs at caudal medullary levels, near the level of the vessels' origin, the dorsal white columns and their respective nuclei

will be damaged. Since the spinothalamic tract is located in the anterolateral aspect of the caudal medulla, it is not affected.

Central or thalamic pain

A lesion of the spinothalamic tract and its nucleus of termination may cause agonizing pain or other unusual sensations

Lesions involving the spinothalamic tract and its nucleus of termination, the ventral posterior lateral nucleus of the thalamus, may initially cause diminished or complete loss of touch, pressure, pain, or temperature sensation, or proprioception from the contralateral side of the body. Spontaneous, inexplicable, agonizing pain and other unusual sensations in the anesthetic parts may follow. This condition is known as central pain (thalamic pain, thalamic syndrome).

Lesions involving the somatosensory cortex

Isolated lesions in the **postcentral gyrus** are uncommon. However, since the postcentral gyrus is supplied by branches of the middle cerebral artery, a vessel which often becomes occluded, this region of the brain may become infarcted. A lesion to the primary somatosensory cortex will result in contralateral loss of:

1 **Two-point discrimination**.
2 **Graphesthesia**, the ability to recognize letters or numbers as they are stroked on the skin.
3 **Stereognosis**, the ability to identify a known object following tactile examination without looking.
4 **Vibratory sense**.
5 **Position sense**.

CLINICAL CONSIDERATIONS (*continued*)

Furthermore, although the individual has a minimal impairment of **pain**, **temperature**, and **touch sensation**, he is unable to *localize* the stimulus. Since pain perception is not only processed in the **somatosensory cortex**, but also in the **anterior cingulate** and **anterior insular cortices**, pain sensation persists following a lesion to the somatosensory cortex as a result of these additional cortical representations of pain.

In recent years, a bilateral **cingulotomy** (transection of the anterior part of the cingulum bundle) has served as an effective treatment in relieving the emotional, agonizing reaction to pain. An isolated lesion in the secondary somatosensory cortex (S-II) results in minimal sensory loss, but since S-II has an important function in memory of somatosensory information and sensory integration, these functions are impaired.

Referred pain

Pain originating in a visceral structure may be referred to and felt in a somatic structure

The actual origin of visceral pain is imprecisely localized. Although pain may originate deep within a visceral structure, such as the heart, the pain may be "referred to," and felt, in another, distant somatic structure such as the left upper limb. Although several explanations have been proposed for this phenomenon, the following two have the most prominence in the field of neuroscience.

Convergence–projection theory of visceral pain

The **convergence–projection theory** of visceral pain, suggests that the central processes of pseudounipolar sensory, general visceral afferent (GVA) neurons supplying visceral structures and the central processes of general somatic afferent (GSA) neurons from a somatic structure, such as the upper limb, enter and terminate at the *same spinal cord level*. Here they converge on and synapse with the same interneurons and/or second order neurons (viscerosomatic neurons) of the ascending pain pathways in the dorsal horn, and the intermediate gray matter. Nociceptive information is transmitted by these GSA pathways to higher brain centers.

Concept of referred pain

Second order GSA projection neurons are continuously being activated by GVA first order neurons, thereby lowering the threshold of stimulation of the second order neurons. Consequently, nociceptive sensory information is relayed by the neurons of the GSA pathway to higher brain centers. Thus, GVA nociceptive input is transmitted via the spinoreticular fibers to the reticular formation, the thalamus, and the hypothalamus. The nociceptive signal is subsequently relayed to the region of the somesthetic cortex that normally receives somatic information from other areas, such as the upper limb, and the brain interprets it as if the pain were coming from that somatic structure (upper limb). Therefore, it is the area(s) of the cerebral cortex, in this case the somatosensory cortex, wherein the signals *terminate*, and not the stimulus, the receptor, or the information, that establishes the localization of the sensation.

Phantom limb pain

Individuals who have had a limb amputated may experience pain or tingling sensations that feel as if they were coming from the amputated limb, just as if that limb were still present

A curious phenomenon has been reported by individuals who have had a limb amputated. These individuals experience pain or tingling sensations that feel as if they were coming from the amputated limb, just as if that limb were still present. Although the mechanism of phantom limb pain is not understood, the following two possible explanations are offered.

If a sensory pathway is activated anywhere along its course, nerve impulses are generated that travel to the CNS where they initiate neural activity. This neural activity ultimately "creates" sensations that feel as though they originated in the nonexistent limb.

Another possibility is that since there is no touch, pressure, or proprioceptive information transmitted to the CNS from the peripheral processes of the sensory neurons that initially innervated the amputated limb, there are no impulses from touch fibers to attenuate the relaying of nociceptive impulses to the nociceptive pathways, enhancing nociceptive transmission and pain sensation (see the gate control theory of pain, below). Since nociception is not as localized, cortical areas corresponding to the phantom limb will be activated.

MODULATION OF NOCICEPTION

The CNS can prevent and/or suppress the flow of some of the incoming nociceptive signals from peripheral structures

Although the CNS is constantly flooded with sensory information, it can prevent and/or suppress the flow of some of the incoming nociceptive signals at the local circuitry level of the spinal cord dorsal horn (and spinal trigeminal nucleus of the brainstem). The CNS can also do this at the level of the descending opioid and nonopioid analgesia-producing pathways that originate in the brainstem, and terminate at the relay sensory nuclei of the ascending sensory systems.

Gate control theory of pain

Nociceptive signals from the periphery are filtered by modulation in the substantia gelatinosa of the dorsal horn

Rubbing a painful area (activation of touch Aδ/Aβ fibers) reduces the sensation of pain. It has been proposed that the **substantia gelatinosa (lamina II)** of the dorsal horn gray matter is the site where pain is filtered by modulation of the sensory nociceptive input to the spinothalamic pain and temperature pathway neurons. The theory proposed to explain this phenomenon, known as the **gate control theory of pain**, suggests that the neural circuitry of the substantia gelatinosa (SG) functions as follows (Fig. 10.25).

The activity of nociceptive unmyelinated C fibers and thinly myelinated Aδ fibers terminating in the SG transmit nociceptive impulses by: (i) inhibiting the SG inhibitory interneuron; and (ii) simultaneously activating the second order spinothalamic tract neuron that projects to the thalamus, "keeping the gate open."

The touch Aδ/Aβ myelinated fibers activate the inhibitory interneuron as well as the second order neuron. However, the inhibitory interneuron, via presynaptic inhibition of the C/Aδ and Aδ/Aβ fibers, prevents impulses from reaching

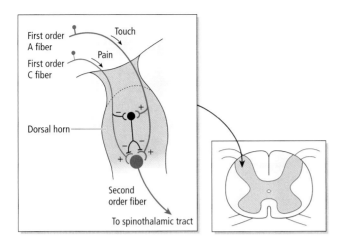

Figure 10.25 ● Gate control theory of pain. Stimulation of the C fibers transmitting nociception keeps the gate to higher brain centers open, whereas stimulation of the large-diameter A fiber closes the gate. (Modified from Heimart, L (1995) *The Human Brain*. Springer-Verlag, New York; fig. 9.2.)

the second order spinothalamic neuron. When someone injures his fingers, for example, he usually rubs the painful area. The rubbing probably stimulates the Aδ/Aβ fibers, which in turn—via the inhibitory interneuron—inhibit the transmission of some of the nociceptive impulses to higher brain centers, providing some relief from pain.

Descending analgesia-producing pathways

Descending analgesia-producing pathways arise from the brainstem and terminate in the spinal cord

Although it was known for many years that opiates, a group of drugs derived from opium (e.g., morphine) provide powerful relief from pain, their mode of action was not understood. It is now known that the opiates bind to "opiate receptors" on specific nerve cells residing in certain areas of the CNS. It was then speculated that, for the nervous system to have "opiate receptors," it must synthesize its own endogenous, opiate-like substances that bind to the "opiate receptors," which probably modulate afferent nociceptive transmission. Three groups of related endogenous opioid peptides have been identified: **enkephalin** (G. enkephalin, "in the head"), **beta-endorphin** ("morphine within"), and **dynorphin** (dynamo + morphine) all of which are known to bind to the same receptors as the opioid drugs.

During a stressful or emotional experience, regions associated with the processing of emotions—namely the telencephalon (frontal cortex), the diencephalon (hypothalamus), and the limbic system—project to and stimulate the enkephalin-releasing neurons of the **periaqueductal gray matter** and other nearby regions of the midbrain. The axons of these enkephalin-releasing neurons form excitatory synapses primarily with the serotonin-releasing neurons of the **raphe nucleus magnus** and the **nucleus gigantocellularis** of the rostral **medullary reticular formation**. Since these neurons release serotonin, they are said to form the **serotonergic-opioid peptide analgesic system**, which modulates nociception. In addition to the serotonergicopioid

peptide analgesic system, there is a **norepinephrine** (adrenergic, nonopioid) **analgesic system** that arises from the **dorsolateral pontine reticular formation** and terminates in the SG of the spinal cord, and also functions in modulating nociception (see discussion below).

Serotonin-releasing neurons

The axons of the **serotonin-releasing neurons** from the raphe nucleus magnus and the nucleus gigantocellularis descend bilaterally in the lateral funiculus of all spinal cord levels to terminate in the SG of the dorsal horn. Here they form excitatory synapses with the inhibitory interneurons, which release the opioid peptides, enkephalin or dynorphin. These interneurons establish axoaxonic synapses with the central processes of the Aδ and C first order nociceptive neurons.

The modulation of nociception occurs in the following fashion. Upon stimulation of the free nerve ending of a pain fiber, the central process of this first order neuron releases substance P, a neurotransmitter believed to function in the transmission of nociceptive information, that excites the second order nociceptive relay neurons in the dorsal horn. If the serotonin-releasing neurons excite the inhibitory interneurons of the SG, these interneurons in turn inhibit the central processes of the first order neurons. Since this inhibition occurs before the impulse reaches the synapse, it is referred to as **presynaptic inhibition** (Fig. 10.26). Thus these nociceptive incoming impulses are filtered by being suppressed at their first relay station in the spinal cord, by the SG inhibitory interneurons releasing enkephalin or dynorphin. This inhibition occurs because the central processes of these first order neurons possess receptors for enkephalin and dynorphin (opioid receptors) in their axolemma.

There is additional evidence suggesting that there are indeed opioid receptors in the axolemma of the central terminals of the first order nociceptive, substance P-releasing neurons terminating in the SG. This evidence is gathered from reports that naloxone, an opioid antagonist, selectively prevents the blocking of substance P release by the central processes of the first order neurons.

Norepinephrine-releasing neurons

Another brainstem region, the **dorsolateral pontine reticular formation** (Fig. 10.27), is the site of origin of a norepinephrine (adrenergic, nonopioid) analgesic pathway that descends in the dorsolateral funiculus of the spinal cord to synapse in the SG (lamina II). Fibers of this pathway make synaptic contact with inhibitory interneurons of the SG (that may release gamma aminobutyric acid (GABA)), thus ultimately leading to the inhibition of the second order projection neurons that reside in lamina V of the dorsal horn of the nociceptive pathway. Unlike the descending opioid analgesic pathways, the effects of the adrenergic (norepinephrine-releasing) pathway are not blocked by naloxone.

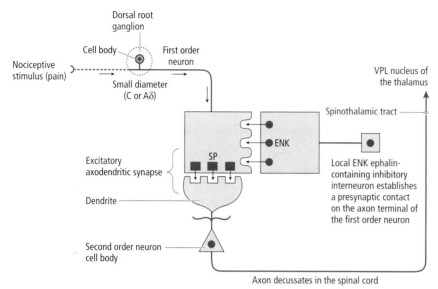

Figure 10.26 ● Opiate-induced suppression of substance P (SP) release in the substantia gelatinosa of the spinal cord dorsal horn. Note the substance P release by the central process of the first order neuron where it synapses with a second order projection neuron of the spinothalamic tract. The local enkephalin-releasing inhibitory interneuron establishes a presynaptic contact on the axon terminal of the first order neuron inhibiting the release of substance P. ENK, enkephalin; VPL, ventral posterior lateral.

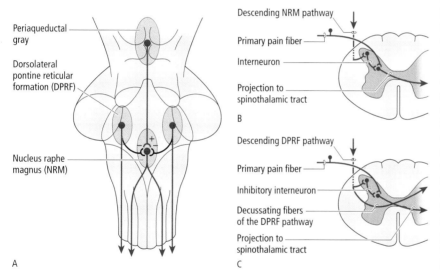

Figure 10.27 ● The descending analgesic pathways. (A) The midbrain periaqueductal gray matter contains enkephalinergic neurons whose axons descend to terminate in the nucleus raphe magnus (NRM) containing serotoninergic neurons. These neurons in turn descend bilaterally to terminate in the dorsal horn of the spinal cord. (B) Descending serotoninergic fibers arising from the NRM terminate on enkephalinergic and dynorphin-containing interneurons in the substantia gelatinosa of the spinal cord. The interneurons inhibit transmission of nociception via presynaptic inhibition of the first order afferent neurons. (C) Descending adrenergic fibers arising from the dorsolateral pontine reticular formation (DPRF) terminate bilaterally on inhibitory interneurons of the substantia gelatinosa of the spinal cord. The interneurons inhibit the second order projection neurons of the spinothalamic tract. (Modified from Burt, AM (1993) *Textbook of Neuroanatomy*. WB Saunders, Philadelphia; fig. 10.25.)

NEUROPLASTICITY

Plastic alterations in neural structures may be induced by a noxious insult that may enhance the magnitude of nociception

Classically, the nociceptive system has been thought of as a sensory system that transmits pain signals from peripheral structures to the spinal cord, brainstem, and higher brain centers. Afferent nociceptive input may be modulated at the dorsal horn level, filtering some of the pain signals, preventing them from being transmitted to higher brain centers.

Recent studies indicate that not only modulation but also "plastic" alterations may be induced in peripheral nerve terminals, the spinal cord, and the brain in response to a noxious insult. These modifications may enhance the magnitude of nociception and may be a factor in the development of pain that may last only days, or may become persistent and last for months, years, or may become permanent.

SYNONYMS AND EPONYMS OF THE ASCENDING SENSORY PATHWAYS

Name of structure or term	Synonym(s)/eponym(s)	Name of structure or term	Synonym(s)/eponym(s)
Astereognosis	Stereoanesthesia	Lamina VII of the dorsal horn of the spinal cord	Nucleus dorsalis
Corpuscle of Ruffini	Ruffini's end organs		Clark's nucleus
Cuneocerebellar tract	Cuneatocerebellar tract		Clark's column
Discriminative tactile sensation	Discriminative touch sensation	Merkel's disc	Merkel's corpuscle
	Fine touch sensation	Muscle spindle	Neuromuscular spindle
Dorsal column nuclei	Nucleus gracilis (NG) and nucleus cuneatus (NC)	Nondiscriminative touch sensation	Crude touch sensation
		Postcentral gyrus	Primary sensory cortex (S-I)
Dorsolateral fasciculus	Tract of Lissauer		Primary somatosensory cortex
	Lissauer's tract		Primary somesthetic cortex
Dynamic proprioception	Kinesthetic sense		Brodmann's areas 3, 1, and 2
External cuneate nucleus	Accessory cuneate nucleus	Projection neuron	Second order neuron
Extrafusal muscle fibers	Skeletal muscle fibers (of gross muscle)	Pseudounipolar neuron	Primary sensory neuron
			First order neuron
Functional component	Functional modality		Afferent neuron
Golgi tendon organ (GTO)	Neurotendinous spindle	Rapidly adapting receptors	Phasic receptors
Hairless skin	Glabrous skin	Secondary somatosensory cortex (S-II)	Secondary somesthetic cortex
Interneuron	Internuncial neuron		Brodmann's area 43
Intrafusal muscle fibers	Skeletal muscle fibers of muscle spindles	Slowly adapting receptors	Tonic receptors
		Spinothalamic tract	Neospinothalamic pathway
Lamina I of the dorsal horn of the spinal cord	Posteromarginal nucleus or zone		Direct pathway of the anterolateral system (ALS)
Lamina II of the dorsal horn of the spinal cord	Substantia gelatinosa (SG)	Static proprioception	Static position sense
		Thalamic pain	Thalamic syndrome
Lamina V of the dorsal horn of the spinal cord	Reticular nucleus	Thermal receptor	Temperature receptor

FOLLOW-UP TO CLINICAL CASE

This woman has a primarily sensory disturbance that involves the distal extremities bilaterally. Severe sensory disturbance, even in the absence of motor deficits or cerebellar abnormality, often leads to gait ataxia or incoordination of the hands depending on whether the feet and/or hands are involved. Therefore, the cerebellum is not necessarily involved, but it may be a good idea to check it with imaging.

The first thing to determine in this case is whether the sensory dysfunction is from pathology in the CNS or the peripheral nervous system (PNS) (e.g. peripheral neuropathy). The PNS can be evaluated by nerve conductions, which reveal how well an electric impulse is conducted by a peripheral nerve. The CNS and the nerve roots can be evaluated by radiologic imaging, particularly MRI. In the present case, nerve conductions were essentially normal. Other tests indicate normal nerve roots. These tests indicate that the CNS should be evaluated closely. The brisk reflexes in the legs, particularly at the ankles, also indicate peripheral neuropathy is unlikely. MRI of the brain and spinal cord is unrevealing.

Laboratory tests to check for a metabolic, or possibly a genetic, cause of pathology to the sensory pathways in the CNS are indicated.

Laboratory tests indicate that this patient has **subacute combined degeneration**, secondary to vitamin B_{12} deficiency. Vitamin B_{12} is a cofactor in enzymatic reactions that are critical for DNA synthesis and neurologic function. Deficiency leads to degeneration of white matter in general, but the posterior columns in the spinal cord tend to be affected early and prominently. The reason for this predilection is not clear. Motor fibers of the corticospinal tract in the spinal cord are also affected relatively early and can lead to bilateral leg weakness. Dementia from degeneration in the brain and visual disturbance from optic nerve involvement may also occur.

Pernicious anemia is an autoimmune disease of gastric parietal cells that ultimately leads to decreased absorption of vitamin B_{12} from the small intestine. Treatment with vitamin B_{12} supplementation is very effective if the disorder is caught early.

5 Is there a peripheral nervous system neuropathy?

6 If this patient's disorder remains undiagnosed and untreated, what other systems are likely to be affected?

QUESTIONS TO PONDER

1. Why is it that an individual responds to a fly walking on the wrist of the right hand, but not to the watch on the left wrist?

2. How do muscle spindles detect a change in muscle length (resulting from stretch or contraction) irrespective of muscle length at the onset of muscle activity?

3. In a simple stretch reflex, what indicates the load placed on a muscle?

4. What is the response of the muscle spindles and Golgi tendon organs during slight stretching and then during further stretching of a muscle?

5. Why does an individual with a lesion in the primary somatosensory cortex still perceive pain?

6. Why is it that when an individual is experiencing a heart attack he feels pain not only in the chest area, but also in the left shoulder and upper limb?

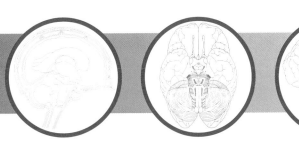

CHAPTER 11

Motor Cortex and Descending Motor Pathways

CLINICAL CASE

A 45-year-old man complains of left foot drop which started 5 months ago. This was very subtle at first, but has been getting progressively worse. The patient can now barely lift his left foot up. He walks with difficulty. More recently he has noticed some clumsiness of his left hand. Upon further questioning he admits to frequent "twitching" of the muscles in his distal lower limbs (particularly in the calf), forearms, and shoulders. His family thinks he has lost some weight. There is no numbness, tingling, pain, or any other neurologic symptom noted. Family history is negative for any neurologic disorder.

Examination shows severe weakness and flaccidity of left ankle dorsiflexion and mild weakness of the intrinsic left hand muscles and left finger extension. Otherwise, strength seems adequate. There is atrophy noted in the muscles of the left hand and the left pretibial muscles. Fasciculations are noted in several muscle groups of the legs, arms, and back. Deep tendon reflexes are pathologically brisk in the arms and legs bilaterally. A Babinski response is present bilaterally. The rest of the neurologic exam was unremarkable.

Motor activity is controlled by intricate interactions of three major regions of the brain: the cerebral cortex, the basal ganglia, and the cerebellum. The **cerebral cortex**, the ultimate command center of the nervous system, is involved in the planning and execution of complex voluntary motor activities. The **basal ganglia** function in the initiation of movement, and modulation of the motor cortex. The **cerebellum** receives information from the cerebral cortex, as well as the visual, auditory, vestibular, and somatosensory systems, which it integrates and utilizes to plan, modify, and coordinate movement. This information enables the cerebellum to play a role in the timing, speed, direction, and precision of motor activ-

ity. The motor cortex relays information to the cerebellum about impending movement. This permits the cerebellum to compare the movement in progress with the movement about to occur. The cerebellum utilizes all of these data to adjust the output of the motor cortex, so that movement is smooth and coordinated. The basal ganglia and the cerebellum exert their influence on the brainstem and spinal cord, and ultimately on motor activity (at a subconscious level), **indirectly** by regulating the output of the motor and premotor cortex, via the thalamus. In contrast, the **primary** and **secondary motor cortex** influence voluntary motor activity via **direct** projections to the brainstem cranial nerve motor nuclei, the reticular formation, and spinal cord, which in turn send commands to the muscular system (basal ganglia and cerebellum → thalamus → motor cortex → brainstem and spinal cord → muscular system → voluntary movement).

CORTICAL AREAS CONTROLLING MOTOR ACTIVITY

Motor activity is controlled by the primary motor and secondary motor cortices

Motor activity is controlled by projections from the primary motor cortex (M-I) and the secondary motor cortex (M-II) of the frontal lobe to the brainstem and spinal cord (Fig. 11.1).

Primary motor cortex

The primary motor cortex functions in the execution of distinct, well-defined, voluntary motor activity of the contralateral side of the body

The **primary motor cortex** (Brodmann's area 4) resides in the **precentral gyrus** of the frontal lobe (Fig. 11.1). It has an important function in the execution of distinct, well-defined, voluntary motor activity. Each precentral gyrus controls movement of the contralateral side of the body. The body is mapped on the primary motor cortex somatotopically, as an upside down homunculus (L., "little person") (Fig. 11.2). Historically, the homunculus was

originally mapped by microstimulation during brain surgery on patients with epilepsy, but in recent years the findings have been confirmed via functional magnetic resonance imaging (fMRI). The part of the precentral gyrus mediating movement of the toes is located near its superior aspect, whereas the part of the precentral gyrus mediating movement of the tongue, lips, and larynx is located near its inferior aspect (bordering the lateral fissure). A striking characteristic of the primary motor cortex in humans is that over half of it is associated with the motor activity of the hands, tongue, lips, and larynx, reflecting the manual dexterity and ability for speech that humans possess. It also influences the motor control of the axial and girdle musculature, specifically the control of the distal muscles of the upper and lower limbs (i.e., the muscles controlling movements of the hands and feet).

In recent years, fMRI studies have provided functional maps of alterations in the oxygen concentration in cerebral vasculature which accompanies neural activity in the brain. Figure 11.3 (for color version, see website) shows the somatotopic organization of the primary motor cortex of eight subjects participating in a study involving the voluntary movement of their fingers, toes, or elbow. The first four subjects (S1–S4) were asked to flex-extend their right fingers, and then their right toes. The second group of four subjects (S5–S8) were asked to flex-extend their right fingers and then their right elbow. The fMRI images of the first four subjects show the region of the primary motor cortex that was active

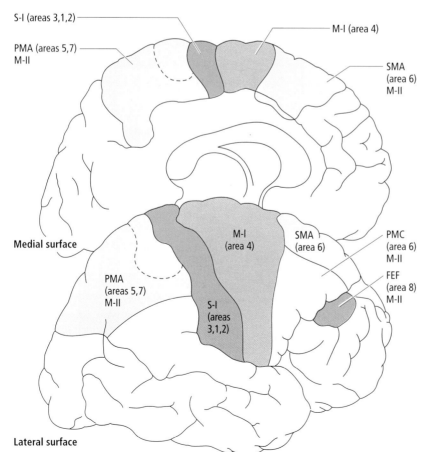

Figure 11.1 ● The motor cortical areas: the primary motor cortex (M-I) and the secondary motor cortex (M-II) consisting of the premotor cortex (PMC), supplementary motor area (SMA), posterior parietal motor area (PMA), and frontal eye fields (FEF). Brodmann's areas are indicated in parentheses.

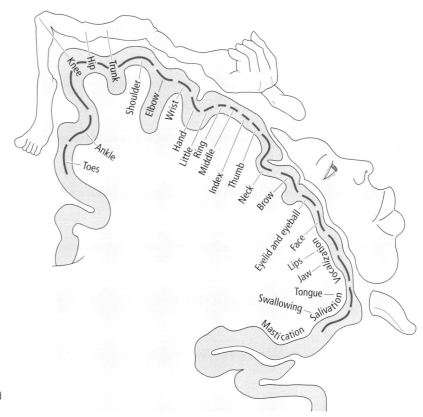

Figure 11.2 ● Coronal section through the primary motor cortex showing the motor homunculus. Note the somatotopic mapping. The cortical area devoted to each body part is proportional to the motor innervation received by the corresponding body part.

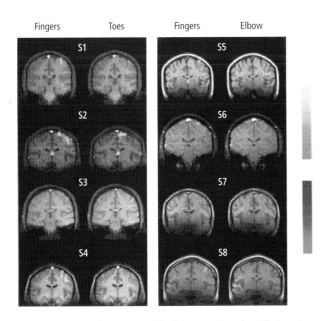

Figure 11.3 ● The fMRI images of the first four subjects (S1–S4) show the region of the primary motor cortex that was active during finger and toe movement, whereas the fMRI images of the second group (S5–S8) show the region of the primary cortex that was active during finger and elbow movement. (From Rao, SM *et al*. (1995) *Neurology* 45, 919–24. Courtesy of Lippincott, Williams & Wilkins, Baltimore.) (For color version, see website.)

during finger and toe movement, whereas the fMRI images of the second group show the region of the primary motor cortex that was active during finger and elbow movement.

Nerve cells in the primary motor cortex are organized into groups, each group sending its axons to the cranial nerve motor nuclei, or the reticular formation in the brainstem, or the spinal cord gray matter, where they control the motor activity of a single muscle. The total cortical area that mediates motor activity of a particular body region, is proportional to the complexity of the motor activity produced in that region.

Secondary motor cortex

The secondary motor cortex functions in the programing of complex motor activity, which is then relayed to the primary motor cortex where the execution of motor activity is initiated

The **secondary motor cortex** consists of four regions: the supplementary motor area, the premotor cortex, the frontal eye field, and the posterior parietal motor area (Fig. 11.1). The first three of these motor cortical areas reside in the frontal lobe (rostral to the central sulcus); the posterior parietal motor area is located in the parietal lobe. The principal function of the **secondary motor cortex** is the programing of complex motor activity, which is then relayed to the primary motor cortex, where the execution of motor activity is initiated. The primary motor cortex then conveys this input mainly to the brainstem or to the spinal cord. Thus, the majority of nerve signals that are generated in the secondary motor cortex cause complex movements produced by groups of muscles performing a task, unlike the discrete muscle contractions elicited by stimulation of the primary motor cortex.

The **supplementary motor area** (SMA) lies in Brodmann's area 6. This area has important functions in the programing phase of the patterns and sequences of elaborate movements, and coordination of movements occurring on the two sides of the body. This cortical area is associated with muscle contractions of the axial (trunk) and proximal limb (girdle) musculature (i.e., muscles controlling movement of the arm and thigh).

The **premotor cortex** (PMC) resides in most of Brodmann's area 6, on the lateral aspect of the frontal lobe. The principal function of this area is the motor control of the axial and proximal limb (girdle) musculature. It also functions in guiding or turning the body and the upper limbs toward a desired (or appropriate) direction. Once an intended movement has begun and is in progress, activity in the PMC decreases, reflecting its key function in the planning phase of motor activity.

The **frontal eye field** (FEF) occupies Brodmann's area 8. This region is located rostral to the premotor area, on the frontal lobe. The FEF functions in the coordination of eye movements, particularly movements mediating voluntary visual tracking of a moving object.

The **posterior parietal motor area** (PMA) corresponds to Brodmann's areas 5 and 7. Area 5 is involved in tactile discrimination (the ability to perceive a subtle distinction by the sense of touch) and stereognosis (the recognition of the three-dimensional shape of an object by the sense of touch). Area 7 is involved with movements that require visual guidance. Thus, when one reaches for a glass of cold water, visual guidance (turning the body and aiming the upper limb in the direction of the glass) and tactile sensation (which in this case helps to realize that the glass is slippery and must be grasped firmly), both play a role in accomplishing a desired motor task.

DESCENDING MOTOR PATHWAYS

The internal pyramidal layer (layer V) of the motor cortex contains the cell bodies of the pyramidal cells, constituting the main output neurons of the cortical descending motor pathways

The cerebral cortex consists of six histologically distinct layers (Fig. 11.4). The **internal pyramidal layer** (layer V), the most conspicuous layer of the motor cortex,

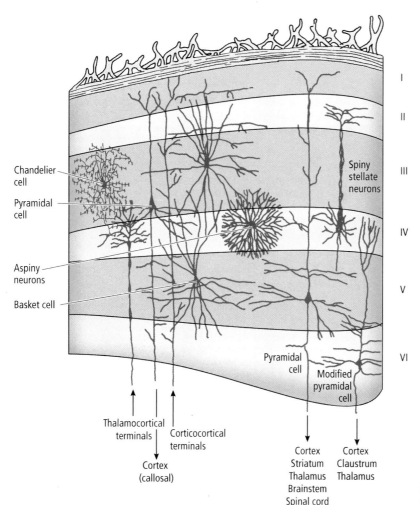

Figure 11.4 ● The six layers of the neocortex and the different cell types located in each layer.

contains the somata of the pyramidal cells. These cells constitute the main output neurons, which contribute to the cortical descending motor pathways, the **corticospinal** and **corticonuclear (corticobulbar) tracts** that terminate in the spinal cord and brainstem, respectively. The older term corticobulbar (cortico, "cortex;" bulbar, "medulla") referred to all of the cortical projections that terminate in the cranial nerve nuclei located in the brainstem. Since not all cranial nerve nuclei are located in the medulla, this older term was replaced with the newer term "corticonuclear" in 1998. The corticonuclear tract includes all cortical projections to the cranial nerve nuclei located in the midbrain, pons, and medulla. Nerve signals arising from the motor cortex elicit skeletal muscle contractions in various parts of the body. All of the pyramidal cell fibers release **glutamate**, an excitatory neurotransmitter, that stimulates excitatory or inhibitory interneurons, or less commonly, lower motoneurons, directly.

There are seven descending motor pathways that ultimately exert their influence on muscle activity (Table 11.1). Three of these pathways, the **lateral corticospinal**, the

Table 11.1 ● The descending motor pathways.

Pathway	Location of cell bodies	Spinal cord/ brainstem location	Ipsilateral / contralateral	Destination / target	Synapses with	Function
Lateral corticospinal tract	Brodmann's areas 4, 6, 5, 7, 3, 1, 2	Lateral funiculus	Pyramidal decussation	All spinal cord levels, primarily cervical and lumbosacral levels	Dorsal horn second order afferent sensory neurons	Sensory modulation
					Lateral intermediate zone interneurons	Execution of rapid, skilled, voluntary movement, especially those of the hand and foot
					Anterior horn interneurons and lower motoneurons	
				Betz cell fibers terminate only at lumbosacral levels	Anterior horn lower motoneurons	Execution of rapid, skilled voluntary movement of the lower limb
Anterior corticospinal tract	Brodmann's areas 4, 6	Anterior funiculus	Ipsilateral	Cervical and thoracic spinal cord levels	Medial aspect of intermediate zone and anterior horn	Voluntary movement of axial and upper limb (girdle) musculature
Corticonuclear (corticobulbar) tract	Brodmann's areas 4, 6, 8, 5, 7, 3, 1, 2	Pons Medulla	Some fibers decussate near termination; others remain ipsilateral	Cranial nerve sensory nuclei	Second order sensory afferent neurons	Sensory modulation
				Brainstem reticular formation	Interneurons	Reflex activity
				Cranial nerve motor nuclei	Interneurons and lower motoneurons	Voluntary movement of muscles of head
Tectospinal tract	Deep layers of the superior colliculus	Anterior funiculus	Decussates at posterior midbrain tegmentum	Cervical and thoracic spinal cord levels	Medial aspect of intermediate zone and anterior horn interneurons	Coordination of eye and neck (head) movements
Rubrospinal tract	Red nucleus	Lateral funiculus	Decussates at anterior midbrain tegmentum	Spinal cord	Lateral aspect of intermediate zone and anterior horn interneurons	Voluntary movement of upper limb muscles
Pontine (medial) reticulospinal tract	Pontine reticular formation	Anterior funiculus	Ipsilateral	Spinal cord	Medial aspect of intermediate zone (interneurons) and anterior horn (lower motoneurons)	Reflex movement of axial (trunk) and limb musculature
Medullary (lateral) reticulospinal tract	Medullary reticular formation	Lateral funiculus	Ipsilateral	Spinal cord	Medial aspect of intermediate zone interneurons	Reflex movement of axial (trunk) and limb musculature
Lateral vestibulospinal tract	Lateral vestibular nucleus	Anterior funiculus	Ipsilateral	Spinal cord	Medial aspect of intermediate zone (interneurons) and anterior horn (lower motoneurons)	Maintenance of posture and balance
Medial vestibulospinal tract	Medial vestibular nucleus	Anterior funiculus	Bilateral, mainly ipsilateral	Cervical and upper half of thoracic spinal cord	Medial aspect of intermediate zone interneurons	Orientation of head

anterior corticospinal, and the **corticonuclear tracts** derive their fibers from the sensorimotor cortex, whereas the other four tracts, the **tectospinal**, **rubrospinal**, **reticulospinal**, and **vestibulospinal tracts**, derive their fibers from the brainstem. All of the descending tracts terminate in the spinal cord with the exception of the corticonuclear tract, which terminates in the brainstem.

Corticospinal tract

Approximately 85–90% of the axons of the corticospinal tract decussate in the caudal medulla, forming the pyramidal decussation

Approximately two-thirds of the **corticospinal tract** fibers (Fig. 11.5) originate from the pyramidal cell layer of the frontal cortex; that is, one-third arise from Brodmann's area 4, and one-third from area 6 (mostly from the supplementary motor area, with some fibers from the premotor cortex). The other third of the corticospinal tract fibers arise from the parietal cortex; specifically from the posterior parietal motor area (Brodmann's areas 5 and 7) and the somatosensory cortex (Brodmann's areas 3, 1, and 2). The pyramidal cells are referred to as the **upper motoneurons** of the descending motor pathways. Their axons descend to synapse in the spinal cord gray matter with:

- interneurons, which in turn synapse with motoneurons;
- alpha motoneurons, which innervate skeletal muscle fibers; or
- gamma motoneurons, which innervate the contractile portion of muscle spindles (muscle stretch receptors).

Unlike the upper motoneurons, the fibers arising from neurons residing in the somatosensory cortex descend to synapse with second order sensory neurons in the somatic relay nuclei of the ascending sensory pathways (and thus are not considered to be upper motoneurons). There they influence motor activity by modulating the transmission of sensory information to higher brain centers (see below). Both the cell bodies and axon terminals of the upper motoneurons (arising from the motor cortical areas) and the somatosensory neurons (arising from Brodmann's areas 3, 1, 2, 5, and 7) reside entirely within the central nervous system (CNS).

As the fibers of the **upper motoneurons** (from the primary and secondary motor cortex) and the **somatosensory fibers** (from the somatosensory cortex) begin their descent, they traverse the **corona radiata** and then course through the **posterior limb of the internal capsule** near its **genu** (Fig. 11.6). As the fibers continue their descent, they gradually come to occupy the posterior half (or posterior third) of the **posterior limb of the internal capsule**. When they reach the mesencephalon, they are located in the middle third of the **crus cerebri (basis pedunculi)**. The corticospinal tract continues inferiorly through the brainstem where it disperses into bundles in the basal pons and then reassembles to form a distinct bundle known as the **pyramid** (a protuberance on the ventral aspect of the medulla).

Approximately 85–90% of the axons of the corticospinal tract **decussate** in the caudal medulla, forming the **pyramidal**

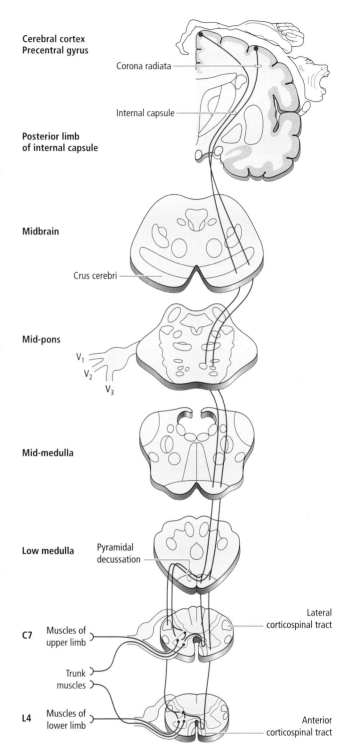

Figure 11.5 ● The origin, course, and termination of the corticospinal tracts. The lateral corticospinal tract synapses with lower motoneurons that innervate the upper and lower limb muscles, whereas the anterior corticospinal tract synapses with the lower motoneurons that innervate the muscles of the trunk. (Modified from Watson, C (1995) *Basic Human Neuroanatomy: an Introductory Atlas.* Little, Brown & Company, Boston; fig. 25.)

decussation (Table 11.1). These axons then descend in the lateral funiculus (L., "cord") of the entire length of the spinal cord, as the **lateral corticospinal tract**, where they terminate

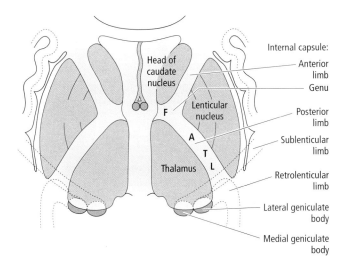

Figure 11.6 ● Horizontal section of the cerebrum showing the anterior limb, genu, and posterior limb of the internal capsule. Note the location of the corticospinal tract axons: A (upper extremity), T (trunk), and L (lower extremity) in the posterior half of the posterior limb of the internal capsule. Fibers carried by the corticonuclear (corticobulbar) tract pass through the genu, F (face).

primarily in the cervical, lumbar, and sacral spinal cord levels (Figs 11.7, 11.8). The remaining 10–15% of the corticospinal tract axons do not decussate but descend ipsilaterally in the anterior funiculus as the smaller, **anterior corticospinal tract**. Axons of the anterior corticospinal tract terminate mainly in the **anterior (ventral) horn gray matter** of the cervical and upper thoracic spinal cord.

Lateral corticospinal tract

> The lateral corticospinal tract mediates the execution of rapid, skilled, voluntary movements of the distal musculature of the upper and lower limbs, especially the intrinsic muscles of the hand

The **lateral corticospinal tract** contains mostly crossed fibers; however, a small percentage of its fibers are uncrossed. This tract contains among its fibers a group of large-diameter myelinated axons arising from the giant Betz cells residing in the primary motor cortex.

Most of the lateral corticospinal tract upper motoneurons projecting to the cervical and lumbosacral spinal cord, end in the **lateral intermediate zone gray matter** (a region of the spinal cord gray matter that is populated by interneurons, and is thus similar to the reticular formation of the brainstem, which also contains interneurons), as well as the **anterior (ventral) horn gray matter** (containing interneurons and lower motoneurons), where they form *excitatory* synapses with **interneurons**. Both the excitatory and inhibitory interneurons synapse with **lower motoneurons**. Excitatory interneurons stimulate the lower motoneurons to cause muscle to contract, whereas the inhibitory interneurons inhibit the lower motoneurons (and may cause muscle to relax). The **first order afferent fibers** transmitting sensory input from the muscle spindles also establish synaptic contacts with the

inhibitory interneurons (receiving input from the corticospinal fibers) in the spinal cord, mediating reflex activity. In contrast, a small number of the lateral corticospinal tract upper motoneurons project to the **anterior (motor) horns** of the spinal cord, where they form *excitatory* synapses directly with lower motoneurons. Many of these monosynaptic connections are with lower motoneurons innervating muscles of the hand.

The giant pyramidal cells, referred to as **Betz cells**, are located exclusively in the primary motor cortex and contribute approximately 3% of the one million fibers in the corticospinal tract. The large-diameter (up to 20 μm) axons of most of the Betz cells descend to synapse only in the lumbar and sacral levels of the spinal cord. Due to their large, myelinated axons, the Betz cells are capable of the fastest nerve impulse transmission to the spinal cord. The remaining (97%) of the corticospinal fibers consist of small-diameter (1–4 μm), slower impulse-conducting fibers. The Betz cell fibers descend to terminate in the lumbar and sacral spinal cord levels where they synapse directly with the lower motoneurons that innervate the musculature of the lower limb. These monosynaptic connections of Betz cells with the lower motoneurons innervating the muscles of the lower limb are actually fewer in number than the monosynaptic connections to lower motoneurons innervating the hand.

Although the lateral corticospinal tract contains mostly crossed fibers, it also contains a minor group of fibers (approximately 2–3%), that do not cross at the pyramidal decussation, but instead descend ipsilaterally. Thus, the lateral corticospinal tract contains both* crossed and uncrossed fibers. At their termination, the uncrossed fibers synapse with the spinal cord **interneurons** mediating movement of the axial (trunk) and proximal limb (girdle) musculature. The uncrossed fibers are associated with the maintenance of upright posture and general orientation of the limbs.

The lateral corticospinal tract mediates the execution of rapid, skilled, voluntary movements of the distal musculature of the upper and lower limbs (i.e., the intrinsic and extrinsic muscles of the hand and foot, especially the muscles of the hand).

Anterior corticospinal tract

> The fibers of the anterior corticospinal tract influence the neurons that innervate the axial and proximal limb (girdle) musculature

The **upper motoneurons** of the **anterior corticospinal tract** do not decussate in the caudal medulla. Instead, they descend in the anterior funiculus of the spinal cord to terminate mainly in the **anterior horn gray matter** of the cervical and upper thoracic spinal cord levels. Near their termination, these fibers decussate to the opposite side of the spinal cord via the anterior white commissure to synapse with **interneurons** that in turn synapse with **lower motoneurons**. Other fibers of the anterior corticospinal tract decussate to the opposite side near their termination and instead synapse directly with lower motoneurons, innervating the axial musculature

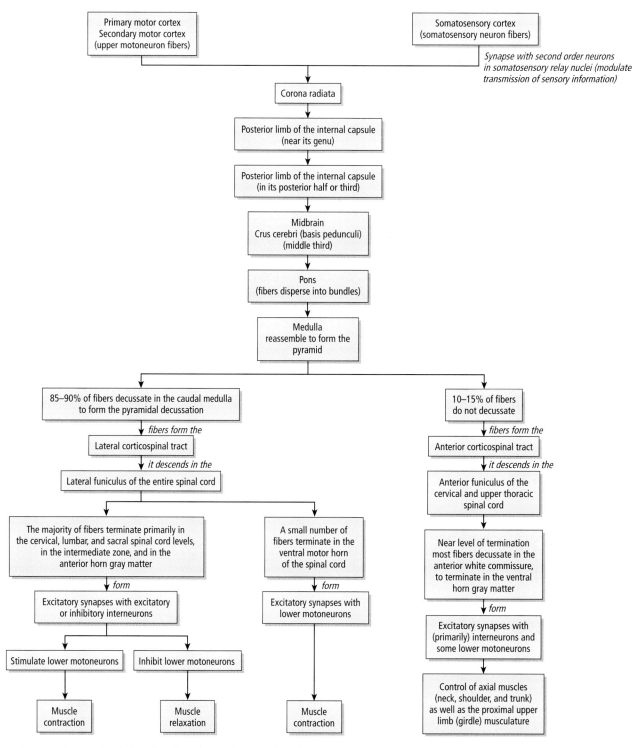

Figure 11.7 ● The origin, course, and termination of the corticospinal tract.

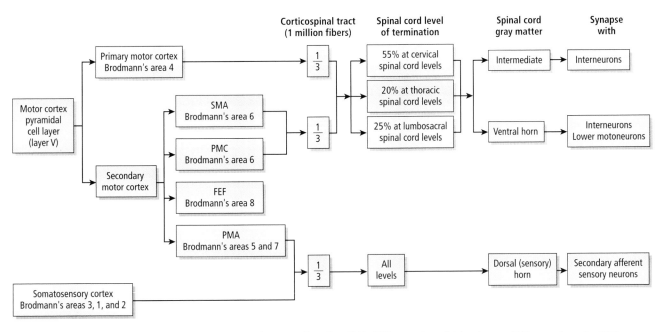

Figure 11.8 ● The origin and termination of the corticospinal tract. FEF, frontal eye fields; PMA, posterior parietal motor area; PMC, premotor cortex; SMA, supplementary motor area.

(such as those of the neck, shoulder, and trunk) as well as the proximal upper limb (girdle) musculature.

Summary of the corticospinal tract

Approximately 55% of the corticospinal tract fibers terminate at cervical spinal cord levels to influence movement of the upper limb musculature, especially the hand

Approximately 55% of all of the corticospinal fibers terminate at cervical levels of the spinal cord, 20% terminate at thoracic levels, and the remaining 25% terminate at lumbar and sacral levels of the spinal cord (Fig. 11.8). The large number of corticospinal fibers terminating at cervical spinal cord levels is an indication of the extensive influence they exert on neurons affecting the motor activity of the upper limb musculature, especially that of the hand.

Corticospinal fibers arising from the somatosensory cortex terminate in the dorsal (sensory) horn of the spinal cord, where they synapse with second order afferent sensory neurons to modulate sensory input (Fig. 11.9). The corticospinal fibers influencing motor activity arise from the motor cortical areas and terminate primarily in the intermediate zone and

Figure 11.9 ● Termination of the corticospinal tracts in the spinal cord. Note that the axons arising from the motor cortex terminate in the ventral horn of the spinal cord where they synapse with interneurons and lower motoneurons that innervate skeletal muscle. In contrast, the axons arising from the sensory cortex terminate in the dorsal horn of the spinal cord where they function in reflexes and modulate the transmission of sensory information to higher brain centers.

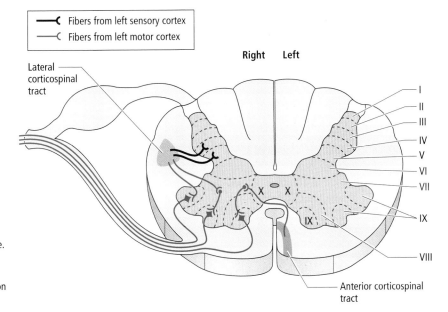

ventral horn gray matter of the spinal cord, where they synapse with interneurons (which in turn synapse with lower motoneurons); whereas a small number of the corticospinal fibers terminate in the ventral horn of the spinal cord, where they synapse directly with lower motoneurons.

The anterior and lateral corticospinal tracts decrease in size at successively lower spinal cord levels, as more and more of their fibers reach their terminations.

The cell bodies of the **lower motoneurons** serving the axial (trunk) and the upper and lower limb musculature, reside in the **anterior (motor) horns** of the spinal cord. More specifically, the cell bodies of the lower motoneurons serving the trunk muscles occupy the medial aspect of the ventral horns, whereas the cell bodies of the lower motoneurons serving the upper and lower limbs reside in the lateral aspect of the ventral horns (Fig. 11.10). The fibers of the lower

motoneurons collect to emerge from the spinal cord as the motor roots of spinal nerves that are a component of the peripheral nervous system.

Although the fibers of the corticospinal tracts terminate principally in the spinal cord, they distribute collaterals to widespread regions of the nervous system in their descent. Collaterals terminate in the ventral nuclei of the thalamus, the basal ganglia, the reticular formation, the red nucleus, the pontine nuclei, the posterior column nuclei, the posterior (sensory) horn of the spinal cord, and the intermediolateral (lateral) cell column (sympathetic) of the spinal cord. Thus, the corticospinal tract probably has more than one function at various levels of the neuronal axis.

Somatosensory fibers influence motor activity

Descending somatosensory fibers synapse with second order sensory neurons in the somatic sensory relay nuclei of the sensory ascending pathways and the sensory nuclei in the dorsal horn of the spinal cord

The **primary somatosensory area**, located in the postcentral gyrus (Brodmann's areas 3, 1, and 2), also projects fibers involved in motor activity to the brainstem and spinal cord. The somatosensory fibers join the upper motoneuron fibers arising from the motor cortex, and accompany them in their descent as the corticospinal tracts, to terminate primarily in the **somatic sensory relay nuclei** of the brainstem and the **dorsal horn** of the spinal cord. The descending somatosensory fibers, however, do not synapse at their termination, with interneurons or motoneurons receiving synapses from the upper motoneurons. Instead, they synapse with the **second order sensory neurons** in the somatic sensory relay nuclei of the sensory ascending pathways (the nucleus gracilis and the nucleus cuneatus of the brainstem), and the sensory nuclei in the dorsal horn of the spinal cord. Their function there is to influence motor activity by modulating the sensory information that is relayed to the brainstem and spinal cord from peripheral structures; thus they are not considered to be upper motoneurons.

Muscle spindle activity

Intrafusal fibers are special stretch receptors dispersed among the extrafusal fibers of a skeletal muscle

Alpha motoneurons innervate the extrafusal fibers of skeletal muscle, whereas gamma motoneurons innervate the intrafusal fibers (housed within the muscle spindles) that are special stretch receptors dispersed among the extrafusal fibers of a muscle. During a normal movement, both the alpha and gamma motoneurons are co-activated. If only the alpha motoneurons innervating a muscle were stimulated, only the extrafusal fibers of the muscle would contract, causing the overall muscle to shorten. Although the intrafusal fibers would passively shorten (because they are attached via connective tissue to the extrafusal fibers), their central

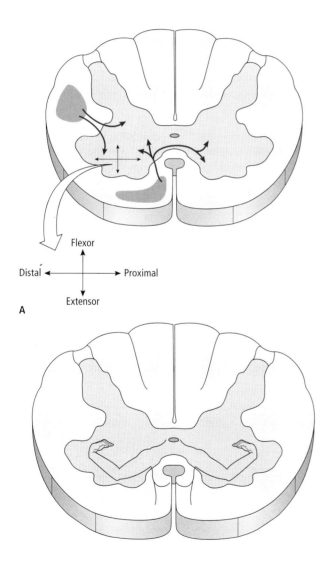

Figure 11.10 ● Somatotopic organization of the anterior horns of the spinal cord. (A) Cross-section of the cervical spinal cord showing the location of motoneurons innervating the upper limb and axial musculature. (B) Cross-section of the cervical spinal cord showing the upper limbs and trunk mapped on the ventral horns of the spinal cord.

noncontractile portion would become slack and be unable to monitor changes in muscle length. Muscle spindles maintain their sensitivity to muscle length, even when the muscle is contracting to a shorter length, via a mechanism known as alpha-gamma co-activation. As the alpha motoneurons stimulate the extrafusal muscle fibers to contract, simultaneously the gamma motoneurons stimulate the contractile portions of the intrafusal fibers to contract. This maintains tension on the central (noncontractile) region of the intrafusal fibers where the sensory endings are located. This alpha-gamma co-activation is necessary to maintain the "stretch sensitivity" of the intrafusal fibers, so that they are ready to detect the slightest stretch at any length (or state of contraction) of the muscle.

Corticonuclear (corticobulbar) tract

The corticonuclear tract fibers terminate not only in their target cranial nerve motor nuclei, but also in the sensory relay nuclei and reticular formation of the brainstem

The corticonuclear tract (Figs 11.11, 11.12; Table 11.1) consists of fibers derived from the primary motor cortex (Brodmann's area 4), the pre-motor cortex (Brodmann's areas 6 and 8), and the somesthetic cortex (Brodmann's areas 3, 1, and 2). The corticonuclear tract, consisting of fibers of **upper motoneurons**, accompanies the corticospinal tract. The two tracts descend in tandem, traversing the **corona radiata** and the **internal capsule** to reach the **crus cerebri (basis pedunculi)** of the midbrain. The corticonuclear tract descends in the internal capsule, but anterior to the corticospinal fibers. The corticonuclear fibers diverge from the corticospinal fibers at various brainstem levels to terminate in their target **cranial nerve somatic motor** or **branchiomotor nuclei**. Similar to the fibers of the corticospinal tracts, some of the corticonuclear fibers synapse directly with motoneurons, but the majority of fibers synapse with **interneurons** housed within the nucleus of termination or with local interneurons of the brainstem reticular formation. The interneurons in turn synapse with the motoneurons of the cranial nerve motor (or branchiomotor) nuclei. The corticonuclear fibers not only terminate in the cranial nerve motor nuclei, but also in the **sensory relay nuclei** (such as the nucleus gracilis, the nucleus cuneatus, the sensory nuclei of the trigeminal nerve, and the nucleus of the solitary tract) and the brainstem **reticular formation**. The corticonuclear fibers affect the motor nuclei of the following cranial nerves: the oculomotor (CN III), trochlear (CN IV), trigeminal (CN V), abducent (CN VI), facial (CN VII), glossopharyngeal (CN IX), vagus (CN X), spinal accessory (XI), and hypoglossal (XII). In general, most cranial nerve motor nuclei receive bilateral projections from the corticonuclear tracts.

Corticonuclear projections to the oculomotor, trochlear, and abducens nuclei

The corticonuclear tract fibers do not project to the oculomotor, trochlear, and abducens nuclei directly. Fibers derived

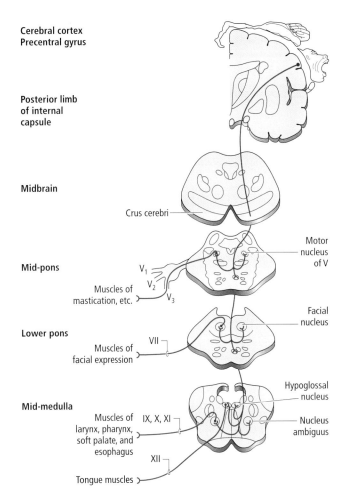

Figure 11.11 ● The origin, course, and termination of the corticonuclear (corticobulbar) tract in the brainstem cranial nerve motor nuclei. (Modified from Watson, C (1995) *Basic Human Neuroanatomy*, 5th edn. Little, Brown & Company, Boston; fig. 22.)

from the **frontal eye field** (Brodmann's area 8) course in the corticonuclear tracts, to terminate in the mesencephalon, specifically in the **superior colliculus**, the **pretectal nuclei**, and the **accessory oculomotor nuclei**. These nuclei then relay inputs to the motor nuclei of the oculomotor, trochlear, and abducent nerves that control eye movements.

Corticonuclear projections to the motor nuclei of the trigeminal and facial nerves

The remaining corticonuclear fibers continue their descent to the pontine and medullary levels (Fig. 11.11), where most of them terminate in the **reticular formation** to synapse with **interneurons** (which in turn synapse with lower motoneurons housed in the cranial nerve motor nuclei). A number of corticonuclear fibers terminate directly and bilaterally in the motor nuclei of the trigeminal and facial nerves.

At the upper pontine levels, some of the fibers diverge from the corticonuclear tract, course into the pontine tegmentum, and terminate bilaterally in the pontine reticular

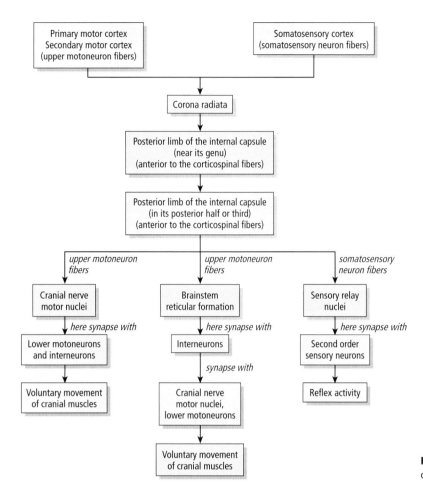

Figure 11.12 ● The origin, course, and termination of the corticonuclear (corticobulbar) tract in the brainstem.

formation and the **motor nucleus of the trigeminal nerve**. The corticonuclear fibers project contralaterally to the lower motoneurons that supply motor innervation to the lateral pterygoid muscle, and bilaterally to the lower motoneurons that innervate the remaining muscles of mastication.

At the midpontine level some of the corticonuclear fibers terminate bilaterally in the facial nucleus, which innervates the muscles of facial expression, the platysma, the posterior belly of the digastric muscle, and the stylohyoid and stapedius muscles. The corticonuclear tract projects bilaterally to the lower motoneurons of the facial nucleus that innervate the muscles of the *upper half* of the face, whereas this same tract projects only contralaterally to the lower motoneurons of the facial nucleus that innervate the muscles of the *lower half* of the face (Fig. 11.13).

Corticonuclear projections to the motor nuclei of the glossopharyngeal, vagus, accessory, and hypoglossal nerves

The remaining corticonuclear fibers terminate in the nucleus ambiguus at caudal pontine levels, the accessory nucleus at

midmedullary levels, and the hypoglossal nuclei at caudal medullary levels.

At the caudal pontine levels and rostral medullary levels, some corticonuclear fibers diverge from the tract to terminate in the **nucleus ambiguus**, a motor nucleus of the glossopharyngeal, vagus, and spinal accessory nerves. These three cranial nerves supply motor innervation to the skeletal muscles of the palate, pharynx, and larynx. The nucleus ambiguus receives bilateral corticonuclear tract projections. A small bundle of corticonuclear fibers, **Pick's bundle**, proceeds inferiorly along with the corticospinal tract to the level of the pyramidal decussation where they cross, then recur and ascend to terminate in the nucleus ambiguus of the opposite side.

At midmedullary levels, some corticonuclear fibers diverge from the corticonuclear tract to terminate primarily in the ipsilateral **accessory nucleus** of the spinal accessory nerve that innervates the sternocleidomastoid and trapezius muscles.

The remaining corticonuclear fibers terminate in the **hypoglossal nuclei** that house the lower motoneurons that innervate the tongue musculature. The corticonuclear fibers project contralaterally on the lower motoneurons that innervate the genioglossus muscle, whereas the remaining

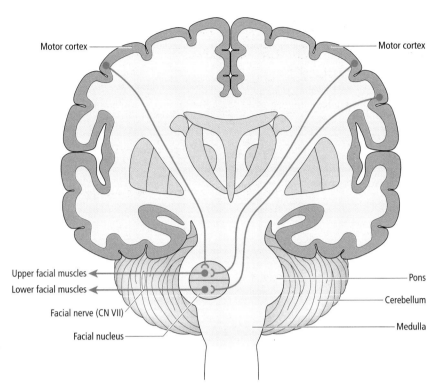

Figure 11.13 ● Corticonuclear (corticobulbar) tract projections to the facial motor nucleus. Note that the upper half of the facial motor nucleus receives bilateral corticonuclear projections, whereas the lower half of the facial motor nucleus receives only contralateral projections.

lower motoneurons that innervate all other tongue musculature receive bilateral projections (with a contralateral predominance).

Corticotectal and tectospinal tracts

The tectospinal tract is involved in the mediation of reflex movements of the eyes, and the cervical and thoracic region of the trunk elicited by visual, auditory, and vestibular stimuli

The visual association areas (Brodmann's areas 18 and 19) give rise to the fibers of the **corticotectal tract** that descend to terminate in the **oculomotor accessory nuclei** (the interstitial nucleus of Cajal, or the nucleus of Darkschewitch) and the deep layers of the **superior colliculus**.

The neurons of the oculomotor accessory nuclei give rise to fibers that join the medial longitudinal fasciculus to terminate in the oculomotor, trochlear, and abducens nuclei, where they influence vertical, rotatory, and smooth pursuit eye movements.

The superior colliculus gives rise to the fibers of the **tectospinal tract** (Fig. 11.14; Table 11.1), which decussates at the level of the red nucleus in the midbrain, and then descends to the medulla, in the medial longitudinal fasciculus. The tectospinal fibers continue their descent in the anterior funiculus of the spinal cord to end at cervical and upper thoracic spinal cord levels where they synapse with interneurons. The tectospinal tract is involved in the mediation of reflex movements of the eyes, and in the cervical and thoracic region of the trunk elicited by visual, auditory, and vestibular stimuli.

Corticorubral, rubrobulbar, and rubrospinal tracts

The rubrospinal tract (and the corticospinal tract) functions in controlling the movement of the hand and digits, by facilitating flexor muscle tone and inhibiting the extensor musculature of the upper limb

The **corticorubral tract** arises from the sensorimotor cortex (similar to the corticospinal tract) and terminates in the ipsilateral red nucleus in the mesencephalon (Fig. 11.15).

The cell bodies in the caudal part of the **red nucleus** give rise to fibers forming the larger **rubrobulbar tract** and the smaller **rubrospinal tract** (which is insignificant in humans). Both of these tracts decussate in the anterior midbrain tegmentum. As the rubrobulbar tract descends, some of its fibers terminate in the principal (main) sensory nucleus of the trigeminal nerve, as well as the subnucleus oralis of the spinal trigeminal nucleus. As other rubrobulbar fibers continue their descent in the brainstem, they terminate in the facial nucleus where they establish synapses with lower motoneurons innervating the muscles of the upper half of the face. Still other rubrobulbar fibers terminate in the lateral reticular nucleus, as well as the nucleus gracilis and nucleus cuneatus in the medulla. The fibers that terminate in the nucleus gracilis and cuneatus modulate the transmission of afferent sensory information to the spinal cord via presynaptic inhibition.

The rubrospinal tract on the other hand, descends in the lateral funiculus of the spinal cord. Its fibers terminate in the lateral intermediate zone and anterior horn of the spinal cord where they synapse with interneurons. The red nucleus facilitates the alpha, beta, and gamma motoneurons that

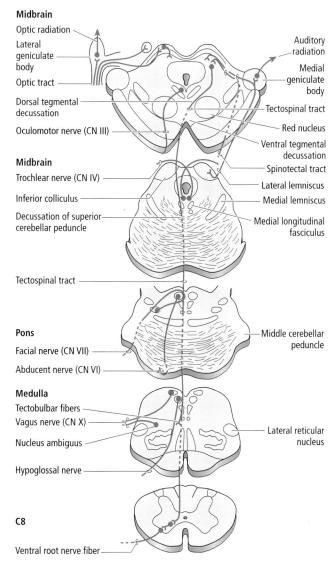

Midbrain
Optic radiation
Lateral geniculate body
Optic tract
Dorsal tegmental decussation
Oculomotor nerve (CN III)

Auditory radiation
Medial geniculate body
Tectospinal tract
Red nucleus
Ventral tegmental decussation
Spinotectal tract

Midbrain
Trochlear nerve (CN IV)
Inferior colliculus
Decussation of superior cerebellar peduncle

Lateral lemniscus
Medial lemniscus
Medial longitudinal fasciculus

Tectospinal tract

Pons
Facial nerve (CN VII)
Abducent nerve (CN VI)

Middle cerebellar peduncle

Medulla
Tectobulbar fibers
Vagus nerve (CN X)
Nucleus ambiguus

Lateral reticular nucleus

Hypoglossal nerve

C8

Ventral root nerve fiber

Figure 11.14 ● The origin, course, and termination of the tectospinal tract. The numbered midbrain structures are: 1, brachium of the superior colliculus; 2, pretectal area; 3, commissure of the superior colliculus; 4, spinotectal tract; 5, fibers from the lateral lemniscus. (Modified from Parent, A (1996) *Carpenter's Human Neuroanatomy*, 9th edn. Williams & Wilkins, Baltimore; fig. 11.18.)

innervate the contralateral upper limb flexor muscles, whereas it simultaneously inhibits those of the extensors, specifically the nerve cells that innervate the distal muscles of the upper limbs. This facilitation and inhibition is mediated by the rubrospinal tract terminating in the spinal cord, and by the rubrobulbar tract which terminates in the flexor region of the medullary reticular formation. The rubrospinal tract (along with the corticospinal tract) functions in controlling the movement of the hand and digits, by facilitating flexor muscle tone and inhibiting the extensor musculature of the upper limb.

Corticoreticular fibers and reticulospinal tracts

The reticulospinal tracts influence the motor control of axial (trunk) and proximal limb musculature and are involved in posture maintenance and orientation of the limbs in an intended direction

The sensorimotor cortex sends bilateral projections via the **corticoreticular fibers** which course with the corticonuclear and the corticospinal tracts to several nuclei dispersed in the brainstem (pontine and medullary) reticular formation. The reticular nuclei also receive an input from the cerebellum, the vestibular nuclei, and nociceptive fibers from the spinal cord.

Neurons in the pontine reticular nuclei (reticularis pontis oralis and caudalis) give rise to fibers that form the **medial (pontine) reticulospinal tract**, which descends ipsilaterally in the anterior funiculus of the spinal cord. These fibers terminate and synapse with spinal cord interneurons and gamma motoneurons at all levels of the spinal cord. The pontine reticular fibers stimulate extensor muscle and inhibit flexor muscle movements (Fig. 11.15).

The **lateral (medullary) reticulospinal tract** arises from the nucleus reticularis gigantocellularis and descends bilaterally in the lateral funiculus of the spinal cord. Nerve fibers terminate at all spinal cord levels, where they synapse mainly with interneurons in the intermediate zone gray matter of the spinal cord. The medullary reticular fibers have an inhibitory effect on extensors and an excitatory affect on flexors. The lateral reticulospinal tract also relays an autonomic input to the sympathetic and parasympathetic neurons of the spinal cord, which mediate autonomic functions such as pupillary dilation, heart rate modulation, and sweating (Fig. 11.15).

These two tracts influence the motor control of axial (trunk) and proximal limb musculature and are involved in posture maintenance and orientation of the limbs in an intended direction.

Vestibulospinal tracts

The lateral vestibulospinal tract is involved in the maintenance of posture and balance; the medial vestibulospinal tract mediates head movement while maintaining gaze fixation on an object

The vestibular nuclei receive sensory input related to head movement from the vestibular apparatus of the inner ear via the vestibular division of the vestibulocochlear nerve (CN VIII) and to balance from the cerebellum. The **lateral vestibulospinal tract** arises from the lateral vestibular nucleus (Fig. 11.16). This tract contains ipsilateral fibers that descend in the anterior funiculus to end at all spinal cord levels, to synapse mainly with excitatory interneurons. These interneurons stimulate motoneurons that innervate axial (trunk) and proximal limb extensor muscles, and simultaneously inhibit lower motoneurons that innervate limb flexor muscles. This tract is involved in the maintenance of posture and balance by specifically facilitating motoneurons that innervate the antigravity muscles (extensor muscle tone of the antigravity muscles). This tract also mediates head and neck movements in response to vestibular sensory input.

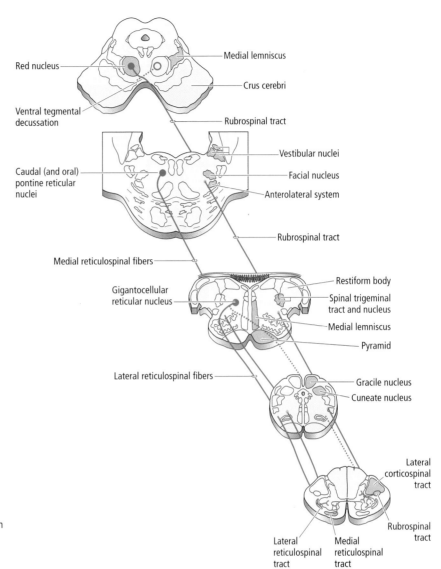

Figure 11.15 ● The origin, course, and termination of the rubrospinal and reticulospinal tracts. (Modified from Haines, DE (2002) *Fundamental Neuroscience*. Churchill Livingstone, Philadelphia; fig. 24.9.)

The **medial vestibulospinal tract** arises from the medial vestibular nucleus (Fig. 11.16). This tract descends mostly ipsilaterally in the medial longitudinal fasciculus of the brainstem, and then in the anterior funiculus of the cervical and upper half of the thoracic spinal cord. Its fibers synapse with interneurons that synapse with alpha and gamma motoneurons. Some fibers terminate on alpha motoneurons directly. These fibers exert their influence on neurons of the cervical spinal cord (maintaining equilibrium elicited by vestibular input), and mediating head movement while maintaining gaze fixation on an object.

Functional classification of the descending motor pathways

The descending motor pathways are classified into three **functional** categories: the ventromedial (anteromedial) group,

the lateral group, and the cortical group. In general, the fibers of each of these functional groups synapse in the gray matter that is in close proximity to their position in the white matter. That is, the fibers of the ventromedial group synapse in the medial aspect and intermediate zone of the spinal cord gray matter, whereas the fibers of the lateral group synapse in the lateral aspect and intermediate zone of the spinal cord gray matter. Furthermore, the lower motoneurons that innervate the flexor muscles occupy a region of gray matter that is posterior to the lower motoneurons innervating the extensor muscles (Figs 11.10A, 11.17).

The ventromedial group of the descending motor pathways controls the axial and proximal limb musculature for balance maintenance and postural adjustment

The **ventromedial group** consists of the anterior corticospinal tract, the medial and lateral vestibulospinal tracts,

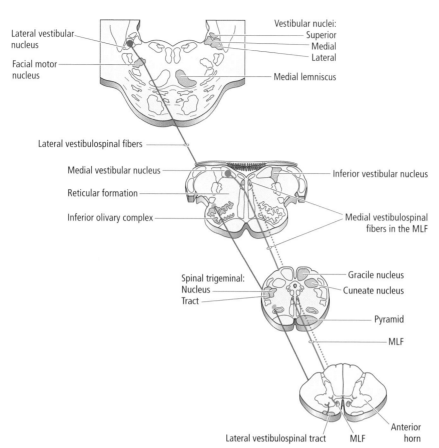

Figure 11.16 ● The origin, course, and termination of the medial and lateral vestibulospinal tracts. MLF, medial longitudinal fasciculus. (Modified from Haines, DE (2002) *Fundamental Neuroscience*. Churchill Livingstone, Philadelphia; fig. 24.7.)

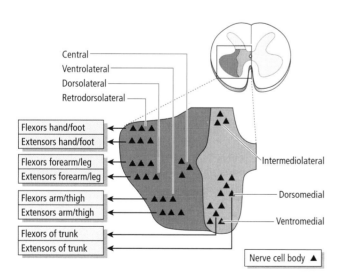

Figure 11.17 ● Somatotopic organization of the ventral horn of the spinal cord. (Modified from Fitzgerald, MJT (1996) *Neuroanatomy Basic and Clinical*, 3rd edn. WB Saunders, Philadelphia; fig. 13.1.)

the medial and lateral reticulospinal tracts, and the tectospinal tract, which are all located in the anterior funiculus of the spinal cord and synapse in the medial aspect of the anterior horn and intermediate zone (Figs 11.9, 11.17). These pathways project bilaterally, controlling the axial and proximal limb musculature of both sides. These tracts function in the bilateral control of gross movements of the axial and proximal limb musculature for balance maintenance and during postural adjustments.

The lateral group of the descending motor pathways controls the proximal, and especially the distal, musculature of the upper and lower limbs

The **lateral group** consists of the lateral corticospinal and the rubrospinal tracts, located mostly in the lateral funiculus of the spinal cord. The fibers of these two tracts synapse in the lateral aspect and intermediate zone of the ventral horn of the spinal cord (Figs 11.10A, 11.17). The rubrospinal tract extends only to the first cervical level of the spinal cord and does not have a very important function in humans. These tracts (mainly the corticospinal tract) function in the control of, in particular, the distal but also of the proximal musculature of the upper and lower limbs, as well as mediating independent digit movements.

The cortical group innervates the distal muscles of the limbs, especially those of the hands

The **cortical group** consists of lateral corticospinal tract fibers that synapse directly with lower motoneurons, particularly the neurons whose fibers innervate the distal muscles of the limbs, such as the intrinsic muscles of the hand. This tract is involved in independent, fractionated movements of the digits.

The lower motoneurons are referred to as the **final common pathway** because they are influenced by the corticospinal, tectospinal, rubrospinal, reticulospinal, vestibulospinal, and reflex neurons. All input is ultimately funneled to the lower motoneurons that innervate the skeletal muscles directly.

Note that the clinical case at the beginning of the chapter refers to a patient who has a motor disturbance in both the upper and lower limbs.

1 Which descending motor pathway has been affected in this patient?

CLINICAL CONSIDERATIONS

Corticospinal and corticonuclear tracts

A lesion in the corticonuclear and/or corticospinal tracts is known as an upper motoneuron lesion

Since the **corticospinal tract** projects from the cerebral cortex through the corona radiata, the internal capsule, the cerebral peduncle, the pons, the medulla, and the entire spinal cord, it is vulnerable to lesions from various sources throughout its path. The most common **corticospinal tract lesion** results from a cerebral vascular accident (a stroke). A stroke can result either from a vascular hemorrhage or a vascular occlusion resulting from a thrombus (loose clot or an air bubble). The middle cerebral artery is buried in the lateral fissure separating the parietal from the temporal lobe, and gives rise to branches that supply structures in the frontal, parietal, and temporal lobes. Many of its branches perforate the cerebral hemisphere to reach deep subcortical structures such as the basal ganglia and the internal capsule. A cerebral vascular accident affecting the internal capsule is referred to as a **capsular stroke**. Since both the corticonuclear and corticospinal tracts course in the internal capsule, a capsular stroke can result in considerable upper motoneuron damage, referred to as an **upper motoneuron (UMN) lesion**. The most prominent physical deficit resulting from damage of the corticospinal tract fibers is a **contralateral hemiplegia (paralysis)** of the upper and lower limbs and extensor plantar response (**Babinski's sign**). Normally, when the plantar surface of the foot is stimulated, the foot reflexly plantarflexes (toes curl down) mediated by the corticospinal tract. In an individual with a corticospinal tract lesion, however, stimulation of the plantar surface of the foot elicits hyperextension of the foot accompanied by dorsiflexion of the great toe and by a fanning of the remaining toes (Babinki's sign). In the absence of the corticospinal tract, this pathologic response is mediated by the descending motor pathways arising from the brainstem. An upper motoneuron lesion also results in **spasticity** in the affected limb(s). Spasticity results following damage to neurons of the primary motor cortex *and* neurons of the secondary motor cortex.

If the **corticonuclear tract** fibers are damaged, the individual will exhibit a weakness of the **contralateral lower face**, and the tongue will deviate toward the impaired side when the patient attempts to protude it. There is weakness of the contralateral lower face because the lower half of the facial motor nucleus receives only contralateral projections from the motor cortex, whereas the upper half of the facial motor nucleus receives bilateral projections from the motor cortex.

Primary motor cortex

A unilateral lesion in the primary motor cortex results in a contralateral flaccid paralysis

An individual who has a **unilateral** lesion confined to the **primary motor cortex (M-I)**, will at first experience a **contralateral flaccid paralysis** in the affected muscles on the contralateral side of the body. After about 2 weeks, the individual will recover function in the affected proximal limb (girdle) muscles; however, the paralysis will persist in the distal muscles of the limbs. This type of lesion will affect mainly the fine movements of the contralateral distal limbs, particularly those of the hand. Although there is recovery of some of the motor functions of the limbs, the individual will not have the fractionated, independent control of the distal muscles of the limbs. When attempting to flex a single finger, all fingers flex concurrently. A lesion confined to the primary motor cortex will not cause a total motor deficit since the tectospinal, reticulospinal, and vestibulospinal tracts and upper motoneurons from the secondary motor cortex will supply motor input to the interneurons and lower motoneurons. Lesions confined to the primary motor cortex are rare. If the lesion also involves Brodmann's area 6, the paralysis will persist and **spasticity** will appear in the distal limb muscles.

Supplementary motor area

A lesion in the supplementary motor area does not cause paralysis, but instead results in the inability to coordinate hand movements bilaterally

A **lesion** confined to the **supplementary motor area** will result in the inability to coordinate hand movements bilaterally. The individual can execute the same motor activity with both hands (concurrently); however, when attempting to simultaneously execute a *different* motor activity with each hand, it may seem complicated and impossible to accomplish.

Premotor cortex

A lesion in the premotor cortex will result in difficulty in performing voluntary movements (apraxia), not paralysis

A lesion confined to the **premotor cortex** typically does not cause paralysis. Instead, an individual with a lesion in the premotor cortex will have difficulty executing voluntary movements with the involved body part, contralateral to the side of the lesion. If the upper limb is affected, the individual will have difficulty in picking up a glass of water or using a fork, in the absence of perceptible changes in muscle tone, spasticity, or paralysis.

Lower motoneuron lesions

A **lower motoneuron (LMN) lesion** is a lesion involving: (i) the cell bodies of the lower motoneurons residing in the cranial nerve motor nuclei or the ventral horn of the spinal cord; or (ii) the axons of the lower motoneurons coursing in a cranial nerve or other peripheral nerve. A LMN lesion results in **flaccid paralysis** and severe **atrophy** and **fasciculations** in the denervated muscle(s).

Note that the clinical case at the beginning of the chapter refers to a patient who has a motor disturbance in both the upper and lower limbs. Symptoms include muscle weakness, flaccidity, atrophy, and fasciculations, and bilateral, pathologically brisk deep tendon reflexes, and a bilateral Babinski response.

2 Based on this patient's symptoms, which neurons have been selectively affected?

3 What are the symptoms following an upper motoneuron lesion?

4 What are the symptoms following a lower motoneuron lesion?

SYNONYMS AND EPONYMS OF THE MOTOR CORTEX AND DESCENDING MOTOR PATHWAYS

Name of structure or term	Synonym(s)/eponym(s)	Name of structure or term	Synonym(s)/eponym(s)
Alpha (α) motoneuron	Lower motoneuron	Layer V of the cerebral cortex	Internal pyramidal layer
Anterior (ventral) horn of the spinal cord	Motor horn of the spinal cord	Gamma (γ) motoneuron	Lower motor neurons
		Medial reticulospinal tract	Pontine reticulospinal tract
Axial	Trunk	Mesencephalon	Midbrain
Basal ganglia	Basal nuclei	Muscle spindle	Neuromuscular spindle
	Deep cerebral nuclei	Oculomotor accessory nuclei	Interstitial nucleus of Cajal and nucleus of Darkschewitch
Central sulcus	Central sulcus of Rolando		
Cerebral vascular accident (CVA)	Stroke	Posterior (dorsal) horns of the spinal cord	Sensory horns of the spinal cord
Corticonuclear tract	Corticobulbar tract (older term)		
Corticoreticular and reticulospinal tracts	Corticoreticulospinal pathway	Posterior parietal motor area (PMA)	Brodmann's areas 5 and 7
		Premotor area	Premotor cortex
Corticorubral and rubrospinal tracts	Corticorubrospinal pathway		Part of Brodmann's area 6
Corticospinal tract	Pyramidal tract (older term)	Primary motor cortex (M-I)	Precentral gyrus
Corticotectal and tectospinal tracts	Corticotectospinal pathway		Brodmann's area 4
Dorsal (posterior) column nuclei	Nucleus gracilis (NG) and nucleus cuneatus (NC)	Primary somatosensory cortex (S-I)	Primary sensory cortex (S-I)
			Primary somesthetic cortex
Extensor plantar response	Babinski's sign		Brodmann's areas 3, 1, and 2
Extrafusal muscle fibers	Skeletal muscle fibers (of gross muscle)		Post central gyrus
		Principal nucleus of the trigeminal nerve	Main nucleus of the trigeminal nerve
Lower motoneurons	Lower motoneuron		
Intermediolateral cell column	Lateral cell column		Chief nucleus of the trigeminal nerve
	Lateral horn	Proximal limb musculature	Girdle musculature
Interneuron	Internuncial neuron	Red nucleus	Nucleus ruber
Intrafusal muscle fibers	Skeletal muscle fibers of muscle spindles	Somatosensory cortex	Somesthetic cortex
		Supplementary motor area (SMA)	Supplementary motor cortex
Lateral reticulospinal tract	Medullary reticulospinal tract		Part of Brodmann's area 6

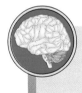

FOLLOW-UP TO CLINICAL CASE

Both the history and the clinical exam are very important for the diagnosis in this case. This patient has **amyotrophic lateral sclerosis** (ALS), commonly known in the USA as Lou Gehrig's disease. This is a neurodegenerative disease affecting only the motor system. Sensory and cognitive functions remain intact throughout the disease. ALS characteristically leads to death of both the upper motoneurons in the motor cortex and also the lower motoneurons in the anterior horns of the spinal cord. It is the most common of the motoneuron diseases—diseases which affect, specifically, the upper and/or lower motoneurons.

The combination of the signs and symptoms of ALS is usually unmistakable. Upper motoneuron loss produces pathologically brisk reflexes, Babinski reflexes (extension of the big toe in response to a scratch of the lateral aspect of the bottom of the foot), and sometimes spasticity or "stiffness" of an extremity. Lower motoneuron loss leads to flaccid weakness, atrophy, and fasciculations. Both types of lesions can cause weakness. Head imaging is typically normal.

Electromyography will confirm or refute the presence of motor neuron disease (that which affects the lower motoneurons). This is an electrical test of muscle fiber physiology, and gives information about the integrity of the motor unit (a lower motoneuron, its axon, and all of the muscle fibers that it innervates).

ALS is a devastating disease. It is more common in older age groups, but the average person affected by it is middle aged or a bit older. This disease leads to relentless progression of muscle weakness, causing the individual to become wheelchair-bound and eventually incapacitated. Distal muscles in one arm or leg, or bulbar muscles (e.g., speech) are affected first. Any muscle group can be a target, and eventually the muscles of breathing become affected. Death from respiratory failure or another intervening illness, such as pneumonia, typically occurs a few or several years from initial diagnosis. The vast majority of cases of ALS are sporadic. A small percentage of cases are hereditary. The pathophysiology is unknown and there is no effective treatment.

5 What tells you that this patient's symptoms are caused by a neurodegenerative disorder and not a stroke?

QUESTIONS TO PONDER

1. How do the intrafusal fibers of muscle spindles maintain sensitivity to detect the slightest stretch of the gross muscle, even during the contracted state?

2. As you are sitting in class looking at the screen in front of the room, you hear a loud, startling noise in the back of the room, as several large books fall from the bookshelf. The entire class turns in unison toward the back of the room to see the source of the noise. Which of the descending motor pathways is involved in the reflex turning of the eyes, head, and upper trunk, in the direction of the source of the noise?

3. Why does an individual who has suffered a stroke from a lesion confined to the primary motor cortex recover some of the crude motor function in the affected part of the body?

4. A capsular stroke damaged the upper motoneuron fibers descending in the posterior half of the posterior limb of the internal capsule, on the right side of the brain. In which parts of the body do you expect to see motor deficits?

5. Which of the three functional groups of the descending motor pathways are involved in mediating independent, fractionated movements of the digits, especially those of the hand?

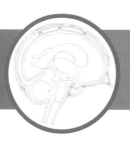
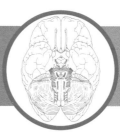
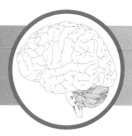

CHAPTER 12

Basal Ganglia

CLINICAL CASE

A 39-year-old man has had abnormal and uncontrollable movements for the past 6 months, as well as forgetfulness, obsessions, and compulsions. His wife notes some mild personality changes as well. He has become somewhat more irritable and withdrawn. These movements are spontaneous, unpredictable, and have become almost continuous. Initially his wife thought he had become "fidgety." Abnormal behaviors as well as the extraneous movements have caused some social embarrassment. The patient's mother died in her fifties at a psychiatric hospital. He has no more information about her. Family history is otherwise unrevealing.

Examination shows obvious chorea consisting of involuntary, nonrhythmic, and persistent jerky movements of the head, neck, and arms that continue during conversation. Memory is mildly diminished. He seems very distractible and has difficulty completing motor tasks. Neurologic exam is otherwise unremarkable. MRI of the brain shows atrophy of the heads of both caudate nuclei.

Normal **motor function** is the result of the intricate interaction of the basal ganglia, cerebellum, and cerebral cortex. The **basal ganglia** initiate motor activity and modulate cortical output related to motor function. The **cerebellum** functions in the coordination of movement, whereas the **cerebral cortex** is involved in the planning and execution of voluntary movement. The basal ganglia and cerebellum exert their influence on the brainstem and spinal cord, and ultimately on motor activity *indirectly*, by regulating the output of the cerebral cortex via the thalamus. The cerebral cortex then influences the execution of motor activity via *direct* projections to the brainstem nuclei (i.e., the cranial nerve motor nuclei, nuclei of the reticular formation, midbrain tectum, and red nucleus) and spinal cord motoneurons.

The function of the basal ganglia is influenced by input arising not only from primary sensory and sensory association areas of the cerebral cortex of all four lobes, but also from the thalamus and brainstem. All four lobes of the cerebrum, the thalamus, and the brainstem project to the input nuclei of the basal ganglia, mainly to the caudate nucleus and putamen. These input nuclei then project to the globus pallidus, which in turn relays basal ganglial output via the thalamus to the motor and other areas of the frontal cortex (Fig. 12.1).

Although more is known about the role of the basal ganglia in motor functions, numerous studies support the finding that they also have other, nonmotor functions as well. Disturbances of the neural connections of the basal ganglia result not only in movement disorders, but also considerable deficits in other, nonmotor functions including cognition, perception, and emotional behaviors.

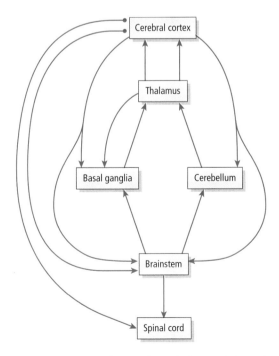

Figure 12.1 ● Connections between the cerebral cortex, thalamus, basal ganglia, cerebellum, brainstem, and spinal cord.

Ultimately, outflow from the basal ganglia reaching the cerebral cortex has an impact not only on motor activity, but also on other functions as diverse as sensorimotor integration, and cognitive and emotional behaviors.

COMPONENTS OF THE BASAL GANGLIA

The caudate nucleus, the putamen, and the nucleus accumbens form the striatum (neostriatum); the striatum and the globus pallidus form the corpus striatum

The term **basal ganglia** is a misnomer since these structures consist of an assortment of subcortical *nuclei*, rather than *ganglia*. The criterion used by early neuroanatomists for the classification of the basal ganglia was any structure composed of gray matter that is embedded deep within, and close to the basal aspect of, the cerebral hemispheres. Thus, previously, the components of the basal ganglia included the caudate nucleus, putamen, nucleus accumbens, globus pallidus, thalamus, subthalamic nucleus, amygdala, and claustrum. In more recent years, however, neuroanatomists include in the basal ganglia only those deep nuclei of the cerebrum which, when damaged, produce movement disorders.

From a clinical perspective, the components of the basal ganglia involved in motor function are the caudate nucleus, putamen, globus pallidus, and subthalamic nucleus (all of which are embedded deep in the cerebral hemispheres), as well as another nucleus, the substantia nigra, which is really located in the midbrain, but is functionally related to the basal ganglia.

The **caudate nucleus** and the **putamen** share an embryologic derivation as well as similar morphological characteristics. Hence they are considered to be a single anatomical structure and are collectively referred to as the **striatum (neostriatum, caudatoputamen)** (Tables 12.1, 12.2). The ventral portions of the head of the caudate nucleus, the putamen, the anterior perforated substance, and the nucleus accumbens together are referred to as the **ventral striatum**.

Anatomically, the striatum (caudate nucleus, putamen, and nucleus accumbens) and the globus pallidus (paleostriatum) collectively form the **corpus striatum**. The putamen is the most massive nucleus of the corpus striatum. The ventral component of the globus pallidus is the **ventral pallidum**.

In addition to the components mentioned so far, the following structures are functionally related to the basal ganglia: the **ventral anterior**, **ventral lateral**, **mediodorsal**, and **intralaminar nuclei of the thalamus**, and the **amygdala** of the limbic system (Table 12.3).

In this chapter, the basal ganglia consist of the **caudate nucleus**, the **lenticular nucleus** with its two components (the **putamen** and **globus pallidus**), and the **nucleus accumbens**; and, since the **subthalamic nucleus** of the ventral thalamus and the **substantia nigra** of the mesencephalon are functionally connected to the corpus striatum, and produce movement disorders when damaged, they are also included. The thalamus, nucleus accumbens, and amygdala do not produce movement disorders when damaged.

Table 12.1 ● Classification of the basal ganglia.

Basal ganglia	Striatum (neostriatum, caudatoputamen)	Ventral striatum	Lenticular (lentiform nucleus)	Corpus striatum
Caudate nucleus Putamen Globus pallidus Subthalamic nucleus (of ventral thalamus) Substantia nigra (of the mesencephalon)	Caudate nucleus Putamen	Ventral portion of caudate nucleus Putamen Anterior perforated substance Nucleus accumbens	Putamen Globus pallidus	Caudate nucleus Putamen Globus pallidus

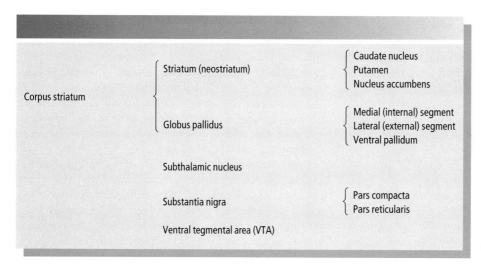

Table 12.2 ● Basal ganglia and associated structures.

Nucleus	Location	Function
Thalamic Ventral anterior (VA) Ventral lateral (VL) Mediodorsal (MD)	Diencephalon	Relay signals related to movement form the basal ganglia to the frontal cortex Relay signals from the basal ganglia to the frontal cortex association areas (which play a role in executive functions) and limbic areas (which play a role in processing of emotions)
Centromedian (CM) Parafascicular (PF)		Relay information from the thalamus (via thalamostriate fibers) to the caudate nucleus, putamen, and ventral striatum
Amygdaloid	Temporal lobe	Emotional and motivational aspects of movement
Claustrum	Between the external and extreme capsules in the telencephalon	Unknown

Table 12.3 ● Nuclei associated with the basal ganglia

It is important to note that the **thalamus** does not only serve as a relay nucleus for *sensory* information to the somatosensory cortex, but also as a relay nucleus for *motor* information that arises from the basal ganglia and the cerebellum that is destined for the motor cortex.

Caudate nucleus

The caudate nucleus consists of a head, body, and tail, and is located in the walls of the lateral ventricle

The **caudate nucleus** (L. cauda, "tail") is a C-shaped structure that is subdivided into a head, body, and tail

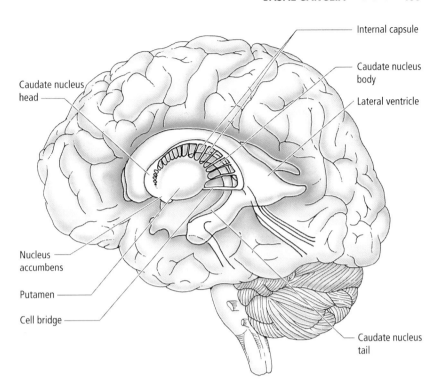

Figure 12.2 ● The caudate nucleus, putamen, and nucleus accumbens and their anatomical relation to the ventricular system.

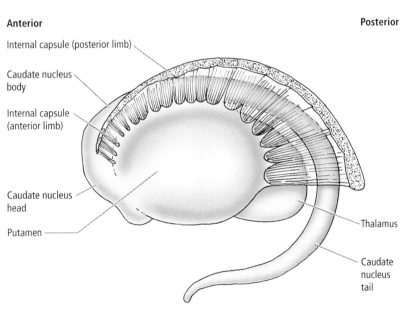

Figure 12.3 ● Lateral view of the corpus striatum and its anatomical relation to the internal capsule.

(Fig. 12.2). Its dilated, somewhat bulbous, rostral end is referred to as the **head of the caudate nucleus**. It is located in the lateral wall of the anterior horn of the lateral ventricle and is continuous ventrally with the putamen (Fig. 12.3). Near the interventricular foramen, the head is continuous with the long, curved **body of the caudate nucleus**, which courses posteriorly and lies on the floor of the lateral ventricle. Near the posterior end of the thalamus, the body decreases in diameter and continues as the long, narrow **tail of the caudate nucleus**. The tail gradually bends ventrally and then anteriorly within the lateral ventricle passing along the roof of its inferior horn and extending into the temporal lobe as far anteriorly as the amygdaloid nucleus. The internal capsule separates the caudate nucleus from the lenticular nucleus.

Lenticular (lentiform) nucleus

The lenticular nucleus is composed of the putamen and the globus pallidus

The biconvex **lenticular nucleus** is located between the insula and the anterior and posterior limbs of the internal capsule. It is separated from the caudate nucleus by the anterior limb of the internal capsule and from the thalamus by the posterior limb of the

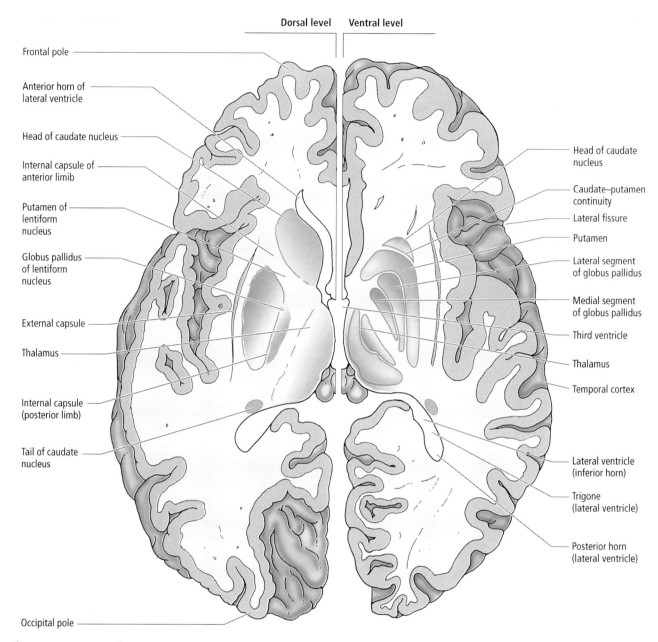

Dorsal level | Ventral level

Frontal pole

Anterior horn of lateral ventricle

Head of caudate nucleus

Internal capsule of anterior limib

Putamen of lentiform nucleus

Globus pallidus of lentiform nucleus

External capsule

Thalamus

Internal capsule (posterior limb)

Tail of caudate nucleus

Occipital pole

Head of caudate nucleus

Caudate–putamen continuity

Lateral fissure

Putamen

Lateral segment of globus pallidus

Medial segment of globus pallidus

Third ventricle

Thalamus

Temporal cortex

Lateral ventricle (inferior horn)

Trigone (lateral ventricle)

Posterior horn (lateral ventricle)

Figure 12.4 ● Horizontal sections through the dorsal level (left) and the ventral level (right) of the corpus striatum.

internal capsule. The lenticular nucleus is divided by myelinated fibers, the lateral (external) medullary lamina, into its two component parts: the laterally positioned, convex putamen and the medially placed globus pallidus (Fig. 12.4).

The **globus pallidus** (L. globus, "globe;" pallidus, "pale") is wedge-shaped on coronal and horizontal sections. Due to its many myelinated fibers it appears paler in fresh specimens than the putamen. A group of myelinated fibers, the medial (internal) medullary lamina, divides the globus pallidus into a medial (internal, inner) segment (GPm) and a lateral (external, outer) segment (GPl). The GPm is embryologically related to the diencephalon and the subthalamus (ventral thalamus), and gives rise to the major output from the basal ganglia.

Although, as indicated above, the lenticular nucleus and the caudate nucleus are separated by the internal capsule, the rostral extent of the **putamen** is connected to the head of the caudate nucleus by bridge-like extensions of gray matter. During early developmental stages, the growing axons of the internal capsule perforated the gray matter of the fused caudate nucleus and putamen (Fig. 12.2). These extensions form a distinct ventral portion of the striatum, the ventral striatum, which via its connections is associated with the limbic system. The intervals between these extensions are traversed by the somewhat vertically oriented, slender but prominent fiber bundles of the anterior limb of the internal capsule (see Fig. 12.3). Thus, in fresh brain sections, the region between

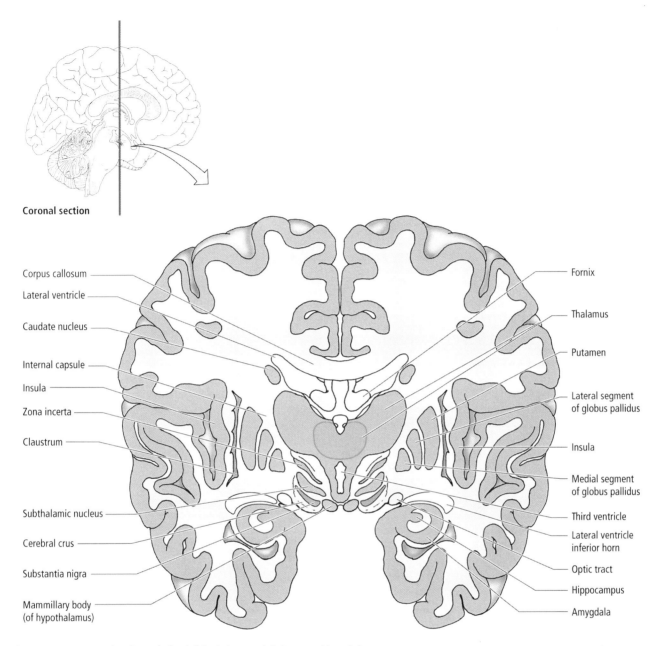

Coronal section

Corpus callosum
Lateral ventricle
Caudate nucleus
Internal capsule
Insula
Zona incerta
Claustrum
Subthalamic nucleus
Cerebral crus
Substantia nigra
Mammillary body (of hypothalamus)

Fornix
Thalamus
Putamen
Lateral segment of globus pallidus
Insula
Medial segment of globus pallidus
Third ventricle
Lateral ventricle inferior horn
Optic tract
Hippocampus
Amygdala

Figure 12.5 ● Coronal section at the level of the thalamus, subthalamus, and hypothalamus.

the caudate nucleus and the lenticular nucleus exhibits alternating stripes of gray matter and white matter. It was named the **corpus striatum** (L., "striped body") based on this striping pattern.

Nucleus accumbens

The nucleus accumbens is associated with the limbic system, and processes the emotional aspects of movement

The **nucleus accumbens** is a component of the striatum. It resides ventral to the anterior limb of the internal capsule and is connected to the caudate nucleus and the putamen. It receives input information from the limbic system and is involved in the processing of the emotional aspects of movement (see Fig. 12.2).

Subthalamic nucleus (nucleus of Luys)

The subthalamic nucleus is a component of the subthalamus

The **subthalamic nucleus**, a component of the subthalamus, is an oval-shaped, biconvex mass of gray matter that lies lateral to the hypothalamus on the medial aspect of the internal capsule (Fig. 12.5). Its function is not known.

Substantia nigra

The substantia nigra is the largest nucleus of the midbrain, and consists of two components: the pars reticulata and pars compacta

The **substantia nigra** (L., "black substance") extends from the rostral end to the caudal end of the mesencephalon dorsal to the

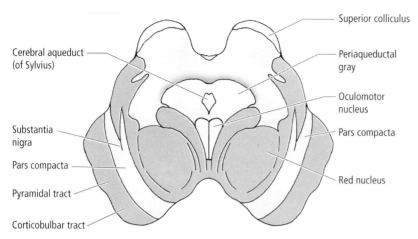

Figure 12.6 ● Transverse section of the rostral midbrain, showing the substantia nigra.

cerebral peduncle. It is composed of two distinct parts: a ventral, cell-sparse, reticular part, the pars reticulata (reticularis) and a dorsal, cellular, compact part, the pars compacta (Fig. 12.6).

The cell-sparse **pars reticulata** consists of: (i) neuron terminals arising from the midbrain raphe nuclei, which release serotonin; and (ii) striatonigral nerve terminals, which release gamma aminobutyric acid (GABA). Although the pars reticulata contains numerous nerve terminals, it is a nuclear structure and also contains nerve cell bodies. The pars reticulata is continuous with, and shares many histologic characteristics with, the **medial segment** of the **globus pallidus**. Furthermore, similar to the globus pallidus, this portion of the substantia nigra receives projections from the striatum and sends its GABAergic neurons to the thalamus. Both the medial segment of the globus pallidus, and the pars reticulata of the substantia nigra, give rise to the *output* of the basal ganglia; due to their similarities and continuity they are considered to be the same structure.

The cellular **pars compacta** consists of pigmented dopaminergic neurons containing neuromelanin. These neurons give rise to the nigrostriatal dopaminergic pathway that projects to the striatum. More over, the dendritic extensions of these dopaminergic neurons extend into the pars reticulata.

NUCLEI ASSOCIATED WITH THE BASAL GANGLIA

Thalamic nuclei

The basal ganglia are interconnected with the ventral anterior, ventral lateral, medial dorsal, and intralaminar nuclei of the thalamus

The **ventral anterior** and the **ventral lateral nuclei of the dorsal thalamus** (often referred to as the "thalamic motor nuclei") relay movement-related signals from the basal ganglia to the frontal cortex.

The **medial dorsal nucleus of the thalamus** relays signals from the basal ganglia to frontal cortex association areas as well as to limbic areas. These areas play a role in cognitive functions and the processing of emotions, respectively.

The **centromedian** and **parafascicular nuclei**, two of the **intralaminar nuclei of the thalamus** representing the rostral extent of the ascending reticular activating system (ARAS), receive inputs from the spinothalamic, trigeminothalamic, and multisynaptic ascending pathways (of the reticular formation) relaying pain sensation. These nuclei relay this information to the somatosensory areas of the cerebral cortex and the caudate nucleus, putamen, and ventral striatum (see Fig. 12.5; Table 12.3). Based on these connections, these nuclei are believed to function in sensorimotor integration. In addition, as a result of their diffuse cortical connections, they are believed to be involved in the maintenance of arousal of the organism as it relates to pain.

Amygdaloid nucleus (amygdala)

The amygdaloid nucleus is a component of the limbic system and is related to the basal ganglia via neural connections

The **amygdaloid nucleus** is located in the temporal lobe, deep to the uncus. Although the amygdaloid nucleus is related to the basal ganglia via neural connections, it is anatomically and functionally part of the limbic system (Fig. 12.7; Table 12.3).

Claustrum

The **claustrum** consists of a slender layer of gray matter, which is separated medially from the convex surface of the putamen by the external capsule, and laterally from the insula by a thin layer of white matter, the extreme capsule. Connections to the basal ganglia have not been established, and its function is as yet unknown (Fig. 12.8; Table 12.3).

INPUT, INTRINSIC, AND OUTPUT NUCLEI OF THE BASAL GANGLIA

The basal ganglia are intricately and extensively interconnected with various regions of the central nervous system (CNS). Viewed from the perspective of their connections, the

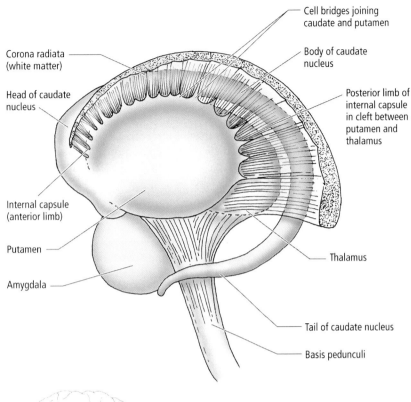

Figure 12.7 ● Lateral view of the corpus striatum, amygdala, thalamus, and internal capsule.

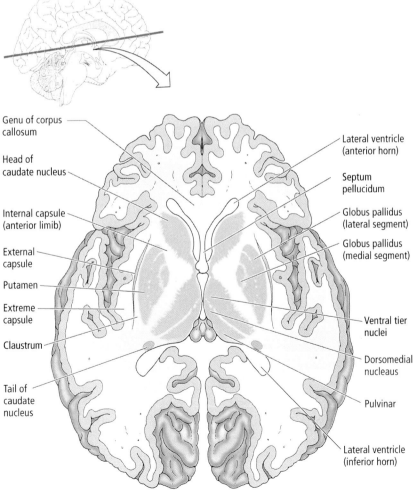

Figure 12.8 ● Horizontal section of the brain at the level of the basal ganglia.

Input nuclei	Intrinsic nuclei	Output nuclei
Caudate nucleus	Globus pallidus (external segment)	Globus pallidus (internal segment)
Putamen	Subthalamic nucleus	Substantia nigra (pars reticulata)
Nucleus accumbens	Substantia nigra (pars compacta)	Ventral pallidum

Table 12.4 ● Input, intrinsic, and output nuclei of the basal ganglia.

component nuclei of the basal ganglia may be assigned into three categories: **input nuclei**, **intrinsic nuclei**, and **output nuclei** (Table 12.4).

Input nuclei

The input nuclei of the basal ganglia are the caudate nucleus, putamen, and nucleus accumbens

The caudate nucleus, putamen, and the nucleus accumbens are the **input nuclei** of the basal ganglia. They receive a prominent *excitatory* input from all four lobes of the cerebral cortex as well as from the thalamus, subthalamus, substantia nigra, and other brainstem structures. Most of the input terminates in the caudate nucleus and the putamen. These input nuclei then relay the information to the intrinsic and output nuclei. The caudate nucleus and the putamen function in the initiation and modulation of gross voluntary movements that are performed at the subconscious level, whereas the nucleus accumbens is associated with the processing of the emotional aspects of movement.

Intrinsic nuclei

The intrinsic nuclei of the basal ganglia are the lateral segment of the globus pallidus, the subthalamic nucleus, and the pars compacta of the substantia nigra

The **intrinsic nuclei** consist of the lateral segment of the globus pallidus, the subthalamic nucleus, and the pars compacta of the substantia nigra. These nuclei are not only interconnected by their local circuit projections, but are also connected with the input and output nuclei. Although the subthalamic nucleus is a source of *excitatory* signals, most local synapses are *inhibitory*.

Both the globus pallidus and the subthalamic nucleus function in the control of the axial and girdle (proximal limb) musculature. The responsibility of these nuclei is to position and stabilize the trunk and proximal parts of the upper and lower limbs, so that the distal limb musculature moving the hands and feet are able to perform the more discreet movements that are controlled by the motor cortex. This concept is consistent with the observation that neural activity in the globus pallidus precedes that of the motor cortex.

Output nuclei

The output nuclei of the basal ganglia are the medial segment of the globus pallidus, the pars reticulata of the substantia nigra, and the ventral pallidum

The **output nuclei** consist of the medial segment of the globus pallidus, the pars reticulata of the substantia nigra, and the ventral pallidum.

Output from the basal ganglia is *inhibitory* (GABAergic), passing from the medial segment of the globus pallidus and from the pars reticulata of the substantia nigra mainly to the thalamus, via the pallidothalamic and nigrothalamic fibers, respectively. However, fibers from these nuclei also project to the subthalamic nuclei, the brainstem, and the cerebral cortex.

The basal ganglia exert their influence on motor activity *indirectly* by controlling the premotor and supplementary motor areas of the cerebral cortex. and *not* by direct projections to the brainstem and spinal cord motoneurons. Note that although all four lobes of the cerebral cortex project to the basal ganglia, output from the basal ganglia terminates exclusively in the frontal lobe of the cerebrum.

CONNECTIONS OF THE BASAL GANGLIA

The basal ganglia have the following characteristics:

* they receive **input fibers** from various sources outside the basal ganglia;
* they are interconnected by **local (intrinsic) fiber projections**; and
* they project **output fibers** to other areas of the brain that are involved in motor function.

Striatum

Afferent fibers (input)

The caudate nucleus and the putamen are the principal input nuclei of the basal ganglia

The caudate nucleus and the putamen are the principal input nuclei of the basal ganglia. The caudate nucleus is associated primarily with cognitive functions and less with motor activity, whereas the putamen is associated primarily with motor functions. The caudate nucleus and putamen receive the following **afferent (input) fibers** (Fig. 12.9; Table 12.5):

* corticostriate fibers;
* thalamostriate fibers;
* nigrostriate fibers;
* fibers from the ventral tegmental area; and
* fibers from the brainstem pedunculopontine tegmental nucleus (PPN).

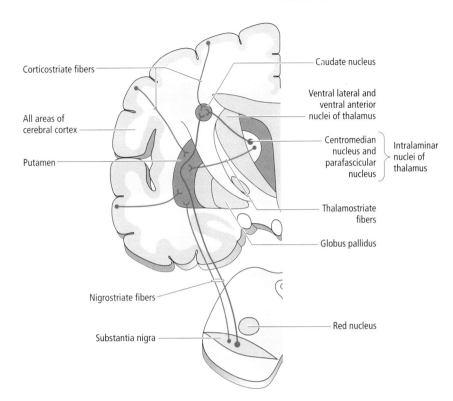

Figure 12.9 ● Afferent (input) projections to the caudate nucleus and putamen. (Modified from Watson, C (1995) *Basic Human Neuroanatomy*, 5th edn. Little, Brown & Company, Boston; fig. 39.)

Table 12.5 ● Afferent (input) fibers to the striatum.

Fibers	Origin	Termination	Neurotransmitter (and type)
Corticostriate	Sensory cortex (Brodmann's areas 3, 1 and 2) Primary motor cortex (Brodmann's area 4) Premotor cortex (Brodmann's area 6) Supplementary motor cortex (Brodmann's area 6)	Putamen	Glutamate (excitatory) *or* Aspartate (excitatory)
	Frontal eye field association areas of arebral cortex	Caudate nucleus	Glutamate (excitatory) Aspartate (excitatory)

Thalamostriate	Intralaminal nuclei of the thalamus
	    Centromedian nucleus
	    Parafascicular nucleus
	Ventral anterior and ventral lateral nuclei of the thalamus
		Caudate nucleus and putamen	Glutamate (excitatory)

Nigrostriate	Substantia nigra
	    Pars compacta
	    Pars reticulata
		Caudate nucleus and putamen	Dopamine (inhibitory)

Other	Ventral tegmental area (VTA) Pedunculopontine tegmental nucleus (PPN)	Ventral striatum Caudate nucleus, putamen, pallidum, and subthalamic nucleus	Dopamine (inhibitory) Serotonin (inhibitory)

Corticostriate fibers

The corticostriate fibers form the principal input to the basal ganglia

The **corticostriate fibers** arise from widespread areas of the cerebral cortex (neocortex), mainly from its motor and somatosensory areas. Each cortical part projects fibers that descend in the internal or external capsules to the **caudate** **nucleus** and the **putamen**, and they release the excitatory neurotransmitters glutamate or aspartate at their termination. Fibers arising from the primary sensory (Brodmann's areas 3, 1, and 2), primary motor (Brodmann's area 4), premotor (Brodmann's area 6), and supplementary motor (Brodmann's area 6) cortex terminate principally in the putamen. Fibers arising from the frontal eye fields (Brodmann's area 8) and association areas of the cortex terminate principally in the caudate nucleus. Moreover, some corticostriate fibers arising from the motor and premotor cortices terminate in the subthalamic nucleus of the striatum.

Thalamostriate fibers

The thalamostriate fibers arise from the intralaminar nuclei of the thalamus and form the second major input to the basal ganglia

The intralaminar (centromedian and parafascicular) nuclei of the thalamus are the cranial continuation of the midbrain reticular formation into the diencephalon and are components of the reticular activating system (RAS). These nuclei receive nociceptive signals via reticulothalamic fibers (of the anterolateral system) and, as components of the RAS, function in alerting the individual and to elicit responses that will enable it to evade painful stimuli.

The **thalamostriate fibers** are excitatory, they terminate mainly in the **putamen** and the **caudate nucleus**, and they release glutamate. In addition, the striatum also receives input fibers from the ventral anterior and ventral lateral nuclei of the thalamus. The function of these latter projections is not yet known.

Nigrostriate fibers

The **nigrostriate fibers** arise from the pars compacta of the substantia nigra and terminate primarily in the **caudate nucleus**, although some fibers terminate in the **putamen**. These predominantly uncrossed fibers are inhibitory or excitatory and release dopamine at their termination.

Fibers from the ventral tegmental area and pedunculopontine tegmental nucleus

The striatum also receives inhibitory dopaminergic nerve fiber terminals from the ventral tegmental area and serotonergic nerve fibers from the pedunculopontine tegmental nucleus

The fibers from the **ventral tegmental area** terminate primarily in the nucleus accumbens of the ventral striatum, and the cerebral cortex. These projections function in the initiation of behavioral responses.

The fibers arising from the brainstem **pedunculopontine tegmental nucleus** terminate in the **caudate nucleus**, **putamen**, **pallidum**, and **subthalamic nucleus**. These inhibitory fibers release serotonin at their termination. The pedunculopontine nucleus may function in the rhythm of movements.

Efferent fibers (output)

Although the caudate nucleus and putamen receive inputs from multiple sources, their output fibers are funneled only to the pallidum and substantia nigra

Although the caudate nucleus and putamen receive inputs from multiple sources such as the cerebral cortex, thalamus, and brainstem, their output fibers are funneled only to the pallidum and substantia nigra.

The **caudate nucleus** and the **putamen** give rise to the following **efferent (output) fibers** (Fig. 12.10; Table 12.6):

- striatopallidal fibers; and
- striatonigral fibers.

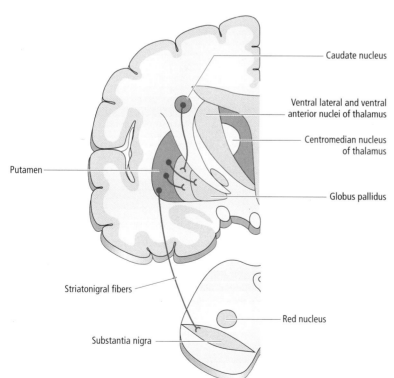

Figure 12.10 ● Efferent (output) projections from the caudate nucleus and putamen. (Modified from Watson, C (1995) *Basic Human Neuroanatomy*, 5th edn. Little, Brown & Company, Boston; fig. 40.)

Fibers	Origin	Termination	Neurotransmitter (and type)

Striatopallidal	Caudate nucleus and putamen	Globus pallidus
		   Internal segment (GPi)
		   External segment (GPe)
			
			GABA and substance P
			GABA and enkephalin

Striatonigral	Caudate nucleus and putamen	Substantia nigra (pars reticulata)	GABA, ACh, or substance P

ACh, acetylcholine; GABA, gamma aminobutyric acid.

Table 12.6 ● Efferent (output) fibers from the striatum.

Striatopallidal fibers

> The striatopallidal fibers terminate in both segments of the globus pallidus

The **striatopallidal fibers** that terminate in the lateral segment of the globus pallidus liberate GABA and enkephalin, whereas those fibers that terminate in the medial segment of the globus pallidus release GABA and substance P.

Striatonigral fibers

The **striatonigral fibers** terminate in the pars reticulata of the substantia nigra. These fibers release GABA, acetylcholine, or substance P.

Globus pallidus

The medial and lateral segments of the **globus pallidus** receive inputs from the same regions but their output projections differ.

Afferent fibers (input)

Both segments of the globus pallidus receive the following **afferent (input) fibers** (Fig. 12.11; Table 12.7):

- striatopallidal fibers; and
- subthalamopallidal fibers.

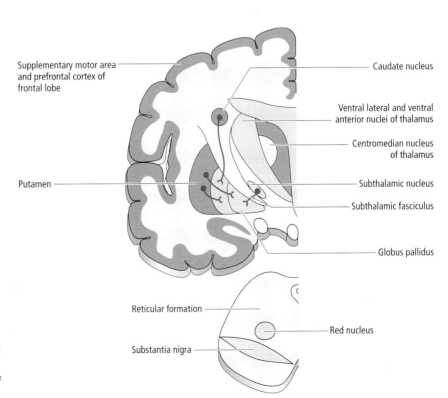

Figure 12.11 ● Afferent (input) projections to the globus pallidus. (Modified from Watson, C (1995) *Basic Human Neuroanatomy*, 5th edn. Little, Brown & Company, Boston; fig. 41.)

Fibers	Origin	Termination	Neurotransmitter (and type)
Striatopallidal	Caudate nucleus Putamen	Globus pallidus (both segments)	GABA and enkephalin (both are inhibitory) *or* GABA (inhibitory) and substance P (excitatory)
Subthalamopallidal	Subthalamic nucleus	Globus pallidus (mainly internal segment)	Glutamate (excitatory)

GABA, gamma aminobutyric acid.

Table 12.7 ● Afferent (input) fibers to the globus pallidus.

Striatopallidal fibers

> The striatopallidal fibers arising from the caudate nucleus and the putamen form the principal input to the globus pallidus

As discussed above, the **striatopallidal fibers** arising from the caudate nucleus and the putamen release GABA and enkephalin or GABA and substance P, and form the *principal input* to the globus pallidus.

Subthalamopallidal fibers

The **subthalamopallidal fibers** arise from the subthalamic nucleus, form the subthalamic fasciculus, and terminate mainly in the medial segment of the globus pallidus. These *excitatory* fibers release glutamate at their termination.

Efferent fibers (output)

> The medial and lateral segments of the globus pallidus each gives rise to well-defined output fibers

Even though the medial and lateral segments of the globus pallidus share both morphological and neurochemical characteristics, each gives rise to well-defined output fibers (Fig. 12.12).

Output from the lateral segment of the globus pallidus

The **lateral segment of the globus pallidus** gives rise to:

- pallidosubthalamic fibers;
- pallidonigral fibers; and
- other fiber projections that terminate in the striatum, reticular thalamic nucleus, and the medial segment of the globus pallidus (Table 12.8).

Pallidosubthalamic fibers

> Pallidosubthalamic fibers arise only from the lateral segment of the globus pallidus

The **pallidosubthalamic fibers** arise only from the lateral segment of the globus pallidus. They join the subthalamic

fasciculus, which terminates in the subthalamic nucleus and sends collateral branches to the pars reticulata of the substantia nigra. These fibers are inhibitory, and release GABA at their terminals.

Pallidonigral fibers

> The pallidonigral fibers arise from the lateral segment of the globus pallidus and terminate in the pars compacta of the substantia nigra

The **pallidonigral fibers** are inhibitory and release GABA at their termination. In addition, the lateral segment of the globus pallidus also relays signals to the reticular nucleus of the thalamus, which assists in the integration of reciprocal connections between the thalamus and the cortex.

Output from the medial segment of the globus pallidus

The **medial segment of the globus pallidus** gives rise to:

- pallidothalamic fibers whose two components are the ansa lenticularis and the lenticular fasciculus (Fig. 12.13);
- pallidotegmental fibers; and
- pallidohabenular fibers (Table 12.8).

The medial segment of the globus pallidus is the main output station of the corpus striatum.

Pallidothalamic fibers

> The pallidothalamic fibers have two main components: the ansa lenticularis and the lenticular fasciculus

The ventral part of the medial segment of the globus pallidus gives rise to a group of the **pallidothalamic fibers** that course ventromedially, and then rostrally, to form a loop, the **ansa lenticularis**, on the medial aspect of the posterior limb of the internal capsule. The ansa lenticularis then courses posteriorly, in the prerubral field (H field of Forel).

The dorsal part of the medial segment of the globus pallidus gives rise to another group of pallidothalamic fibers that course medially, traversing the posterior limb of the internal capsule. Medial to the subthalamus, these fibers assemble to form the **lenticular fasciculus** (H_2 field of Forel).

The pallidothalamic fibers coursing in the lenticular fasciculus subsequently join the pallidothalamic fibers of the ansa lenticularis, to form a prominent fiber bundle known as the

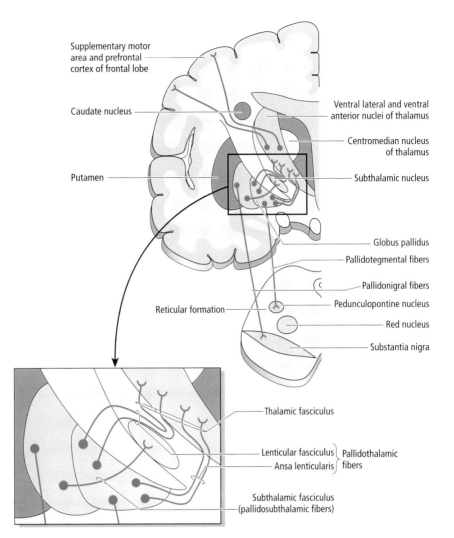

Figure 12.12 ● Efferent (output) projections from the globus pallidus. (Modified from Watson, C (1995) *Basic Human Neuroanatomy*, 5th edn. Little, Brown & Company, Boston; fig. 42.)

Fibers	Origin	Termination	Neurotransmitter (and type)
Pallidosubthalamic	Globus pallidus (external segment)	Subthalamic nucleus and collateral branches to the substantia nigra (pars reticulata)	GABA
Pallidonigral	Globus pallidus (external segment)	Substantia nigra (pars compacta)	GABA
Pallidothalamic Ansa lenticularis Lenticular fasciculus	Globus pallidus (internal segment)	Thalamic nuclei: ventral anterior (VA) ventral lateral (VL) mediodorsal (MD) centromedian (CM) parafascicular (PF)	
Pallidotegmental	Globus pallidus (internal segment)	Pedunculopontine tegmental nucleus (PPN)	
Pallidohabenular	Globus pallidus (internal segment)	Lateral habenular nucleus	
Other	Globus pallidus (external segment)	Striatum Reticular thalamic nucleus Globus pallidus (internal segment)	

Table 12.8 ● Efferent (output) fibers from the globus pallidus.

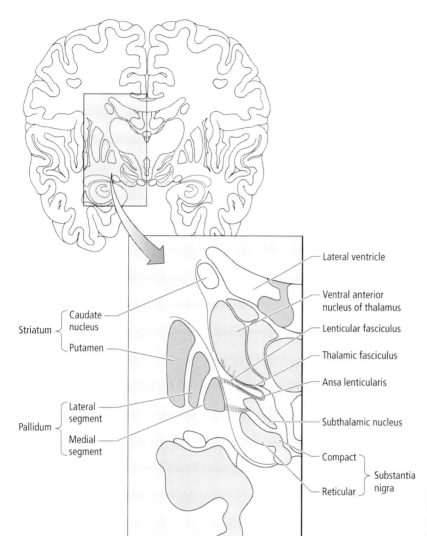

— Lateral ventricle

— Ventral anterior
nucleus of thalamus

— Lenticular fasciculus

— Thalamic fasciculus

— Ansa lenticularis

— Subthalamic nucleus

Caudate
nucleus

Striatum

Putamen

Lateral
segment

Pallidum

Medial
segment

Compact ⎤
⎬ Substantia
Reticular ⎦ nigra

Figure 12.13 ● Principal output connections of the basal ganglia arising from the globus pallidus: the ansa lenticularis and lenticular fasciculus. These two fasciculi merge to form the thalamic fasciculus.

H_1 field of Forel. This bundle proceeds medially and caudally to the prerubral field (H field of Forel) rostral to the red nucleus. The fibers then form a loop and course to the thalamus collectively as the **thalamic fasciculus** (H_1 field of Forel). The thalamic fasciculus terminates in the ventral anterior, ventral lateral, medial dorsal, centromedian, and parafascicular nuclei of the thalamus. The thalamus in turn projects to the primary motor cortex as well as to the supplementary motor area and premotor cortex of the secondary motor cortex, all of which contribute fibers to the corticonuclear, corticospinal, and corticopontocerebellar tracts. The signals arising from the basal ganglia that are relayed to the spinal cord via the contralateral lateral corticospinal tracts are involved in limb movements. Recall that the ventral anterior and ventral lateral nuclei of the thalamus are considered to be the "thalamic motor nuclei" since they receive signals related to motor function and send signals to the motor areas of the cortex.

Note that the output fibers arising from the basal ganglia and the fibers arising from the cerebellum that are destined for the ventral anterior and ventral lateral nuclei of the thalamus,

do not overlap at their terminations. They terminate in distinct areas of these thalamic nuclei.

Pallidotegmental fibers

The pallidotegmental fibers arise from the medial segment of the globus pallidus and terminate in the pedunculopontine nucleus (PPN) in the inferior tegmentum of the mesencephalon

The pallidotegmental fibers arise from the medial segment of the globus pallidus and terminate in the PPN in the inferior tegmentum of the mesencephalon. The PPN, a nucleus of the reticular formation, is associated with the reticulospinal tract cells, which terminate on lower motoneurons and affect motor function.

Pallidohabenular fibers

Pallidohabenular fibers course in the ansa lenticularis and lenticular fasciculus, and then the stria medullaris

The pallidohabenular fibers arise from the medial segment of the globus pallidus, course in the ansa lenticularis and lenticular fasciculus in the H field of Forel, and then join the stria medullaris to terminate in the lateral habenular nucleus.

The habenular nucleus, a component of the habenular nuclear complex of the epithalamus, is associated with the limbic system.

CIRCUITS CONNECTING THE BASAL GANGLIA, THALAMUS, AND CEREBRAL CORTEX

The four separate systems of circuits of the basal ganglia are arranged in parallel

The four separate systems of circuits (paths) of the basal ganglia are arranged in parallel. Each circuit relays distinct input from various areas of the cerebral cortex to the basal ganglia where information is integrated. The integrated information is relayed to the thalamus and then to different areas of the frontal cortex where the execution of motor activity is initiated.

Each **circuit** consists of "closed loop" and "open loop" components. In the "closed loop" component, information arising from a particular cortical area is relayed through the circuit back to its initial cortical source. In the "open loop" component, information (arising from cortical areas that have a similar function as the initial cortical area of the closed loop), is relayed to the cortical source of the closed loop.

Although in the previous paragraphs careful attention was paid to maintain a difference between "circuits" and "loops," in reality these terms are used synonymously. The four loops described below are really circuits, each with closed loop and open loop components.

Each system of circuits consists of many distinct parallel circuits, with each circuit having a specific function. One circuit within a particular system may be associated with a specific movement of the foot, whereas another circuit in the same system may be associated with the same type of movement of the hand.

The following circuits (loops) have been identified: a motor loop, an oculomotor loop, an association loop, and a limbic loop.

Sensory-motor loop

The basal ganglia influence motor activity by projections to the motor cortex

Signals from the basal ganglia are relayed to the motor cortical areas via the motor loop where they influence the upper motoneurons of the corticospinal, corticonuclear, and other descending motor tracts, which in turn influence the lower motoneurons of the brainstem and spinal cord, and ultimately motor activity.

The motor areas, as well as various other cortical areas, give rise to a massive number of **corticostriate fibers**, which terminate in the **caudate nucleus** and **putamen** (Fig. 12.14).

In the **closed loop**, a stream of corticostriate fibers arising from the **supplementary motor cortex** (Brodmann's area 6) project mostly to the putamen, the "sensory-motor area" of the striatum as well as to the caudate nucleus. The putamen projects to both the medial and lateral segments of the **globus**

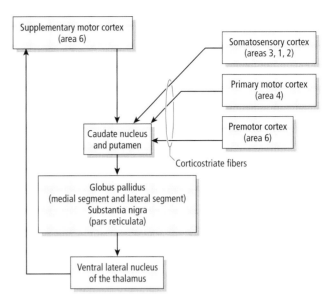

Figure 12.14 ● Sensory–motor loops. In the closed loop, information flows from the supplementary motor cortex to the caudate nucleus and putamen, and from there to the globus pallidus and the substantia nigra, continuing to the thalamus and then back to the supplementary motor cortex. In the open loop, input is contributed by the somatosensory cortex, primary motor cortex, and premotor cortex to the closed loop. (Modified from Noback, CR *et al.* (1996) *The Human Nervous System*, 5th edn. Williams & Wilkins, Baltimore; fig. 24.5.)

pallidus and the pars reticulata of the **substantia nigra**, all of which in turn project to the **ventral lateral nucleus of the thalamus**. Thalamocortical fibers from the ventral lateral nucleus of the thalamus project back to the **supplementary motor cortex**, completing the loop.

In the **open loop**, corticostriate fibers arising from the **primary motor cortex** (Brodmann's area 4), the **premotor cortex** (Brodmann's area 6), and the **somatosensory cortex** (Brodmann's areas 3, 1, and 2) are channeled to the putamen. From there the information continues through the motor circuit to terminate in the **supplementary motor cortex**, which is the origin of the closed loop.

In the **sensory-motor loop**, signals from the basal ganglia are relayed to the motor cortical areas of the **frontal lobe**. There they exert their influence by planning the sequence of actions in order to execute learned motor activities. This influence is exerted on the upper motoneurons, which in turn influence (via the corticonuclear and corticospinal tracts) the lower motoneurons of the brainstem and spinal cord, and ultimately motor activity.

Oculomotor loop

The oculomotor loop has an important function in the control of voluntary saccadic ocular movements

In the **closed loop**, **corticostriate fibers** arising from the **frontal eye field** (Brodmann's area 8) of the cerebral cortex project to the body of the **caudate nucleus** (Fig. 12.15). The caudate nucleus projects to the medial segment of the **globus pallidus** and the pars reticulata of the **substantia nigra**.

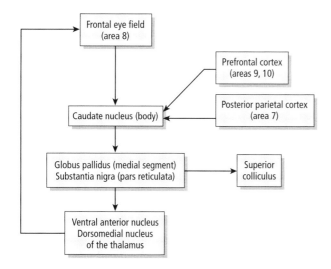

Figure 12.15 • Oculomotor loops. In the closed loop, information flows from the frontal eye field to the caudate nucleus and then to the globus pallidus and the substantia nigra and from there to the thalamus and then back to the frontal eye field. In the open loop, input is contributed by the prefrontal cortex and the posterior parietal cortex to the closed loop. (Modified from Noback, CR *et al*. (1996) *The Human Nervous System*, 5th edn. Williams & Wilkins, Baltimore; fig. 24.7.)

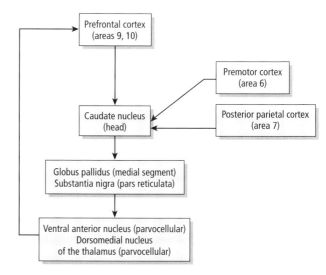

Figure 12.16 • Association loops. In the closed loop, information flows from the prefrontal cortex to the caudate nucleus and then to the globus pallidus and the substantia nigra and from there to the thalamus and then back to the prefrontal cortex. In the open loop, input is contributed by the premotor and posterior parietal cortex to the closed loop. (Modified from Noback, CR *et al*. (1996) *The Human Nervous System*, 5th edn. Williams & Wilkins, Baltimore; fig. 24.6.)

Pallidothalamic and nigrothalamic fibers project to the **ventral anterior** and **dorsomedial nuclei of the thalamus**. Thalamocortical fibers project back to the **frontal eye field**, closing the loop.

In the **open loop**, corticostriate fibers arising from the **prefrontal cortex** (Brodmann's areas 9 and 10) and the **posterior parietal cortex** (Brodmann's area 7) terminate in the body of the caudate nucleus. The signals are relayed through the circuit to terminate in the frontal eye field, which is the origin of the closed loop. The globus pallidus and the substantia nigra also relay this information to the deep layers of the **superior colliculus**.

The **oculomotor loop** has an important function in the control of voluntary saccadic ocular movements.

Association (cognitive) loop

The association loop functions in the planning of motor activity and determining the direction of movement

In the **association loop** various association cortical areas of all four lobes project mainly to the ipsilateral head of the **caudate nucleus**, which is the "association area" of the striatum (Fig. 12.16).

In the **closed loop**, **corticostriate fibers** arising from the **prefrontal cortex** (Brodmann's areas 9 and 10), project to the head of the caudate nucleus, which in turn projects to the medial segment of the **globus pallidus** and to the pars reticulata of the **substantia nigra**. They in turn project to the **ventral anterior** and **dorsomedial nuclei of the thalamus**. Thalamocortical fibers terminate in the prefrontal cortex, closing the loop.

In the **open loop**, corticostriate fibers arising from the **premotor cortex** (Brodmann's area 6) and the **posterior parietal motor area** (Brodmann's area 7) project to the head of the caudate nucleus. The signals are relayed through the circuit to the prefrontal cortex, the origin of the closed loop.

The association (cognitive) loop functions in the planning of motor activity and determining the direction of movement.

Limbic loop

The limbic loop functions in the emotional and motivational aspects of movement, manifested as various facial expressions or other body movements

In the **closed loop**, **corticostriate fibers** arising from the **anterior cingulate gyrus** (Brodmann's area 24) and the **orbitofrontal cortex** (Brodmann's areas 10 and 11) project to the **ventral striatum (nucleus accumbens)** and the head of the **caudate nucleus** (Fig. 12.17). They, in turn, project to the **ventral pallidum**, the medial segment of the **globus pallidus**, and the pars reticulata of the **substantia nigra**. Fibers arising from these areas project to the **ventral anterior** and **dorsomedial nuclei of the thalamus**. Thalamocortical fibers terminate in the anterior cingulate gyrus and the orbitofrontal cortex, closing the loop.

In the **open loop**, corticostriate fibers arising from the **medial** and **lateral temporal lobe**, the **hippocampus**, the **amygdala**, and the **entorhinal area** project to the ventral striatum (nucleus accumbens) and to the head of the caudate nucleus. The signals are relayed through the circuit to terminate in the anterior cingulate gyrus and the orbitofrontal cortex, which is the origin of the closed loop.

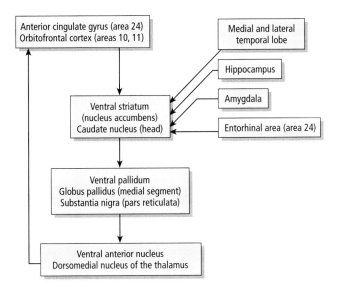

Figure 12.17 ● Limbic loops. In the closed loop information flows from the anterior cingulate gyrus and orbitofrontal cortex to the ventral striatum and the caudate nucleus and then to the ventral pallidum, globus pallidus, and substantia nigra, and from there to the thalamus and then back to the anterior cingulate gyrus and orbitofrontal cortex. In the open loop, input is contributed by the medial and lateral temporal lobe, hippocampus, amygdale, and entorhinal area to the closed loop. (Modified from Noback, CR *et al.* (1996) *The Human Nervous System*, 5th edn. Williams & Wilkins, Baltimore; fig. 24.8.)

The **limbic loop** functions in the emotional and motivational aspects of movement, manifested as various facial expressions or other body movements.

OTHER CIRCUITS OF THE BASAL GANGLIA

Other circuits of the basal ganglia involve the substantia nigra, subthalamic nucleus, and the pedunculopontine nucleus (Table 12.9).

Substantia nigra

Afferent fibers (input)

The two regions of the **substantia nigra**, the pars reticulata and the pars compacta, both receive **afferents (input)** from:

- the striatum, via striatonigral fibers;
- the globus pallidus, via pallidonigral fibers; and
- the subthalamic nucleus.

Efferent fibers (output)

The substantia nigra sends fibers to:

- the ventral lateral, ventral anterior, and medial dorsal nuclei of the thalamus; and
- the striatum.

The former is via inhibitory GABAergic nigrothalamic fibers arising from the pars reticulata—which also sends collateral branches to the midbrain superior colliculus and tegmental area. The latter sends inhibitory dopaminergic nigrostriatal fibers arising from the pars compacta.

Subthalamic nucleus

Afferent fibers (input)

The **subthalamic nucleus** receives **afferents (input)** from:

- the lateral segment of the globus pallidus that provides GABAergic fibers, the most prominent subcortical input to the subthalamic nucleus;
- the motor cortex; and
- the pedunculopontine nucleus (PPN), whose fibers are cholinergic.

Nucleus	Afferents	Efferents
Substantia nigra	Striatum Globus pallidus Subthalamic nucleus	Ventral anterior (VA), ventral lateral (VL), and mediodorsal (MD) nuclei of the thalamus Striatum
Subthalamic nucleus	External segment of the globus pallidus Motor cortex Pedunculopontine nucleus Midbrain raphe nucleus Ventral median nucleus of the thalamus	Internal segment of the globus pallidus External segment of the globus pallidus Pars reticulata of the substantia nigra Ventral pallidum
Pedunculopontine nucleus	Globus pallidus	Globus pallidus Substantia nigra

Table 12.9 ● Other circuits of the basal ganglia.

In addition, a smaller number of input fibers arise from the midbrain raphe nuclei (serotonergic) and the ventral median nucleus of the thalamus (glutaminergic).

Efferent fibers (output)

The subthalamic nucleus sends projections that terminate in both the medial and lateral segments of the globus pallidus, as well as in the pars reticulata of the substantia nigra, and in the ventral pallidum. All of these fibers release glutamate and are excitatory.

It is evident, based on the above projections, that the globus pallidus and the subthalamic nucleus are interconnected via the subthalamic fasciculus. The subthalamic nucleus modulates the output of the globus pallidus and the substantia nigra, regions which contribute to the output of the basal ganglia.

Pedunculopontine nucleus

The **pedunculopontine nucleus** receives GABA-releasing **input** fibers from the globus pallidus, and gives rise to glutaminergic **output** fibers, which terminate in the globus pallidus and the substantia nigra.

NEUROTRANSMITTERS OF THE BASAL GANGLIA

The neurons of the basal ganglia release the following neurotransmitters: glutamate, GABA, dopamine, acetylcholine, and neuropeptides (Table 12.10).

Glutamate-releasing neurons

The cerebral cortex and subthalamic nucleus give rise to glutamate-releasing fibers

Various regions of the **cerebral cortex** and the **subthalamic nucleus** give rise to corticostriate and subthalamopallidal **glutamate-releasing fibers**, which project to the **striatum** and the **globus pallidus**, respectively. The glutamate-releasing neurons are excitatory to the GABAergic and cholinergic neurons of the striatum (Fig. 12.18).

GABA-releasing neurons

GABA-releasing neurons are the principal neurons of the striatum

Gamma aminobutyric acid (GABA)-releasing neurons are inhibitory neurons. They are the principal neurons of the **striatum**, thus making GABA the principal neurotransmitter of the basal ganglia. Additionally, the **globus pallidus** and the pars reticulata of the **substantia nigra** also house GABA-releasing neurons. The fibers of these neurons form the striatopallidal, striatonigral, pallidothalamic, and nigrothalamic pathways (Fig. 12.18).

Dopamine-releasing neurons

Dopamine-releasing neurons are located in the pars compacta of the substantia nigra and their degeneration are the cause of Parkinson's disease

Dopamine-releasing neurons are located in the pars compacta of the **substantia nigra**. Their axons form the **dopaminergic nigrostriatal pathway**, which terminates in the caudate nucleus and the putamen. These axons have an *inhibitory* affect on these striatal GABAergic neurons that project to the lateral segment of the globus pallidus. However, they have an *excitatory* affect

Table 12.10 • Neurotransmitters of the basal ganglia.

Neurotransmitter	Excitatory/inhibitory	Region	Fiber pathways	Termination
Glutamate	Excitatory	Cerebral cortex Subthalamic nucleus	Corticostriatal fibers Subthalamopallidal fibers	Striatum Globus pallidus
Gamma aminobutyric acid (GABA)	Inhibitory	Striatum	Striatopallidal fibers Striatonigral fibers	Globus pallidus Substantia nigra
		Globus pallidus Substantia nigra	Pallidothalamic fibers Nigrothalamic fibers	Thalamus Thalamus
Dopamine	Inhibitory	Substantia nigra (pars compacta)	Nigrostriatal fibers	Putamen where they synapse with GABAergic neurons, which project to the lateral segment of the globus pallidus
	Excitatory	Substantia nigra (pars compacta)	Nigrostriatal fibers	Putamen where they synapse with GABAergic neurons, which project to the medial segment of the globus pallidus and the pars reticulata of the substantia nigra
Acetylcholine	Excitatory	Striatum	Intrastriatal	Striatum
Neuropeptides (enkephalin, dynorphin, substance P, somatostatin, neurotensin, neuropetide Y, cholecystokinin)				

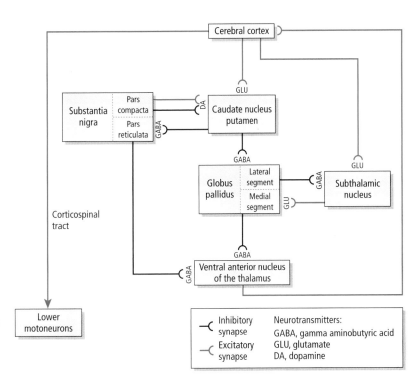

Figure 12.18 ● Neural circuitry and neurotransmitters of the basal ganglia. (Modified from Young, PA & Young, PH (1997) *Basic Clinical Neuroanatomy*. Williams & Wilkins, Baltimore; fig. 8.10.)

on those striatal GABAergic neurons that project to the medial segment of the globus pallidus and the pars reticulata of the substantia nigra. These diametrically opposite effects of dopamine at different terminations are due to differential reactions of the dopamine receptors (Fig. 12.18).

Acetylcholine-releasing neurons

The acetylcholine-releasing neurons consist of local circuit intrastriatal neurons (interneurons)

Acetylcholine-releasing neurons are inhibited by the dopaminergic nigrostriatal neurons, and in turn are excitatory to the GABAergic output neurons of the striatum (Fig. 12.19).

Neuropeptide-releasing neurons

Neuropeptide-releasing neurons of the basal ganglia may contain the following neurotransmitters: enkephalin, dynorphin, substance P, somatostatin, neurotensin, neuropeptide Y, and cholecystokinin. These neurotransmitters are present concurrently with other neurotransmitters in the same neuron (for example, both GABA and enkephalin are located in the same neuron) (Fig. 12.19).

"DIRECT" AND "INDIRECT" LOOPS (PATHWAYS) OF THE BASAL GANGLIA

Output signals from the basal ganglia are relayed to the thalamus by flowing via direct and indirect loops

Widespread areas of the cerebral cortex project (via corticostriate fibers) to the caudate nucleus, putamen,

and ventral striatum of the basal ganglia. Output signals arising from the basal ganglia (i.e., in the pallidothalamic and nigrothalamic fibers) are relayed to the thalamus. In turn the thalamus projects to specific cortical areas of the frontal cortex. The information flows between the basal ganglia and the cerebral cortex via "**direct loops**" and "**indirect loops**," which are wiring patterns depicting the main circuits of the basal ganglia (motor, oculomotor, association, and limbic loops) discussed earlier. To demonstrate the direct loop and indirect loop, the motor loop is used as an example.

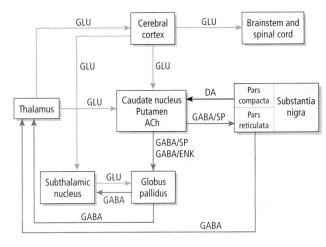

Figure 12.19 ● Major pathways of the basal ganglia and their neurotransmitters. ACh, acetylcholine; DA, dopamine; ENK, enkephalin; GABA, gamma aminobutyric acid; GLU, glutamate and/or aspartate; SP, substance P. (Modified from Fix, JD (1995) Neuroanatomy, 2nd edn. Williams & Wilkins, Baltimore; fig. 21.4.)

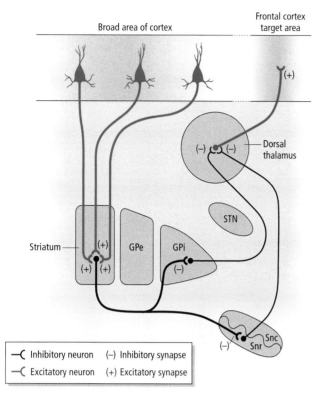

Figure 12.20 • The direct loop of the basal ganglia. GPe, globus pallidus (external segment); GPi, globus pallidus (internal segment); Snc, substantia nigra (pars compacta); Snr, substantia nigra (pars reticulata); STN, subthalamic nucleus. (Modified from Burt, AM (1993) *Textbook of Neuroanatomy*. WB Saunders, Philadelphia; fig. 16.3.)

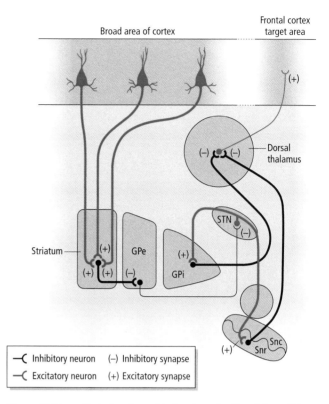

Figure 12.21 • The indirect loop of the basal ganglia. GPe, globus pallidus (external segment); GPi, globus pallidus (internal segment); Snc, substantia nigra (pars compacta); Snr, substantia nigra (pars reticulata); STN, subthalamic nucleus. (Modified from Burt, AM (1993) *Textbook of Neuroanatomy*. WB Saunders, Philadelphia; fig. 16.4.)

The motor loop of the basal ganglia consists of two distinct pathways that connect it to the cerebral cortex. Through these two pathways signals from the **input station**, the **putamen** (associated with motor activity), are transmitted to the **output stations**, the **medial segment of the globus pallidus (GPm)** and the **substantia nigra pars reticulata (SNr)**. One pathway is referred to as the direct loop and the other is referred to as the indirect loop. Although these pathways are in parallel, one has an *excitatory* while the other has an *inhibitory* influence on the cerebral cortex. It is via these pathways that the basal ganglia regulate the output of the motor cortex and thus regulate motor activity indirectly.

In the direct loop (Fig. 12.20), **corticostriate (glutaminergic, excitatory) fibers** terminate in the **striatum** (mostly to the **putamen**), where they *excite* a group of **GABAergic inhibitory neurons** (also containing substance P). These neurons in turn send their fibers to the GPm and the SNr where they have an inhibitory influence on the **GABAergic inhibitory pallidothalamic** and **nigrothalamic neurons**, respectively. The inhibition of the inhibitory projection neurons housed in the GPm and the SNr results in *disinhibition* (excitation) of the **thalamocortical excitatory fibers** to the cerebral cortex, and ultimately *stimulation* of the motor cortex.

In the indirect loop (Fig. 12.21), corticostriate (glutaminergic, excitatory) fibers terminate in the striatum (mostly to the putamen), where they *stimulate* another group of GABAergic

inhibitory neurons (also containing enkephalin). These neurons in turn send their fibers to the **GPl** where they have an inhibitory influence on the **GABAergic inhibitory pallidosubthalamic neurons**. The subthalamic nucleus houses glutaminergic excitatory neurons that project to the GPm and the SNr. The GPm and the SNr project GABAergic inhibitory pallidothalamic and nigrothalamic fibers, respectively, to the thalamus, which in turn projects **glutaminergic excitatory thalamocortical fibers** to the cortex. Usually, the inhibitory pallidosubthalamic neurons cause a reduction of the excitatory influence that the subthalamic nucleus has on the GPm and the SNr. Enhanced stimulation of the indirect loop results in *disinhibition* of the subthalamic nucleus, and thus stimulation of the inhibitory GABAergic neurons in the GPm and SNr. The GPm and SNr, via pallidothalamic and nigrothalamic fibers, inhibit the thalamocortical neurons, resulting in *inhibition* of the motor cortex.

CIRCUITS THAT MODULATE ACTIVITY OF THE BASAL GANGLIA

Activity of the basal ganglia is modulated by the dopaminergic nigrostriatal pathway and by the thalamostriatal fibers

The **dopaminergic nigrostriatal pathway** arises from the **substantia nigra pars compacta** and terminates in the **striatum**. **Dopaminergic** fibers arising from the pars compacta of the substantia nigra and the retrorubral nucleus form the nigrostriatal pathway whose fibers terminate in the caudate nucleus or the putamen, where they synapse with GABAergic neurons. Dopamine is usually an inhibitory neurotransmitter; however, it has a different effect on different populations of neurons housed in the putamen. It is believed that the putamen contains neurons with up to five different types of dopamine receptors, two of which are D_1 and D_2 receptors.

The dopaminergic neurons from the substantia nigra pars compacta synapse with striatal GABAergic–substance P neurons of the direct loop, which possess D_1 receptors and project directly from the putamen to the GPm and SNr. These synapses have an *excitatory effect* on the **direct loop GABAergic–substance P neurons** of the putamen, which terminate in the GPm and in the SNr.

The dopaminergic neurons from the **retrorubral nucleus** synapse with striatal GABAergic–enkephalin neurons of the indirect loop, which possess D_2 receptors. These striatal neurons project to the GPl which in turn projects to the subthalamic nucleus, which then projects to the GPm. These synapses with the striatal neurons with D_2 receptors have an *inhibitory effect* on the **indirect loop GABAergic–enkephalin neurons** of the putamen.

The nigrostriatal pathway strengthens corticostriate fiber input to the striatum concerning motor activity by stimulation of the direct loop and by inhibition of the indirect loop. The cholinergic intrastriatal interneurons, however, counteract the cortical input on the dopaminergic neurons. These cholinergic neurons stimulate the GABAergic–enkephalin striatal output fibers of the indirect loop, which has an inhibitory influence on the thalamocortical fibers. The net effect of the basal ganglia is inhibitory.

The neurons that project directly to GPm possess D_1 receptors, whereas those that project to the GPl and the pars reticulata of the substantia nigra have D_2 receptors.

The **thalamostriatal fibers** arise from the **intralaminar (centromedian** and **parafascicular) nuclei of the thalamus** and terminate primarily in the striatum, although some fibers terminate in the globus pallidus and in the subthalamic nucleus. The function of these fibers is unknown.

CLINICAL CONSIDERATIONS

Disorders involving the basal ganglia include hypertonicity and dyskinesias

Hypertonicity

Hypertonicity is an abnormal increase of muscle tone in response to passive stretch. Severe hypertonicity is referred to as rigidity. One of the normal functions of the basal ganglia, when stimulated, is to relay signals to the motor cortex and brainstem, which ultimately inhibit muscle tone. Following a lesion of the basal ganglia, this inhibitory influence is lost and symptoms of hypertonicity are manifested contralateral to the side of the lesion.

Dyskinesias

Dyskinesias may be classified into hyperkinesias or hypokinesias

Dyskinesias include unintentional, disorderly, purposeless movements. The disorders of the basal ganglia may be classified into hyperkinetic disorders or hypokinetic disorders. Dyskinesias "occur at rest," that is without volitional intent.

Hyperkinetic disorders

The symptoms of hyperkinetic disorders are characterized by abnormal involuntary movements, displayed by affected individuals as tremor, chorea, athetosis, or ballism

The symptoms of hyperkinetic disorders are characterized by abnormal involuntary movements, displayed by affected individuals as tremor, chorea, athetosis, or ballism. Hyperkinetic disorders are caused by a disturbance of the excitatory subthalamopallidal neurons of the indirect loop.

Tremor is a rhythmic, low amplitude movement that may be manifested as rhythmic nodding of the head, or in the hands and feet.

Chorea (G. choros, "dance") consists of a sequence of rapid, jerky, somewhat agile and flowing movements involving mainly the hands and feet, the tongue, and facial muscles.

Athetosis (G. athetos, "not fixed") is a condition in which the individual displays slow, vermicular ("worm-like") involuntary movements, which usually affect the hands and feet. This condition results following degeneration of the lateral segment of the globus pallidus. Since the globus pallidus becomes silent, the ventrolateral nucleus of the thalamus can send signals spontaneously to the motor cortex.

Ballismus (G. ballismos, "jumping about") is the most extreme type of dyskinesia.

Hemiballismus (G. hemi, "half;" ballismos, "jumping about" or "to throw") is a rare condition most often affecting older individuals, who exhibit involuntary ballistic (violent striking) movements on only one side of the body, that affect only the proximal muscles of a limb. It results following a cerebral vascular lesion of the ganglial branch of the posterior cerebral artery, which involves the contralateral subthalamic nucleus. The subthalamic nucleus functions in the integration of flowing movements produced by different parts of the body. Normally, the subthalamic nucleus projects glutaminergic (excitatory) fibers to the two output nuclei of the basal ganglia, the GPm, and the SNr, which in turn send inhibitory projections to the thalamus. Thalamocortical fibers that are excitatory project to the motor cortex. Projections thus far are ipsilateral, however the upper motoneurons arising from the cortex decussate in the pyramids, thus affecting the opposite side of the body. A lesion in the subthalamic nucleus would result in disinhibition of the thalamus, which in turn becomes overactive, overstimulating the motor cortex which in turn results in hyperkinetic symptoms in the opposite side of the body (Fig. 12.22). Although hemiballismus may occur following destruction of the subthalamic nucleus, it most often occurs following destruction of the striatal neurons that normally inhibit the lateral segment of the globus pallidus, which in turn

exert an inhibitory influence on the subthalamic nucleus. Whatever the case may be, the inhibitory effect exerted by the medial segment of the globus pallidus on the thalamus is reduced, which in turn overstimulates the motor areas of the cortex. In this condition, the thalamocortical pathway, arising from the ventral lateral nucleus of the thalamus projecting to the supplementary motor area of the secondary motor cortex, is affected. Hemiballismus may be alleviated either with chemical substances, such as dopamine-blocking drugs or GABA-mimetic agents, or by surgical removal of the ventral lateral nucleus of the thalamus. Hemiballismus usually disappears several weeks after treatment.

Hyperkinetic disorders are caused by a disturbance of the excitatory subthalamopallidal neurons of the **indirect loop** (Fig. 12.22). This creates an imbalance between the direct loop (where pallidothalamic neurons are stimulated) and the indirect loop (where pallidothalamic neurons are inhibited). This causes underinhibition of the thalamic neurons, which ultimately results in excess cortical activity and movement.

Huntington's disease

Huntington's disease is a rare, genetic disorder; the neurons that degenerate to produce this disease are part of the indirect loop

Huntington's disease is a rare, inherited, autosomal dominant genetic disorder, which is associated with a gene defect on chromosome 4. The symptoms of Huntington's disease become perceptible in the fourth or fifth decade of life as a result of degeneration of the GABAergic, substance P, and cholinergic-releasing neurons housed in the striatum, and simultaneous degeneration of the cerebral cortex (Fig. 12.23).

At its early stages, the neurons that degenerate are the striatal GABAergic neurons that project to the lateral segment of the globus pallidus, but as the disease progresses, eventually the entire striatal neuron population degenerates.

As a consequence of the loss of the GABAergic inhibitory influence, which is normally exerted by the striatum via the striatonigral pathway on the dopaminergic neurons of the substantia nigra (pars compacta, SNc), the SNc dopaminergic nigrostriatal neurons become overactive. This results in the dopaminergic nigrostriatal inhibitory pathway (over)inhibiting and thus depressing the function of the striatum. This imbalance is responsible for the abnormal movements displayed by affected individuals. The choreiform movements are reduced following treatment with antidopaminergic drugs. As a result of the degeneration (atrophy) of the caudate nuclei that occupy the lateral ventricles, radiographs reveal distended lateral ventricles resulting in **hydrocephalus ex vacuo**.

In the early stages of Huntington's disease, the cells affected are mainly the GABAergic inhibitory neurons that project from the striatum to the lateral segment of the globus pallidus (GPl). This results in a decrease of inhibitory influence on the GPl. Since the GPl normally exerts a tonic inhibitory influence on the subthalamic nucleus, this neural loss will result in an increase of the tonic inhibitory influence exerted on the subthalamic nucleus by the globus pallidus. The subthalamic nucleus normally sends excitatory projections to the output stations of the basal ganglia, the GPm and the SNr. The output from the (output stations of the) basal ganglia is normally inhibitory to the thalamus, whose output in turn is excitatory to the motor cortex. This neural loss will result in overinhibition of the subthalamic nucleus, which will in turn understimulate the GPm and the SNr. The output nuclei will relay reduced inhibitory signals to the thalamus and brainstem terminations. Inhibition of an inhibitory target results in what is referred to as **disinhibition**, which is really excitation. Thus the thalamus and brainstem terminations are disinhibited following the loss of the GABAergic neurons, which results in overstimulation of the motor cortex, and ultimately of the lower motoneurons, producing involuntary movements.

CLINICAL CONSIDERATIONS (*continued*)

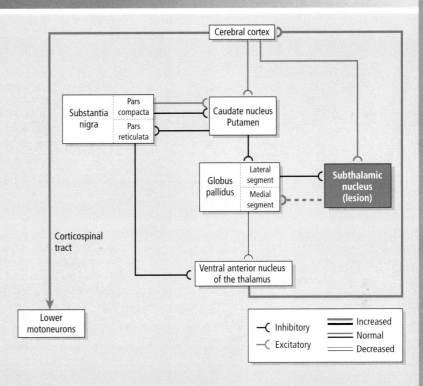

Figure 12.22 ● Subthalamic nucleus lesion. Note the neural circuitry modifications resulting in hyperkinetic disorders. (Modified from Young, PA & Young, PH (1997) *Basic Clinical Neuroanatomy*. Williams & Wilkins, Baltimore; fig. 8.11.)

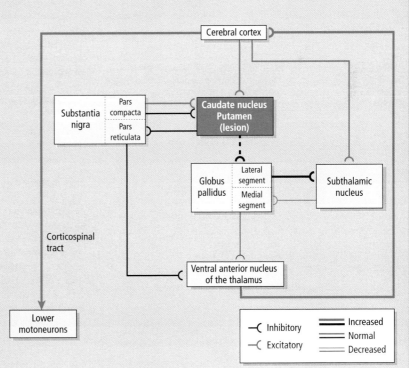

Figure 12.23 ● Striatal lesion. Note the neural circuitry modifications resulting in hyperkinetic disorders. (Modified from Young, PA & Young, PH (1997) *Basic Clinical Neuroanatomy*. Williams & Wilkins, Baltimore; fig. 8.12.)

During the early stages of the disease, involuntary, choreiform movements of the limbs and sudden movements of the face appear. As the disease progresses, additional muscles become affected, and the individual is incapable of moving, speaking, or swallowing (Fig. 12.24). These symptoms are accompanied by advancing dementia and cognitive impairment due to degeneration of the caudate nucleus and the cerebral cortex.

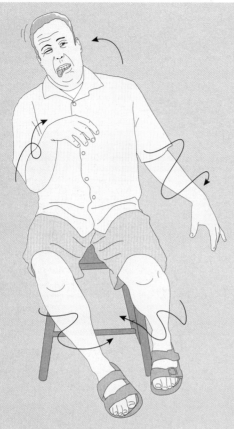

Figure 12.24 ● An individual with Huntington's chorea. Symptoms include choreic movements of the limbs and smacking of the lips and tongue. (Modified from Young, PA & Young, PH (1997) *Basic Clinical Neuroanatomy*. Williams & Wilkins, Baltimore; fig. 8.9.)

Sydenham's chorea (St Vitus' dance)

Sydenham's chorea appears as a consequence of childhood rheumatic fever

Sydenham's chorea results from a bacterial infection. The infectious bacteria contain antigens that are comparable to the protein receptors located in the cell membrane of the neurons housed in the caudate nucleus and the putamen. The individual infected by this bacterium produces antibodies that bind to the bacterial antigens as well as to the receptors of the striatal neurons. These neurons act as if they were stimulated by neurotransmitter substances and fire, resulting in choreiform movements, involving the face, trunk, and extremities. This condition, however, is temporary and the child will recover completely.

Tardive dyskinesia

Tardive dyskinesia is a condition that affects some individuals who are chronically treated with antipsychotic drugs

In **tardive dyskinesia**, an affected individual displays repetitive movements of the face, mouth, and tongue, as well as choreoathetotic movements of the trunk and limbs.

The antipsychotic drugs (phenothiazines and butyrophenones) block the transmission of dopamine in the brain. These drugs are aimed at the neurons

housed in the ventral tegmental area whose axons form the mesolimbic dopaminergic pathway, but cause the dopamine receptors (D_3 receptors) to become hypersensitive. This results in an imbalance of the effect of the nigrostriatal pathway on the motor loop, causing abnormal movements. In recent years newer antipsychotic drugs have become available that do not produce such symptoms.

Hypokinetic disorders

Hypokinetic disorders are characterized by bradykinesia or akinesia, and result from neuronal degeneration in the neostriatum

Hypokinetic disorders are characterized by **bradykinesia** (slowness of execution of a movement) or akinesia. **Akinesia** is a disorder in which the affected individual is unable to plan or to direct a movement toward a desired position or target.

Hypokinetic disorders result from neuronal degeneration in the neostriatum, disrupting the **direct loop** of the basal ganglia. That is, the **GABAergic inhibitory neurons** of the neostriatum, which normally send their fibers to the **medial segment of the globus pallidus**, degenerate, eliminating their *inhibitory* influence on the **GABAergic inhibitory pallidothalamic neurons**. Consequently, this permits (frees) the tonically active pallidothalamic neurons to continually (without restraint) overinhibit the **thalamocortical excitatory neurons** whose fibers terminate in the cerebral cortex. In other words, the thalamus is not disinhibited. This paucity of thalamic input to the cerebral cortex understimulates the corticospinal and corticonuclear tracts. The components of the **indirect** pathway though are undisturbed, thus creating an imbalance between the direct and indirect loops. The subthalamopallidal projections (of the indirect loop) stimulate the pallidothalamic neurons that in turn overinhibit the thalamus. Thus the insufficient thalamic disinhibition (excitation) via the direct loop is augmented by the overinhibition of the thalamus via the indirect loop, diminishing normal cortical activity, and increasing abnormal cortical activity. This discrepancy in the funneling of input to the cerebral cortex via the direct and indirect loops ultimately causes an increase in the stimulation of antagonist muscles, and not a decrease in muscular activity.

Parkinson's disease (parkinsonism, "paralysis agitans")

Parkinson's disease occurs following degeneration of the dopaminergic neurons of the pars compacta of the substantia nigra

Parkinson's disease is the most prevalent disorder associated with the basal ganglia, affecting approximately 1% of individuals over the age of 50. It results following **degeneration** of the **dopaminergic neurons** of the pars compacta of the **substantia nigra** (Fig. 12.25). Due to the degeneration of these neurons, dopamine is not produced, thus there is a **reduction of dopamine** levels in the **caudate nucleus** and the **putamen**, where the **nigrostriatal neurons** terminate. Symptoms usually do not appear until about 80% of the dopaminergic neurons of the substantia nigra have degenerated. The reduction of dopamine levels in the striatum results in an increase of acetylcholine release by intrastriatal neurons, and ultimately in the increase of the inhibitory influence exerted by the basal ganglia on the thalamus. An inhibited thalamus understimulates the motor cortex and brainstem terminations, which result in slowness, or loss of movement, characteristic of Parkinson's disease.

Although individuals affected by this disease may have a resting tremor, muscle rigidity, hypokinesia, bradykinesia, or impairment of postural reflexes, not all symptoms are necessarily expressed in the same individual (Fig. 12.26). These individuals have no paralysis. However, the akinesia gives one the impression that an individual with Parkinson's disease is paralyzed. The akinesia and the tremor generated the term "paralysis agitans."

CLINICAL CONSIDERATIONS (*continued*)

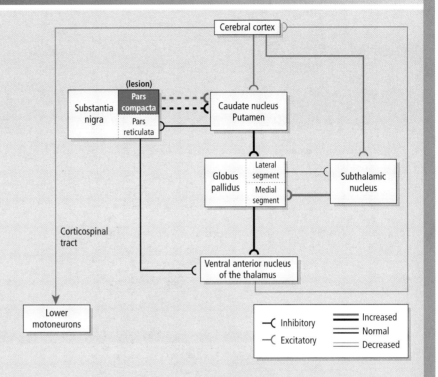

Figure 12.25 ● Decreased dopamine. Note the neural circuitry modifications resulting in hypokinetic disorders. (Modified from Young, PA & Young, PH (1997) *Basic Clinical Neuroanatomy*. Williams & Wilkins, Baltimore; fig. 8.13.)

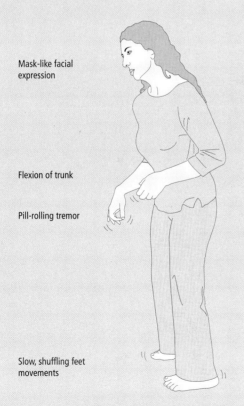

Mask-like facial expression

Flexion of trunk

Pill-rolling tremor

Slow, shuffling feet movements

Figure 12.26 ● Individual with Parkinson's disease. Symptoms include mask-like facial expression, flexed head and trunk, arms close to trunk, pill-rolling tremor of the hands, and slow, shuffling movements of the feet.

Individuals with this disease have a **resting tremor** affecting the hands, which is exhibited as a "pill-rolling tremor," where the index finger rubs on the thumb—in a manner similar to the way that pills were made many years ago. Interestingly, this tremor, caused by the regular interchange in contraction of the agonist and antagonist muscles, is not evident when the affected individual is asleep, during voluntary movement, or during general anesthesia. In contrast, cerebellar tremor is expressed during movement ("intention tremor"), and is absent at rest (see Chapter 13). Also present is muscular **rigidity**, which results from widespread increased muscle tone. Rigidity worsens during the advanced stages of Parkinson's disease. If the rigidity is continuous during a movement, it is referred to as "lead-pipe rigidity," whereas if the rigidity is discontinuous resulting from intermittent muscle relaxations during a movement, it is referred to as "cog-wheel rigidity." Rigidity of all flexors results in the affected individual having a stooped posture.

Parkinson's disease is also characterized by **hypokinesia** (G. hypo, "few;" kinesia, "movement") and **bradykinesia** (G. brady, "slow") in which the affected individual has trouble in both initiating and executing voluntary movements. These are exhibited by a blank, expressionless, mask-like face, slow blinking, slurred speech, and lack of upper limb movements that usually accompany walking. An affected individual has difficulty getting up from a chair, walking, picking up objects, etc. A shuffling gait may also develop, in which the individual takes short steps. These movements begin with great effort, followed by an increase in speed, although it is difficult to stop a movement in progress. However, muscle strength and deep tendon reflexes are not influenced by this disease.

In humans, melanin begins to appear in the substantia nigra around the fourth or fifth year of childhood. Autopsy of the midbrain of individuals who had Parkinson's disease reveals an absence of melanin.

Since dopamine does not cross the blood–brain barrier, patients with Parkinson's disease are treated with dihydroxyphenylalanine (L-DOPA, which

CLINICAL CONSIDERATIONS (*continued*)

can cross this barrier to restore the missing dopamine) along with dopamine agonists, an L-DOPA uptake inhibitor (carbidopa), and monoamine oxidase (MAO) inhibitors.

In addition to pharmacologic treatment, the signs and symptoms of Parkinson's disease have in recent years been alleviated by surgical procedures that involve lesions of the thalamus (thalamotomy) or the medial segment of the globus pallidus (pallidotomy). An alternative surgical procedure includes stimulation electrodes aimed at target nuclei such as the thalamus, globus pallidus, or the subthalamic nucleus.

Patients receiving pharmacologic or surgical treatment experience relief from some of the symptoms associated with Parkinson's disease; however, the progression of the disease can not be halted.

Parkinson's disease (a hypokinetic disorder) and Huntington's disease (a hyperkinetic disorder), are two severe disorders of the basal ganglia reflecting two opposite ends of basal ganglial dysfunction spectrum. If excessive L-DOPA is administered to an individual with Parkinson's disease, the individual will manifest choreic movements. L-DOPA administered to a patient with Huntington's disease will intensify the choreic movements.

Wilson's disease (hepatolenticular degeneration)

Wilson's disease, an autosomal recessive genetic disorder, is localized on chromosome 13 and is associated with an error in the body's metabolism of copper

Wilson's disease is seen in young adults (10–25 years of age), and results following degeneration mostly of the putamen and the globus pallidus, although other structures such as the cerebral cortex, thalamus, red nucleus, and cerebellum may also be involved. Degeneration is characterized by the loss of nerve cells and accumulation of protoplasmic astrocytes. Consequently, the nerve tissue exhibits small spaces, giving it a spongy appearance. Lenticular degeneration is usually accompanied by cirrhosis of the liver.

An individual with this disease manifests symptoms such as tremor, rigidity, and choreiform or athetotic movements, as well as speech disorders and a loss of facial expression. The tremor manifested by an affected individual is not tremor at rest, as that seen in other basal ganglial disease. The tremor here is referred to as **asterixis**, characterized as a "wing-beating" tremor, manifested following extension of the upper limbs. The tremor may affect the hands at the wrist, or the entire upper limb.

Individuals affected by this disorder experience relief from symptoms following treatment, which includes decreasing the concentration of copper in the body.

Note that the clinical case at the beginning of the chapter refers to a patient with abnormal, uncontrollable choreiform movements, motor deficits, forgetfulness, and abnormal behaviors. An MRI scan shows atrophy of the head of the caudate nucleus, bilaterally.

1 What neurodegenerative disease produces the unique combination of choreiform movements and progressive deterioration of mental function exhibited by this patient?

2 Which nuclei of the basal ganglia are usually affected in this disease?

3 What do you expect genetic testing results to reveal?

SYNONYMS AND EPONYMS OF THE BASAL GANGLIA

Name of structure or term	Synonym(s)/eponym(s)	Name of structure or term	Synonym(s)/eponym(s)
Acetylcholine-releasing fibers	Cholinergic fibers	Medial segment of the globus pallidus (GPm)	Internal segment of the globus pallidus (GPi)
Amygdala	Amygdaloid nucleus		Inner segment of the globus pallidus (GPi)
Basal ganglia	Basal nuclei		
	Deep cerebral nuclei		Globus pallidus internus (GPi)
Corticonuclear tract	Corticobulbar tract (older term)	Mesencephalon	Midbrain
Corticospinal tract	Pyramidal tract (older term)	Paralysis agitans	Parkinson's disease
Dopamine-releasing fibers	Dopaminergic fibers		Parkinsonism
Frontal eye field (FEF)	Brodmann's area 8	Premotor cortex	Premotor area
Gamma aminobutyric acid-releasing fibers	GABAergic fibers		Part of Brodmann's area 6
Globus pallidus (GP)	Paleostriatum	Primary motor cortex (M-I)	Precentral gyrus
Glutamate-releasing fibers	Glutaminergic fibers		Brodmann's area 4
Hepatolenticular degeneration	Wilson's disease	Primary somatosensory cortex (S-I)	Primary sensory cortex (S-I)
Huntington's disease	Huntington's chorea (older term)		Primary somesthetic cortex
Interneuron	Internuncial neuron		Postcentral gyrus
Lateral medullary lamina	External medullary lamina		Brodmann's areas 3, 1, and 2
Lateral segment of the globus pallidus (GPl)	External segment of the globus pallidus (GPe)	Proximal limb musculature	Girdle musculature
	Outer segment of the globus pallidus	Red nucleus	Nucleus ruber
		Striatum	Neostriatum
	Globus pallidus externus (GPe)	Substantia nigra pars reticulata	Substantia nigra pars reticularis
Lenticular nucleus	Lentiform nucleus	Subthalamic nucleus	Nucleus of Luys
Lower motoneuron	Lower motor neuron	Supplementary motor area (SMA)	Part of Brodmann's area 6
Medial medullary lamina	Internal medullary lamina	Sydenham's chorea	St Vitus' dance
		Thalamic fasciculus	H_1 field of Forel

FOLLOW-UP TO CLINICAL CASE

This patient has **Huntington's disease**, confirmed by genetic testing. This patient has typical symptoms of Huntington's disease. Chorea is the most identifiable and specific characteristic, but the most problematic and disabling symptoms are psychiatric disturbances and dementia.

Chorea is a Greek term for "dance." It is characteristic of lesions or pathology in the basal ganglia, especially of the caudate nucleus and putamen. However, the exact localization and pathophysiology of chorea is uncertain. Many lesions involving the caudate and putamen do not produce choreiform or similar movement disorders. Chorea may be generalized, as in Huntington's disease, or unilateral, in which case it is called hemichorea. The most common cause of hemichorea is a stroke in the contralateral basal ganglia, although it may be caused by any lesion involving certain parts of the contralateral basal ganglia. A number of different conditions, genetic or acquired, can produce chorea. Certain medications such as levodopa, prescribed for the treatment of Parkinson's disease, can produce choreiform movements if excess dosages are taken.

Huntington's disease is an autosomal dominant neurodegenerative disease. Therefore an affected parent has a 50% chance of passing the disease to his/her children. It affects the caudate and putamen early and most prominently, but other parts of the basal ganglia and the cerebral cortex are also affected. The disease often presents itself when the affected individual is in his thirties or forties. Usually by that time the individual has had children already and may have passed the gene to his children. The abnormal gene is on chromosome 4 and contains an expanded trinucleotide sequence. This gene produces the Huntingtin protein. The normal function of this protein, and how the mutated protein causes the death of neurons, is unclear. Genetic testing is available for this disease. Huntington's disease causes progressive and relentless deterioration of mental function, which leads to incapacity and death 10–20 years after onset. Chorea and psychosis can be treated by antidopaminergic medication; however, there is no effective treatment for the progressive dementia.

4 In addition to abnormal choreiform movements, what are the most disabling symptoms of Huntington's disease?

QUESTIONS TO PONDER

1. Why are the basal ganglia and the limbic system interconnected?

2. What causes hypertonicity following a lesion of the basal ganglia?

3. One of the causes of hemiballismus is a lesion to the subthalamic nucleus; it is manifested as violent flinging movements of the proximal limb muscles on the opposite side of the body. How do you account for the symptoms appearing contralateral to the side of the lesion?

4. What is the underlying cause of hyperkinetic and hypokinetic disorders?

5. What is likely to occur if excessive L-DOPA is administered to an individual with Parkinson's disease and to an individual with Huntington's disease?

CHAPTER 13

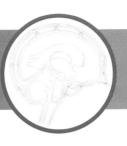
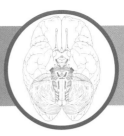
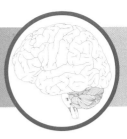

Cerebellum

CLINICAL CASE

A 72-year-old woman developed sudden severe vertigo about 5 hours prior to presentation in the emergency room. The vertigo has persisted and remained severe. She became nauseated and vomited a few times. She has not been able to walk, and cannot even sit on the side of the bed without falling over. There was initially some double vision but this has since resolved. She complains that her left arm is "weak" and heavy. Her speech is mildly slurred. She feels that she is being pulled to the left when she attempts to stand or sit up.

Exam shows mild dysarthria (slurred speech), but language function is normal. Bilateral end gaze nystagmus is present, which is much more prominent toward the left. Facial strength and sensation is normal. Despite the patient's complaint, exam shows strength throughout to be normal. However, there is dysmetria and ataxia involving the left arm, but the right arm is normal. The patient cannot stand or even sit up in bed on her own. Sensation is normal throughout. Head CT in the emergency room was normal.

Movement is produced by complex interactions of the **basal ganglia**, the **cerebellum**, and the **cerebral cortex** (Table 13.1). The basal ganglia *initiate* motor activity and *modulate* cortical output related to motor function, the cerebellum functions in the *coordination* of movement, whereas the cerebral cortex is involved in the *planning* and *execution* of voluntary movement. The cerebellum and basal ganglia exert their influence on the brainstem and spinal cord and ultimately on motor activity at the subconscious level, *indirectly*, by regulating the output of the primary motor cortex and premotor areas of the secondary motor cortex. The motor cortex influences the execution of motor activity via *direct* projections to the brainstem nuclei (i.e., cranial nerve motor nuclei, nuclei of the reticular formation, midbrain tectum, and red nucleus) and spinal cord motoneurons.

Input from the motor cortex, and the visual, auditory, vestibular, and somatosensory systems is funneled into the cerebellum where it is integrated, and then utilized to plan and coordinate motor activity; that is, the cerebellum plays a key function in the execution of a motor task as it relates to the timing, speed, direction, and precision of muscular activity, whether of a single muscle or groups of muscles. Additionally, the cerebellum receives information about upcoming motor activity from the motor cortex, thus it is able to monitor the commands arising from the motor cortex that are relayed to the lower motoneurons of the brainstem

Structure	Function(s)
Cerebral cortex	
Premotor cortex	Planning of voluntary movement
Primary motor cortex	Execution of voluntary movement
Basal ganglia	Modulate premotor and primary motor cortex output
Cerebellum	Coordinates movements
	Maintenance of posture, balance (equilibrium), and muscle tone
	Learning of motor tasks
	Processes memory of skilled motor activity

Table 13.1 ● Role of the cerebral cortex, basal ganglia, and cerebellum in the production of movement.

and spinal cord. This capability enables the cerebellum to compare the impending movement with the movement in progress. It also plays an active role in voluntary movement by continuously adjusting the outflow of the motor and premotor cortex, so that movement is modified to be precise, smooth, flowing, and coordinated.

The cerebellum is the conductor behind a specific movement, since it not only determines its speed, but with the aid of projections from the visual and other systems, it also orchestrates its course. The cerebellum has important functions in **proprioception**, **muscle tone**, **maintenance of posture**, **balance (equilibrium)**, and **coordination of skilled voluntary movements**, as well as in the **learning and memory of motor tasks**, such as playing a musical instrument and riding a bicycle. All of these functions are performed at the subconscious level.

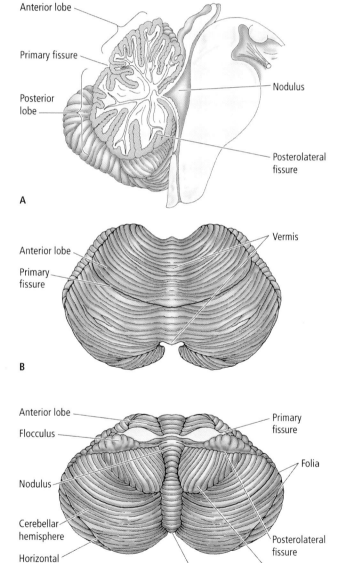

MORPHOLOGY OF THE CEREBELLUM

The cerebellum displays alternating, slender, parallel elevations known as folia, and depressions known as sulci, that facilitate a great increase in the surface area of the cerebellar cortex

The **cerebellum** (L., "little brain") is composed of two **cerebellar hemispheres** and the intervening **vermis** (L., "worm"), which is separated from each hemisphere by shallow longitudinally disposed furrows (Fig. 13.1). The surface of the cerebellum displays alternating, slender, parallel elevations (ridges) known as **folia** and depressions (grooves) known as **sulci**, that facilitate a great increase in the surface area of the cerebellar cortex (Fig. 13.1C). The cerebellum is connected to the dorsal aspect of the brainstem by three pairs of prominent fiber bundles, the **superior**, **middle**, and **inferior cerebellar peduncles** (see Fig. 13.8). On its ventral surface, near the middle cerebellar peduncle, a small, bulb-like region of each cerebellar hemisphere, known as the **flocculus**, is connected to a region of the vermis known as the **nodulus**.

Gray matter and white matter

The cerebellum consists of an outer shell of gray cortex, and a core of white matter containing deep gray nuclei

Like the cerebrum, the cerebellum consists of gray matter and white matter, organized into an outer shell

Figure 13.1 ● The cerebellum: (A) midsagittal view, (B) dorsal view, and (C) ventral view.

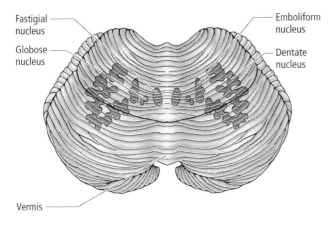

Fastigial
nucleus

Globose
nucleus

Emboliform
nucleus

Dentate
nucleus

Vermis

Figure 13.2 ● The deep nuclei of the cerebellum.

of gray cortex, and a core of white matter containing deep gray nuclei. The **gray matter** is distributed in two regions, as the three-layered outer **cerebellar cortex** and the **deep cerebellar nuclei (cerebellar nuclei)** (Figs 13.2), which are embedded within the white matter. The greater part of the cerebellum is composed of **white matter**, also referred to as the **medullary center** or **medullary white matter**, consisting of myelinated axons and neuroglia. There are three categories of these axons (fibers): intrinsic, afferent, and efferent (Fig. 13.3).

1 The **intrinsic (local, association) fibers** arise from the Purkinje cells of the cerebellar cortex and terminate in the deep cerebellar nuclei.
2 The **afferent (input) fibers** arise from extracerebellar sources and terminate in the deep cerebellar nuclei and/or the cortex.
3 The **efferent (output) fibers** principally originate in the deep cerebellar nuclei (although some arise from the cortex) and exit the cerebellum.

When sectioned in the sagittal plane through the vermis or cerebellar hemispheres, the gray and white matter of the cerebellum are recognizable with the unaided eye. Due to the presence of the deep sulci and the extensive folding of the cerebellar surface, the arborization of the white matter resembles the branching of a tree. Thus early neuroanatomists referred to this image as the **arbor vitae** (L., "tree of life") (Fig. 13.4).

Folding of the cerebellar cortex

Approximately 85% of the cerebellar cortex lines the banks of the sulci and fissures of the cerebellum, and is hidden from the cerebellar surface

As the cerebellum develops, the **cerebellar cortex** undergoes considerable folding resulting in the formation of the cerebellar **folia**, **sulci**, and **fissures**. The cerebellar cortex laminates the underlying white matter of the cerebellum. Each folium consists of a thin layer of gray matter containing nerve cell bodies, as well as a white matter center, composed mostly of myelinated axons and neuroglia. As a result of this folding, approximately 85% of the cerebellar cortex becomes buried (tucked), lining the banks of the sulci and fissures of the cerebellum, whereas the remaining cortex covers the exposed cerebellar surface.

Layers of the cerebellar cortex

The number of neurons in the cerebellar cortex far outnumber those of the much larger cerebral hemispheres

The cerebellar cortex is simpler than the cerebral cortex, in that it is composed of only three layers (as opposed to six layers) (Table 13.2). The number of neurons of the cerebellar cortex far outnumber those of the much larger cerebral hemispheres and the neuronal organization of the cerebellar

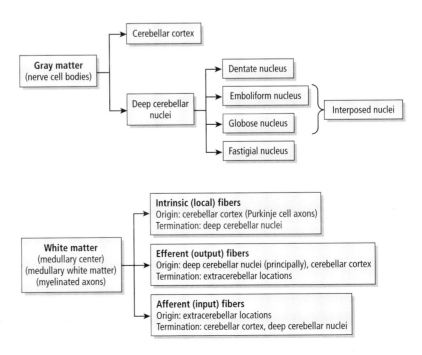

Figure 13.3 ● Organization of the gray and white matter of the cerebellum.

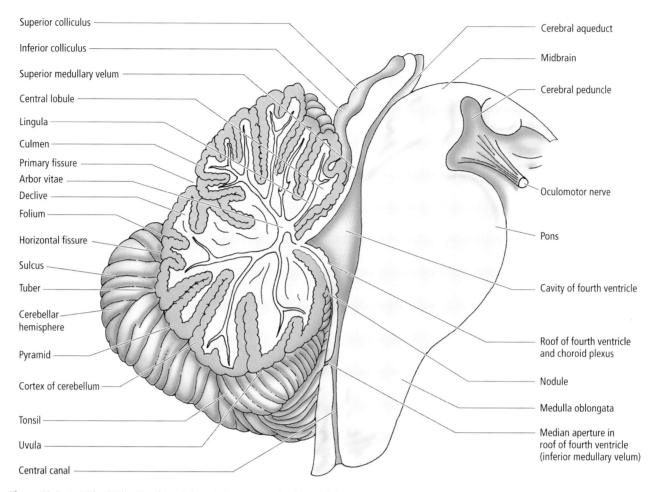

Figure 13.4 ● Midsagittal section through the brainstem and vermis of the cerebellum.

Table 13.2 ● The cerebellar cortex.

Layer	Contents	Neurotransmitter	Synapses
Molecular	Cells		
	Outer stellate cells	Taurine	Receive excitatory synapses from parallel fibers
			Form inhibitory synapses with Purkinje cells
	Basket cells	GABA	Receive excitatory synapses from parallel fibers
			Form inhibitory synapses with Purkinje cells
	Fibers		
	Purkinje cell dendrites		
	Granule cell parallel fibers		
Purkinje	Cells		
	Purkinje cell bodies (their axons form the principal output of the cerebellar cortex)	GABA	Form inhibitory synapses in: deep cerebellar nuclei vestibular nuclei
Granular	Cells		
	Granule cells	Glutamate	Form excitatory synapses with Purkinje, outer stellate, basket, and Golgi cells
	Golgi cells (inner stellate cells)	GABA	Receive excitatory synapses from mossy fibers, climbing fibers, and parallel fibers
			Form inhibitory synapses in glomeruli; modulate mossy fiber signal transmission to granule cells

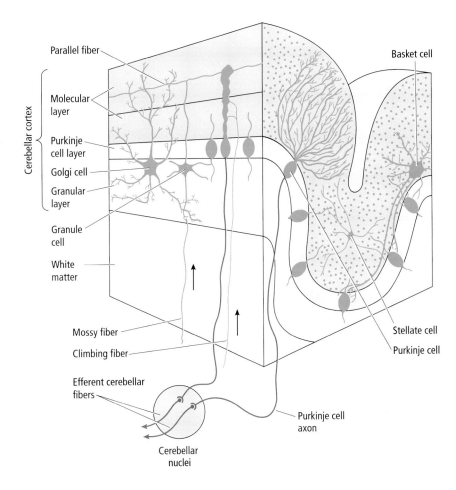

Labels on figure:
- Parallel fiber
- Molecular layer
- Cerebellar cortex
- Purkinje cell layer
- Golgi cell
- Granular layer
- Granule cell
- White matter
- Mossy fiber
- Climbing fiber
- Efferent cerebellar fibers
- Cerebellar nuclei
- Basket cell
- Stellate cell
- Purkinje cell
- Purkinje cell axon

Figure 13.5 ● The cerebellar cortex and its component cell layers.

cortex, unlike that of the cerebrum, is homogeneous through-out the various regions of the cerebellum.

The cerebellar cortex consists of an outer molecular layer that lies deep to the pia mater, a middle Purkinje cell layer, and an inner granular layer that lies on the surface of the cerebellar white matter (Fig. 13.5). The cerebellar cortex contains five distinct types of nerve cells: stellate cells, basket cells, Purkinje cells, granule cells, and Golgi cells (inner stellate cells).

Although the **molecular layer** houses **stellate cells** and the **basket cells**, both of which are inhibitory interneurons, it is mostly occupied by the **dendrites of the Purkinje cells**, and the **parallel fibers of the granule cells** (see discussion below).

The **Purkinje cell layer**, the intermediate layer of the cerebellar cortex, lies between the molecular and granular layers. It is occupied by the cell bodies of **Purkinje cells**, which are only found in the cerebellum.

The **granular layer** is the deepest and thickest layer of the cerebellar cortex. It houses mostly **granule cells** and some **Golgi cells**. In addition, this layer also contains synaptic complexes, known as **cerebellar glomeruli**.

The cerebellar cortex receives two special types of fibers: **climbing fibers** and **mossy fibers**. Climbing fibers are the axons of neurons whose cell bodies are located in the inferior olivary nucleus. Mossy fibers include the majority of the remaining afferents to the cerebellum that arise from wide-spread areas of the nervous system (see discussion below).

Deep to the cerebellar cortex is the cerebellar white matter, which contains myelinated axons made up of **afferent fibers**, **efferent fibers**, and **intrinsic (local) fibers** of the cerebellum.

Neurons of the cerebellar cortex

The cerebellar cortex has five distinct cell types

The cerebellar cortex has five distinct cell types (Fig. 13.5; Table 13.3). We will begin with the cells of the deep (granular) layer and work up through the Purkinje layer to the cells in the superficial (molecular) layer. The interrelationships among them are discussed later in this chapter under "Functional organization of the cerebellum" (see p. 236).

Granule cells

Granule cells are the only excitatory neurons of the cerebellar cortex, and their axons bifurcate in the molecular layer to form parallel fibers

Granule cells are the most numerous cells of the cerebellar cortex; in fact there are so many granule cells that their number exceeds the total neuron population of the cerebral cortex.

Table 13.3 ● Neurons of the cerebellar cortex.

Cell	Cell body location	Axon location	Dendrite location	Axon synapse type and neurotransmitter	Axon synapses with	Miscellaneous
Granule	Granular layer	Molecular layer where they form parallel fibers		Excitatory (glutamate)	Dendrites of Purkinje cells, and outer stellate, basket, and Golgi cells	Only intrinsic excitatory cells of cerebellar cortex. Axons form parallel fibers
Golgi (inner stellate)	Granular layer	Granular layer	All three layers of cortex	Inhibitory (GABA)	Glomeruli to modulate mossy fiber signal transmission to granule cells	Are inhibitory interneurons. Parallel fibers, mossy fibers, and climbing fibers form excitatory synapses with Golgi cells
Purkinje	Purkinje layer	White matter of cerebellum	Molecular layer; in a single plane; run perpendicular to parallel fibers	Inhibitory (GABA)	Deep cerebellar nuclei (especially dentate); also some project to vestibular nucleus	Only extracerebellar projection from the cerebellar cortex
Outer stellate	Molecular layer	Purkinje cell layer		Inhibitory (taurine)	Purkinje cells	Are inhibitory interneurons. Parallel fibers form excitatory synapses with outer stellate cells
Basket	Molecular layer	Purkinje and molecular layer		Inhibitory (GABA)	Form basket-like junctions with Purkinje cell body	Are inhibitory interneurons. Parallel fibers of granule cells establish excitatory synapses with basket cells

GABA, gamma aminobutyric acid.

Although the cell bodies of granule cells (the smallest neuron cell bodies of the nervous system) reside in the granular layer, their axons continue into the molecular layer where they bifurcate to form a T-shaped configuration. These are known as **parallel fibers** because they are oriented parallel not only to the cerebellar surface but also to the longitudinal axis of the folium in which they are embedded. Within the molecular layer, these unmyelinated parallel fibers course through the bushy dendrites of a series of Purkinje cells, like telephone wires running through branches of a series of trees. A single parallel fiber establishes synapses with thousands of Purkinje cells, and any one Purkinje cell receives synaptic contacts from thousands of parallel fibers.

Each granule cell, via its parallel fibers, forms glutamate-releasing **excitatory synapses** with the dendrites of Purkinje cells, as well as with stellate cells, basket cells, and Golgi cells. Note that the *granule cells are the only intrinsic excitatory nerve cells of the cerebellar cortex.*

Golgi cells

Golgi cells are inhibitory (GABAergic) interneurons

The **Golgi cells**, also known as **inner stellate cells**, are **inhibitory interneurons**; their cell bodies occupy the granular layer and their dendritic trees ramify in the molecular layer of the cerebellar cortex. Golgi cells form **gamma aminobutyric acid (GABA)**-releasing inhibitory synapses with mossy fibers within the glomeruli. Glomeruli are synaptic complexes of Golgi cells and their terminals, mossy fibers, and granule cell dendrites. They are located in the granular layer of the cerebellar cortex. It should be recalled that parallel fibers of the granule cells as well as mossy and climbing fibers to the cerebellum form excitatory synapses with the Golgi cells.

Purkinje cells

The primary target of the Purkinje cell axons are the deep cerebellar nuclei

Purkinje cells are multipolar neurons that have a large cell body and an extensive dendritic tree; in fact, they are the *largest* neurons of the central nervous system (CNS). Their flask-shaped cell bodies are located in the single-layered Purkinje cell layer, whereas their striking, flattened bushy dendrites, reside and ramify in the molecular layer. The Purkinje cell dendrites are aligned in a single plane (similar to the fanned-out feathers of a peacock's tail), and are arranged perpendicular to the parallel fibers and the longitudinal axis of the folium in which they are embedded. The axon of each Purkinje cell courses through the granular layer to reach the underlying white matter core of the cerebellum containing the deep cerebellar nuclei. These axons, which become

Zone	Cortical region	Cerebellar nucleus
Vermal (median)	Vermis	Fastigial nucleus
Paravermal (intermediate)	Medial region of cerebellar hemispheres	Interposed nuclei
Lateral (hemispheric)	Lateral region of cerebellar hemispheres	Dentate nucleus

Table 13.4 ● The three zones of the cerebellum and associated cortical region and cerebellar nucleus/nuclei.

myelinated upon entering the white matter, terminate principally in the ipsilateral **deep cerebellar nuclei**, particularly the dentate nucleus, where they establish **GABAergic inhibitory synapses**. However, axons of some Purkinje cells (of the flocculonodular lobe) go right past the deep cerebellar nuclei, leave the cerebellum, and synapse in the **vestibular nuclei**. This Purkinje cell projection to the vestibular nuclei is the *only* extracerebellar projection *from* the **cerebellar cortex**. Via these projections, the Purkinje cells regulate the activity of the deep cerebellar nuclei and the vestibular nuclei.

Stellate cells

Stellate cells are inhibitory interneurons

Stellate (L. stella, "star," "star-shaped") **cells** are **inhibitory interneurons** that occupy the molecular layer of the cerebellar cortex. The stellate cells are believed to form **taurine-releasing inhibitory synapses** with the dendrites of the Purkinje cells. Recall that the **parallel fibers** of the granule cells form excitatory synapses with the stellate cells.

Basket cells

Basket cells are inhibitory interneurons

Basket cells are **inhibitory interneurons** and occupy the molecular layer of the cerebellar cortex. Within the molecular layer, axons of numerous basket cells form "basket-like" configurations that cover the cell body of a Purkinje cell. **GABA** is released at these synapses, inhibiting the Purkinje cells from firing. Recall that parallel fibers of the granule cells establish excitatory synapses with the basket cells.

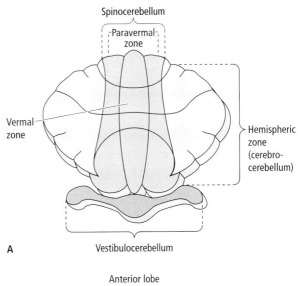

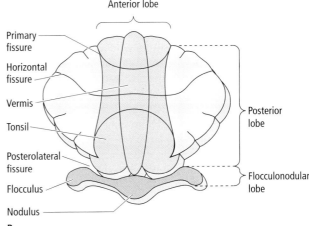

Figure 13.6 ● (A) The zones and phylogenetic classification of the cerebellum. (B) The lobes and fissures of the cerebellum.

Zones of the cerebellum

The zones of the cerebellum are composed of cortex, white matter, and the associated deep cerebellar nucleus (or nuclei)

Four pairs of deep cerebellar nuclei, the **fastigial nucleus**, **dentate nucleus**, **emboliform nucleus**, and **globose nucleus** (the last two are frequently referred to as the **interposed nuclei**), are embedded within the cerebellar white matter (see Fig. 13.2). Based on the connections between the regions of the cortex and the deep cerebellar nuclei, the cerebellum is divisible into functional zones, namely the **vermal (median)**, **paravermal (intermediate)**, and **hemispheric (lateral) zone** (Fig. 13.6A). These functional zones are composed of cortex, white matter, and the associated deep cerebellar nucleus (or nuclei), as listed in Table 13.4.

Lobes of the cerebellum

The cerebellum consists of the anterior, posterior, and flocculonodular lobes

As the cerebellum increases in size during development, its cortex is compacted and forms alternating folia and sulci. Three of these sulci are

Table 13.5 ● Lobes of the cerebellum.

Lobe	Phylogenetic name	Other name	Components	Function
Anterior	Paleocerebellum	Spinocerebellum	Vermis, paravermal zone, most of anterior lobe	Controls posture, muscle tone, and executes as well as coordinates muscle activity of the trunk and limbs during stereotyped activity. Vermis controls axial and girdle musculature, whereas the intermediate hemisphere controls limb musculature
Posterior (middle)	Neocerebellum	Cerebrocerebellum Pontocerebellum	(Lateral) cerebellar hemispheres	Planning, coordination, and execution of rapid, fine, nonstereotyped (skilled) movement
Flocculonodular	Archicerebellum	Vestibulocerebellum	Nodulus and right and left flocculi	Balance and posture maintenance, coordination of head and eye movements

especially deep and are known as the **primary**, **horizontal**, and **posterolateral fissures** (Fig. 13.6B). These fissures permit the horizontal division of the cerebellum into three lobes: the **anterior**, **posterior** (also known as **middle lobe**), and **flocculonodular lobes**. The flocculonodular lobe is composed of the right and left flocculi and the unpaired nodulus. The anterior lobe is separated from the posterior lobe by the primary fissure. The posterior lobe is divided into two regions by the horizontal fissure and is separated from the flocculonodular lobe by the posterolateral fissure.

Interestingly, these lobes also correspond to the phylogenetic development of the cerebellum (Table 13.5). The posterior lobe is phylogenetically the newest portion of the cerebellum, and is therefore also known as the **neocerebellum** (G. neo, "new"). The oldest portion of the cerebellum is the flocculonodular lobe, and is also referred to as the **archicerebellum** (G. archi, "beginning"). The **paleocerebellum** (G. paleo, "ancient") is intermediate in phylogenetic development and corresponds to the anterior lobe.

Flocculonodular lobe (vestibulocerebellum, archicerebellum)

The flocculonodular lobe is reciprocally connected with the vestibular system

The paired **flocculi** (L. flocculus, "tuft of wool") and the **nodulus** (of the vermis) together form a small lobe, the **flocculonodular lobe**.

Since this lobe is associated via its connections to the vestibular system, functionally it is referred to as the **vestibulocerebellum** (Fig. 13.6). The vestibulocerebellum is unique since it receives direct projections (first order neuron fibers) from the vestibular division of the vestibulocochlear nerve (CN VIII). Some of the second order neurons housed in the vestibular nuclei also project to the vestibulocerebellum. Note that all vestibular projections (first and second order neuron fibers) to the vestibulocerebellum are ipsilateral. The

vestibulocerebellum (via its influence on the descending vestibulospinal tracts) is associated with balance and posture maintenance. Additionally due to its projections to, and the influence it exerts on, the vestibular nuclei, it is also responsible for the coordination of head and eye movements.

Anterior lobe (spinocerebellum, paleocerebellum)

The anterior lobe is reciprocally connected with the spinal cord

The second part of the cerebellum to develop phylogenetically arose later in evolution and is known as the **paleocerebellum**. It is composed of the greater part of the vermis, the **paravermal zone (paravermis, intermediate hemisphere)**, and most of the **anterior lobe**. This part of the cerebellum developed in relation to, and therefore has reciprocal projections with, the brainstem and spinal cord, and is functionally referred to as the **spinocerebellum** (see Fig. 13.6). Sensory (proprioceptive and exteroceptive) input from the muscle spindles and Golgi tendon organs of the limbs and trunk is relayed to the spinocerebellum via the **spinocerebellar tracts**, and from the head via the **trigeminocerebellar fibers**. These tracts and fibers carry proprioceptive information to the cerebellum as a movement that is being performed advances towards completion. This input is then processed by the spinocerebellum, which makes adjustments if necessary. The spinocerebellum controls posture and muscle tone. It also executes and coordinates muscle activity of the trunk and limbs (particularly of the hands and feet) during stereotyped movements, such as walking. Stereotyped movements consist of repetitive movements lacking variation. The spinocerebellum is somatotopically organized; that is, the vermis controls axial musculature (head and trunk), whereas the paravermal hemisphere functions in the control of the limb musculature (mainly the hands and feet) (Fig. 13.7). The inferior portion of the vermis is associated with crude motor coordination, whereas its superior portion is associated with precise motor coordination.

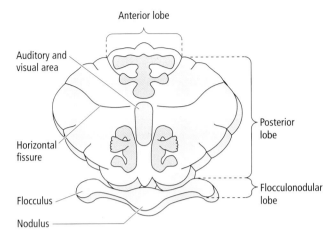

Figure 13.7 ● Sensory depiction in the cerebellar cortex. Note that visual and auditory information is relayed to the central region of the vermis. Somatosensory information is relayed to the vermal and paravermal zones of the anterior lobe, and the paravermal zone of the posterior lobe.

Posterior lobe (cerebrocerebellum, pontocerebellum, neocerebellum)

> The posterior lobe is reciprocally connected to the cerebral cortex

The most prominent lobe of the cerebellum is the most recent phylogenetically and is thus referred to as the **neocerebellum**. It consists of the **cerebellar hemispheres** but does not include the paravermal zone. Since the neocerebellum has a vast number of reciprocal connections with the cerebral cortex, it is functionally referred to as the **cerebrocerebellum (or pontocerebellum)** (see Fig. 13.6). The cerebellar hemispheres do not exhibit any perceptible anatomical landmark separating the paravermal cortex from the hemispheres. Due to the influence it exerts on the motor cortex, the cerebrocerebellum is associated with the planning, coordination, and execution of rapid, fine, nonstereotyped (learned, skilled) movements such as ice skating. Nonstereotyped movement is characterized as nonrepetitive, variable, and of diverse pattern.

CEREBELLAR PEDUNCLES

The cerebellum is attached to the posterior aspect of the brainstem by three pairs of prominent fiber bundles: the **superior**, **middle**, and **inferior cerebellar peduncles** (L. ped, "foot") (Fig. 13.8; Table 13.6). These peduncles are major (and the only) communication highways whereby afferent (input) and efferent (output) fibers enter or exit the cerebellum.

Superior cerebellar peduncle

> The superior cerebellar peduncle consists predominantly of efferent pathways arising from the cerebellar cortex, and the deep cerebellar nuclei

The **superior cerebellar peduncle** attaches the cerebellum to the caudal midbrain and the pons (Table 13.6). This peduncle consists predominantly of **efferent** pathways arising from the cerebellar cortex and the deep cerebellar nuclei—especially from the dentate, emboliform, and globose nuclei—with some fibers arising from the fastigial nucleus. The efferent pathways have four components:

- the dentorubrothalamic pathway;
- the interpositorubrothalamic pathway;
- the fastigiothalamic tract; and
- the fastigiovestibular tract.

The fibers of the first two pathways form a bundle of axons known collectively as the **brachium conjuctivum** (L. brachium, "arm;" conjuctivum, "joining"), which conveys the principal cerebellar efferent (output) pathway.

The superior cerebellar peduncle also carries **afferent** pathways to the cerebellum. The input pathways are:

- the anterior spinocerebellar tract, transmitting proprioceptive input from the lower limb and trunk;
- the tectocerebellar fibers, transmitting visual input from the superior colliculus;
- the rubrocerebellar fibers, transmitting information from the red nucleus;
- the trigeminocerebellar fibers, transmitting sensory information from the head; and
- the ceruleocerebellar fibers from the locus ceruleus that regulate cerebellar activity.

Middle cerebellar peduncle (brachium pontis)

> The massive middle cerebellar peduncle contains afferent fibers from the pons—the pontocerebellar fibers

The middle cerebellar peduncle joins the cerebellum to the dorsal aspect of the pons. The majority of fibers arising from the pontine nuclei destined for the cerebellum are the pontocerebellar fibers (transverse fibers of the pons) (Table 13.6). These fibers decussate and then pass into the cerebellum via the contralateral **middle cerebellar peduncle**, the largest of the cerebellar peduncles, which is also known as the **brachium pontis**. This peduncle consists of almost entirely of pontocerebellar fibers.

Since signals arising in the cerebral cortex are transmitted via corticopontine fibers to the pontine nuclei, the corticopontine and the pontocerebellar fibers collectively form the corticopontocerebellar pathway, which relays **afferents** to the **cerebrocerebellum (neocerebellum)**.

Inferior cerebellar peduncle

> The inferior cerebellar peduncle contains mostly afferent pathways to the cerebellum from the spinal cord and brainstem

The **inferior cerebellar peduncle** connects the cerebellum to the medulla. It carries mostly **afferent** pathways to the cerebellum from the spinal cord and brainstem (Table 13.6). This peduncle consists of two divisions: the more prominent, laterally positioned, restiform body, and the slender, medially located, juxtarestiform body.

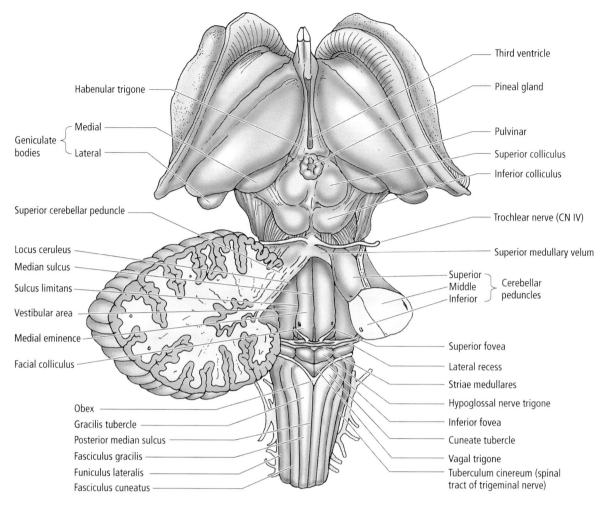

Figure 13.8 ● Posterior view of the brainstem and part of the left lobe of the cerebellum. Note the superior, middle, and inferior cerebellar peduncles.

Table 13.6 ● The cerebellar peduncles.

Cerebellar peduncle	Connects cerebellum to	Afferents (input) fibers	Efferents (output) fibers arise from

Superior (mostly efferent fibers)	Caudal midbrain and pons	Anterior spinocerebellar tract
		Tectocerebellar fibers
		Rubrocerebellar fibers
		Trigeminocerebellar fibers
		Ceruleocerebellar fibers
			Cerebellar cortex
			Deep cerebellar nuclei
			  Dentorubrothalamic pathway
			  Interpositorubrothalamic pathway
			  Fastigiothalamic tract
			  Fastigiovestibular tract

Middle (brachium pontis) (afferent fibers)	Pons	Pontocerebellar fibers	
Inferior (mostly afferent fibers) Restiform body (laterally)	Medulla	Dorsal spinocerebellar tract Rostral spinocerebellar tract Cuneocerebellar tract Olivocerebellar fibers Trigeminocerebellar fibers Reticulocerebellar fibers	
Juxtarestiform body (medially)		Vestibulocerebellar fibers	Cerebellovestibular fibers Cerebelloreticular fibers

The **restiform body** includes proprioceptive **afferent fibers** from the spinal cord and brainstem to the cerebellum carried in the following tracts or fibers:

- the dorsal spinocerebellar tract;
- the rostral spinocerebellar tract;
- the cuneocerebellar tract;
- the trigeminocerebellar fibers;
- the olivocerebellar fibers; and
- the reticulocerebellar fibers.

The first four tracts/fibers terminate in the **spinocerebellum (paleocerebellum)**, whereas the olivocerebellar fibers terminate *throughout* the **cerebellar cortex**, but mainly in the **neocerebellum**. The reticulocerebellar fibers, emerging from the nuclei of the pontine and medullary reticular formation, terminate in the **spinocerebellum** and **vestibulocerebellum**.

The **juxtarestiform body** includes mostly **afferent fibers** to the cerebellum, but also some efferent fibers from the cerebellum. The afferent fibers arise from first order and second order vestibular neurons and reach the **vestibulocerebellum** and the vermis of the **spinocerebellum** as vestibulocerebellar fibers. The only efferent fibers that leave the cerebellum via the juxtarestiform body are the cerebellovestibular (fastigiovestibular, fastigiobulbar) fibers and the cerebelloreticular fibers.

DEEP CEREBELLAR NUCLEI

The cerebellum has four pairs of nuclei embedded deep in its white matter core

As mentioned above, there are four pairs of intra-cerebellar nuclei, collectively known as the **deep cerebellar nuclei**. These are embedded deep in the cerebellar medullary white matter, and from lateral to medial, they are the **dentate nucleus**, the **emboliform nucleus**, the **globose nucleus**, and the **fastigial nucleus**. Recall that the emboliform and globose nuclei are collectively known as the **interposed nuclei**.

The deep cerebellar nuclei receive collaterals of cerebellar afferents and Purkinje cell axon terminals from the overlying cerebellar cortex; they are the main source of cerebellar output

Each of the deep cerebellar nuclei (Table 13.7) receives input from the collaterals of afferents destined for the corresponding region of the cerebellar cortex, permitting the deep cerebellar nuclei to be informed of input as it is being relayed to the cerebellar cortex. The fastigial nucleus also receives vestibulocerebellar fibers, which include axons of first order neurons of the vestibular nerve (CN VIII), as well as axons of second order neurons from the vestibular nuclei. The vestibulocerebellar fibers transmit sensory input directly from the vestibular apparatus of the inner ear. These connections play a role in the maintenance of equilibrium.

Although the deep cerebellar nuclei project to different parts of the brain, each one also has projections to the **inferior olivary nucleus (inferior olive)** as well as to the brainstem **reticular formation**. Furthermore, each deep cerebellar nucleus sends reciprocal projections to the same region of the **cerebellar cortex** that projects to it. It should be understood that although output from the cerebellum arises from the cerebellar cortex and the deep cerebellar nuclei, the *deep cerebellar nuclei are the main source of cerebellar output*. The deep cerebellar nuclei influence the descending motor pathways and ultimately the motoneurons of the brainstem and spinal cord (Fig. 13.9).

Nucleus	Afferents (input)	Efferents (output) to
Dentate nucleus	Collateral branches of pontocerebellar afferents Purkinje cell axons from cortex of cerebrocerebellum	Ventral lateral (VL) nucleus of the thalamus Red nucleus Oculomotor nucleus Cerebellar cortex Reticular formation Inferior olivary nucleus
Interposed nuclei (emboliform and globose)	Collateral branches of cerebellar afferents Purkinje cell axons from cortex of spinocerebellum Anterior spinocerebellar tract	Red nucleus Ventral lateral (VL) nucleus of the thalamus Cerebellar cortex Reticular formation Inferior olivary nucleus
Fastigial nucleus	Collateral branches of cerebellar afferents Purkinje cell axons from cortex of vestibulocerebellum Vestibulocerebellar fibers First order neurons of CN VIII Second order neurons from vestibular nuclei	Lateral vestibular nucleus Medial vestibular nucleus Inferior vestibular nucleus Ventral lateral (VL) nucleus of the thalamus Cerebellar cortex Reticular formation

Table 13.7 ● The deep cerebellar nuclei.

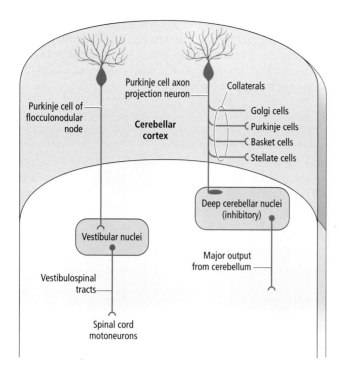

Figure 13.9 ● Purkinje cell projections from the cerebellar cortex to the deep cerebellar nuclei and the vestibular nuclei.

Dentate nucleus

The dentate nucleus is associated with the cerebrocerebellum

The **dentate nucleus** (L. dens, "tooth," "tooth-shaped") is the largest, the most laterally positioned, and the most conspicuous of the deep cerebellar nuclei. It appears similar to the inferior olivary nucleus since it resembles a "collapsed bag." It receives input from the collaterals of pontocerebellar afferents and the Purkinje cell terminals originating from the **cerebrocerebellum (pontocerebellum)** (Table 13.7).

The dentate nucleus gives rise to efferent fibers that join the **brachium conjuctivum**, the major component of the superior cerebellar peduncle. These efferent fibers, joined by fibers from the **interposed nuclei**, decussate and project to the contralateral **ventral lateral** (VL) **nucleus of the thalamus**. This thalamic projection is the major output of the dentate nucleus. The VL nucleus gives rise to fibers that ascend to terminate predominantly in the **premotor cortex** and the **primary motor cortex**. One of the outputs of both the premotor and primary motor cortices is the **anterior corticospinal tract**, which has an important function in the maintenance of muscle tone of the trunk and proximal (girdle) muscles. Although the cerebellum receives afferents (input) from both the *motor* and the *sensory* areas of the cerebral cortex about intended motor activity via the **corticopontocerebellar pathway**, the cerebellum projects via a relay in the thalamus to the motor cortical areas, particularly of the primary motor area, where it influences upcoming motor activity.

Additionally, a few fibers arising from the dentate nucleus exit the cerebellum via the same route but project to the parvocellular division of the **red nucleus**, and the **oculomotor**

nucleus of the opposite side. The parvocellular division of the red nucleus sends fibers to the ipsilateral inferior olivary nucleus, which projects heavily to the cerebellum. The fibers terminating in the oculomotor nucleus synapse with the lower motoneurons that innervate the superior rectus muscle. Since the dentate nucleus neurons, whose axons teminate in the oculomotor nucleus, receive an input from the vestibular primary fibers, they may serve as a connection of a vestibulo-oculomotor pathway.

Globose and emboliform nuclei (interposed nuclei)

The interposed nuclei are associated with the spinocerebellum

Together, the **globose** (L., "globe-shaped") and **emboliform** (G. emballein, "to insert") **nuclei** are referred to as the **interposed nuclei**. Afferents to these nuclei include: Purkinje cell terminals arising from the **spinocerebellum (paravermal cortex)**, as well as collaterals of input fibers arriving in the cerebellum by way of the restiform body and via the anterior spinocerebellar tract (Table 13.7).

Axons arising from the interposed nuclei join the brachium conjuctivum, *cross* to the opposite side, and project to the contralateral **red nucleus**. Other axons project to the ipsilateral **VL nucleus of the thalamus**. The projection to the red nucleus is the major output of the interposed nuclei. The red nucleus gives rise to the **rubrospinal tract**, whereas the VL nucleus projects to the premotor and primary motor cortex, which give rise to the **lateral corticospinal tract**. Recall that the rubrospinal and lateral corticospinal tracts together form the descending lateral systems and are involved in the control of the distal musculature of the upper and lower limbs (see Chapter 11 for more detail).

Fastigial nucleus

The fastigial nucleus is associated with the vestibulocerebellum

The **fastigial nucleus** (L. fastigius, "summit" since it is located in the roof of the fourth ventricle) receives Purkinje cell fibers arising from the **vestibulocerebellum**, and first order afferent collaterals arising from the vestibular apparatus and second order fibers from the vestibular nuclei (Table 13.7).

The fastigial nucleus gives rise to efferent fibers that leave the cerebellum via the juxtarestiform body of the inferior cerebellar peduncle. These are the fastigiovestibular (cerebellovestibular) fibers and the fastigioreticular fibers.

The **fastigiovestibular fibers** terminate principally in the lateral and inferior vestibular nuclei where they influence the vestibulospinal tracts, bilaterally. The **fastigioreticular fibers** terminate in the pontine and medullary reticular formation where they influence the reticulospinal tracts bilaterally (but mainly contralaterally). Recall that the vestibulospinal and reticulospinal tracts (collectively referred to as the descending medial systems) have an important function in balance and posture maintenance as well as in the motor activity of the proximal limb (girdle) musculature (see Chapter 11 for more detail).

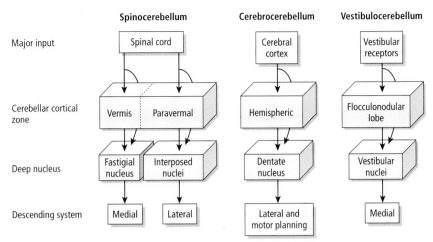

Figure 13.10 ● Functional organization of the spinocerebellum, cerebrocerebellum, and vestibulocerebellum. (Modified from Martin, JH (1996) *Neuroanatomy, Text and Atlas*, 2nd edn. Appleton & Lange, Connecticut; fig. 10.6.)

AFFERENTS (INPUT) TO THE CEREBELLUM

Afferent fibers to the cerebellum terminate primarily in the cerebellar cortex, but also send collaterals to the appropriate or corresponding deep cerebellar nucleus

The **afferent (input) fibers** to the cerebellum outnumber the efferent (output) fibers from the cerebellum by three to one. Afferent fibers pass primarily into the **cerebellar cortex** and they do so mainly via the inferior and middle cerebellar peduncles, although a number of fibers may enter via the superior cerebellar peduncle.

Afferent signals to the cerebellum arise from three main sources (Fig. 13.10; Table 13.8).

1 The **vestibular system** (vestibular ganglion and nuclei), which terminates in the vestibulocerebellum.
2 The **spinal cord**, which terminates in the spinocerebellum.
3 The **cerebral cortex**, mostly via the corticopontocerebellar pathway but also via the corticoreticulocerebellar and the cortico-olivocerebellar pathways, all of which terminate in the cerebrocerebellum.

In addition to these main sources, the cerebellar cortex also receives afferents from the hypothalamus, superior colliculi, ventral midbrain tegmentum, locus ceruleus, pontine raphe nuclei, trigeminal nerve nuclei, cochlear nuclei, and the deep cerebellar nuclei.

Afferents to the cerebellum arrive as:

- **mossy fibers**;
- **climbing fibers**;
- **monoaminergic fibers**; or
- other fibers.

Mossy fibers

Most of the afferent fibers to the cerebellum are mossy fibers

Mossy fibers include most of the afferents to the cerebellum which terminate in the **cerebellar cortex**. They are **excitatory**, release **glutamate**, and arise from the vestibular system, spinal cord, and cerebral cortex via the brainstem (Table 13.8). On their way to the cerebellar cortex to influence the Purkinje cells, the mossy fibers send collaterals to the **deep cerebellar nuclei**, where they also form **excitatory synapses**.

Mossy fiber afferents from the vestibular system

Afferents from the vestibular system terminate in the vestibulocerebellum as mossy fibers

Sensory information about changes in head position and orientation of the head relative to gravity is transmitted from the vestibular apparatus of the inner ear by the peripheral processes of first order bipolar neurons whose cell bodies are housed in the ipsilateral **vestibular ganglion**. The central processes of these neurons form the root of the vestibular division of the vestibulocochlear nerve (CN VIII), and enter the brainstem. Most of these central processes terminate in the **vestibular nuclei** to synapse with second order neurons. However, a small number of these central processes join the juxtarestiform body (part of the inferior cerebellar peduncle) and terminate ipsilaterally as **mossy fibers** in the **vestibulocerebellum**.

Cell bodies of second order neurons housed in the vestibular nuclei give rise to fibers that form a larger pathway than the fibers of the first order neurons. They also join the juxtarestiform body to terminate bilaterally as mossy fibers in the vestibulocerebellum.

The afferents from the vestibular system that terminate in the vestibulocerebellum (flocculonodular lobe) also send collaterals to the **fastigial nucleus**.

Mossy fiber afferents from the spinal cord

Afferents from the spinal cord terminate in the spinocerebellum as mossy fibers

Input from the spinal cord to the cerebellum consists of: the anterior (ventral) spinocerebellar tract, the posterior (dorsal) spinocerebellar tract, the cuneocerebellar tract, and

Table 13.8 • Afferents to the cerebellum.

Types of fibers	Fibers/tract/pathway	Origin	Termination
Mossy fibers	Vestibulocerebellar fibers	Vestibular ganglion Vestibular nuclei	Cortex of vestibulocerebellum and part of vermis
	Spinocerebellar fibers:		
	Anterior (ventral) spinocerebellar tract	Spinal cord	Cortex of spinocerebellum (vermis)
	Posterior (dorsal) spinocerebellar tract	Spinal cord	Cortex of spinocerebellum (vermis)
	Cuneocerebellar tract	Accessory cuneate nucleus	Cortex of spinocerebellum (paravermal zone)
	Rostral spinocerebellar tract	Spinal cord	Cortex of spinocerebellum
	Corticopontocerebellar pathway:		
	Corticopontine fibers	Primary motor cortex, secondary motor cortex, somesthetic cortex	Pontine nuclei
	Pontocerebellar fibers (transverse fibers of the pons)	Pontine nuclei	Cortex of cerebrocerebellum
	Corticoreticulocerebellar pathway:		
	Corticoreticular fibers	Various areas of the cerebral cortex	Pontine and medullary reticular formation nuclei
	Reticulocerebellar fibers	Pontine and medullary reticular formation nuclei	Cortex of cerebrocerebellum
	Cochleocerebellar fibers	Cochlear nuclei	Cortex of vermis
	Tectocerebellar fibers	Superior colliculus	Cortex of vermis
	Trigeminocerebellar fibers	Trigeminal nuclei	Cortex of cerebellum
	Rubrocerebellar fibers	Red nucleus	
Climbing fibers	Cortico-olivocerebellar pathway:		
	Cortico-olivary fibers	Primary motor cortex, secondary motor cortex, somesthetic cortex	Inferior olivary nucleus
	Olivocerebellar fibers	Inferior olivary nucleus	All layers of cerebellar cortex, mainly in cerebrocerebellum
Monoaminergic fibers		Ventral midbrain tegmentum	All layers of the cerebellar cortex (as diffuse fibers)
		Pontine raphe nuclei	Granular and molecular layers of cerebellar cortex
		Locus ceruleus	All layers of cerebellar cortex (as diffuse fibers)
Other fibers		Hypothalamus	All layers of cerebellar cortex
		Deep cerebellar nuclei	Cerebellar cortex

the rostral spinocerebellar tract. All of these tracts relay proprioceptive information (from muscles, tendons, joints, and skin) and terminate in the cortex of the **spinocerebellum** as **mossy fibers** (see Chapter 10 for more detail).

The **anterior (ventral) spinocerebellar tract** relays proprioceptive information from the lower trunk and lower limb. This tract ascends contralaterally in the spinal cord, and its fibers enter the cerebellum via the superior cerebellar peduncle and terminate in the cortex of the **vermis**. It is interesting to note that these fibers *cross twice* (once in the spinal cord, and then again in the cerebellar white matter), so that they terminate in the cerebellar hemisphere ipsilateral to the origin of the information.

The **posterior (dorsal) spinocerebellar tract** relays proprioceptive input from the lower trunk and lower limb. This tract ascends in the spinal cord ipsilaterally, and passes through the inferior cerebellar peduncle to enter the cortex of the vermis.

The **cuneocerebellar tract** (cuneatocerebellar tract) relays information from the upper trunk and upper limb, and passes through the inferior cerebellar peduncle to terminate in the ipsilateral **paravermal zone** cortex of the anterior lobe of the cerebellum.

The **rostral spinocerebellar tract** relays information from the upper limb. It passes through the inferior cerebellar peduncle to terminate in the cortex of the ipsilateral vermis.

The afferents from the spinal cord that terminate in the **spinocerebellum (anterior lobe)** also send collaterals to the **globose** and **emboliform nuclei**.

A striking characteristic of the spinocerebellar tracts is that they relay signals to the cerebellum at a conduction velocity unparalleled by any other tract of the CNS. These tracts owe

Table 13.8 ● *Continued.*

Collaterals	Neurotransmitter	Excitatory/inhibitory	Function(s)
Deep cerebellar nuclei	Glutamate	Excitatory	Transmit sensory input about changes in head position and orientation
Deep cerebellar nuclei	Glutamate	Excitatory	
	Glutamate	Excitatory	Relay proprioceptive input from trunk and lower limb
	Glutamate	Excitatory	Relay proprioceptive input from lower trunk and lower limb
	Glutamate	Excitatory	Relay proprioceptive input from upper trunk and upper limb
	Glutamate	Excitatory	Relay proprioceptive input from upper limb
Deep cerebellar nuclei	Glutamate	Excitatory	Relays signals that keep cerebellum informed of an actual movement in progress and an impending movement
Deep cerebellar nuclei	Glutamate	Excitatory	Functions in feedback systems
	Glutamate	Excitatory	Relay sensory input about the location and direction of a sound or object in space
	Glutamate	Excitatory	
	Glutamate	Excitatory	Relay sensory input from orofacial structures and stretch receptors of the muscles of mastication
	Aspartate	Excitatory	Functions in feedback systems
Interposed and dentate nuclei	Dopamine	Inhibitory	Modulate cerebellar activity
	Serotonin	Inhibitory	Modulate cerebellar activity
	Norepinephrine (noradrenaline)	Inhibitory	Modulate cerebellar activity
	Histamine		Coordinate somatic and visceral motor functions

their rapid conduction velocity to their wide-diameter, heavily myelinated axons. This keeps the cerebellum continually informed of the current position and movement of body parts, and it enables it to make rapid adjustments of upcoming motor activity if necessary.

Mossy fiber afferents from the cerebral cortex

Afferent signals from the cerebral cortex are relayed (via the pontine nuclei) to the cerebrocerebellum by mossy fibers

Signals arising from the cerebral cortex are transmitted to the cerebellum via the **corticopontocerebellar pathway** and the **corticoreticulocerebellar pathway**. These pathways terminate in the **cerebrocerebellum (posterior lobe)**.

The **primary motor cortex**, the **secondary motor cortex**, and the **somatosensory cortex** of each cerebral hemisphere give rise to more than 20 million axons that descend in the corona radiata, the internal capsule, and the cerebral peduncle to the pons and spinal cord. Approximately 1 million of these axons form the corticospinal tracts. The other 19 million axons are destined for the pontine nuclei (i.e., as corticopontine fibers of the corticopontocerebellar pathway), the reticular formation, and, via the corticonuclear (corticobulbar) fibers, to the cranial nerve motor nuclei in the brainstem.

Corticopontocerebellar pathway

The corticopontocerebellar pathway is the largest pathway associated with the cerebellum

Most of the 19 million fibers arising from the **cerebral cortex** are the **corticopontine fibers**, and as their name indicates, they terminate *ipsilaterally* in the **pontine nuclei**. Fibers arising from the pontine nuclei, known as **pontocerebellar fibers**, decussate (then referred to as the **transverse fibers of the pons** as they decussate) and gather to form the middle cerebellar peduncle to enter the cerebellum and terminate in the cerebellar cortex as **mossy fibers**. The pontocerebellar fibers form the *largest* mossy fiber input to the cerebellum. The pontocerebellar fibers send collaterals to the **dentate nucleus** and terminate throughout the cerebellar cortex— with the exception of the flocculonodular lobe—in the following manner: (i) signals originating from the primary motor cortex are relayed via the corticopontocerebellar pathway to the **vermal** and **paravermal zones** of the cerebellum; and (ii) signals originating from the premotor, somatosensory, and association cortical areas are relayed via the corticopontocerebellar pathway to the **hemispheric zone** of the cerebellum.

The **corticopontocerebellar pathway** is the largest pathway associated with the cerebellum as evidenced by the massive **middle cerebellar peduncles** connecting the pons to the cerebellum. Based on information relayed to the somesthetic cortex from muscle receptors, this pathway transmits signals that keep the cerebellum informed about a movement in progress. Additionally, based on commands of the primary and secondary motor cortices relayed to the lower motoneurons of the brainstem and spinal cord, it also keeps the cerebellum informed about upcoming movement. Thus these signals enable the cerebellum to monitor and adjust motor activity continuously, so that muscular movement is precise, smooth, flowing, and coordinated.

Corticoreticulocerebellar pathway

The cerebral cortex alerts the cerebellum to the initiation of a movement via the corticoreticulocerebellar pathway

Various regions of the cerebral cortex give rise to **corticoreticular fibers** that descend to synapse, mostly ipsilaterally, in the nuclei of the pontine and medullary **reticular formation**. **Reticulocerebellar fibers** pass via the ipsilateral inferior and middle cerebellar peduncles into the **vermis** of the cerebellum to terminate as **mossy fibers** where they function in feedback systems. Via this pathway, the cerebral cortex alerts the cerebellum of the initiation of a movement. The cerebellum then monitors motor activity and makes any necessary modifications.

Climbing fibers

Fibers arising from the inferior olivary nucleus (the olivocerebellar fibers) destined for the cerebellum, are referred to as "climbing fibers" when they reach the cerebellar cortex

The cerebral cortex, in addition to projecting to the pons via **corticopontine fibers** (part of the corticopontocerebellar pathway) and to the reticular formation via **corti-coreticular fibers** (part of the **corticoreticulocerebellar pathway**), as discussed above, also projects to the **inferior olivary nucleus** via **cortico-olivary fibers**.

The fibers arising from the pons and the reticular formation destined for the cerebellum (pontocerebellar and reticulocerebellar fibers, respectively), are referred to as mossy fibers when they reach the cerebellar cortex. In contrast, the fibers arising from the **inferior olivary nucleus** (the **olivocerebellar fibers**) destined for the cerebellum, are referred to as **climbing fibers** when they reach the cerebellar cortex (see Table 13.8).

Cortico-olivocerebellar pathway

The inferior olivary nucleus, a relay nucleus of the cortico-olivocerebellar pathway, is believed to play an important instructing role when one learns to perform a new motor skill

The **cortico-olivocerebellar pathway** originates from the primary motor cortex, the secondary motor cortex, and the somatosensory cortex and follows the same path to the brainstem as does the corticopontocerebellar pathway. The **cortico-olivary fibers**, however, terminate *bilaterally* in the **inferior olivary nuclei**. Input from the spinal cord, the red nucleus (major input), the cerebral cortex (mainly the motor cortex), and the deep cerebellar nuclei, is funneled into the inferior olivary nucleus, which is a cerebellar relay nucleus. The **inferior olivary nucleus** gives rise to a group of fibers that are destined for the contralateral cerebellar cortex. These are the **olivocerebellar fibers**, the sole efferents from the inferior olivary nucleus, that, as mentioned above, terminate in the cerebellar cortex as **climbing fibers**. On their way to the cerebellum, the olivocerebellar fibers decussate, course through the inferior cerebellar peduncle, enter the cerebellar white matter, send collaterals to the **deep cerebellar nuclei**, and "climb" to the cortical granular layer where they form **aspartate-releasing excitatory synapses** with granule cells and Golgi cells. The climbing fibers then continue their course through the Purkinje cell layer, where they terminate in the molecular layer as unmyelinated fibers to form powerful aspartate-releasing excitatory synapses with **Purkinje cell dendrites**. The inferior olivary nucleus is believed to play an important instructing role when one learns to perform a new motor skill.

Monoaminergic fibers

Monoaminergic fibers (dopaminergic, norepinephrine, or serotonergic fibers) projecting to the cerebellum arise from the ventral midbrain tegmentum, the locus ceruleus, and the pontine raphe nuclei

The **ventral midbrain tegmentum** gives rise to **dopaminergic fibers** that terminate in the interposed and dentate nuclei as well as in the cerebellar cortex. These dopaminergic *inhibitory* fibers function in the regulation of cerebellar activity (see Table 13.8).

The **norepinephrine (noradrenergic) fibers** arising from the **locus ceruleus** pass into the cerebellum via the superior and middle cerebellar peduncles to terminate in the cerebellar cortex where they form *inhibitory synapses* with dendrites of Purkinje cells and granule cells. These noradrenergic inhibitory fibers function in the regulation of cerebellar activity.

The fibers arising from the **pontine raphe nuclei** pass into the cerebellum via the middle cerebellar peduncle where they release **serotonin** in the granular and molecular layers of the cerebellar cortex. These fibers *inhibit* Purkinje cells, and function to regulate cerebellar activity.

Afferents from other sources

In addition to the above afferent projections, the cerebellum also receives afferents from the following sources: (i) the hypothalamus; (ii) the cochlear nuclei; (iii) the superior colliculi; and (iv) the trigeminal nerve nuclei (see Table 13.8).

The fibers arising from the **hypothalamus** release **histamine** at their terminals distributed throughout the cerebellar cortex. These fibers function to coordinate somatic and visceral motor responses.

The **cochlear nuclei** (which process auditory information) as well as the **superior colliculi** (which process information associated with the tracking of a moving object) relay sensory input to the dorsal aspect of the vermis regarding the location and shift in position of a sound or object.

The **trigeminal nerve nuclei** also send projections (trigeminocerebellar fibers) relaying sensory input from orofacial structures and the stretch receptors of the muscles of mastication. These fibers pass into the cerebellum via the inferior cerebellar peduncle where they terminate as mossy fibers.

EFFERENTS (OUTPUT) FROM THE CEREBELLUM

Efferent fibers from the cerebellum arise from the Purkinje cells of the cerebellar cortex and the cells of the deep cerebellar nuclei

Efferent fibers from the cerebellum arise from two sources (see Fig. 13.9):

1 **Purkinje cells**, which constitute the ultimate integrating terminal within the cerebellar cortex.
2 Cells of the **deep cerebellar nuclei**. These nuclei house the nerve cells whose *axons form the principal cerebellar output* (see discussion below, pp. 235–6).

Efferent fibers from Purkinje cells

The majority of the Purkinje cell axons terminate locally in the deep cerebellar nuclei. A small extracerebellar projection terminates in the vestibular nuclei

The **Purkinje cell axons** of the cerebellar cortex have two destinations. The only **extracerebellar** destination is as follows: the axons of the Purkinje cells located in the cortex of the **vestibulocerebellum** go past the deep cerebellar nuclei, exit the cerebellum, to end in the **vestibular nuclei**. The majority of Purkinje cell axons, though, terminate **locally** at their main targets (destination)—the **deep cerebellar nuclei**. The Purkinje cell axons always form *inhibitory synapses*.

It is important to note that Purkinje cell axons arising from the cerebellar cortex of the vermis, paravermal zone, or the hemispheric zone overlying the deep cerebellar nuclei project to the corresponding deep cerebellar nucleus (see Fig. 13.10 and discussion below).

All of the Purkinje cells that project to the deep cerebellar nuclei send collaterals to Golgi cells, as well as to other Purkinje cells, basket cells, and stellate cells of the cerebellar cortex.

Output from the flocculonodular lobe to the vestibular nuclei

Purkinje cells of the flocculonodular lobe project to the vestibular nuclei

Purkinje cell axons arising from the cortex of the **flocculonodular lobe (vestibulocerebellum)** form a small extracerebellar projection as they exit the cerebellum via the juxtarestiform body to terminate in the **vestibular nuclei** (see Fig. 13.10). **Vestibulospinal tracts** originate in the vestibular nuclei and terminate on those motoneurons of the spinal cord that control posture and balance.

Note that the flocculonodular lobe projects primarily to the vestibular nuclei (which are located outside the cerebellum) and sends only a few Purkinje cell fibers to the fastigial nucleus.

Based on the projections of the cerebellum to the vestibular nuclei, and since both the deep cerebellar nuclei and the vestibular nuclei receive *excitatory afferent fibers* from the inferior olivary nucleus in addition to receiving *inhibitory afferent fibers* from Purkinje cells, the vestibular nuclei are considered by some to be anatomically analogous to the deep cerebellar nuclei. Thus, the vestibular and deep cerebellar nuclei share two common sources of afferent fibers.

Output from the vermal zone and the fastigial nucleus

Purkinje cells of the vermal zone cortex project to the fastigial nucleus

Purkinje cell axons arising from the cortex of the **vermal zone** project to the ipsilateral **fastigial nucleus** (see Fig. 13.10). The fastigial nucleus gives rise to fibers that exit the cerebellum via the inferior cerebellar peduncle to terminate bilaterally in the **lateral vestibular nucleus** and in the contralateral brainstem **reticular formation**.

The vestibular nuclei give rise to the **vestibulospinal tracts**, and the reticular nuclei give rise to the **reticulospinal tracts**. Collectively these tracts form the **medial descending system**, which terminates in the spinal cord and has an important function in the maintenance of posture, balance, and muscle tone of extensor muscles.

Recall that the cortex of the vermis receives an input from the spinal cord. The fastigial nucleus also gives rise to a small number of fibers that pass into the superior cerebellar peduncles and ascend bilaterally to the VL nucleus of the **thalamus**. The thalamus in turn projects to the premotor and primary motor cortex. The neurons of the premotor and primary motor cortices, whose axons form the **anterior corticospinal tract**, control motor activity of the axial and proximal limb (girdle) musculature.

Output from the paravermal zone and the interposed nuclei

Purkinje cells of the paravermal zone cortex project to the interposed nuclei

The **Purkinje cell axons** arising from the cortex of the **paravermal zone** project to the **interposed nuclei** (see Fig. 13.10), which are associated with the execution and modification of movements. These nuclei in turn, project, via the superior cerebellar peduncle, to the magnocellular component of the contralateral **red nucleus**. The red nucleus gives rise to the **rubrospinal tract** that terminates in the spinal cord contralaterally and functions in regulating motor activity by facilitating the muscle tone of the ipsilateral flexors. The interposed nuclei also send some fibers, via the superior cerebellar peduncle, to the VL nucleus of the **thalamus**, which projects to the premotor and primary motor cortex. One of the outputs of these cortices is the **lateral corticospinal tract**. The rubrospinal tract and the lateral corticospinal tract together form the **lateral descending system**, which controls the motor activity of the distal musculature of the limbs, especially the hands.

Output from the hemispheric zone and the dentate nucleus

Purkinje cells of the hemispheric zone cortex project to the dentate nucleus

Purkinje cell axons arising from the cortex of the **hemispheric zone** of the cerebellum project to the **dentate nucleus**, which is associated with the *planning* of movements (see Fig. 13.10). Fibers arising from neurons of the dentate nucleus form the **dentorubrothalamic pathway**. These fibers exit the cerebellum by joining the superior cerebellar peduncle, decussate, and terminate to synapse in two places: the parvocellular component of the red nucleus and the VL nucleus of the thalamus (most fibers terminate here). *This projection to the VL nucleus of the thalamus is the principal efferent projection of the cerebellum.* The majority of the fibers in the superior cerebellar peduncle originate from the dentate nucleus.

The **parvocellular component of the red nucleus** gives rise to fibers that join the **central tegmental tract** to terminate in the ipsilateral **inferior olivary nucleus**.

The **VL nucleus of the thalamus** gives rise to fibers that ascend to terminate in the ipsilateral **primary motor** and **premotor cortex**, which give rise to the **lateral corticospinal tract**. Via its influence on the lateral corticospinal tract, the cerebellum plays an important role in the planning phase, initiation, timing, and precision of discrete movements, specifically the reciprocal contractions of agonist and antagonist muscles of the limbs (especially of the hands).

FUNCTIONAL ORGANIZATION OF THE CEREBELLUM: INTRINSIC CIRCUITRY

As discussed above, the histologic organization of the **cerebellar cortex** is identical throughout the cerebellum (see Fig. 13.5). It contains **Purkinje cells** whose functions are *inhibitory*, and four types of **interneurons**, three of which are *inhibitory*—namely **basket cells**, **stellate cells**, and **Golgi cells**—whereas the fourth type, the **granule cells**, are *excitatory*.

Excitatory inputs to the cerebellar cortex

The climbing and mossy fibers provide the major excitatory input to the cerebellum

Excitatory inputs to the **cerebellar cortex** are derived from both extrinsic fibers and intrinsic fibers. The **extrinsic fibers** are composed of **climbing fibers** and **mossy fibers**. The **intrinsic fibers** are the axons of **granule cells** of the granular cell layer of the cerebellar cortex. An additional source of excitatory synapses are the **deep cerebellar nuclei**, which send their axons into the cerebellar cortex as nucleocortical connections.

Climbing fibers

Climbing fibers are the axon terminals of neurons whose cell bodies reside exclusively in the inferior olivary nucleus

The **inferior olivary nucleus** gives rise to the **olivocerebellar fibers**. On their way to the cerebellum they decussate, and when they reach the cerebellar white matter they branch, send **excitatory collaterals** to the **deep cerebellar nuclei**, and proceed by "climbing" towards the granular layer of the cerebellar cortex as **climbing fibers**. There, a climbing fiber gives rise to about 10 branches that extend into the molecular layer of the cerebellar cortex where they synapse with Purkinje cells. Each terminal of a climbing fiber forms 300–500 **direct, excitatory** synaptic contacts with the dendrites of an individual **Purkinje cell** (see Fig. 13.5). Each individual Purkinje cell receives synaptic contacts from only a single climbing fiber. *An impulse transmitted from a climbing fiber to the dendrites of a Purkinje cell generates a prolonged, oscillatory-type, powerful depolarization* of that Purkinje cell.

Additionally, the climbing fibers also depolarize the Golgi, stellate, and basket cells. These inhibitory interneurons attenuate Purkinje cell activity, which has a more potent effect on cerebellar cortical outflow than does the limited, intense depolarization of a small population of Purkinje cells that are depolarized directly by a climbing fiber.

Mossy fibers

Most of the afferents to the cerebellum consist of mossy fibers

Most of the afferents to the cerebellum consist of **mossy fibers** (see Fig. 13.5). Mossy fibers relay information to the cerebellum from various sources: (i) the spinal cord; (ii) the vestibular ganglion and vestibular nuclei; (iii) the pontine nuclei; (iv) the reticular nuclei; and (v) the trigeminal nuclei. Afferent fibers enter the cerebellum by passing through all three cerebellar peduncles; they then course through the cerebellar white matter where they branch, and prior to their termination in the cerebellar cortex, send **excitatory collaterals** to the **deep cerebellar nuclei**. When they reach their destination they terminate in synaptic complexes, known as **glomeruli**, within the granular layer of the cerebellar cortex.

A glomerulus has the following components: a **mossy fiber**, which establishes *excitatory synapses* with the dendrites of a **granule cell**, and a **Golgi cell** and its terminals, which form inhibitory synapses with **granule cell** dendrites. A mossy fiber activates a granule cell within a glomerulus.

It takes a large number of simultaneously stimulated mossy fibers to activate a granule cell. The axon of each granule cell bifurcates in the molecular layer to form parallel fibers, which form **excitatory synapses** with the dendrites of Purkinje cells, basket cells, stellate cells, and Golgi cells (all of which are inhibitory).

A single parallel fiber synapses with thousands of Purkinje cells in succession (as a single electrical wire can pierce through and contact the branches of many trees in succession). The dendritic tree of a single Purkinje cell is traversed by thousands of parallel fibers, which establish synapses with dendritic terminals (as multiple telephone wires can pass among the branches of a single tree). Each parallel fiber establishes only a few synapses with each Purkinje cell. Recall that, in contrast, a climbing fiber forms several hundred direct synaptic contacts with a Purkinje cell. Consequently as a result of the greater number of synaptic contacts, the climbing fiber input exerts a stronger excitatory influence on Purkinje cells than does the mossy fiber input. Thus it takes a multitude of concurrently stimulated mossy fibers to trigger a nerve impulse in a single Purkinje cell. Interestingly, mossy fiber stimulation triggers recurring Purkinje cell action potentials, rather than the single, sustained, powerful depolarization generated by climbing fibers.

It should therefore be noted that a Purkinje cell may be stimulated either by: (i) a climbing fiber, directly, resulting in a very specific output signal; or (ii) mossy fibers, indirectly, via granule cell parallel fibers, resulting in a less specific but tonic output signal.

Basket cells, stellate cells, and Golgi cells are all inhibitory. The basket cells and the stellate cells form inhibitory synapses with the Purkinje cells. The Golgi cells are stimulated by mossy fibers within the glomeruli and by the parallel fibers that form synapses on their apical dendrites. The stimulated Golgi cells then respond by inhibiting the granule cells back in the glomeruli; that is, they prevent further excitability of the granule cells by upcoming excitatory impulses from the mossy fibers.

Inhibitory inputs to the cerebellar cortex

Inhibitory inputs to the cells of the cerebellar cortex are derived from **Golgi cells**, **Purkinje cells**, **basket cells**, and **stellate cells**. All four types of cells are **intrinsic** modulator cells and they all release **GABA**.

Inhibitory output from the cerebellar cortex

The single output from the cerebellar cortex is via the axons of Purkinje cells and is excitatory

There is only a single output from the **cerebellar cortex**— the axons of the **Purkinje cells (inhibitory)**. These cells transmit integrated information from the cerebellar cortex to the **vestibular nuclei** and to the **deep cerebellar nuclei**.

Output from the deep cerebellar nuclei

Output from the deep cerebellar nuclei is excitatory

The neurons housed in the deep cerebellar nuclei are continually under *excitatory* influences exerted on them by the collaterals of climbing and mossy fibers and *inhibitory* influences exerted on them by Purkinje cell axons. The effect that these excitatory and inhibitory influences have on cerebellar input during motor activity, however, is still uncertain.

These excitatory and inhibitory influences exerted on the cells of the deep cerebellar nuclei are constantly balanced, hence the intensity of the efferent signals from the cells of the deep cerebellar nuclei remains the same during moderate levels of prolonged excitation. However, during intense motor activity (e.g., when running), the excitatory influence is exerted on the cells of the deep cerebellar nuclei *prior* to the inhibitory influence. Thus the **deep cerebellar nuclei** first relay an *excitatory* output signal to the motor system in order to adjust the motor activity in progress, and then relay an *inhibitory* output signal to ultimately inhibit the motor activity. Thus, once a movement is initiated, the deep cerebellar nuclear excitatory output modifies the motor activity and, shortly thereafter, it is inhibited so as to prevent overshooting (missing the mark) of the movement in progress. An increase in the firing rate of the cells of the deep cerebellar nuclei assures that the cerebellum provides an excitatory output signal, whereas a decrease in the firing rate of these cells provides an inhibitory output signal.

Influence of mossy and climbing fibers on cerebellar output

The cerebellum processes information derived from the ipsilateral side of the body and from the contralateral cerebral cortex

The **mossy fibers** form the principal conduit of excitatory signals to the deep cerebellar nuclei by a **direct** projection (mossy fibers →

cells of the deep cerebellar nuclei). The mossy fibers simultaneously form an **alternate pathway**, which also ultimately projects to the deep cerebellar nuclei, but first relays in the cerebellar cortex. The mossy fiber stimulates a granule cell that, via its parallel fibers, stimulates Purkinje cells. The Purkinje cells then project primarily to the deep cerebellar nuclei, thus completing the alternate pathway of mossy fiber output to the deep cerebellar nuclei. (Purkinje cells also have a small extracerebellar projection to the vestibular nuclei.)

Stellate cells, basket cells, and Golgi cells modulate Purkinje cell excitation generated by both mossy fibers and climbing fibers. Consequently, Purkinje cells have a strong inhibitory influence on the cells of the deep cerebellar and vestibular nuclei, modulating their output. It is the processing of the afferent input to the cerebellum, and its modulation via Purkinje cells, that ultimately determines the smoothing of movements in progress.

It is important to remember that the cerebellum processes information derived from the *ipsilateral* side of the body, and from the *contralateral* cerebral cortex.

CLINICAL CONSIDERATIONS

A lesion confined to one cerebellar hemisphere results in symptoms that appear on the ipsilateral side of the body

It is well known that electrical stimulation of the cerebellum does not produce any type of sensation or movement. This led early neuroanatomists to refer to the cerebellum as a "silent area" of the brain. The cerebellum plays a role in cognitive functions in part via its projections to the frontal lobe, and has an important function in motor learning. It is clear that a lesion involving the cerebellum results in the abnormal execution of voluntary and involuntary motor activities, motor learning, and other cognitive dysfunction. Now that its internal circuitry is better understood, it has helped us understand the source of these effects.

Since the intrinsic circuitry of the cerebellar cortex is identical throughout the cerebellum, it is difficult to correlate a function with a particular region of the cerebellar cortex. Instead, it is the origin and destination of the afferent and efferent fibers that facilitates functional identification in the cerebellum.

Although the cerebellum is subdivided into three functionally distinct zones, each including cortex, white matter, and one or two deep cerebellar nuclei, lesions are rarely confined to one zone only. Generally speaking, lesions involving the deep cerebellar nuclei (the major source of cerebellar output) or the superior cerebellar peduncles (which convey most of the cerebellar output fibers) result in more serious symptoms than lesions that are confined to the cerebellar cortical region. Furthermore, although the cerebellum is involved in motor function, a lesion in the cerebellum results in **abnormal execution** of a motor task and *not* deficits in motor function such as paralysis or paresis. A lesion confined to one cerebellar hemisphere results in symptoms that appear on the body on the **same side as the lesion**. The reason why this occurs is due to the fact that the cerebellar efferent connections and the descending motor pathways upon which the cerebellum exerts its influence are crossed. Additionally, the main afferent pathways from the spinal cord to the cerebellum, namely the cuneocerebellar and posterior spinocerebellar tracts, are ipsilateral.

The most common symptoms attributed to cerebellar malfunction are **hypotonia** (decrease in muscle tone) and **ataxia** (G. atactos, "disorderly," "uncoordinated").

Severe trauma to the cerebellum results in serious symptoms; however, after a variable amount of time, full recovery may follow. It is believed that other parts of the brain may "take over" and compensate for any cerebellar deficits. Persistent conditions, however, such as the prolonged, slow growth of a tumor, cause milder symptoms. In this case, the growing lesion and the damage produced are accompanied by continuous compensation for the cerebellar deficits.

Flocculonodular syndrome

Flocculonodular syndrome has been characterized by the inability to maintain equilibrium

Flocculonodular syndrome has been characterized by the **inability to maintain equilibrium**—without an accompanying ataxia of the limbs, hypotonia, or tremor—and unsteady walking and swaying from side to side. The individual may also experience **nystagmus**, presented by rhythmic oscillations of the eyes. Since lesions involving the flocculonodular lobe may include midline cerebellar components, the symptoms may be bilateral.

Disorders resulting following a lesion in the vermal and paravermal zones

A lesion involving the vermal and paravermal zones of the cerebellum results in abnormal stance and gait (abnormal standing or walking/running)

Following a lesion in the **vermal** or **paravermal zones**, standing is characterized by the feet positioned far apart, providing a compensatory broad base. While walking, the individual is unable to "walk in tandem." The affected individual also exhibits **titubation**, a condition characterized by a rhythmic tremor (involuntary oscillation) of the trunk or head when sitting or standing, and postural changes of the head, in which the head may be held in a rotated position or tilted towards one side. Due to the lesion's midline proximity, the side in which the head is rotated or tilted may not be a reflection of the side of the lesion.

Cerebellar disease may be manifested in various abnormal movements of the eyes. The most conspicuous abnormal eye movement is spontaneous **nystagmus** that occurs without stimulation of the vestibular apparatus. Nystagmus is characterized by rhythmic oscillation of one or both eyes, and is manifested when the eyes are deviated laterally in the horizontal plane towards the side of the lesion.

Disorders resulting following lesions in the hemispheric zone

A lesion affecting one cerebellar hemisphere is exhibited primarily as ataxia and tremor on the ipsilateral side of the body

A lesion involving the **hemispheric zone** may result in numerous disorders, as described below. A lesion affecting one cerebellar hemisphere is exhibited primarily as ataxia and tremor on the ipsilateral side of the body.

Ataxia (G. atactos, "disorderly") is the lack of coordination of movements. The timing and precision of motor tasks are impaired, resulting in awkard movement.

CLINICAL CONSIDERATIONS (*continued*)

Ocular movement disorders, of which the most common is **nystagmus**, is most noticeable when the individual deviates his eyes towards the side of the lesion. Ocular movement disorders result as a consequence of asynergic (uncoordinated) activity of the extraocular muscles.

Tremor is characterized by the exhibition of **static** and **kinetic tremors**. **Intention tremor** is manifested during a voluntary movement, and is especially apparent towards the end of a movement, such as when putting glasses on.

Delayed initiation and termination of motor activity. The affected individual has difficulty initiating a motor activity, and once the activity is ongoing, he then has difficulty stopping it.

Abnormal stance and gait is also seen in individuals with hemispheric lesions. The individual stands with feet apart, and tends to sway forward, backward, or to the side, resembling a state of intoxication. Ataxia may also be evident when moving the lower limbs.

Decomposition of movement may occur following cerebellar disease. Movements are jerky, awkward, and inaccurate. An individual with such a lesion attempts to compensate for the awkward movements by making gradual movements such as moving one part (arm, forearm, hand, finger) of the body at a time.

Hypotonia (diminished muscle tone) may be exhibited following manipulation of the limbs at a joint. A decrease occurs in resistance to this passive manipulation, resulting in excess movement of the limbs referred to as "loose jointed" or "rag-doll appearance," since the damaged cerebellum does not exert its influence on the stretch reflex. Hypotonia is velocity independent. This condition gradually diminishes over time.

Dysarthria (G. dys, "abnormal," "disorderly;" arthroun, "to utter distinctly") is characterized by impaired speech that is slow and slurred. It is caused from lack of coordination of the muscles used to produce speech and is referred to as "scanning" speech, because of the excess and equal stress on all syllables.

Dysmetria (G. dys, "abnormal," "disorderly;" metron, "measure") is a disorder in which the individual is unable to estimate the distance between the moving body part and a target ("past pointing").

Dysdiadochokinesia (adiadochokinesia) (G. diadocho, "alternating;" kinesis, "movement") is the inability to carry out rapid alternating movements regularly (example rapid pronation and supination of the forearm).

Dysrhythmokinesis is the inability to maintain rhythm while performing alternating movements at a fast pace.

Impaired check and rebound is a condition which results from loss of cerebellar input to the stretch reflex. When a limb is displaced from a certain position against resistance (e.g., trying to straighten an individual's flexed arm against resistance), its abrupt release does not result in its return to its initial position, but instead it is displaced beyond its previous position. The individual is unable to stop a movement suddenly.

Note that the clinical case in the beginning of the chapter refers to a patient whose symptoms include sudden-onset severe vertigo, nausea, dysarthria, nystagmus, dysmetria, and ataxia in the left arm.

1 A cerebellar stroke is suspected. Which side of the cerebellum has been affected?

2 Which zone or zones of the cerebellum have been affected?

3 Which vessel may have been occluded in this patient?

SYNONYMS AND EPONYMS OF THE CEREBELLUM

Name of structure or term	Synonym(s)/eponym(s)
Anterior lobe of the cerebellum	Spinocerebellum Paleocerebellum
Cuneocerebellar tract	Cuneatocerebellar tract
Deep cerebellar nuclei	Cerebellar nuclei
Basal ganglia	Deep cerebral nuclei Basal nuclei
Fastigiovestibular fibers	Cerebellovestibular fibers
Flocculonodular lobe	Vestibulocerebellum Archicerebellum
Gamma aminobutyric acid-releasing fibers	GABAergic fibers
Golgi cells	Inner stellate cells
Hemispheric zone	Lateral zone
Inferior olivary nucleus	Inferior olive Olive
Lower motoneuron	Lower motor neuron
Middle cerebellar peduncle	Brachium pontis
Olivocerebellar fiber terminals	"Climbing fibers"
Paravermal zone	Intermediate zone
Pontocerebellar fibers	Transverse fibers of the pons
Posterior lobe of the cerebellum	Middle lobe of the cerebellum Cerebrocerebellum Pontocerebellum Neocerebellum
Premotor area	Premotor cortex Part of Brodmann's area 6
Primary motor cortex (M-I)	Precentral gyrus Brodmann's area 4
Proprioception	Position sense
Vermal zone	Median zone

FOLLOW-UP TO CLINICAL CASE

This patient had a **left cerebellar stroke** in the distribution of the **left posterior inferior cerebellar artery** (PICA). This is a common type of stroke and is therefore important for all physicians to know about, not just neurologists. The inferior and lateral cerebellum as well as the dorsolateral medulla are supplied by the PICA. However, many infarctions involve only part of the PICA territory and may involve only the cerebellum. The PICA arises most commonly from the vertebral artery just proximal to the basilar artery. Thrombosis of the PICA or the vertebral artery or emboli to the vertebral artery are the commonest causes of this stroke syndrome.

The symptoms in the case above are typical. The cerebellum, specifically the cerebellar vermis and surrounding parts of the inferior midline cerebellum, have important connections with the vestibular nuclei. Therefore, vertigo or dizziness is common. Gait is often severely disturbed and gait testing is critical. In fact, sometimes it is the only abnormality in cerebellar disease. Focal cerebellar pathology causes *ipsilateral* ataxia or dysmetria of the limbs, as opposed to the contralateral dysfunction caused by most other brain lesions. Ocular dysfunction is common. Complaints of blurry or double vision, nystagmus towards the side of the lesion, ipsilateral gaze paresis, or other ocular paresis are common. Additional symptoms can occur with involvement of the dorsolateral medulla, according to the structures in that region of the brainstem.

An initial head CT is usually normal unless there is some hemorrhage present. After a day or two it will show the stroke. MRI gives an exquisite view of the cerebellum and brainstem.

Often the most distressing and disabling symptom, along with the inability to walk, is vertigo. This can be relieved with antidopamine or similar medication. Symptoms will usually improve or resolve over time (days, weeks, or months).

QUESTIONS TO PONDER

1. Why is it that a cerebellar lesion confined to one cerebellar hemisphere results in symptoms that appear on the same side of the body?

2. Distinguish between the tremor resulting following a lesion in the basal ganglia and a lesion involving the cerebellum.

3. An individual who is inebriated stands with feet apart and waves his arms in different directions to maintain his balance, and tends to sway forward, backward, or to the side. These are also symptoms exhibited by an individual who has a lesion in which of the three cerebellar zones?

4. Based on your knowledge of the intrinsic circuitry of the cerebellum, what is the net output of the cerebellum—inhibitory or excitatory?

5. What causes the hypotonia exhibited (following manipulation of the limbs at a joint) by individuals following a lesion in the hemispheric zone of the cerebellum?

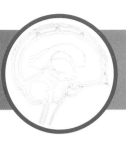
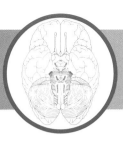
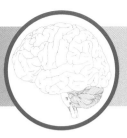

CHAPTER 14

Reticular Formation

CLINICAL CASE

A 58-year-old man presented with sudden onset of complete left-sided paralysis and slurred speech. The head CT in the ER demonstrated evidence of early edematous changes in the distribution of the right middle cerebral artery (MCA). A head CT 2 days later showed a very large right hemisphere infarction involving the entire right MCA territory. He had been somewhat drowsy but easily aroused during the first few days of hospitalization. He also had a right gaze preference, left hemineglect, and severe left hemiplegia. He became more lethargic after the first few days, and then could not be aroused. He was placed on mechanical ventilation due to respiratory difficulties.

Examination in the ICU revealed that he was comatose (a sleep-like state from which one cannot be aroused). His right pupil was fixed and dilated. Other brainstem reflexes were intact. There was no movement elicited on the left side, but there was some movement following stimulation on the right. However, there was a Babinski reflex (extensor plantar response) present on the right (indicating dysfunction of the descending motor tracts controlling the right side of the body).

There was subsequent deterioration of the patient's condition. He eventually lost all his brainstem reflexes (pupils became unresponsive to light, eye blink to corneal touch was lost, spontaneous respiratory effort ceased, etc.). All limb movement was lost. Brain death was confirmed.

The **reticular formation** (L. reticulum, "little net") consists of various distinct populations of cells embedded in an intricate polysynaptic network of cell processes occupying the central core of the brainstem. From an evolutionary perspective, the reticular formation is phylogenetically an ancient neural complex that is closely associated with two other ancient neural systems, the **olfactory system** which mediates the visceral sense of smell, and the **limbic system** which functions in the visceral and behavioral responses to emotions. The reticular formation and the olfactory and limbic systems are interrelated as a result of their participation in *visceral functions* and *behavioral responses*. The reticular formation is continually informed of activity occurring in almost all areas of the nervous system and responds by influencing the following:

skeletal muscle motor activity; somatic and visceral sensation; autonomic nervous system activity; endocrine functions; biological rhythms, via reciprocal connections to the hypothalamus, and the level of consciousness.

MORPHOLOGY OF THE RETICULAR FORMATION

Each subdivision of the reticular formation has its own distinct cytoarchitecture, specific connections, and functions

The **reticular formation** is most prominent in the brainstem, where it forms the central core gray matter of the midbrain, pons, and medulla. The spinal cord also contains throughout its entire length an analogue of the reticular formation, the intermediate zone of gray matter. However, this intermediate zone of gray matter, consisting of interneurons, is not as extensive as the brainstem reticular formation. The brainstem reticular formation extends from the diencephalon almost as far caudally as the pyramidal decussation.

The reticular formation contains fibers that are oriented in all planes, thus in histologic sections it appears as an interlacing structure that fills the area among various ascending and descending pathways, cranial nerve nuclei, and other gray matter. Although it appears scattered, indistinct, and ambiguous, the reticular formation, in fact, consists of numerous different histologic subdivisions each having its own distinct cytoarchitecture, specific connections, and functions.

Neurons of the reticular formation

The structure of the neurons of the reticular formation facilitates the collection of information from ascending and descending fibers

The neurons of the reticular formation possess elaborate dendritic trees whose branches radiate in all directions (Fig. 14.1). Some neurons give rise to an ascending or descending axon, with numerous collateral branches. Other neurons give rise to a primary axon, which bifurcates forming an ascending and a descending branch, both of which then give rise to collateral branches. The dendrites are oriented perpendicular to the long axis of the brainstem. The elaborate radiating dendritic trees, and the axons and their collaterals, facilitate the ability of the neurons of the reticular formation to collect information from ascending and descending fibers arising from various sources, as these fibers traverse the brainstem tegmentum. Information converging on the reticular formation is integrated, and the reticular formation, via its output, influences nerve cell activity at all levels of the central nervous system (CNS). As a result of its central location and cytoarchitecture, a single neuron of the reticular formation can exert its influence on various somatic or visceral functions via direct or indirect projections to higher brain centers, local brainstem centers, and the spinal cord. Many neurons of the reticular formation are involved in local multisynaptic and reflex circuits.

Based on its connections (input and output), the reticular formation can be thought of as the CNS "command center" where surveillance of activities occurring in distant sites of the CNS takes place. It is as a result of its diverse connections that the reticular formation can integrate and modulate various activities and functions of almost all areas controlled by the CNS.

Nuclei of the reticular formation

More than 100 nuclei scattered throughout the tegmentum of the midbrain, pons, and medulla have been identified as being part of the brainstem reticular formation

More than 100 nuclei scattered throughout the tegmentum of the midbrain, pons, and medulla have been identified as being part of the brainstem reticular formation (Fig. 14.2).

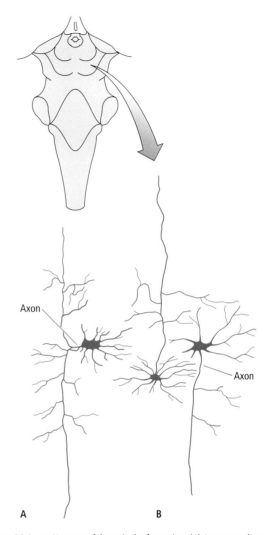

Figure 14.1 ● Neurons of the reticular formation. (A) A neuron whose primary axon divides into an ascending and a descending branch. (B) Note the intermingling of neuronal dendrites and axonal collateral branches.

Most of the nuclei of the reticular formation are not as clearly defined as are other nuclei of the CNS. Although the nuclei of the reticular formation have a number of diverse functions, they are classified according to the following four general functions:

1 The regulation of the level of consciousness, and ultimately cortical alertness.
2 The control of somatic motor movements.
3 The regulation of visceral motor or autonomic functions.
4 The control of sensory transmission.

ZONES OF THE RETICULAR FORMATION

Anatomically, the reticular formation is divided into four longitudinal zones (columns) on the basis of their mediolateral location in the brainstem

The zones of the reticular formation are: the unpaired median zone, the paired paramedian zone, the paired medial zone, and the paired

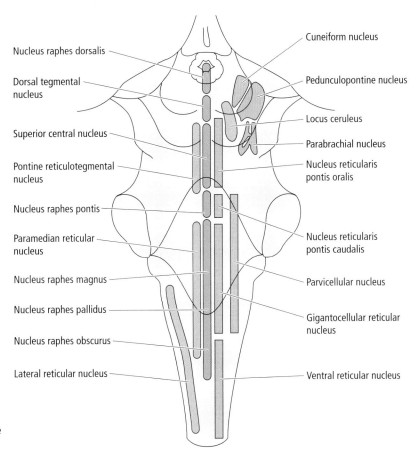

Figure 14.2 ● The nuclei of the reticular formation in the brainstem.

Table 14.1 ● Zones of the reticular formation and their component nuclei.

Brainstem location	Median zone	Paramedian zone	Medial zone ("motor" or "efferent" zone)	Lateral zone ("sensory" or "afferent" zone)
Midbrain	Nucleus raphes dorsalis (nucleus linearis) Dorsal tegmental nucleus			Cuneiform nucleus Parabrachial nucleus Pedunculopontine nucleus
Pons	Superior central nucleus Nucleus raphes pontis Nucleus raphes magnus	Pontine reticulotegmental nucleus Paramedian reticular nucleus	Nucleus reticularis pontis oralis Nucleus reticularis pontis caudalis	Parabrachial nucleus Pedunculopontine nucleus Parvicellular nucleus
Medulla	Nucleus raphes pallidus Nucleus raphes obscurus	Paramedian reticular nucleus	Gigantocellular reticular nucleus Ventral reticular nucleus	Parvicellular nucleus

lateral zone (Table 14.1). Some authors consider the median and paramedian zones to be one zone.

Median zone (also known as the median column, midline raphe)

The neurons of the median zone that project to higher brain centers are associated with sleep

The unpaired **midline raphe** (G. raphe, "seam") nuclei consist of intermediate-size neurons. These nuclei are present along much of the ventral aspect of the brainstem, except in areas of the basis pontis and the medulla that are occupied by various bundles of decussating fibers such as the pyramidal and lemniscal decussations.

The neurons that project to the spinal trigeminal nucleus and the dorsal horn of the spinal cord modulate or suppress the transmission of nociception

The raphe nuclei of the midbrain are the **dorsal tegmental nucleus** and the **nucleus raphes dorsalis (nucleus linearis)**; those of the pons are the **nucleus raphes magnus**, the

nucleus raphes pontis, and the **superior central nucleus**; in the medulla they are the **nucleus raphes obscurus** and the **nucleus raphes pallidus** (Fig. 14.2).

Numerous neurons of the raphe nuclei synthesize serotonin. The serotonergic neurons that project to higher brain centers are associated with sleep; those neurons that project to the spinal trigeminal nucleus and the dorsal horn of the spinal cord modulate or suppress the transmission of nociception.

Paramedian zone (also known as the paramedian column, paramedian reticular nuclei, paramedian reticular nuclear group)

Via their connections with the cerebral cortex, cerebellum, vestibular nuclei, and spinal cord, the nuclei of the paramedian zone function in feedback systems associated with intricate movements

The **paramedian zone**, located lateral to the midline, receives primarily uncrossed afferent (input) fibers from the cerebral cortex, the fastigial and dentate nuclei of the cerebellum, the vestibular nuclei, and the spinal cord (Fig. 14.2). Efferent (output) fibers from this zone project to the vermis, uvula, and fastigial nucleus of the cerebellum. This nuclear group functions in feedback systems associated with intricate patterns of movement.

Medial zone (also known as the medial column, magnocellular reticular formation, central group of reticular nuclei)

The neurons of the medial zone influence the autonomic nervous system, level of arousal, and motor control of the axial and proximal limb musculature

The **medial zone** also referred to as the "motor," "efferent," or "effector" zone, consists of large-size neurons. The nuclei of the medial zone are the **ventral reticular** (nucleus reticularis ventralis, central medullary nucleus), **gigantocellular reticular** (nucleus reticularis gigantocellularis), and the **pontine reticular nuclei** (nucleus reticularis pontis oralis and nucleus reticularis pontis caudalis) (Fig. 14.2).

These medial zone nuclei contain neurons whose axons bifurcate to give rise to long ascending and descending branches, each with collaterals. The *ascending fibers* of these neurons course in the central tegmental tract to terminate in the hypothalamus, which controls the autonomic nervous system, and in the intralaminar nuclei of the thalamus, which function in arousal. The *descending fibers* extend inferiorly to the spinal cord by joining the pontine and medullary **reticulospinal tracts**. These fibers are involved in motor control of the axial (trunk) and proximal limb musculature (shoulder, hip, and proximal lower limb muscles).

In addition, the medial zone of the pontine reticular formation and the rostral medullary reticular formation also give rise to the **reticulobulbar tract**, which terminates in the motor and sensory cranial nerve nuclei, where they function

in motor control and modulation of the transmission of sensory information.

Other fibers include the **reticulocerebellar fibers**, which project from the medial zone to the cerebellum (with the exception of those arising from the ventral reticular nucleus).

The medial zone of the caudal pons and the rostral medullary reticular formation contains small, medium, and a considerable number of very large neurons, and is called the **gigantocellular (magnocellular) reticular nucleus**.

Lateral zone (also known as the lateral column, parvicellular reticular formation, lateral nuclear group)

The lateral zone receives sensory information, integrates it, and then relays it to the medial zone. The medial zone then mediates the modulation of sensory afferent input and maintenance of alertnes

The **lateral zone** also referred to as the "sensory" or "afferent" zone, consists of a group of nuclei containing small-size interneurons, the most numerous type of cells in the reticular formation. These small-sized interneurons have short ascending and descending branches that project mainly locally to the medial zone of the reticular formation. Other interneurons of the lateral zone terminate in the brainstem cranial nerve motor nuclei.

The lateral zone extends primarily into the pons and medulla of the brainstem, and is continuous inferiorly with the spinal cord intermediate zone of gray matter, which is also heavily populated by interneurons. The intermediate zone of gray matter should not be confused with the intermediolateral (lateral) horn of the spinal cord, which contains the cell bodies of preganglionic neurons of the sympathetic nervous system.

The nuclei of the lateral zone are the parvicellular nucleus, which extends into the medulla and pons; the parabrachial nucleus, which extends into the pons and mesencephalon; the pedunculopontine nucleus, which is located in the rostral pons and caudal midbrain; and the cuneiform nucleus, which lies entirely in the mesencephalon.

The **parvicellular nucleus** (L. parvus, "small") is located medial to the spinal trigeminal nucleus and ventral to the vestibular nuclei. It receives sensory information from the cerebrum, cranial nerves, cerebellum, and the spinal cord via collateral branches of various somatosensory pathways relaying touch, pressure, pain, temperature, and general proprioception. The lateral zone integrates the sensory information and then relays it to the medial zone. Via the **reticulobulbar** and descending **reticulospinal tracts** (all of which arise from the medial zone), the reticular formation functions in the modulation of sensory afferent input, and in the maintenance of alertness.

The **parabrachial nucleus** is associated with visceral and limbic functions. The **pedunculopontine** and the **cuneiform nuclei** send fibers to brain centers such as the motor cortex, caudate nucleus, putamen, globus pallidus (internal segment), subthalamus, substantia nigra (pars compacta), and the cerebellum, all of which are associated with motor functions.

NUCLEI ASSOCIATED WITH THE RETICULAR FORMATION

A number of brainstem nuclei are associated with, but are not considered part of, the reticular formation. These nuclei are the **red nucleus**, the **inferior olivary nucleus**, and the **precerebellar reticular nuclei**. In addition, the **periaqueductal gray matter** of the midbrain also has extensive connections with the reticular formation.

Precerebellar reticular nuclei

The precerebellar reticular nuclei function in the coordination of muscle activity

The **precerebellar reticular nuclei** (see Fig. 14.2) consist of the **paramedian reticular nucleus**, the **pontine reticulotegmental nucleus**, and the **lateral reticular nucleus**. These nuclei are functionally separate from the other reticular nuclei, send fibers to the cerebellum, and function in the coordination of muscle activity.

Periaqueductal gray matter

The periaqueductal gray matter functions in the processing of autonomic and limbic activities, as well as modulation of nociception

The **periaqueductal gray matter** of the midbrain receives afferent fibers from the cerebral cortex, the hypothalamus, the limbic system, the parabrachial nucleus of the reticular formation, the solitary nucleus, as well as from the ascending sensory systems. Efferent fibers arising from the periaqueductal gray matter project back to the above regions, as well as to the medullary raphe nuclei. Based on its connections, and its association with the reticular formation, it is believed that the periaqueductal gray matter functions in the processing of autonomic and limbic activities as well as the modulation of nociception.

INPUT TO AND OUTPUT FROM THE RETICULAR FORMATION

Afferents (input) to the reticular formation

The reticular formation receives input via collateral branches of the ascending and descending pathways from widespread regions of the CNS. Input sources include the somatosensory, visual, auditory, and vestibular systems, the premotor and primary motor cortices, cranial nerve nuclei, the diencephalon, basal ganglia, the cerebellum, and the amygdala.

Efferents (output) from the reticular formation

The reticular formation gives rise to output fibers that project to the following areas of the CNS: widespread areas of the cerebral cortex, the diencephalon, basal ganglia, the red nucleus, the substantia nigra, the midbrain tectum, cranial nerve motor nuclei, the cerebellum, nuclei of the autonomic nervous system, and the spinal cord.

FUNCTIONS OF THE RETICULAR FORMATION

The reticular formation, via its vast number of connections to widespread areas of the CNS, is involved in a broad spectrum of activities

The reticular formation receives a continuous flow of somatosensory, auditory, visual, and visceral sensory information through these vast connections and in turn exerts its influence by processing, controlling, and/or modulating the following:

- skeletal muscle motor activity, including muscle tone and reflexes;
- somatic sensation;
- visceral sensation;
- autonomic nervous system activity;
- endocrine functions;
- biological rhythms, via reciprocal connections to the hypothalamus; and
- level of consciousness.

Control of motor activity

Motor activity is controlled by fibers traveling within the following fiber tracts: the corticoreticular fibers, pontine reticulospinal tract, and medullary reticulospinal tract (Table 14.2).

Corticoreticular fibers

The corticoreticular fibers terminate bilaterally in the medial zone of the pontine and medullary reticular formation where they modulate the activity of the reticulobulbar and reticulospinal neurons

The **corticoreticular fibers** arise from the premotor cortex and from the supplementary motor area of the secondary motor cortex. In their descent to the brainstem, they accompany the corticonuclear and corticospinal tracts. The corticoreticular fibers terminate bilaterally in the medial zone of the pontine and medullary reticular formation in the nuclei that give rise to the reticulospinal tracts. In addition to receiving corticoreticular fibers from the motor cortex, the medial zone of the pontine and medullary reticular formation also receives fibers arising from other sources involved in motor function such as the basal ganglia, red nucleus, and substantia nigra via the central tegmental tract. All of the above fibers terminating in the medial zone of the pontine and medullary reticular formation modulate the activity of the reticulobulbar and reticulospinal neurons.

The corticoreticular fibers, their **nuclei** of termination, and the **medial** and **lateral reticulospinal tracts** are referred to as the **corticoreticulospinal pathway (system)**. The descending

Table 14.2 ● The reticular formation and associated tracts.

Fibers/tract	Origin	Destination	Function
Corticoreticular fibers	Premotor cortex Supplementary motor area	Medial zone of pontine and medullary reticular formation (nucleus reticularis pontis oralis, nucleus reticularis pontis caudalis, and gigantocellular reticular nucleus)	Modulate the activity of the reticulobulbar and reticulospinal neurons
Pontine (medial) reticulospinal tract	Nucleus reticularis pontis oralis	Ipsilateral spinal cord to synapse with interneurons and motoneurons	Stimulation of extensor and Inhibition of flexor muscles of the trunk and proximal limb
	Nucleus reticularis pontis caudalis	Ipsilateral spinal cord to synapse with first order muscle spindle afferents	Prevent transmission of muscle spindle afferent signals, which has an inhibitory effect on stretch reflexes
Medullary (lateral) reticulospinal tract	Gigantocellular reticular nucleus Ventral reticular nucleus	Spinal cord (primarily ipsilateral) to synapse with interneurons and motoneurons	Inhibition of extensor and stimulation of flexor muscles of the trunk and proximal limb
Central tegmental tract	Basal ganglia Red nucleus Substantia nigra	Medial zone of pontine and medullary reticular formation	Modulates the activity of the reticulobulbar and reticulospinal neurons

fibers of the medial and lateral reticulospinal tracts synapse primarily with spinal cord interneurons, which in turn synapse with lower motoneurons, although some synapse directly with lower motoneurons. The medial and lateral reticulospinal tracts function in locomotion and postural control.

Pontine (medial) reticulospinal tract

The pontine (medial) reticulospinal tract stimulates the extensors and inhibits the flexors of the axial and proximal limb musculature

The **medial zone** is the motor (efferent) zone of the **pontine reticular formation**. This zone consists of the **nucleus reticularis pontis oralis** and **nucleus reticularis pontis caudalis**. The medial zone of the pontine reticular formation gives rise to the **pontine (medial) reticulospinal tract** (Fig. 14.3), which descends in the ipsilateral anterior funiculus of the spinal cord. This tract synapses with interneurons and gamma motoneurons at all levels of the spinal cord stimulating the extensors and inhibiting the flexors of the axial and proximal limb musculature. Furthermore, many medial reticulospinal tract fibers synapse with propriospinal interneurons that function in reflexes involving multiple spinal cord segments. These propriospinal interneurons synapse with lower motoneurons that innervate the axial and proximal limb musculature.

In addition, a few medial reticulospinal tract fibers establish inhibitory synaptic contacts with the termination of the central processes of those first order neurons whose peripheral processes innervate muscle spindles, thus preventing the transmission of afferent input from those muscle spindles. This mechanism has an inhibitory effect on stretch reflexes, with resultant smoothing of voluntary movement.

Medullary (lateral) reticulospinal tract

The medullary (lateral) reticulospinal tract fibers have an inhibitory effect on extensors and an excitatory effect on flexors of the axial and proximal limb musculature

The **medial zone** of the rostral **medullary reticular formation** (nucleus reticularis gigantocellularis and the nucleus reticularis ventralis) gives rise to the **medullary (lateral) reticulospinal tract** (Fig. 14.3). Similar to the medial reticulospinal tract, this tract descends (primarily) in the ipsilateral anterolateral funiculus of the spinal cord. Nerve fibers of this tract terminate at all spinal cord levels, where they synapse primarily with interneurons in the intermediate zone of gray matter. The lateral reticulospinal tract fibers have an opposite effect to that of the medial reticulospinal tract fibers, in that they have an inhibitory effect on extensors and an excitatory effect on flexors of the axial and proximal limb musculature.

Additionally, some fibers of the lateral reticulospinal tract synapse with those lower motoneurons of the spinal cord that supply motor innervation to the distal muscles of the upper and lower limbs. These fibers exert primarily an inhibitory influence on the lower motoneurons that innervate axial extensor muscles, and a facilitatory influence on those lower motoneurons that innervate limb flexors. Recall that the lateral corticospinal tract functions in the execution of fine, skilled movements of the hands and feet (see Chapter 11 for more detail).

Note that the descending fibers of the medial and lateral reticulospinal tracts relay signals that arise from the areas mentioned above (premotor cortex, supplementary motor area, basal ganglia, red nucleus, substantia nigra, and cerebellum), as well as signals arising from other areas of the reticular formation. All of these signals are integrated and then influence the activity of the alpha and gamma motoneurons innervating skeletal muscle. Furthermore, these tracts

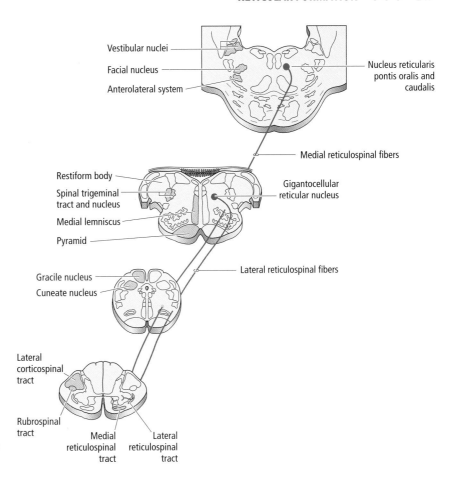

Figure 14.3 ● The origin, course, and termination of the medial and lateral reticulospinal tracts.

also control muscle tone and reflex activity. Since the reticular formation functions in reciprocal inhibition, during contraction of flexor muscles there is simultaneous relaxation of the antagonistic extensor muscles. The medial and lateral reticulospinal tracts, with the contribution of the lateral vestibulospinal tract, function in balance maintenance and in making postural adjustments. Muscle tone, balance maintenance, and postural adjustments form a necessary background upon which voluntary movement is executed.

Control of eye movements

The PPRF of the medial zone of the pontine reticular formation functions in mediating conjugate horizontal eye movements elicited by head movements

The **nucleus reticularis pontis oralis**, **nucleus reticularis pontis caudalis**, and **nucleus reticularis gigantocellularis** receive sensory information from the visual, auditory, and vestibular systems, and function in head and eye coordination.

The **paramedian pontine reticular formation (PPRF)** (Fig. 14.4) of the medial zone of the pontine reticular formation is not a nucleus *per se*, but instead is a subset of neurons of the nucleus reticularis pontis oralis and caudalis that functions in mediating conjugate *horizontal* eye movements elicited by head movements. It receives afferent fibers from the frontal eye fields, the superior colliculus, and the vestibular nuclei, as well as from other regions of the reticular formation. Efferent fibers from the PPRF terminate mainly in the abducens nucleus of the same side that innervates the ipsilateral lateral rectus muscle, and, via the medial longitudinal fasciculus, to the contralateral oculomotor nucleus to synapse specifically with the motoneurons that supply the contralateral medial rectus muscle.

The **rostral interstitial nucleus of the medial longitudinal fasciculus** located at the cranial end of the midbrain at the level of the superior colliculus contains a collection of nerve cells that function in controlling conjugate *vertical* eye movements (Fig. 14.4A).

Control of pain sensation

The raphe nuclei suppress or modulate the transmission of nociceptive signals from first order neurons to second order projection neurons that terminate in higher brain centers

As a result of its location in the brainstem, the reticular formation is in a position to exert its influence on ascending sensory and descending motor pathways, as well as on other pathways.

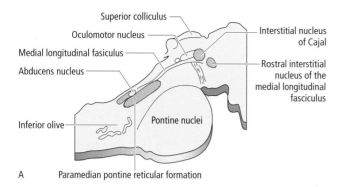

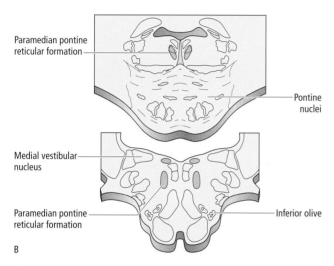

Figure 14.4 ● The location of the horizontal and vertical gaze centers in the brainstem in (A) sagittal, and (B) transverse sections.

The fibers of the trigeminothalamic tract transmit nociceptive signals from visceral and somatic structures of the head, whereas the spinothalamic and spinoreticular tracts transmit nociceptive signals from visceral and somatic structures of the body to their target thalamic nuclei. As these fibers traverse the brainstem reticular formation on their way to the thalamus, they give rise to collateral branches that terminate in the lateral zone (the "sensory" or "afferent" zone) of the reticular formation. These signals not only activate the **ascending reticular activating system** (ARAS), which relays information to the cerebral cortex alerting the individual, but also relays information to the hypothalamus, the limbic system, the serotonergic raphe nucleus magnus, and the raphe nucleus gigantocellularis of the medial zone of the reticular formation. The hypothalamus and the limbic system function in the manifestation of visceral and emotional/behavioral responses to sensory stimuli (such as pain). The serotonergic neurons of the raphe nuclei give rise to fibers that join the reticulobulbar and the reticulospinal tracts to descend to their target termination, the spinal trigeminal nucleus and the dorsal horn of the spinal cord, respectively (Fig. 14.5). The **serotonin** liberated by these descending fibers at their axon terminals stimulates inhibitory enkephalinergic interneurons, each of which forms a presynaptic contact (axoaxonic synapse) on the terminals of the central processes of the first order nociceptive neurons. By this mechanism, the raphe nuclei suppress or modulate the transmission of nociceptive signals from the first order neurons to the second order projection neurons that terminate in higher brain centers, specifically the thalamus, where nociceptive signals reach consciousness. For a more detailed description see Chapter 10.

Modulation of the autonomic nervous system

Visceral information arrives at the reticular formation from the cerebral cortex, hypothalamus, and limbic system. Sensory information from visceral structures that modulate the cardiovascular and respiratory systems is transmitted to the reticular formation via collateral branches derived from the ascending sensory pathways and via the **solitary tract**, which relays baroreceptor (from the carotid sinus, aortic sinus), chemoreceptor (from the carotid body, aortic body), volume receptor (from the heart atria), and stretch receptor (from the lungs) information from the glossopharyngeal and vagus nerves. The sensory information is processed in vasopressor and vasodepressor centers located in the reticular formation, which are believed to be involved in the control of vital functions such as respiration and the control of heart rate. The response from these centers is conveyed via the **reticulobulbar** and **reticulospinal tracts**, to the autonomic nuclei of the brainstem and spinal cord.

The **vasopressor center** that corresponds to the **rostral ventrolateral medullary reticular formation** and the **parvicellular nucleus** of the lateral zone nuclei, gives rise to fibers that join the **reticulospinal tract** to descend to the spinal cord. Here fibers synapse with preganglionic sympathetic neurons of the intermediolateral column, which in turn synapse with postganglionic sympathetic neurons that accelerate the heart rate. Postganglionic sympathetic neurons also cause peripheral vasoconstriction, and thus increase blood pressure.

The **vasodepressor center** that corresponds to the **caudal ventromedial medullary reticular formation** includes the **raphe nuclei** and the **gigantocellular reticular nucleus** of the medial zone nuclei. This center gives rise to fibers that join the **reticulobulbar tract** to terminate in the dorsal motor nucleus of the vagus. Here, fibers synapse with preganglionic parasympathetic neurons, which in turn synapse with postganglionic parasympathetic neurons in the wall of the heart, which decelerate the heart rate and lower blood pressure.

Stimulation of the **gigantocellular nucleus** of the brainstem reticular formation induces *inspiration*, whereas stimulation of the **parvicellular nucleus** induces *expiration*. The cardiovascular centers and the respiratory centers are thought to be overlapping. In addition, the neurons of the pontine parabrachial nucleus give rise to fibers that terminate in the brainstem and spinal cord where they exert their influence on the preganglionic parasympathetic neurons of the vagus nerve, the preganglionic sympathetic neurons of the intermediolateral column of the spinal cord, and the lower motoneurons of the phrenic and intercostal nerves that

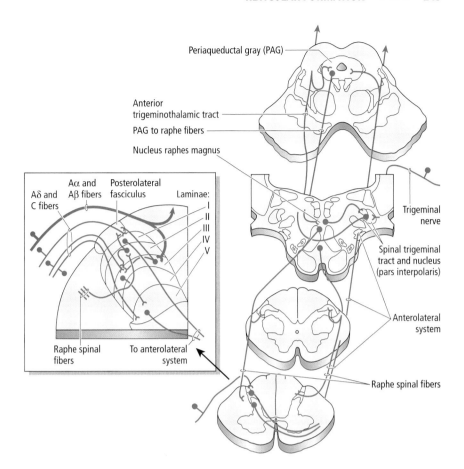

Figure 14.5 ● Descending pathways that modulate the transmission of nociception from the brainstem and spinal cord to higher brain centers. (Modified from Haines, DE (2002) *Fundamental Neuroscience*. Churchill Livingstone, Philadelphia; fig. 18.16.)

innervate the diaphragm and the intercostal muscles associated with breathing movements.

Coordination of cranial nerve function

The brainstem reticular formation contains interneurons that are located near the cranial nerve nuclei and participate in the coordination of reflex activity associated with the cranial nerves

Interneurons located in the **lateral reticular formation** project locally to the nearby cranial nerve nuclei. The **ventrolateral reticular formation** contains neurons that participate in the coordination of the visceral functions of the vagus nerve. The vagus nerve innervates the gastrointestinal, respiratory, and cardiovascular systems, and via its connections with the reticular formation plays a role in eliciting reflex responses associated with swallowing, coughing, breathing, and changes in blood pressure.

Interneurons of the lateral reticular formation are also associated with the trigeminal, facial, and hypoglossal nerve nuclei, which innervate structures of the mouth and face. The motor control exerted by these cranial nerves on structures they innervate in the orofacial region is coordinated by the reticular formation. Although motor control of the muscles of mastication—those of the tongue, lips, soft palate, and upper pharynx—is under voluntary control, during chewing the

action of all of these structures is automated and is executed without our being aware of it. The branches of the trigeminal nerve transmit general proprioceptive information from the temporomandibular joint, teeth, and muscles of mastication, and general sensation information from the mouth (thermal sensation and information about food consistency) to the sensory nuclei of the trigeminal nerve. These nuclei in turn project to the motor nuclei of the trigeminal and facial nerves and to the reticular formation, which in turn coordinates the movements of orofacial structures during chewing.

One of the most interesting associations of the reticular formation is its participation in the control of the muscles of facial expression during emotional responses. When an individual smiles while posing for a photograph, the imitation smile is voluntarily produced by descending input from the motor cortex (i.e., the corticonuclear tract) to the cranial nerve motor nuclei (i.e., the facial motor nucleus). This is sometimes referred to as a "pyramidal smile" (named after the pyramidal cells of the motor cortex forming the corticonuclear tract). In contrast, a sincere, heartfelt "emotional" smile is elicited by an alternate pathway, circumventing the primary motor cortex. This pathway includes descending motor input from accessory motor areas of the frontal lobe and the basal ganglia that reaches the facial nerve motor nuclei via relays in the reticular formation. This is often referred to as the "Duchenne smile" after the French neurologist and physiologist Duchenne de Boulogne who studied facial expressions. Individuals who have suffered a stroke that damaged the descending corticonuclear tract fibers, paralyzing the muscles of facial expression on one side of the face, are unable to smile voluntarily. However, when they hear pleasant news, a genuine happy facial expression is elicited. This may be hard to believe, but there is a neuroanatomical basis for this phenomenon. Although voluntary control via descending projections from the motor cortex to the lower half of the facial motor nucleus is unilateral, activation of the reticular formation by higher brain centers (i.e., accessory motor areas and basal ganglia) that are involved in eliciting emotional facial expressions, is bilateral.

Influence on the endocrine system

The reticular formation also influences the activities of the hypothalamus, modulating the formation or release of hypothalamic releasing hormones (or release-inhibiting hormones), which in turn influence the activities of the pituitary gland.

Control of consciousness

Waking up in the morning, remaining awake all day, and falling asleep at night, are all functions of the brainstem reticular formation

On their way to higher brain centers, the ascending sensory pathways (the trigeminothalamic, spinothalamic, and spinoreticular tracts) relaying general and nociceptive sensation, give rise to collateral branches that terminate in the parvicellular nucleus of the lateral zone of the reticular formation. The lateral zone gives rise to fibers that terminate in the medial zone of the reticular formation. The medial zone then projects via the central tegmental tract to the hypothalamus and the intralaminar nuclei of the thalamus. A spray of thalamocortical fibers arising from the thalamus project to widespread areas of the cerebral cortex. These fibers are referred to as the **ascending reticular activating system** (ARAS), the arousal system that functions in the sleep–wake cycle. Sensory information must be continually funneled to the cerebral cortex in order to maintain consciousness. Various levels of *wakefulness* are contingent upon the level of reticular formation activation. Waking up in the morning, remaining awake all day, and falling asleep at night, are all functions of the brainstem reticular formation. It is interesting to note that without a continuous stream of sensory input from the ARAS portion of the reticular formation to serve as an arousal system, which in turn activates the cerebral cortex, the cerebral cortex alone is unable to maintain *consciousness* and to function normally. Planning our day, going about our normal daily activities, and interacting with the stimuli in the environment are all mediated by the cerebral cortex.

Pain signals that may awaken an individual from sleep are relayed to the cortex via the ARAS. The ARAS stimulates the hypothalamus and limbic system, which are involved in visceral functions and the emotional and behavioral responses to the painful stimulus.

Sensory stimuli (visual, auditory, olfactory, or somatic) that startle or surprise an individual, such as a snake, siren, strong odors, or unexpected contact with an unknown object, activate the ARAS, and evoke an alerting response. We usually awaken in the morning following the sudden sound of an alarm clock, a loud noise coming from the street, or the smell of coffee. The ARAS has to be adequately stimulated in order to activate or "awaken" the cerebral cortex. On the contrary, lack of or inadequate stimulation of this system, can result in dozing off, as may occur when sitting in a dark, quiet room.

It is interesting to note that whereas anesthetics block the transmission of sensory signals that are relayed via the ascending sensory pathways through the ARAS to the cerebral cortex, they have no effect on the transmission of auditory signals. This may explain a curious phenomenon reported by patients that while they are under general anesthesia they are able to hear conversations by individuals in the operating room.

CLINICAL CONSIDERATIONS

Consciousness can be altered following head trauma, drug intoxication, anesthesia, or metabolic disturbances. A lesion anywhere along the path of the ARAS that affects the transmission of ARAS signals to the cerebral cortex, can result in various disorders of consciousness.

Frequently, head trauma can result in increased intracranial pressure. Since the brain is surrounded by the bony skull, intracranial pressure has no outlet, and it compresses the soft brain tissue. An increase in intracranial pressure may push the cerebellar tonsils toward the foramen magnum, which will then apply pressure on or compress the medulla. This will damage the respiratory centers in the medulla causing a central apnea (absence of breathing).

The midbrain is quite vulnerable and lesions damaging the reticular formation can cause hypersomnia associated with slow respiration. When the midbrain is compressed, with consequent extensive damage of the ARAS pathways, a comatose state ensues.

An upper spinal cord lesion at T6 or above will damage the descending hypothalamospinal and reticulospinal tracts that terminate in the sympathetic intermediolateral horn of the spinal cord. Normally these tracts synapse with the preganglionic sympathetic neurons residing in the intermediolateral horn, and control autonomic activities. This type of lesion will at first cause a reduction in sympathetic activity such as a lowering of blood pressure, orthostatic hypotension, and slowed heart rate. A gradual sympathetic reflex hyperactivity appears in response to denervation hypersensitivity of the sympathetic neurons. This is exhibited as sympathetic responses such as high blood pressure, sweating, piloerection, urinary retention, and a decrease in peripheral blood flow.

Note that the clinical case at the beginning of the chapter refers to a patient who presented with complete unilateral paralysis, slurred speech, ocular deviation, Babinski reflex, respiratory difficulties, and drowsiness, which progressed to a lethargic and comatose state and loss of all brainstem reflexes.

1 Which descending motor tracts have been damaged in this patient to initially cause a complete unilateral paralysis, slurred speech, and Babinski reflex?

2 Which neural system has been damaged to cause lethargy, respiratory difficulties, a comatose state, and loss of all brainstem reflexes?

3 What do unilateral pupillary dilation and fixed pupil indicate?

SYNONYMS AND EPONYMS OF THE RETICULAR FORMATION

Name of structure or term	Synonym(s)/ eponym(s)
Axial musculature	Trunk musculature
Babinski reflex	Extensor plantar response
Basal ganglia	Basal nuclei
	Deep cerebral nuclei
Corticoreticulospinal pathway	Corticoreticulospinal system
Corticospinal tract	Pyramidal tract (older term)
Gigantocellular reticular nucleus	Nucleus reticularis gigantocellularis
	Magnocellular reticular nucleus
Inferior olivary nucleus	Inferior olive
	Olive
Intermediolateral horn	Lateral horn
Lateral zone of the reticular formation	Lateral column of the reticular formation
	Parvicellular reticular formation
	Lateral nuclear group
Medial zone of the reticular formation	Medial column of the reticular formation
	Magnocellular reticular formation
	Central group of the reticular formation
Median zone of the reticular formation	Median column of the reticular formation
	Midline raphe
Medullary reticulospinal tract	Lateral reticulospinal tract

FOLLOW-UP TO CLINICAL CASE

This patient had a massive **stroke**. The above scenario is a typical progression indicative of **brain herniation** secondary to progressive edema from the stroke. The edema causes swelling of the brain and since the skull is rigid the swelling follows the route of least resistance downward, and consequently causes compression of other structures. With severe edema there is a shift of the midline structures of the brain to the normal side, opposite the stroke (midline shift), a downward shift of the diencephalon and brainstem, and herniation of the ipsilateral medial temporal lobe through the tentorium cerebelli into the posterior cranial fossa.

Impairment of consciousness occurs with diffuse dysfunction of the cerebral cortex (i.e., metabolic derangements), diencephalic lesions, or upper brainstem lesions. The latter two structures are the locale of the ARAS, which is critical for maintaining consciousness. Lesions involving the ARAS result in coma. In contrast, a focal brain lesion affecting only part of the cerebral cortex and subcortical white matter will cause no or minimal impairment of consciousness. Advancing lethargy with a focal brain lesion, such as stroke or tumor, often indicates progressive brain herniation leading to brainstem function impairment (assuming metabolic problems are ruled out as the cause).

Other signs besides progressive lethargy and coma are also important. Stretching and compression of the ipsilateral oculomotor nerve (CN III) over the tentorial notch leads to ipsilateral pupillary dilation and fixed pupil. Compression or ischemia of the contralateral cerebral peduncle causes ipsilateral weakness or pathologic reflexes (Babinski sign). Other brainstem reflexes such as the corneal blink reflex, oculovestibular or oculocephalic reflexes, gag reflex, and respiratory effort can be lost. Loss of all brainstem reflexes indicates brain death.

Name of structure or term	Synonym(s)/ eponym(s)
Nucleus linearis	Nucleus raphes dorsalis
Paramedian zone of the reticular formation	Paramedian column of the reticular formation
	Paramedian reticular nuclei
	Paramedian reticular nuclear group
Pontine reticulospinal tract	Medial reticulospinal tract
Premotor cortex	Part of Brodmann's area 6
Proximal limb musculature	Girdle musculature
Supplementary motor area	Part of Brodmann's area 6
Trigeminothalamic tracts	Trigeminal lemnisci
Ventral reticular nucleus	Nucleus reticularis ventralis
	Central medullary nucleus

QUESTIONS TO PONDER

1. With your knowledge of the ascending sensory pathways and the cranial nerves, describe how nociceptive information is relayed to the reticular formation.

2. What is the general structure of the neurons of the reticular formation and how does their structure facilitate their collection of information from ascending and descending pathways?

3. What is the function of the medial zone of the reticular formation?

4. Why is it that when we are chewing we (fortunately) do not bite our tongues?

5. If a lesion in the midbrain damages the ARAS what is likely to happen?

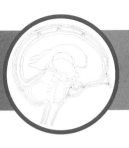
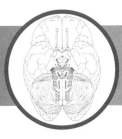
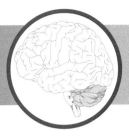

CHAPTER 15

Cranial Nerves

CLINICAL CASE

A 70-year-old male has excruciating pain in the lower left part of his face. This began 1 month ago. He describes it as being like a jolt of lightning that radiates from his left ear, down to his jaw, and to the side of his mouth. These jolts of pain occur numerous times each day. Between attacks his face seems normal. He denies any numbness or tingling sensations. There is no hearing abnormality. The pain is triggered by talking, chewing, or touch of the lower left part of his face. He is unable to eat or brush his teeth, particularly on the left side, since he fears triggering another painful attack. He can only drink his meals through a straw and cannot lie in bed on his left side. He had the same symptoms about 2 years ago. At that time he was treated with a medication which helped; symptoms subsided, but he stopped taking the medicine. The pain is so distressing that the patient admits to contemplating suicide.

The general and neurologic exam is normal, except that he withdraws and will not let anyone touch the left side of his face.

There are 12 pairs of cranial nerves emerging from the brain and radiating from its surface (Fig. 15.1). They pass through skull foramina, fissures, or canals to exit the cranial vault and then distribute their innervation to their respective structures in the head and neck. One of the cranial nerves, the vagus (L.,

"wanderer") continues into the trunk where it innervates various thoracic and abdominal organs.

In addition to being named, the cranial nerves are numbered sequentially with Roman numerals in the order in which they arise from the brain, rostrally to caudally. The

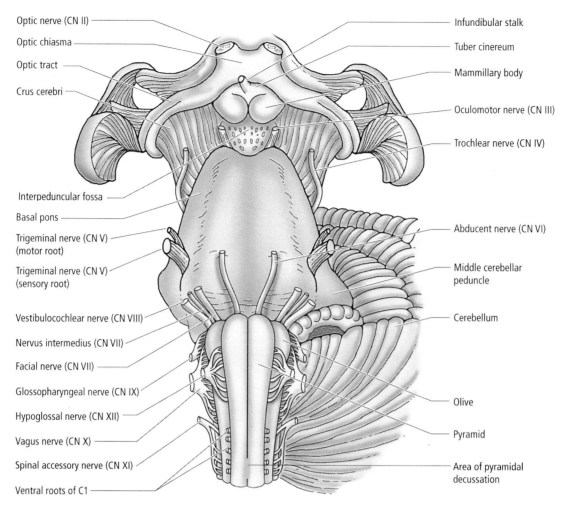

Figure 15.1 ● Ventral view of the brainstem showing the cranial nerves.

following list includes their names and corresponding numbers.

I   Olfactory nerve.
II   Optic nerve.
III   Oculomotor nerve.
IV   Trochlear nerve.
V   Trigeminal nerve.
VI   Abducent nerve.
VII   Facial nerve.
VIII Vestibulocochlear nerve.
IX   Glossopharyngeal nerve.
X   Vagus nerve.
XI   Spinal accessory nerve.
XII   Hypoglossal nerve.

Although the cranial nerves and their sensory and parasympathetic ganglia (Tables 15.1, 15.2) form part of the peripheral nervous system, the optic nerve is really an out-growth of the brain that emerges from the prosencephalon (not the brainstem as other cranial nerves), and is therefore not a typical cranial nerve. Moreover, part of the spinal accessory nerve arises from the cervical spinal cord; thus

Table 15.1 ● Sensory ganglia of the cranial nerves

Ganglion	Cranial nerve association
Trigeminal (semilunar, Gasserian)	Trigeminal (V)
Geniculate	Facial (VII)
Cochlear (spiral)	Cochlear (VIII)
Vestibular (Scarpa's)	Vestibular (VIII)
Superior glossopharyngeal	Glossopharyngeal (IX)
Inferior glossopharyngeal	Glossopharyngeal (IX)
Superior vagal	Vagus (X)
Inferior vagal (nodose)	Vagus (X)

there are only nine pairs of cranial nerves that emerge from the brainstem.

The main sensory and motor nuclei of the cranial nerves are shown in Fig. 15.2.

In describing the various functional components (modalities) of the cranial nerves, the definition of the following terms should be kept in mind: *afferent* is sensory input; *efferent* is motor output that may be *somatic* to skeletal muscles or *visceral* to smooth muscle, cardiac muscle, and glands, and

Ganglion association	Cranial nerve association	Trigeminal	Function(s)
Ciliary	Oculomotor (III)	Ophthalmic division	Constricts pupil; lens accommodation
Pterygopalatine	Facial (VII)	Maxillary division	Lacrimation; nasal gland, and minor salivary gland secretion
Submandibular	Facial (VII)	Mandibular division	Salivation (parotid gland)
Otic	Glossopharyngeal (IX)	Mandibular division	Salivation (submandibular and sublingual glands)
Intramural	Vagus (X)		Gland secretion; peristalsis

Table 15.2 ● Parasympathetic ganglia of the cranial nerves.

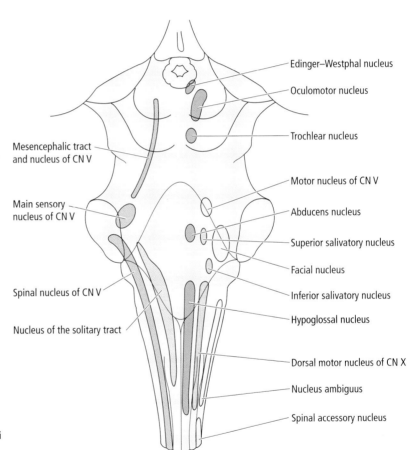

Figure 15.2 ● The nuclei of the cranial nerves. The sensory nuclei are illustrated on the left, and the motor nuclei on the right.

special visceral efferent to striated muscles derived from the branchial arches; *general* refers to those components that may be carried by cranial nerves as well as spinal nerves; *special* refers to functional components that are carried by cranial nerves only. The following categories describe the functional components carried by the various cranial nerves (Table 15.3).

1 **General somatic afferent** (GSA). These fibers carry general sensation (touch, pressure, pain, and temperature)

from cutaneous structures and mucous membranes of the head, and **general proprioception** (GP) from somatic structures such as muscles, tendons, and joints of the head and neck. The trigeminal, facial, glossopharyngeal, and vagus nerves transmit GSA input to the spinal nucleus of the trigeminal nerve.

2 **General somatic efferent** (GSE). These fibers provide general motor innervation to skeletal muscles derived from embryonic somites. The oculomotor, trochlear, and abducent nerves innervate the extraocular muscles that

Modality	Cranial nerves	Function(s)
General somatic afferent (GSA)	V, VII, IX, X	General sensation and general proprioception
General somatic efferent (GSE)	III, IV, VI XII	Motor supply to extraocular muscles Motor supply to tongue
General visceral afferent (GVA)	VII, IX, X	General sensation from viscera
General visceral efferent (GVE)	III, VII, IX, X	Parasympathetic fibers to viscera
Special somatic afferent (SSA)	II VIII	Special sensory input from retina Special sensory input from vestibulocochlear apparatus
Special visceral afferent (SVA)	I VII, IX, X	Special sense of smell Special sense of taste
Special visceral efferent (SVE)	V, VII, IX, X	Motor innervation to muscles of branchiomeric origin: mandibular, hyoid, 3rd, 4th, and 6th branchial arches

Table 15.3 ● Cranial nerve functional components.

control eye movements, whereas the hypoglossal nerve supplies motor innervation to the muscles of the tongue, mediating movement of the tongue.

3 **General visceral afferent** (GVA). General sensation from the viscera is transmitted by the facial, glossopharyngeal, and vagus nerves.

4 **General visceral efferent** (GVE). These fibers provide visceral motor (parasympathetic) innervation to the viscera. The only cranial nerves that transmit parasympathetic fibers are the oculomotor, facial, glossopharyngeal, and vagus nerves.

5 **Special somatic afferent** (SSA). These fibers carry special sensory input from the eye (retina), for vision, and from the ear (vestibular apparatus for equilibrium, and cochlea for hearing). The only nerves transmitting this component are the optic and vestibulocochlear nerves.

6 **Special visceral afferent** (SVA). These are special sensory fibers from the viscera. These fibers convey the special sense of smell transmitted by the olfactory nerve and the special sense of taste transmitted by the facial, glossopharyngeal, and vagus nerves.

7 **Special visceral efferent** (SVE). These motor fibers are special because they supply motor innervation to skeletal muscles of branchial arch origin. These fibers are carried by the nerves of the branchial arches, which are the trigeminal, facial, glossopharyngeal, and vagus nerves.

Table 15.4 summarizes the modalities, nuclei, ganglia, and functions of the cranial nerves.

OLFACTORY NERVE (CN I)

The olfactory receptor cells reside in the olfactory epithelium, and not in a sensory ganglion as is typical of other cranial nerves

The **bipolar olfactory receptor cells** (first order sensory neurons) of the olfactory apparatus reside not in a sensory ganglion, but instead in the **olfactory epithelium (neuroepithelium)** of the modified nasal mucosa lining the roof and adjacent upper walls of the nasal cavities (see Fig. 19.1). The axons of these bipolar neurons are **SVA fibers** transmitting *olfactory* sensation. These axons assemble to form bundles, the **olfactory fila** (L., "threads"), which collectively form **cranial nerve I**. The olfactory fila traverse the fenestrations of the cribriform plate of the ethmoid bone to terminate in the olfactory bulb where they synapse with **second order relay neurons** and **interneurons** (see Chapter 19).

OPTIC NERVE (CN II)

The optic nerve consists of the myelinated axons of the retinal ganglion cells

The **optic nerve** mediates the special sense of *vision* via its **SSA fibers**. Light entering the eye activates cells known as rods and cones, the photoreceptors of the retina. Electrical signals generated by the photoreceptors are transmitted to other cells of the retina that process and integrate sensory input. The **first order sensory bipolar neurons** of the visual pathway reside in the retina and transmit electrical signals of visual sensory input to the **multipolar second order ganglion cells** of the retina. The ganglion cells give rise to unmyelinated axons that converge at the optic disc and traverse the lamina cribrosa, a sieve-like perforated area of the sclera, to emerge from the back of the eyebulb. At this point, the ganglion cell axons acquire a myelin sheath and assemble to form the optic nerve. This nerve, an outgrowth of the diencephalon, leaves the orbit via the optic canal to enter the middle cranial fossa. There, the optic nerves of the right and left sides join each other to form the **optic chiasma** (G., "optic crossing") where partial decussation of the optic nerve fibers of the two sides takes place. All ganglion cell axons arising from the **nasal half** of the retina *decussate* (through the central region of the chiasma) to the opposite optic tract. All ganglion cell axons arising from the **temporal half** of the

Table 15.4 ● Sensory receptors.

Cranial nerve	Functional component (modality)	Nucleus	Location of cranial nerve nuclei	Ganglion	Distribution	Function(s)
I Olfactory	SVA	–	Telencephalon	–	Olfactory mucosa	Smell
II Optic	SSA	–	Diencephalon	–	Ganglion cells of retina	Vision
III Oculomotor	GSE	Oculomotor	Mesencephalon (tegmentum)	–	All extraocular muscles except the lateral rectus and superior oblique	Eye movement
	GVE (parasympathetic)	Edinger–Westphal	Mesencephalon (tegmentum)	Ciliary (parasympathetic)	Sphincter pupillae muscle Ciliary muscle	Pupillary constriction Lens accommodation
	GP	Mesencephalic nucleus of the trigeminal	Mesencephalon	–	All extraocular muscles except the lateral rectus and superior oblique	Kinesthetic sense
IV Trochlear	GSE	Trochlear	Mesencephalon (tegmentum)	–	Superior oblique	Eye movement
	GP	Mesencephalic nucleus of the trigeminal	Mesencephalon	–	Superior oblique	Kinesthetic sense
V Trigeminal	SVE	Motor nucleus of the trigeminal	Metencephalon	–	Muscles of mastication: temporalis masseter medial pterygoid lateral pterygoid Mylohyoid, anterior belly of the digastric	Chewing
					Tensor tympani	Tenses tympanic membrane
					Tens veli palatini	Tenses soft palate
	GSA	Main (chief, principal) nucleus of the trigeminal	Metencephalon (pons)	Trigeminal	Scalp, anterior two-thirds of the dura, cornea, conjunctiva, face, paranasal sinuses, teeth, gingiva, and anterior two-thirds of the tongue	General sensation
		Spinal nucleus of the trigeminal	Metencephalon (pons to C3)			
	GP	Mesencephalic nucleus of the trigeminal	Mesencephalon	–	Muscles of mastication Periodontal ligament	Muscle stretch sensation Pressure sensation
VI Abducent	GSE	Abducens	Metencephalon (pons)	–	Lateral rectus	Eye movement
	GP	Mesencephalic nucleus of the trigeminal	Mesencephalon	–	Superior oblique	Kinesthetic sense
VII Facial	SVE	Facial	Metencephalon (pons)	–	Muscles of facial expression, platysma, posterior belly of the digastric, and stylohyoid	Facial expression
					Stapedius	Tension on stapes
	GVE (parasympathetic)	Superior salivatory	Myelencephalon	Pterygopalatine (parasympathetic)	Lacrimal gland Glands of the nasal cavity and palate	Lacrimation Mucous secretion
				Submandibular (parasympathetic)	Submandibular and sublingual glands	Salivation
	SVA	Solitarius	Myelencephalon	Geniculate	Anterior two-thirds of the tongue	Taste
	GVA	Solitarius	Myelencephalon	Geniculate	Middle ear, nasal cavity, and soft palate	Visceral sensation

Table 15.4 ● *Continued.*

Cranial nerve	Functional component (modality)	Nucleus	Location of cranial nerve nuclei	Ganglion	Distribution	Function(s)
	GSA	Spinal nucleus of the trigeminal	Metencephalon (pons)	Geniculate	External auditory meatus and area posterior to ear	General sensation
VIII Vestibulocochlear						
Cochlear	SSA	Dorsal and ventral cochlear	Myelencephalon	Spiral	Organ of Corti (inner ear)	Hearing
Vestibular	SSA	Vestibular complex	Myelencephalon	Vestibular	Utricle Saccule Semicircular canal ampullae (inner ear)	Equilibrium
X Glossopharyngeal	SVE	Ambiguus	Myelencephalon	–	Stylopharyngeus and pharyngeal constrictors	Swallowing
	GVE (parasympathetic)	Inferior salivatory	Myelencephalon	Otic (parasympathetic)	Parotid gland	Salivation
	SVA	Solitarius	Myelencephalon	Inferior ganglion of the glossopharyngeal	Posterior one-third of the tongue and adjacent pharyngeal wall	Taste
	GVA	Ambiguus Solitarius	Myelencephalon	Inferior ganglion of the glossopharyngeal	Middle ear, pharynx, tongue, carotid sinus	Visceral sensation
	GSA	Spinal nucleus of the trigeminal	Myelencephalon	Superior ganglion of the glossopharyngeal	Posterior one-third of the tongue, soft palate, upper pharynx, and auditory tube	General sensation
X Vagus	GVE (parasympathetic)	Dorsal motor nucleus of the vagus	Myelencephalon	Thoracic and abdominal submucosal and myenteric autonomic plexuses	Thoracic and abdominal viscera	Gland secretion, peristalsis
	SVE	Ambiguus	Myelencephalon	–	Muscles of the larynx and pharynx	Phonation
	SVA	Solitarius	Myelencephalon	Inferior (nodose)	Epiglottis	Taste
	GVA	Solitarius	Myelencephalon	Inferior (nodose)	Thoracic and abdominal viscera Carotid body	Visceral sensation
	GSA	Spinal nucleus of the trigeminal	Myelencephalon	Superior (jugular)	Area posterior to the ear, external acoustic meatus, and posterior part of meninges	General sensation
XI Spinal accessory	SVE	Ambiguus	Myelencephalon	–	Laryngeal muscles To sternocleidomastoid and trapezius	Phonation Head and shoulder movements
XII Hypoglossal	GSE	Hypoglossal	Myelencephalon	–	Muscles of the tongue	Tongue movement

retina proceed (through the lateral aspect of the chiasma) *without decussating* and join the optic tract of the same side. The ganglion cell axons coursing in each optic tract curve around the cerebral peduncle to terminate and relay visual input in one of the following four regions of the brain: the **lateral geniculate nucleus**, a thalamic relay station for vision; the **superior colliculus**, a mesencephalic relay station for vision associated with somatic reflexes; the **pretectal area**, a mesencephalic region associated with autonomic reflexes; and the **hypothalamus** (see Figs 16.5, 16.7, 16.9).

OCULOMOTOR NERVE (CN III)

The oculomotor nerve provides motor innervation to four of the six extraocular muscles and the levator palpebrae superioris, and parasympathetic innervation to the sphincter pupillae and ciliary muscles

The **oculomotor nerve** supplies **skeletal motor (somatomotor)** innervation to the superior rectus, medial rectus, inferior rectus, and inferior oblique muscles (which move the bulb of the eye) and the levator palpebrae superioris muscle (which elevates the upper eyelid). It also provides **parasympathetic** (visceromotor) innervation to the ciliary and sphincter pupillae muscles, two intrinsic smooth muscles of the eye.

The triangular-shaped **oculomotor nuclear complex** is located in the mesencephalon. It is situated ventral to the periaqueductal gray, adjacent to the midline at the level of the superior colliculus. The oculomotor nucleus consists of several **subnuclei** representing each of the extraocular muscles. These subnuclei are composed of groups of nerve cell bodies of the **GSE neurons** that innervate the listed extraocular muscles and the levator palpebrae superioris muscle. The cell group innervating the levator palpebrae superioris is located in the midline, sending motor fibers to this muscle bilaterally (both right and left upper eyelids). The cell group innervating the superior rectus sends projections to the opposite side; whereas the cell group innervating the medial rectus, inferior oblique, and inferior rectus sends projections to the same side.

The **Edinger–Westphal nucleus**, a subnucleus of the oculomotor nuclear complex is located dorsally, medially, and rostral to the GSE nuclear complex. It contains the cell bodies of **GVE preganglionic parasympathetic neurons** whose axons join the GSE fibers as they converge and pass ventrally in the midbrain to emerge from the ventral aspect of the brainstem in the interpeduncular fossa as the oculomotor nerve.

The oculomotor nerve proceeds anteriorly within the cranial vault, travels within the cavernous sinus, and by passing through the superior orbital fissure, enters the ipsilateral orbit. Within the orbit, the oculomotor nerve gives rise to branches carrying the GSE fibers that innervate the levator palpebrae superioris muscle and all but two of the extraocular muscles. The preganglionic parasympathetic fibers of the oculomotor nerve terminate in the **ciliary ganglion** where they synapse with postganglionic parasympathetic nerve cell bodies. Postganglionic parasympathetic fibers exit the ganglion and reach the sphincter pupillae and ciliary muscles via the short ciliary nerves to provide them with parasympathetic innervation. The parasympathetic fibers, when stimulated, cause contraction of the sphincter pupillae muscle, which results in constriction of the pupil. Pupillary constriction reduces the amount of light that impinges on the retina. Stimulation of the parasympathetic nervous system causes pupillary constriction (whereas stimulation of the sympathetic nervous system, which innervates the dilator pupillae muscle, causes pupillary dilation). Ciliary muscle contraction releases the tension on the suspensory ligaments of the lens, changing its thickness to become more convex. This accommodates the lens for near vision.

GSA pseudounipolar neurons, whose cell bodies reside within the **mesencephalic nucleus** of the trigeminal nerve, send their peripheral processes to terminate in the muscle spindles of the extraocular muscles. These fibers travel via the branches of the ophthalmic division of the trigeminal nerve. GSA (GP) sensory input is transmitted from the muscle spindles via the spindle afferents centrally to the trigeminal nuclear complex, mediating coordinated and synchronized eye movements by reflex and voluntary control of muscles.

CLINICAL CONSIDERATIONS

Unilateral damage to the oculomotor nerve results in deficits in the *ipsilateral* eye. The following ipsilateral muscles will be paralyzed: the levator palpebrae superioris, resulting in **ptosis** (G., "drooping") of the upper eyelid; the superior and inferior recti, resulting in an inability to move the eye vertically; and the medial rectus, resulting in an inability to move the eye medially. The eye deviates laterally (due to the unopposed lateral rectus), resulting in **lateral strabismus**. This causes the eyes to become misaligned as one eye deviates from the midline, resulting in **horizontal diplopia** (double vision). The inferior oblique is also paralyzed. Since the innervation to the lateral rectus (CN VI) and superior oblique (CN IV) muscles is intact and these two muscles are functional, the eye ipsilateral to the lesion deviates inferiorly and laterally (Fig. 15.3).

The sphincter pupillae muscle becomes nonfunctional due to interruption of its parasympathetic innervation. The pupil ipsilateral to the lesion will remain dilated (**mydriasis**) and does not respond (constrict) to a flash of light. This may be the first clinical sign of intracranial pressure on the GVE fibers of the oculomotor nerve. The ciliary muscle is also nonfunctional due to interruption of its parasympathetic innervation, and cannot accommodate the lens for near vision (that is, cannot focus on near objects).

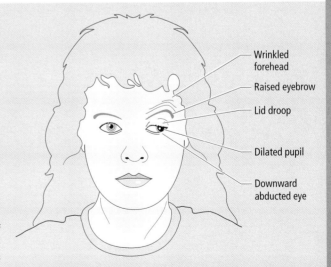

Wrinkled forehead

Raised eyebrow

Lid droop

Dilated pupil

Downward abducted eye

Figure 15.3 ● A lesion involving the left oculomotor nerve results in the following symptoms ipsilateral to the side of the lesion: (i) lateral strabismus, (ii) ptosis (drooping of the upper eye lid), (iii) pupillary dilation, (iv) loss of accommodation of the lens, and (v) downward and outward deviation of the eye.

TROCHLEAR NERVE (CN IV)

The trochlear nerve is the smallest (thinnest) cranial nerve and the only one whose fibers originate totally from the contralateral nucleus

The **trochlear nerve** provides motor innervation to only one of the extraocular muscles of the eye, the **superior oblique muscle** (a common mnemonic is SO$_4$).

The nerve cell bodies of **GSE neurons** reside in the **trochlear nucleus**, which lies adjacent to the midline in the tegmentum of the caudal midbrain. Fibers arising from this nucleus initially descend for a short distance in the brainstem and then course dorsally in the periaqueductal gray matter. The fibers *decussate* posteriorly and emerge from the brainstem at the junction of the pons and midbrain, just below the inferior colliculus.

The trochlear nerve is unique because it is the only cranial nerve whose fibers originate totally from the contralateral nucleus, it surfaces on the *dorsal* aspect of the brainstem, and it is the smallest (thinnest) of the cranial nerves. As the trochlear nerve emerges from the brainstem, it curves around the cerebral peduncle and proceeds anteriorly within the cavernous sinus to pass into the orbit via the superior orbital fissure. Consequently, this cranial nerve has the longest intracranial course and is highly susceptible to increased intracranial pressure.

CLINICAL CONSIDERATIONS

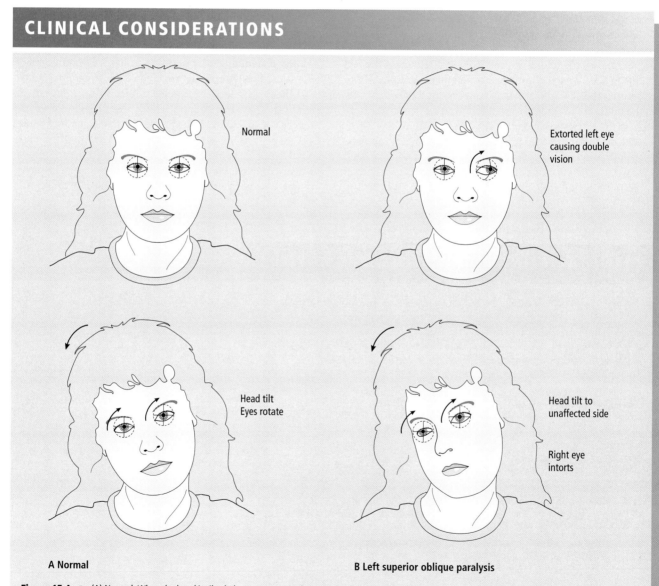

Normal

Extorted left eye causing double vision

Head tilt Eyes rotate

Head tilt to unaffected side

Right eye intorts

A Normal

B Left superior oblique paralysis

Figure 15.4 ● (A) Normal: When the head is tilted, the eyes rotate in the opposite direction. (B) Left superior oblique paralysis following a lesion to the trochlear nerve: the affected eye becomes extorted with consequent double vision. To minimize the double vision, the individual tilts her head toward the unaffected side which intorts the normal eye.

CLINICAL CONSIDERATIONS (*continued*)

Damage to the trochlear nucleus results in **paralysis** or **paresis** of the *contralateral* superior oblique muscle, whereas damage to the **trochlear nerve** results in the same deficits but in the *ipsilateral* muscle.

Normally, contraction of the superior oblique muscle causes the eye to *intort* (rotate inward) accompanied by simultaneous *depression* (downward) and *lateral* (outward) movement of the bulb of the eye. This is sometimes referred to as the "Salvation Army muscle" ("down and out"). Intorsion of the eyeball is the turning of the eyeball around its axis, so that the superior pole of the eyeball turns inward. Imagine that extreme intorsion (which we really cannot do) will bring the superior pole of the eye facing the medial wall of the orbit. When the superior oblique muscle is paralyzed, the ipsilateral eye will *extort* (rotate outward) accompanied by simultaneous *upward* and *outward* movement of the eye (Fig. 15.4B). This is caused by the unopposed inferior oblique muscle and results in **external strabismus.**

Since the eyes become misaligned following such a lesion, an individual with **trochlear nerve palsy** experiences **vertical diplopia** (double vision), accompanied by weakness of downward movement of the eye, most notably in an effort to adduct the eye (turn medially). The diplopia is most apparent to the individual when descending stairs or while reading (looking down and inward). To counteract the diplopia and to restore proper eye alignment, the individual realizes that the diplopia is reduced as he tilts his head towards the side of the unaffected eye (Fig. 15.4B). Normally, tilting of the head to one side elicits a reflex rotation about the anteroposterior axis of the eyes in the opposite direction (Fig. 15.4A), so that the image of an object will remain fixed on the retina. Tilting of the head toward the *unaffected* side causes the unaffected eye to rotate inward and become aligned with the affected eye which is rotated outward. Also, pointing the chin downward ("chin tuck") rolls the normal eye upward.

TRIGEMINAL NERVE (CN V)

The trigeminal nerve, the largest of the cranial nerves, provides the major general sensory innervation to part of the scalp, most of the dura mater, and the orofacial structures

The trigeminal system consists of the trigeminal nerve, ganglion, nuclei, tracts, and central pathways. The trigeminal sensory pathway, which transmits *touch, nociception,* and *thermal sensation,* consists of a three neuron sequence (first, second, and third order neurons) from the periphery to the cerebral cortex respectively (Figs 15.5, 15.6). The peripheral processes of the first order neurons radiating from the trigeminal ganglion gather to form three separate nerves, the three divisions of the trigeminal nerve whose peripheral endings terminate in sensory receptors of the orofacial region. Their cell bodies are housed in the trigeminal ganglion. The central processes of these neurons enter the pons, join the spinal tract of the trigeminal, and terminate in the trigeminal nuclei where they establish synaptic contacts with second order neurons housed in these nuclei. The trigeminal nuclei, with the exception of the mesencephalic nucleus, contain second order neurons as well as interneurons. The second order neurons give rise to fibers that may or may not decussate in the brainstem and join the ventral or dorsal trigeminal lemnisci. These lemnisci ascend to relay

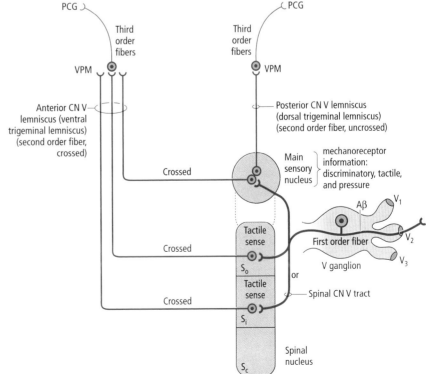

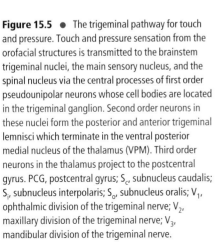

Figure 15.5 ● The trigeminal pathway for touch and pressure. Touch and pressure sensation from the orofacial structures is transmitted to the brainstem trigeminal nuclei, the main sensory nucleus, and the spinal nucleus via the central processes of first order pseudounipolar neurons whose cell bodies are located in the trigeminal ganglion. Second order neurons in these nuclei form the posterior and anterior trigeminal lemnisci which terminate in the ventral posterior medial nucleus of the thalamus (VPM). Third order neurons in the thalamus project to the postcentral gyrus. PCG, postcentral gyrus; S_c, subnucleus caudalis; S_i, subnucleus interpolaris; S_o, subnucleus oralis; V_1, ophthalmic division of the trigeminal nerve; V_2, maxillary division of the trigeminal nerve; V_3, mandibular division of the trigeminal nerve.

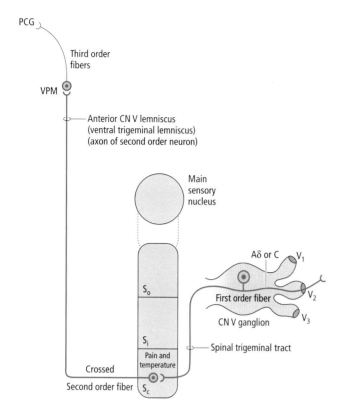

Figure 15.6 • The trigeminal pathway for pain and temperature. Pain and temperature sensation from the orofacial structures is transmitted to the brainstem subnucleus caudalis (S_c) of the spinal trigeminal nucleus via the central processes of first order pseudounipolar neurons whose cell bodies are located in the trigeminal ganglion. Second order neurons from the subnucleus caudalis join the anterior trigeminal lemniscus to terminate in the ventral posterior medial nucleus of the thalamus (VPM). Third order neurons from the VPM terminate in the postcentral gyrus (PCG). For other abbreviations, see Fig. 15.5.

trigeminal sensory input to the ventral posterior medial (VPM) nucleus of the thalamus, where they synapse with third order neurons. The third order neurons then relay sensory information to the postcentral gyrus (somesthetic cortex) of the cerebral cortex for further processing.

The **trigeminal nerve** is the largest cranial nerve. It provides the major **GSA** innervation (touch, pressure, nociception, and thermal sense) to part of the scalp, most of the dura mater, the conjuctiva and cornea of the eye, the face, nasal cavities, paranasal sinuses, palate, temporomandibular joint, lower jaw, oral cavity, and teeth. It also provides **SVE (branchiomotor)** innervation to the muscles of mastication (temporalis, masseter, medial pterygoid, lateral pterygoid), and the mylohyoid, anterior belly of the digastric, tensor tympani, and tensor veli palatini muscles.

The trigeminal nerve is the only cranial nerve whose sensory root enters and motor root exits at the ventrolateral aspect of the pons (see Fig. 15.1). The larger, **sensory root** consists of the central processes (axons) of the pseudounipolar sensory neurons of the trigeminal ganglion. These axons enter the pons to terminate in the trigeminal sensory nuclear complex of the brainstem. The **motor root** is smaller and consists of the axons of motor (branchiomotor) neurons exiting

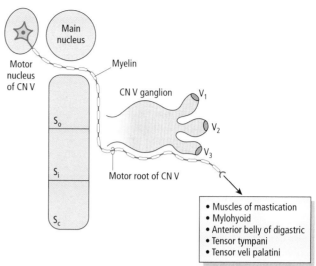

Figure 15.7 • Branchiomotor innervation of the trigeminal nerve. The motor nucleus of the trigeminal nerve contains the motoneurons whose axons assemble to form the motor root of the trigeminal nerve. The motor root exits the pons and joins the mandibular division of the trigeminal nerve and distributes to the muscles of mastication, the mylohyoid, the anterior belly of the digastric, the tensor tympani, and the tensor veli palatini muscles to provide them with motor innervation. For abbreviations, see Fig. 15.5.

the pons (Fig. 15.7). The motor root joins the sensory portion of the mandibular division of the trigeminal nerve just outside the skull, to form the mandibular trunk. Before the motor root joins it, the trigeminal nerve displays a swelling, the **trigeminal ganglion**, which lies in a bony depression of the petrous temporal bone on the floor of the middle cranial fossa. Since this is a sensory ganglion there are no synapses occurring here. As the peripheral processes of the pseudounipolar neurons exit the ganglion, they form three divisions (hence "trigeminal," meaning the "three twins"). These divisions traverse the foramina of the skull to exit the cranial vault on their way to reach the structures they innervate. The **ophthalmic division** is purely sensory and innervates the upper part of the face; the **maxillary division** is also purely sensory (although there may be some exceptions) and innervates the middle part of the face. The **mandibular division** is mixed, that is it carries sensory innervation to the lower face and branchiomotor innervation to the muscles listed above.

Trigeminal nuclei

The trigeminal system includes four nuclei: one *motor* nucleus, the motor nucleus of the trigeminal; and three *sensory* nuclei, the main (chief, principal) sensory nucleus of the trigeminal, the mesencephalic nucleus of the trigeminal, and the spinal nucleus of the trigeminal (see Fig. 15.2; Table 15.5).

Motor nucleus

The motor nucleus of the trigeminal nerve contains the cell bodies whose axons form the motor root of the trigeminal nerve, which provides motor innervation to the muscles of mastication

Table 15.5 ● The trigeminal nuclei.

Motor nucleus

Sensory nuclei:
- Main (chief, principal) nucleus of the trigeminal
- Mesencephalic nucleus of the trigeminal
- Spinal nucleus of the trigeminal:
  - Subnucleus oralis
  - Subnucleus interpolaris
  - Subnucleus caudalis

The **motor nucleus of the trigeminal** is located at the midpontine levels, medial to the main sensory nucleus. It contains interneurons and the cell bodies of **multipolar** alpha and gamma motor (**branchiomotor**) neurons whose axons form the **motor root** of the trigeminal nerve as they exit the pons. The branchiomotor fibers join the mandibular division of the trigeminal nerve and are distributed to the muscles of mastication as well as to the mylohyoid, anterior belly of the digastric, tensor tympani, and tensor veli palatini muscles.

Sensory nuclei

The sensory nuclei of the trigeminal nerve transmit sensory information from the orofacial structures to the thalamus

The **sensory nuclei** consist of a long cylinder of cells, which extends from the mesencephalon to the first few cervical spinal cord levels. Two of these nuclei—the main sensory nucleus and the spinal nucleus of the trigeminal—receive the first order afferent terminals of pseudounipolar neurons whose cell bodies are housed in the trigeminal ganglion. These nuclei serve as the **first sensory relay station** of the trigeminal system.

The **main (chief, principal) sensory nucleus of the trigeminal nerve** is located in the midpons. Based on its anatomical and functional characteristics, it is homologous to the nucleus gracilis and nucleus cuneatus. It is associated with the transmission of mechanoreceptor information for *discriminatory (fine) tactile* and *pressure sense*.

The **mesencephalic nucleus of the trigeminal** is unique, since it is a true "sensory ganglion" (and not a nucleus), containing cells that are both structurally and functionally ganglion cells. During development, neural crest cells are believed to become embedded within the CNS, instead of becoming part of the peripheral nervous system, as other sensory ganglia. This nucleus houses the cell bodies of **sensory** (first order) **pseudounipolar neurons**, thus there are *no synapses* in the mesencephalic nucleus. The peripheral large-diameter myelinated processes of these neurons convey **GP** input from the muscles innervated by the trigeminal nerve and the extraocular muscles, as well as from the periodontal ligament of the teeth.

The **spinal nucleus of the trigeminal** is the largest nucleus of the three nuclei. It extends from the midpontine region

to level C3 of the spinal cord, and is continuous inferiorly with the dorsal-most laminae (substantia gelatinosa) of the dorsal horn of the spinal cord. This nucleus consists of three subnuclei: the rostral-most subnucleus oralis (pars oralis), the caudal-most subnucleus caudalis (pars caudalis), and the intermediate subnucleus interpolaris (pars interpolaris).

The **subnucleus oralis** merges with the main sensory nucleus superiorly and extends to the pontomedullary junction inferiorly. It is associated with the transmission of discriminative (fine) tactile sense from the orofacial region.

The **subnucleus interpolaris** is also associated with the transmission of tactile sense, as well as dental pain, whereas the **subnucleus caudalis** is associated with the transmission of nociception and thermal sensations from the head. The subnucleus caudalis extends from the level of the obex (medulla) to the C3 level of the spinal cord. It is the homologue of the substantia gelatinosa since their neurons have similar cellular morphology, synaptic connections, and functions. Since the subnucleus caudalis lies immediately superior to the substantia gelatinosa of the cervical spinal cord levels, it is also referred to as the "**medullary dorsal horn**."

The trigeminal nerve does not have any parasympathetic nuclei in the CNS, or parasympathetic ganglia in the peripheral nervous system. However, it is anatomically associated with the parasympathetic ganglia of other cranial nerves (oculomotor, facial, and glossopharyngeal) and carries their autonomic "hitchhikers" to their destination.

Trigeminal tracts

The trigeminal system includes three tracts: the spinal tract of the trigeminal, the ventral trigeminal lemniscus, and the dorsal trigeminal lemniscus

The **spinal tract of the trigeminal** nerve consists of ipsilateral first order afferent fibers of sensory trigeminal ganglion neurons and mediates *tactile, thermal*, and *nociceptive sensibility* from the orofacial region to the spinal nucleus of the trigeminal. The spinal tract of the trigeminal also carries first order sensory axons of the facial, glossopharyngeal, and vagus nerves. These nerves terminate in the spinal trigeminal nucleus, conveying GVA or GSA sensory input from their respective areas of innervation to be processed by the trigeminal system. The spinal tract descends lateral to the **spinal nucleus of the trigeminal**, its fibers synapsing with neurons at various levels along the extent of this nucleus. Inferiorly this tract overlaps the dorsolateral fasciculus of Lissauer at upper cervical spinal cord levels.

The **ventral trigeminal lemniscus (ventral trigeminothalamic tract)** consists of mainly crossed nerve fibers from the main sensory and spinal nuclei of the trigeminal. This tract relays mechanoreceptor input for *discriminatory tactile* and *pressure sense* (from the main nucleus) as well as *sharp, well-localized pain* and *temperature* and *nondiscriminatory (crude) touch* sensation (from the spinal nucleus) to the contralateral **ventral posterior medial** (VPM) **nucleus** of the thalamus.

The **dorsal trigeminal lemniscus (dorsal trigeminothalamic tract)** carries uncrossed nerve fibers from the main sensory nucleus of the trigeminal, relaying *discriminatory* *tactile* and *pressure sense* information to the ipsilateral VPM nucleus of the thalamus.

The thalamus also receives indirect trigeminal nociceptive (dull, aching pain) input via the reticular formation (reticulo-thalamic projections).

Trigeminal pathways

Touch and pressure sense

Nearly half of the sensory fibers in the trigeminal nerve are Aβ myelinated discriminatory touch fibers. As the central processes of pseudounipolar (first order) neurons enter the pons, they bifurcate into short ascending fibers, which synapse in the **main sensory nucleus**, and long descending fibers, which terminate and synapse mainly in the **subnucleus oralis** and less frequently in the **subnucleus interpolaris** of the spinal nucleus of the trigeminal. These fibers descend in the spinal trigeminal tract to reach their target subnuclei. Some second order fibers from the main sensory nucleus cross the midline and join the ventral trigeminal lemniscus to ascend and terminate in the contralateral VPM nucleus of the thalamus. Other second order fibers from the main sensory nucleus do not cross. They form the dorsal trigeminal lemniscus, and then ascend and terminate in the ipsilateral VPM nucleus of the thalamus. Descending fibers terminating in the subnucleus oralis or interpolaris synapse with second order neurons whose fibers cross the midline and ascend in the ventral trigeminal lemniscus to the contralateral VPM nucleus of the thalamus. The VPM nucleus of the thalamus houses third order neurons that give rise to fibers relaying touch and pressure information to the postcentral gyrus of the cerebral cortex.

Pain and thermal sense

> The subnucleus caudalis is involved in the transmission of pain and thermal sensation from orofacial structures

The remaining half of the sensory fibers in the trigeminal nerve are similar to the Aδ and C nociceptive and temperature fibers of the spinal nerves. As the central processes of pseudounipolar neurons enter the pons, they descend in the **spinal tract** of the trigeminal and most of them synapse in the **subnucleus caudalis** of the spinal nucleus of the trigeminal. Nociceptive sensory input relayed in the subnucleus caudalis is modified, filtered, and integrated prior to its transmission to higher brain centers.

Interneurons located in the subnucleus caudalis project superiorly to the subnucleus oralis and interpolaris of the spinal nucleus and to the main sensory nucleus of the trigeminal, where they modulate the synaptic activity and relay of sensory input from all of these nuclei to higher brain centers. Furthermore, interneurons residing in the subnucleus oralis and interpolaris project to the subnucleus caudalis where they may in turn modulate the neural activity there.

Most of the second order fibers from the subnucleus caudalis cross the midline and join the contralateral ventral trigeminal lemniscus, whereas others join the ipsilateral ventral trigeminal lemniscus. All the fibers ascend to the VPM nucleus of the thalamus where they synapse with third order neurons in that nucleus. The fibers of third order neurons ascend in the posterior limb of the internal capsule to relay somatosensory information from the trigeminal system to the **postcentral gyrus** of the somatosensory cortex for further processing.

Electrophysiological observations have indicated that electrical stimulation of the midbrain periaqueductal gray matter, the medullary raphe nuclei, or the reticular nuclei, has an inhibitory effect on the nociceptive neurons of the subnucleus caudalis.

Substance P, a peptide in the axon terminals of small-diameter first order neurons, has been associated with the transmission of nociceptive impulses. A large number of substance P axon terminals have been located in the subnucleus caudalis. Opiate receptors have also been found in the subnucleus caudalis, which can be blocked by opiate antagonists. These findings indicate that there may be an endogenous opiate analgesic system that could modulate the transmission of nociceptive input from the subnucleus caudalis to higher brain centers.

Motor pathway

> The motor root fibers of the trigeminal nerve innervate the muscles of mastication

Branchiomotor neurons housed in the **motor nucleus of the trigeminal** give rise to fibers which, upon exiting the pons, form the **motor root** of the trigeminal nerve (see Fig. 15.7). This short root joins the sensory fibers of the mandibular division of the trigeminal nerve outside the skull. Motor fibers are distributed peripherally via the motor branches of the mandibular division, providing motor innervation to the muscles of mastication (temporalis, masseter, medial pterygoid, lateral pterygoid) and the mylohyoid, anterior belly of the digastric, tensor tympani, and tensor veli palatini muscles.

Mesencephalic neural connections

> Pseudounipolar neurons of the mesencephalic nucleus transmit general proprioception input to the main sensory and motor nuclei of the trigeminal and reticular formation

The peripheral processes of the pseudounipolar neurons housed in the **mesencephalic nucleus of the trigeminal** accompany the motor root of the trigeminal as they both exit the pons. These peripheral processes follow: (i) the motor branches of the mandibular division to the muscle spindles of the muscles of mastication; (ii) the orbital branches of the ophthalmic division to the muscle spindles of the extraocular muscles; and (iii) the dental branches of the maxillary and mandibular divisions to the sensory receptors of the periodontal ligament of the maxillary and mandibular teeth, respectively. The central processes of the neurons transmitting general proprioceptive input from all the muscles and from the periodontal ligament synapse in the **main sensory nucleus** and in the **motor nucleus** of the trigeminal, as well as in the reticular formation to mediate reflex responses.

Jaw jerk (masseteric) reflex

The afferent and efferent limbs of the jaw jerk reflex are formed by the branches of the trigeminal nerve

The **jaw jerk reflex** is a monosynaptic, myotatic (G., "muscle stretch") reflex for the masseter and temporalis muscles. A hammer gently tapped on the chin causes the intrafusal muscle fibers within the muscle spindles of the (relaxed) masseter and temporalis muscles to stretch, which stimulate the sensory nerve fibers innervating them. The cell bodies of these sensory pseudounipolar neurons are located in the **mesencephalic nucleus of the trigeminal** (Fig. 15.8). Their peripheral processes, which terminate in the muscle spindles (and are carried by branches of the trigeminal mandibular division), form the afferent limb of the reflex arc. The central processes of these neurons synapse in the motor nucleus of the trigeminal bilaterally, as well as in the main sensory nucleus and the reticular formation. The efferent limb of this reflex arc is formed by the motoneuron fibers traveling to the masseter and temporalis muscles (bilaterally, via motor branches of the trigeminal mandibular division) to cause them to contract and compensate for the stretch.

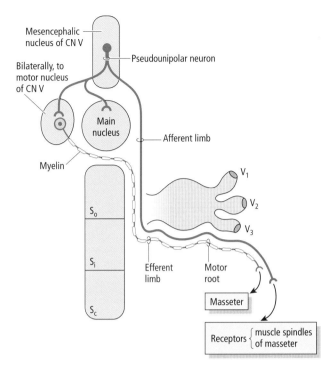

Figure 15.8 ● The jaw jerk reflex. The mesencephalic nucleus of the trigeminal nerve contains the nerve cell bodies of pseudounipolar neurons whose peripheral processes terminate in the muscle spindles of the masseter muscle. Sensory information (about muscle stretch) is carried by the central processes of these neurons to the ipsilateral main sensory and bilaterally to the motor nucleus of the trigeminal nerve. The motor neurons innervating the masseter muscle cause its contraction. For abbreviations, see Fig. 15.5.

CLINICAL CONSIDERATIONS

Skull fractures may cause a unilateral lesion of the branchiomotor fibers to the muscles of mastication, which will result in a **flaccid paralysis** or **paresis** with subsequent muscle **atrophy** of the ipsilateral muscles of mastication. This becomes apparent upon muscle palpation when the patient is asked to clench his jaw. When depressing the lower jaw it deviates *towards* the affected side (weak side) primarily due to the unopposed action of the lateral pterygoid muscle of the unaffected side. This impairs chewing on the lesion side due to muscle paralysis.

Damage to the fibers innervating the tensor tympani muscle results in **hyperacusis** (acute sense of hearing) and impaired hearing on the ipsilateral side.

Damage to the GSA fibers of the mandibular division will result in loss of sensation from the areas supplied by the branches of this division. Although the trigeminal nerve has an extensive distribution in the head, there is minimal overlapping of the areas innervated by its three divisions, especially in the central region of the face. Lesions in the peripheral branches of the trigeminal nerve can be located by testing for sensory deficits in the areas that are innervated by each of the three trigeminal divisions. If a lesion is located distal to the joining of the autonomic fibers that hitchhike with the trigeminal branches to the lacrimal gland or the salivary glands, then both sensory and autonomic innervation are interrupted.

Infection of the trigeminal ganglion by herpes zoster virus (known as shingles) causes a significant amount of pain as well as damage to the sensory fibers of the three trigeminal divisions (the ophthalmic division is most commonly infected). This results in loss of sensation on the affected side. Damage to the sensory fibers innervating the cornea (via the ophthalmic division) results in a loss of the corneal reflex when the ipsilateral eye is stimulated (afferent limb damage of the corneal reflex).

Trigeminal neuralgia (trigeminal nerve pain, tic douloureux)

A common clinical concern regarding the trigeminal nerve is **trigeminal neuralgia**. This condition results from idiopathic etiology (unknown cause) and is manifested as intense, sudden onset, and recurrent unilateral pain in the distribution of one of the three divisions of the trigeminal nerve, most commonly the maxillary division. There may be a trigger zone in the distribution of the affected trigeminal division, and if it is stimulated it may trigger an attack that usually lasts for less than a minute. This condition may be treated pharmacologically or surgically. Surgical treatment includes sectioning of the affected trigeminal division as it emerges from the trigeminal ganglion or producing a lesion in the trigeminal ganglion. Although these procedures may alleviate the excruciating pain experienced by patients, they also abolish tactile sensation from the affected area. Sectioning of the descending spinal trigeminal tract proximal to its termination in the subnucleus caudalis selectively obliterates the afferents relaying nociception but spares the fibers relaying tactile sensation from the orofacial region.

Note that the clinical case at the beginning of the chapter refers to a patient suffering from intermittent excruciating unilateral pain in the lower half of the left side of his face.

1 Which cranial nerve provides sensory innervation to the lower half of the face?

2 Pain sensation from the lower half of the face is relayed to the brainstem by sensory neurons whose cell bodies are located in which ganglion?

3 In which brainstem nucleus is pain sensation from the lower half of the face relayed to?

4 Name the thalamic nucleus where pain sensation from the lower half of the face is relayed to.

ABDUCENT NERVE (CN VI)

The abducent nerve innervates only one extraocular muscle, the lateral rectus

The **abducent nerve** supplies motor innervation to the lateral rectus muscle, which abducts the eye (a common mnemonic is LR_6). The abducent nerve exits the brainstem at the pontomedullary junction, then courses anteriorly, traverses the cavernous sinus, and upon leaving the sinus it passes via the superior orbital fissure into the orbital fossa where it innervates the ipsilateral lateral rectus muscle.

Normally, both eyes move together regardless of the direction of gaze. This is achieved by precise coordinated action of all the extraocular muscles of both eyes. The oculomotor, trochlear, and abducens nuclei are interconnected and are controlled by higher brain centers of the cerebral cortex as well as by the brainstem. During horizontal gaze, when looking to one side, the lateral rectus muscle of one side and the medial rectus muscle of the contralateral side contract simultaneously.

Abducens nucleus

The abducens nucleus mediates conjugate horizontal movement of the eyes

The **abducens nucleus** and the internal genu of the facial nerve form an elevation, known as the facial colliculus (L., "little hill") in the floor of the fourth ventricle. Axons emerging from the abducens nucleus belong to **GSE nerve cell bodies**. The axons course ventrally in the pontine tegmentum to exit in the ventral aspect of the brainstem at the pontomedullary junction.

The abducens nucleus contains two different populations of neurons (Fig. 15.9). One group (which makes up 70% of the nucleus neurons) consists of the GSE motoneurons, whose axons form the abducent nerve and project to the ipsilateral

lateral rectus muscle. The second group consists of internuclear neurons. Their axons emerge from the nucleus, immediately decussate and project via the contralateral medial longitudinal fasciculus (MLF) to the contralateral oculomotor nucleus. There the internuclear neuron terminals synapse with motoneurons that project to and innervate the medial rectus muscle. The MLF interconnects the abducens, trochlear, and oculomotor nuclei so that the two eyes move in unison. Thus the abducens nucleus mediates conjugate horizontal movement of the eyes.

When higher brain centers stimulate the abducens nucleus the following occur simultaneously:

1 Stimulation of the GSE motoneurons of the abducens nucleus that cause the ipsilateral lateral rectus muscle to contract, causing the eye to *abduct*.

2 Stimulation of the internuclear neurons of the same abducens nucleus that project, via the contralateral MLF, to the contralateral oculomotor nucleus. Here they form excitatory synapses with the motoneurons projecting to the contralateral medial rectus muscle causing it to contract so that the opposite eye *adducts*, resulting in coordinated lateral gaze.

GSA input from the lateral rectus muscle is transmitted centrally to the trigeminal nuclear complex via the processes of pseudounipolar neurons whose cell bodies are believed to reside in the mesencephalic nucleus of the trigeminal nerve.

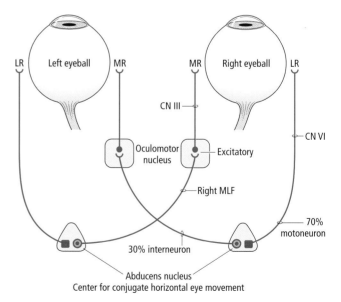

Figure 15.9 ● The connections of the abducens nucleus with the oculomotor nucleus. Note that the abducens nucleus is the center for conjugate horizontal eye movement. It contains two populations of neurons: (i) lower motoneurons whose axons form the abducent nerve that innervates the lateral rectus muscle (LR); and (ii) interneurons whose axons cross the midline and join the contralateral medial longitudinal fasciculus (MLF) to synapse in the oculomotor nucleus with the motoneurons that innervate the medial rectus muscle (MR).

CLINICAL CONSIDERATIONS

Abducent nerve lesion

A lesion in the abducent nerve causes paralysis of the lateral rectus muscle, resulting in medial strabismus and horizontal diplopia

A lesion in the abducent nerve (GSE, motor fibers) results in **paralysis** of the lateral rectus muscle that normally *abducts* the eye. The eye will then deviate medially as a result of the unopposed action of the medial rectus (Fig. 15.10). The individual can turn the ipsilateral eye from its medial position to the center (looking straight ahead), but not beyond it. This paralysis results in **medial strabismus (convergent, internal strabismus, esotropia)**. Since the eyes become misaligned, the individual experiences **horizontal diplopia** (double vision; i.e., a single object is perceived as two separate objects next to each other). The diplopia is greatest in an effort to look toward the side of the lesion and it is reduced by looking towards the unaffected side since the visual axes become parallel. The individual realizes that the diplopia is reduced by turning his head slightly so that his chin is pointing toward the side of the lesion. Bilateral abducent nerve lesion results in the individual becoming "cross-eyed."

Abducens nucleus lesion

A lesion involving the abducens nucleus results in medial strabismus, horizontal diplopia, and lateral gaze paralysis

A lesion involving the abducens nucleus (Fig. 15.11) results in the same deficiency as a lesion to the abducent nerve, with the addition of the inability to turn the opposite eye medially as the individual attempts to gaze toward the side of the lesion. This condition, referred to as **lateral gaze paralysis**, occurs because the damaged abducens nucleus no longer provides excitatory input to the opposite oculomotor nucleus neurons that innervate the medial rectus muscle.

Unilateral medial longitudinal fasciculus lesion: internuclear ophthalmoplegia

A lesion to one MLF results in internuclear ophthalmoplegia

If the oculomotor, trochlear, and abducent nerves and their nuclei are intact, but there is a **unilateral MLF lesion**, eye movements in all directions are possible. However, since the connections between the nuclei of these nerves are interrupted, horizontal ocular movements will not occur in a conjugate fashion.

When there is a lesion of the right MLF, and the individual attempts to gaze to the right, the lesion is not apparent, since both eyes can move simultaneously to the right. However, when attempting to gaze to the left, the right eye cannot move inward (medially beyond the midline) but the left eye, which should move outward (laterally) in this lateral gaze, does since it is not affected. If you ask this same individual to look at a near object placed directly in front of him, which necessitates that both eyes adduct (converge), he is able to do so. This indicates that: (i) both oculomotor nerves (which innervate the medial recti) are intact; and (ii) the upper motoneurons arising from the motor cortex (which stimulate the motoneurons of the oculomotor nuclei) are also intact. Therefore, a unilateral lesion of the MLF becomes apparent only during conjugate horizontal eye movement, when gazing away from the side of the lesion.

"One-and-a-half"

A rare condition resulting from a lesion near the abducens nucleus, involving the ipsilateral abducens nucleus and decussating MLF fibers arising from the contralateral abducens nucleus

A rare condition referred to as "one-and-a-half" results following a lesion in the vicinity of the abducens nucleus, which involves the entire ipsilateral

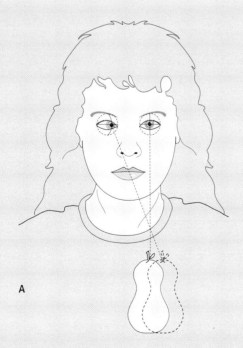

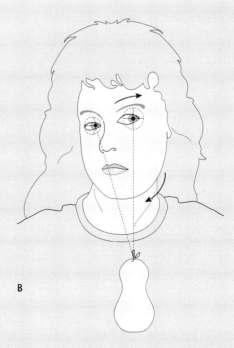

Figure 15.10 ● (A) Medial strabismus of the right eye due to paralysis of the lateral rectus muscle, resulting in diplopia (double vision). (B) To minimize the diplopia, the individual turns her head toward the side of the lesion, which abducts the normal eye.

CLINICAL CONSIDERATIONS (*continued*)

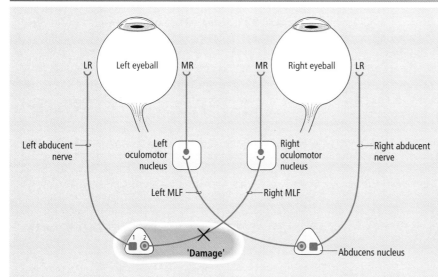

Figure 15.11 ● A lesion of the left abducens nucleus will damage: (i) the lower motoneurons of the abducent nerve, paralyzing the left lateral rectus muscle (LR); and (ii) the interneurons that synapse with the lower motoneurons of the oculomotor nucleus that innervate the right medial rectus muscle (MR). The affected individual is unable to gaze to the side of the lesion (left) during conjugate horizontal eye movement. MLF, medial longitudinal fasciculus.

abducens nucleus as well as the decussating MLF fibers arising from the contralateral abducens nucleus. If a lesion is present in the vicinity of the left abducens nucleus the following things happen:

1 The **GSE motoneurons**, whose axons form the left abducent nerve innervating the left lateral rectus, are damaged. Therefore, the left lateral rectus muscle is paralyzed.
2 The **internuclear neurons** housed in the left abducens nucleus are also damaged. Their crossing fibers (coursing in the right MLF) do not, therefore, form excitatory synapses with the motoneurons of the contralateral oculomotor nucleus that innervate the right medial rectus muscle.
3 The crossing fibers of the internuclear neurons arising from the contralateral (right) abducens nucleus are also damaged; thus they do not

form excitatory synapses with the motoneurons of the left oculomotor nucleus that innervate the left medial rectus.

Therefore, when attempting to gaze to the left, the left eye will not abduct and the right eye will not adduct during conjugate horizontal gaze to the left. When attempting to gaze to the right, the right eye responds normally, that is it is able to abduct, whereas the left eye will not be able to adduct during conjugate horizontal gaze to the right. It is important to note that the innervation to all the extraocular muscles of both eyes is intact, except one—the left lateral rectus. If you ask this individual to look at a near object placed directly in front of him, both eyes will converge, since both medial recti and their innervation (branches of the oculomotor nerve) are intact. Thus this type of lesion becomes apparent only during conjugate horizontal eye movement.

FACIAL NERVE (CN VII)

The facial nerve provides motor innervation to the muscles of facial expression

The **facial nerve** (Fig. 15.12) provides **branchiomotor** innervation to the muscles of facial expression, the platysma, the posterior belly of the digastric muscle, the stylohyoid muscle, and the stapedius muscle. It also transmits *taste sensation* from the anterior two-thirds of the tongue, as well as **parasympathetic** (secretomotor) innervation to the lacrimal, submandibular, and sublingual glands. Additionally, it provides *general sensation* to the back of the ear, pinna, and external auditory meatus, as well as *visceral sensation* from the nasal cavity and the soft palate.

The facial nerve consists of two parts: the **facial nerve proper** and the **nervus intermedius**. The facial nerve proper is the motor root of the facial nerve consisting of the axons of **SVE (branchiomotor) neurons** whose cell bodies reside in the **facial nucleus**. This nucleus contains subnuclei, each supplying specific muscles or groups of muscles. The nervus

intermedius is sometimes referred to as the "sensory root," which is a misnomer since in addition to sensory fibers it also carries parasympathetic fibers. The nervus intermedius consists of the axons of the **GVE (secretomotor) parasympathetic neurons**, whose cell bodies reside in the superior salivatory nucleus. It also contains the central processes of first order, sensory pseudounipolar neurons whose cell bodies are housed in the **geniculate** (L., "bent like a knee") **ganglion**, the only sensory ganglion of the facial nerve. Some of these pseudounipolar neurons transmit SVA (taste) sensation from the anterior two-thirds of the tongue, others convey GSA sensation from the area posterior to the ear, whereas others carry GVA sensation from the nasal cavity and soft palate.

Both nerve roots (motor root and nervus intermedius) emerge from the brainstem at the cerebellopontine angle. Near their exit from the brainstem, the two roots of the facial nerve accompany one another to the internal acoustic meatus of the petrous portion of the temporal bone and

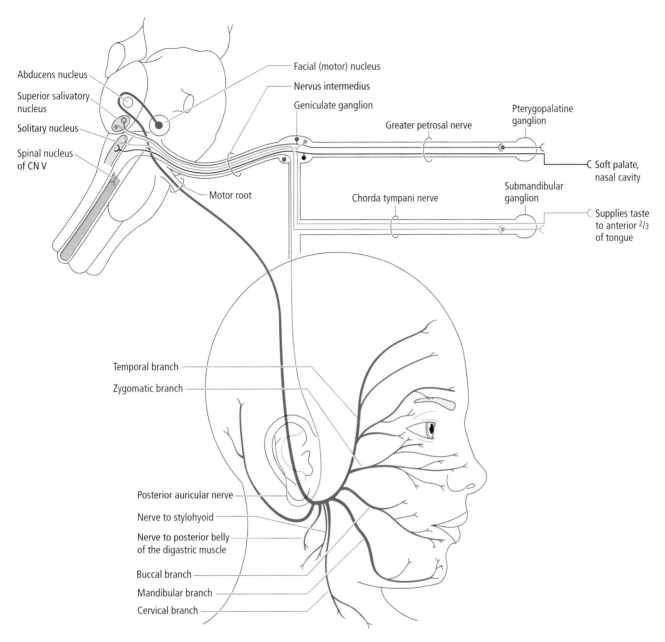

Figure 15.12 ● The origin and distribution of the facial nerve and its major branches.

proceed to the facial canal where the nervus intermedius presents a swelling—the **geniculate ganglion**.

The facial nerve gives rise to three of its branches in the facial canal: the greater petrosal nerve, the nerve to the stapedius muscle (which innervates the stapedius muscle in the middle ear), and the chorda tympani nerve. The facial nerve exits the facial canal via the stylomastoid foramen and courses to the parotid bed where its main trunk gives rise to numerous muscular branches, which radiate from within the substance of the gland to innervate their respective muscles (muscles of facial expression, platysma, posterior belly of the digastric, and stylohyoid muscles).

The **superior salivatory nucleus** contains GVE preganglionic parasympathetic nerve cell bodies (Figs 15.12, 15.13)

whose axons leave the brainstem via the nervus intermedius. These preganglionic fibers are distributed by the greater petrosal and chorda tympani nerves. The fibers in the greater petrosal nerve subsequently join the nerve of the pterygoid canal to enter the pterygopalatine fossa where they terminate and synapse in the **pterygopalatine ganglion**, one of the two parasympathetic ganglia of the facial nerve. Postganglionic parasympathetic fibers from this ganglion are distributed to the lacrimal gland and the glands of the nasal and oral cavity to provide them with secretomotor innervation. The **chorda tympani nerve** joins the lingual nerve, a branch of the mandibular division of the trigeminal nerve. The chorda tympani carries preganglionic parasympathetic fibers to the **submandibular ganglion** (the second parasympathetic

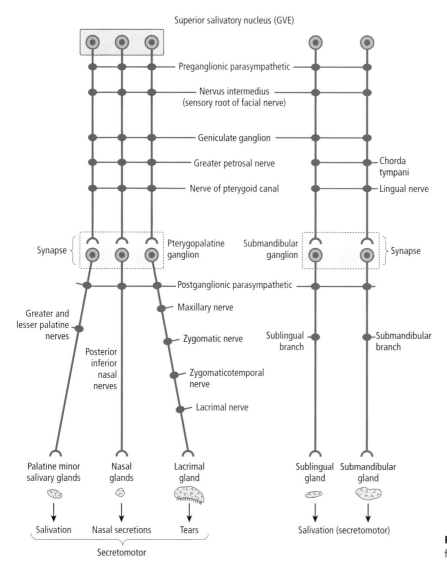

Superior salivatory nucleus (GVE)

Preganglionic parasympathetic

Nervus intermedius
(sensory root of facial nerve)

Geniculate ganglion

Greater petrosal nerve — Chorda tympani

Nerve of pterygoid canal — Lingual nerve

Synapse — Pterygopalatine ganglion — Submandibular ganglion — Synapse

Postganglionic parasympathetic

Maxillary nerve

Greater and lesser palatine nerves

Zygomatic nerve

Posterior inferior nasal nerves

Zygomaticotemporal nerve

Lacrimal nerve

Sublingual branch — Submandibular branch

Palatine minor salivary glands — Nasal glands — Lacrimal gland — Sublingual gland — Submandibular gland

Salivation — Nasal secretions — Tears — Salivation (secretomotor)

Secretomotor

Figure 15.13 ● Parasympathetic innervation of the facial nerve. GVE, general visceral efferent.

ganglion of the facial nerve), where the fibers synapse with its postganglionic parasympathetic neurons. The postganglionic parasympathetic fibers from this ganglion course to the submandibular and sublingual glands providing them with secretomotor innervation.

The geniculate ganglion houses the cell bodies of the SVA neurons, which are responsible for transmission of taste sensation from the anterior two-thirds of the tongue (Fig. 15.14). The peripheral processes of these neurons run in the chorda tympani, and reach the tongue via the lingual nerve of the mandibular division of the trigeminal nerve. The central processes of the SVA neurons enter the brainstem via the nervus intermedius to join the ipsilateral **solitary tract** and terminate in the **solitary nucleus**.

Other pseudounipolar neurons of the geniculate ganglion mediate GVA sensation. Their peripheral processes run in the greater petrosal nerve and terminate in the nasal cavity and the soft palate. Their central processes course in the nervus intermedius, join the ipsilateral solitary tract, and terminate in the solitary nucleus.

Still other pseudounipolar neurons of the geniculate ganglion are responsible for pain, temperature, and touch sensation from the pinna and the external auditory meatus (GSA fibers). The peripheral processes of these neurons terminate in the pinna and the external auditory meatus. Their central processes course in the nervus intermedius and join the **spinal tract of the trigeminal**, and terminate to synapse in the **spinal nucleus of the trigeminal**.

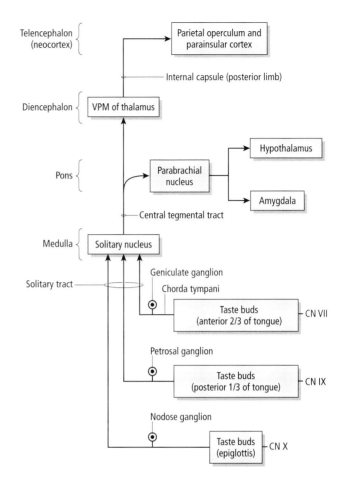

Figure 15.14 ● The gustatory pathway. Taste sensation is transmitted by cranial nerves VII (from the anterior two-thirds of the tongue), IX (from the posterior one-third of the tongue), and X (from the epiglottis). Taste sensation is relayed via the solitary tract to the solitary nucleus. The central tegmental tract arising from the solitary nucleus projects to the parabrachial nucleus and to the ventral posterior medial (VPM) nucleus of the thalamus, hypothalamus, and amygdala. The VPM nucleus of the thalamus projects to the gustatory cortex residing in the parietal operculum and the parainsular cortex. (Modified from Fix, JD (1995) *Neuroanatomy*. Williams & Wilkins, Media; fig. 20.2.)

CLINICAL CONSIDERATIONS

A lesion to the facial nerve within the facial canal or near its exit from the stylomastoid foramen causes Bell's palsy

A unilateral lesion of the facial nerve near its root or in the facial canal prior to giving off any of its branches (thus damaging all of its fibers), results in the following conditions *ipsilateral* to the lesion: damage to the SVE (branchiomotor fibers), results in a **flaccid paralysis** or **paresis** (impairment) of the muscles of facial expression, the platysma, stylohyoid, and posterior belly of the digastric muscles with subsequent muscle **atrophy**. The stapedius muscle will also be **paralyzed** and the individual will experience **hyperacusis** (an acute sense of hearing). Usually the stapedius muscle dampens vibrations of the ossicles, but when it is paralyzed, vibrations from the tympanic membrane are transmitted to the ossicles and subsequently to the inner ear receptors for hearing. Furthermore, damage of the SVA fibers relaying taste results in a **loss of taste** from the anterior two-thirds of the tongue. Damage of the GVE parasympathetic fibers causes **decreased salivary secretion** from the submandibular and sublingual glands. Since both parotid glands (innervated by a different cranial nerve) and the contralateral sublingual and submandibular glands remain functional, it is difficult to determine from salivary action alone

whether there is an interruption of the parasympathetic innervation to the ipsilateral submandibular and sublingual glands. In addition, the efferent limb of the corneal blink reflex will be damaged.

Bell's palsy may be idiopathic, or result following trauma or viral infection of the facial nerve within the facial canal or near its exit from the stylomastoid foramen. This condition is characterized by a paresis or paralysis of the muscles of facial expression ipsilateral to the lesion. **Bell's phenomenon** is exhibited by individuals with a Bell's palsy. As the individual attempts to close the eyes, the eye on the affected side deviates up and out.

A unilateral lesion of the facial nerve proximal to the geniculate ganglion causes loss of tear formation by the ipsilateral lacrimal gland. A condition referred to as **"crocodile tear syndrome"** (lacrimation while eating) may result as follows. As the preganglionic parasympathetic ("salivation") fibers originating from the superior salivatory nucleus are regenerating, they may be unsuccessful at finding their way to their intended destination, the submandibular ganglion, and instead take a wrong route to terminate in the pterygopalatine ganglion. The fibers then establish inappropriate synaptic contacts with postganglionic ("lacrimation") neurons whose fibers project to the lacrimal gland.

VESTIBULOCOCHLEAR NERVE (CN VIII)

The vestibular division of CN VIII transmits information about position sense and balance, whereas the cochlear division mediates the sense of hearing

The **vestibulocochlear nerve** consists of two distinct and separate nerves enclosed within one connective tissue sheath, the **vestibular nerve** (concerned with *position sense* and *balance*) and the **cochlear nerve** (concerned with *hearing*). Both nerves transmit **SSA** information from specialized peripheral ciliated mechanoreceptors ("hair cells").

The vestibular nerve is the only cranial nerve to send the central processes of some of its first order neurons to synapse directly in the cerebellum

The cell bodies of the **sensory first order bipolar neurons** of the **vestibular nerve** reside within the **vestibular ganglion of Scarpa** (see Fig. 18.6). Their peripheral processes terminate in special receptors, the **cristae** in the ampullae of the semicircular ducts and the **maculae** of the utricle and saccule, housed within the petrous temporal bone (see Figs 18.2–18.4). The central processes of these neurons enter the brainstem to synapse not only in the vestibular nuclear complex, where they synapse with **second order neurons** of the vestibular pathway, but also in the cerebellum (see Fig. 18.6). The vestibular nerve is unique since it is the only cranial nerve that sends the central processes of some of its first order neurons to synapse *directly* in the cerebellum.

The cell bodies of the sensory first order bipolar neurons of the **cochlear nerve** are housed within the **spiral (cochlear) ganglion** (see Fig. 17.3). Their peripheral processes terminate and synapse in the organ of Corti, containing the special receptors that transduce sound waves into electric impulses. The spiral ganglion and the organ of Corti lie within the cochlea, a snailshell-shaped structure of the inner ear, embedded within the petrous temporal bone (see Fig. 17.3). The central processes of these neurons accompany the seventh vestibular nerve to synapse in the **cochlear nuclei** in the brainstem with second order neurons of the auditory pathway (see Fig. 17.4).

GLOSSOPHARYNGEAL NERVE (CN IX)

The glossopharyngeal nerve provides parasympathetic innervation to the parotid gland

The **glossopharyngeal nerve**, one of the smallest cranial nerves, carries five functional components. These are: (i) SVA (taste) and (ii) GVA sensation from the posterior one-third of the tongue, the adjacent pharyngeal wall, and the carotid sinus (a baroreceptor or blood pressure receptor located near the bifurcation of the common carotid artery), (iii) GSA sensation from the external ear, (iv) SVE (branchiomotor) innervation to the stylopharyngeus muscle, and (v) GVE parasympathetic innervation to the parotid gland.

The glossopharyngeal nerve exits the brainstem as a group of rootlets posterior to the olive in the dorsolateral sulcus. These rootlets immediately collect to form the main trunk of the glossopharyngeal nerve, which shortly exits the cranial vault via the jugular foramen where it presents two swellings, its **superior** and **inferior ganglia** (Fig. 15.15). The superior ganglion contains GSA, and the inferior ganglion contains GVA and SVA, cell bodies of **first order pseudounipolar** neurons.

The inferior ganglion of the glossopharyngeal nerve houses the cell bodies of the **SVA (taste)** neurons. Their peripheral processes course with the trunk of the glossopharyngeal nerve to the tongue where they supply the posterior one-third of the tongue and adjacent pharyngeal wall with taste sensation. The central processes of the SVA neurons pass into the brainstem via the glossopharyngeal nerve root, join the **solitary tract** and terminate in the **solitary nucleus** (Fig. 15.16A).

GVA first order nerve cell bodies reside in the **inferior ganglion** of the glossopharyngeal nerve. Their peripheral processes terminate in the mucosa of the posterior one-third of the tongue, tonsil and adjacent pharyngeal wall, tympanic cavity, and auditory tube (Fig. 15.16B). Unilateral stimulation of the pharyngeal wall elicits a bilateral contraction of the pharyngeal muscles and soft palate (**gag reflex**). The glossopharyngeal nerve serves as the afferent limb (GVA peripheral fibers whose cell bodies are housed in the inferior ganglion), whereas the vagus nerve provides the efferent limb of the reflex arc. The central processes of the afferent fibers enter the solitary tract and synapse in the **nucleus ambiguus**. The nucleus ambiguus sends motor fibers via the vagus nerve to the muscles of the palate and pharynx. Many individuals in the general population do not have a gag reflex.

Baroreceptor fibers terminate in the carotid body and sinus, which form the afferent limb of the reflex arc that controls blood pressure. The central processes of the GVA neurons enter the brainstem via the glossopharyngeal nerve root, join the solitary tract and terminate in the solitary nucleus. The solitary nucleus relays sensory input to the reticular formation, the brainstem GVE (autonomic) motor nuclei, and the intermediolateral horn (containing preganglionic sympathetic neurons) of the spinal cord for reflex activity related to the control of arterial lumen diameter and blood pressure.

The glossopharyngeal nerve also provides **GSA** touch, pain, and temperature innervation to the pinna of the ear and the external auditory meatus. The cell bodies of these sensory neurons are located in the superior ganglion of the glossopharyngeal nerve. The central processes of these neurons course in the glossopharyngeal nerve root, enter the brainstem, and join the **spinal tract of the trigeminal nerve** to terminate and synapse in the **spinal nucleus of the trigeminal nerve**. Recent clinical evidence supports that fibers transmitting nociceptive sensory input from the pharyngeal wall and posterior one-third of the tongue enter the brainstem and descend in the spinal tract of the trigeminal and terminate in the spinal nucleus of the trigeminal. Furthermore, sensation from oral structures is transmitted via the glossopharyngeal afferent terminals to the **main sensory nucleus** of the trigeminal.

The nucleus ambiguus contains the **SVE branchiomotor** nerve cell bodies whose axons emerge from the brainstem along with rootlets of the glossopharyngeal nerve, and course with the trunk of the glossopharyngeal nerve (Fig. 15.16C). These axons then leave the glossopharyngeal nerve as the

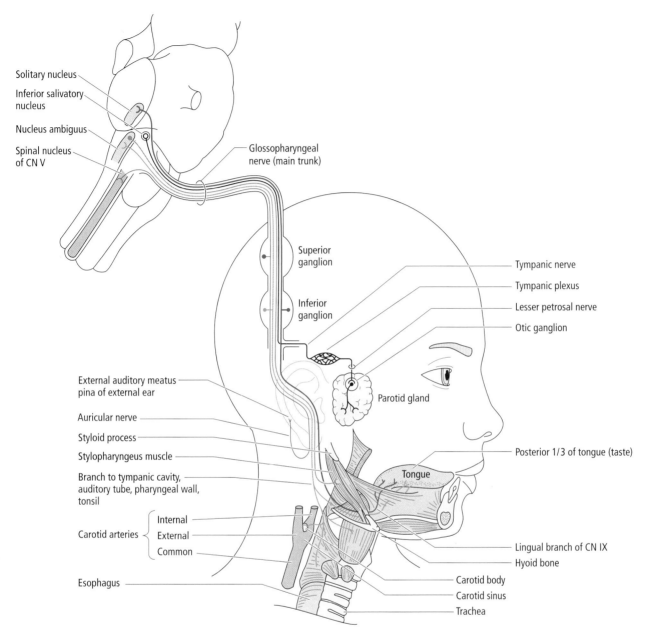

Figure 15.15 ● The origin and distribution of the glossopharyngeal nerve and its major branches.

nerve to the stylopharyngeus muscle, the only muscle innervated by the glossopharyngeal nerve.

The **inferior salivatory nucleus**, located in the medulla, contains the **GVE** cell bodies of preganglionic parasympathetic neurons whose axons exit the brainstem as part of the glossopharyngeal nerve (Fig. 15.16D). These fibers then branch off as the tympanic nerve and subsequently spread out to form the tympanic plexus in the tympanic cavity. The preganglionic parasympathetic fibers course to the **otic ganglion**, the parasympathetic ganglion of the glossopharyngeal nerve (located in the infratemporal fossa), where they synapse with postganglionic parasympathetic neurons whose fibers join the auriculotemporal branch of the trigeminal nerve to reach the parotid gland, providing it with secretomotor innervation.

CLINICAL CONSIDERATIONS

A unilateral lesion to the glossopharyngeal nerve near its exit from the brainstem, damaging all of its fibers, will result in damage to the SVA fibers relaying taste sensation and will cause **ipsilateral loss of taste sensation** from the posterior one-third of the tongue. Damage to the GVE parasympathetic fibers will cause a **reduction in salivary secretion** of the parotid gland; and damage to the GVA fibers will result in **diminished visceral sensation** from the pharyngeal mucous membrane, **loss of the gag reflex** (due to damage of the afferent limb of the reflex arc), and **loss of the carotid sinus reflex**. The stylopharyngeus muscle, which elevates the pharynx during swallowing, will be paralyzed.

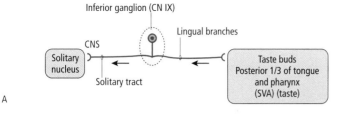

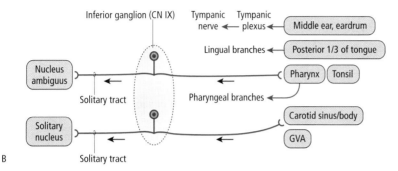

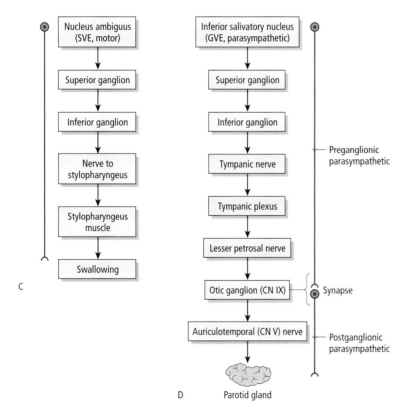

Figure 15.16 ● Innervation by the glossopharyngeal nerve: (A) special visceral afferent (SVA; taste); (B) general visceral afferent (GVA); (C) special visceral efferent (SVE; skeletal motor); and (D) general visceral efferent (GVE; parasympathetic).

VAGUS NERVE (CN X)

The vagus nerve has the most extensive distribution in the body, innervating structures in the head but also the neck, thorax, and abdomen

The **vagus** (L., "wanderer") **nerve** (Fig. 15.17) is a large cranial nerve that has the most extensive distribution in the body. Although it is a cranial nerve, its innervation is not limited to the structures in the head, but also extends into the neck, thorax, and abdomen. The vagus nerve carries five functional components: (i) SVA; (ii) GVA; (iii) GSA; (iv) SVE; and (v) GVE (the same functional components carried by the facial and glossopharyngeal nerves). A group of fine rootlets surface in the medulla in the dorsolateral sulcus, inferior to the glossopharyngeal nerve and superior to the spinal accessory nerve. The rootlets join to form two distinct bundles—a smaller inferior and a larger superior that collectively form the vagus nerve. The inferior bundle joins the spinal accessory nerve and accompanies it for a short distance, but then the two diverge to go their separate ways. The smaller vagal bundle joins the main trunk of the vagus to exit the cranial vault via the

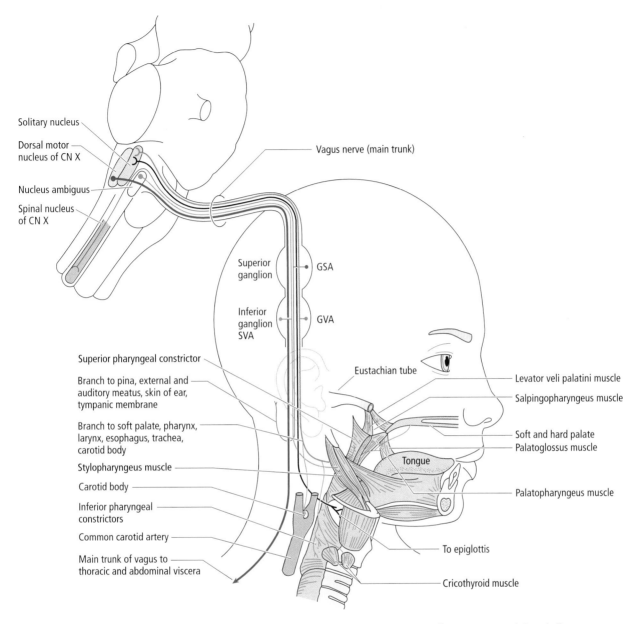

Figure 15.17 ● The origin and distribution of the vagus nerve and its major branches. GSA, general somatic afferent; GVA, general visceral afferent; SVA, special visceral afferent.

jugular foramen. Inferior to the jugular foramen, the vagus nerve displays two swellings, the superior (jugular) and inferior (nodose) ganglia. The **superior ganglion** houses the cell bodies of pseudounipolar first order sensory neurons carrying GSA information from the pinna of the ear and external auditory meatus and the dura of the posterior cranial fossa. The **inferior ganglion** contains the pseudounipolar first order nerve cell bodies transmitting GVA sensory innervation from the mucosa of the soft palate, pharynx, and larynx, and a minor SVA (taste) sensation from the epiglottis.

SVA (taste) pseudounipolar neuron cell bodies located in the inferior ganglion of the vagus nerve send their peripheral fibers to terminate in the scant taste buds of the epiglottis. Their central processes enter the brainstem along with the

other vagal fibers to terminate in the **solitary nucleus** (Fig. 15.18A).

GVA pseudounipolar neuron cell bodies housed in the inferior ganglion distribute their peripheral processes in the mucous membranes of the soft palate, and those lining the pharynx, larynx, esophagus, and trachea. Chemoreceptor fibers (GVA also) terminate in the carotid body where they monitor blood carbon dioxide concentration. The central processes of all of the GVA neurons enter the brainstem, course in the **solitary tract** and terminate in the solitary nucleus (Fig. 15.18A).

GSA pseudounipolar neuron cell bodies conveying pain, temperature, and touch sensation reside in the superior ganglion and send their peripheral processes to the pinna,

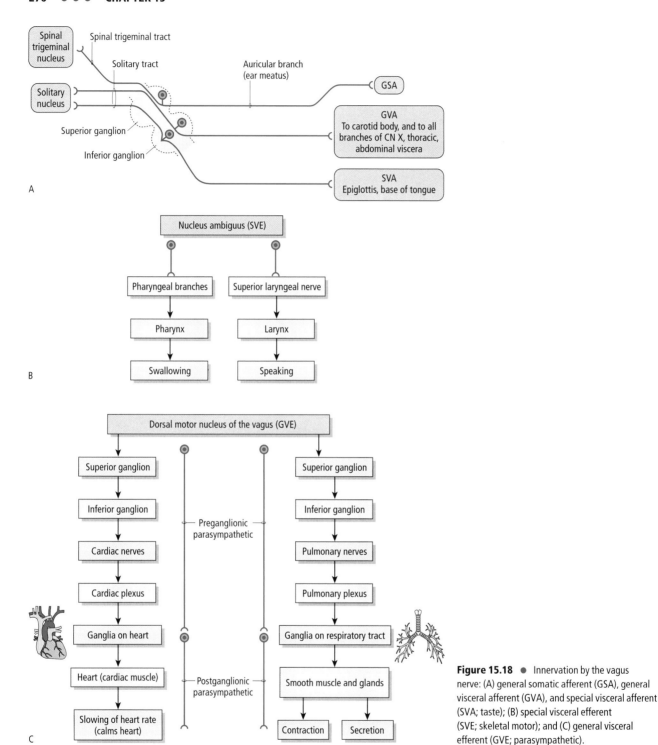

Figure 15.18 ● Innervation by the vagus nerve: (A) general somatic afferent (GSA), general visceral afferent (GVA), and special visceral afferent (SVA; taste); (B) special visceral efferent (SVE; skeletal motor); and (C) general visceral efferent (GVE; parasympathetic).

external auditory meatus, skin of the ear, and tympanic membrane. Their central processes enter the brainstem, join the **spinal tract of the trigeminal** and terminate in the **spinal nucleus of the trigeminal** (Fig. 15.18A).

The cell bodies of the **SVE branchiomotor neurons** are located in the **nucleus ambiguus**. The fibers of these neurons innervate all of the laryngeal and pharyngeal muscles with the exception of the stylopharyngeus and the tensor veli palatini muscles (Fig. 15.18B).

The vagus nerve has a very extensive **GVE** distribution. It supplies parasympathetic innervation to the laryngeal mucous glands and all of the thoracic and most of the abdominal organs. The **dorsal motor nucleus of the vagus** houses the nerve cell bodies of preganglionic parasympathetic neurons whose fibers accompany the other vagal fibers upon their exit from the brainstem. These fibers run in the main trunk of the vagus into the thorax where they leave the main trunk and join the autonomic plexuses scattered throughout the thoracic and abdominal cavities. The preganglionic fibers terminate and synapse in the terminal parasympathetic ganglia or ganglia near or within the viscera. Parasympathetic innervation decreases the heart rate (calms the heart), reduces adrenal gland secretion, activates peristalsis, and stimulates glandular activity of various organs (Fig. 15.18C).

CLINICAL CONSIDERATIONS

Unilateral damage of the vagus nerve near its emergence from the brainstem results in a number of deficiencies on the ipsilateral side. Damage to the SVE branchiomotor fibers will cause **flaccid paralysis** or **weakness** of: (i) the pharyngeal muscles and levator veli palatini of the soft palate, resulting in **dysphagia** (difficulty swallowing); (ii) the laryngeal muscles, resulting in **dysphonia** (hoarseness) and **dyspnea** (difficulty breathing); and (iii) **loss of the gag reflex** (efferent limb). Damage to the GVA fibers will cause **loss of general sensation** from the soft palate, pharynx, larynx, esophagus, and trachea. Damage to the GVE fibers will cause **cardiac arrhythmias**.

A bilateral lesion of the vagus nerve is incompatible with life, due to the interruption of parasympathetic innervation to the heart.

SPINAL ACCESSORY NERVE (CN XI)

The spinal accessory nerve supplies motor innervation to the sternocleidomastoid, trapezius, and many of the intrinsic laryngeal muscles

The **spinal accessory nerve** (Fig. 15.19) supplies motor innervation to the sternocleidomastoid, trapezius, and many of the intrinsic laryngeal muscles. In the early literature this nerve was described as consisting of two distinct parts: a cranial (bulbar) and a spinal root. It is now understood that the "cranial root" of the accessory nerve is composed of *aberrant* **vagal fibers** arising from the **nucleus ambiguus** in the medulla. These vagal fibers collectively form a distinct root as they emerge from the brainstem. On the other hand, the **spinal accessory nerve** derives its fibers from the **spinal accessory nucleus** residing in the posterolateral aspect of the ventral horns of cervical spinal cord levels **C2–C5** (or **C6**). This nucleus is continuous superiorly with the nucleus ambiguus of the medulla. Delicate rootlets emerging from the surface of the lateral funiculus of the spinal cord (interposed between the dorsal and ventral spinal roots) converge and assemble to form the spinal accessory nerve. This nerve trunk ascends, enters the cranial vault through the foramen magnum, and proceeds on the lateral aspect of the medulla to join the aberrant vagal fibers as they emerge from the medulla. The two groups of fibers accompany one another for a short distance but then diverge to go their separate ways. The aberrant vagal fibers join the main trunk of the vagus nerve and follow those fibers of the vagus that are destined to supply most of the intrinsic laryngeal muscles. The spinal accessory nerve exits the cranial vault via the jugular foramen. It courses inferiorly to the deep surface of the sternocleidomastoid muscle providing it with motor innervation. It continues its inferior course to the posterior triangle of the neck and then proceeds to the deep aspect of the upper part of the trapezius muscle to supply it with motor innervation. In view of its origin, many neuroanatomists no longer consider the accessory nerve to be a true cranial nerve, but instead a unique type of spinal nerve.

Additionally, there are differences of opinion relating to the classification of the functional components of the spinal accessory nerve. Some authors consider that this nerve carries **branchiomotor SVE** fibers since neurons of the spinal accessory nucleus develop in a manner characteristic of SVE, not GSE, neurons; whereas others believe that they are **somatomotor**, that is GSE.

Recent literature supports that **GSA** proprioceptive fibers are carried by the spinal accessory nerve from the upper cervical spinal cord levels to the structures it innervates, but questions the branchial arch origins of the trapezius and sternocleidomastoid muscles.

CLINICAL CONSIDERATIONS

A unilateral lesion confined to the spinal accessory nucleus or the nerve proximal to its muscular distribution results in an **ipsilateral flaccid paralysis** and subsequent **atrophy** of the sternocleidomastoid and upper part of the trapezius muscles. An individual with such a lesion is unable to turn his or her head away from the lesion. Normally, unilateral contraction of the sternocleidomastoid muscle draws the mastoid process inferiorly, bending the head sideways (approximating the ear to the shoulder), which is accompanied by an upward turning of the chin towards the opposite side. If the upper part of the trapezius is paralyzed, the upper border of the scapula is rotated laterally and inferiorly with its inferior angle pointing towards the spine. This results in slight drooping of the ipsilateral shoulder, accompanied by a weakening of the shoulder when attempting to raise it.

HYPOGLOSSAL NERVE (CN XII)

The hypoglossal nerve provides motor innervation to the muscles of the tongue

The **hypoglossal nerve** (Fig. 15.20) provides motor innervation to the muscles of the tongue. The cell bodies of the **GSE** lower motoneurons of the hypoglossal nerve reside in the **hypoglossal nucleus**, a cell column in the medulla. This nucleus, located ventral to the floor of the fourth ventricle near the midline, forms a triangular elevation—the **hypoglossal trigone**—in the floor of the midline of the ventricle. The nerve cell bodies of the hypoglossal nucleus give rise to axons that course ventrally to arise as a series of tiny rootlets on the ventral surface of the medulla in the sulcus separating the pyramid and the olive. These rootlets collect to form the hypoglossal nerve, which exits the cranial vault through the hypoglossal foramen. The nerve then

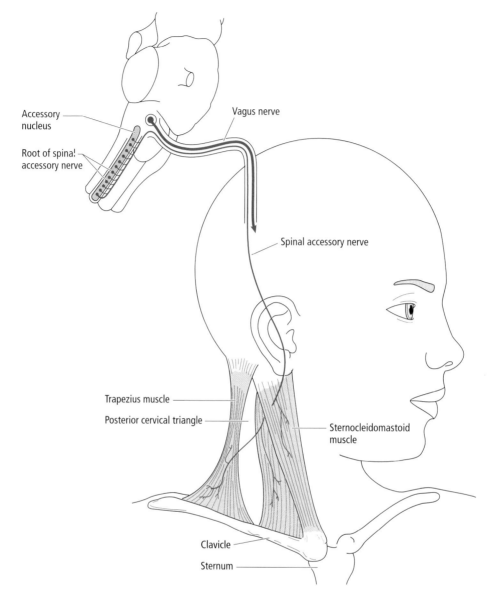

Figure 15.19 ● The origin and distribution of the spinal accessory nerve and its major branches.

courses to the submandibular region to serve the *ipsilateral* side of the tongue. The hypoglossal nerve innervates the intrinsic muscles (transverse, longitudinals, and vertical) and all the extrinsic muscles of the tongue (styloglossus, hyoglossus, and genioglossus) with the exception of the palatoglossus. Recent studies indicate that **GSA** fibers terminating in muscle spindles of the tongue musculature transmit proprioceptive sensation to the trigeminal system involved in reflex activity of mastication. Some investigators believe that the cell bodies of these GSA pseudounipolar neurons are located in the mesencephalic nucleus of the trigeminal nerve, whereas others maintain that they are dispersed along the hypoglossal nerve.

CLINICAL CONSIDERATIONS

A unilateral lesion of the hypoglossal nerve will cause the tongue to deviate toward the side of the lesion (impaired side)

A lesion in the hypoglossal nucleus or nerve results in **flaccid paralysis** and subsequent **atrophy** of the ipsilateral tongue musculature. **Hemiparalysis** of the tongue causes creasing (wrinkling) of the dorsal surface of the tongue ipsilateral to the lesion. Normally, the simultaneous contraction of the paired genioglossi muscles causes the tongue to protrude straightforward. During examination of the patient it is important to remember that a unilateral lesion of the hypoglossal nerve will cause the tongue to deviate towards the *side of the lesion* (impaired side) since the functional genioglossus on the intact side is unopposed by the paralyzed, inactive genioglossus on the lesion side.

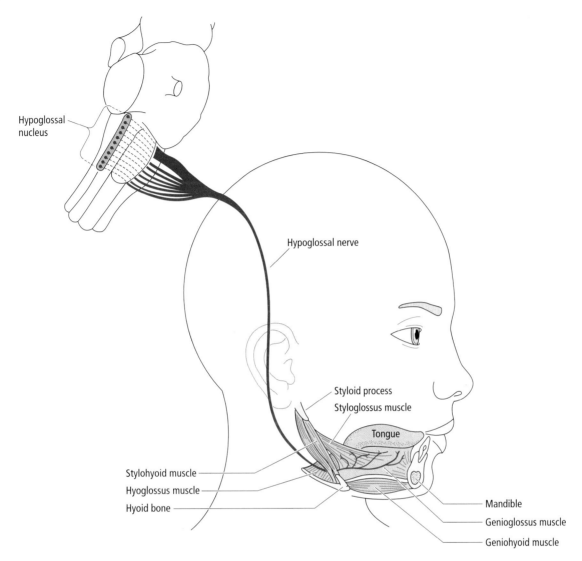

Figure 15.20 ● The origin and distribution of the hypoglossal nerve.

SYNONYMS AND EPONYMS OF THE CRANIAL NERVES

Name of structure or term	Synonym(s)/eponym(s)	Name of structure or term	Synonym(s)/eponym(s)
Cochlear ganglion	Spiral ganglion	Postcentral gyrus	Primary sensory cortex (S-I)
Discriminatory tactile sense	Fine touch sensation		Primary somatosensory cortex
Dorsal trigeminal lemniscus	Dorsal trigeminothalamic tract		Primary somesthetic cortex
Functional components of cranial nerves	Modalities of cranial nerves		Brodmann's areas 3, 1, and 2
		Pseudounipolar neurons	Unipolar neuron
General somatic efferent (GSE)	Somatic motor	Special visceral efferent (SVE)	Branchiomotor
	Somatomotor	Sphincter pupillae muscle	Constrictor pupillae muscle
General visceral efferent (GVE)	Visceral motor	Spinal nucleus of the trigeminal	Descending nucleus of the trigeminal
	Visceromotor	Spinal tract of the trigeminal	Descending tract of the trigeminal
	Secretomotor	Subnucleus caudalis of the spinal trigeminal nucleus	Pars caudalis of the spinal trigeminal nucleus
Inferior ganglion of the vagus nerve	Nodose ganglion		
Internuclear neurons	Interneurons	Subnucleus interpolaris of the spinal trigeminal nucleus	Pars interpolaris of the spinal trigeminal nucleus
Main nucleus of the trigeminal	Chief nucleus of the trigeminal		
	Principal nucleus of the trigeminal	Subnucleus oralis of the spinal trigeminal nucleus	Pars oralis of the spinal trigeminal nucleus
Mandibular division of the trigeminal nerve	Mandibular nerve		
		Superior ganglion of the vagus nerve	Jugular ganglion
Maxillary division of the trigeminal nerve	Maxillary nerve	Trigeminal neuralgia	Trigeminal nerve pain
			Tic douloureaux
Medial strabismus	Internal strabismus	Ventral trigeminal lemniscus	Ventral trigeminothalamic tract
	Convergent strabismus	Vestibular ganglion	Vestibular ganglion of Scarpa
	Esotropia	Vestibulocochlear nerve	Acoustic nerve (older term)
Ophthalmic division of the trigeminal nerve	Ophthalmic nerve		

FOLLOW-UP TO CLINICAL CASE

This patient has **trigeminal neuralgia**, also called **tic douloureux**. This is a purely clinical diagnosis, and tests are usually normal. This is a very common disorder, and this is a typical presentation. The pain is indeed excruciating and should be taken very seriously, as suicide is not an uncommon result!

This condition is most common in the elderly, though it can occur in younger age groups. The common etiology is thought to be from ephaptic transmission of nerve impulses, or in other words "short circuiting." The most common cause is from vascular "loops" that develop and surround one of the divisions of the trigeminal nerve at its root, most commonly affecting the ophthalmic and sometimes the maxillary divisions. This causes compression of the nerve, demyelination, and ephaptic

transmission. This condition is usually spontaneous and comes "out of the blue." Trigeminal neuralgia in a young person brings up the specter of multiple sclerosis. Multiple sclerosis is a disease of the central nervous system, and can be a cause of trigeminal neuralgia. This is thought to result from demyelination of the trigeminal nerve root as it enters the brainstem.

There are effective treatments for this condition. Carbamazepine, an antiseizure medication, is the most effective. Other antiseizure medications have been used. Trigeminal neuralgia from vascular loops can be treated, if refractory to medications, by microvascular decompression surgery. This surgical procedure generated much skepticism when it was first introduced, but has produced excellent results for refractory cases and has now become widely accepted.

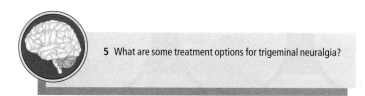

5 What are some treatment options for trigeminal neuralgia?

QUESTIONS TO PONDER

1. What is the first clinical sign of intracranial pressure on the GVE (parasympathetic fibers) of the oculomotor nerve?

2. What are the functional deficits caused by a lesion to the trochlear nucleus or to the trochlear nerve?

3. What are the functional deficits following a lesion to the right abducens nucleus?

4. What eye movement functional deficits result following a lesion to one medial longitudinal fasciculus?

5. What eye movement deficits result following a lesion in the vicinity of the abducens nucleus?

6. What is the cause of the "crocodile tear syndrome"?

7. Which cranial nerves are likely to be damaged from a growing pituitary tumor?

8. Name the cranial nerves that are susceptible to damage from a tumor growing in the vicinity of the cerebellopontine angle.

Retinal ve

Fovea cer

Macula lu

Optic disc

Dura of o
nerve she

Central re
artery and

Optic ner

Cerebros|

Choroid

Sclera —

Extraocul

Figure 16.1 ● Ana
covers the remainder
The inner layer is form
converge at the poste

a protective rigi
one-sixth of the
parent avascula
not only permits
it also refracts it
cornea, is appare
sclera permits th
region, the **lami**

Middle layer

The middle layer of th
the choroid, ciliary bo

cells. Since it res
the **uvea** (L. u
middle layer, kr
the eye. The cho
tion for the retin
that has passed
and glare inside
merges with a t

C H A

Vis

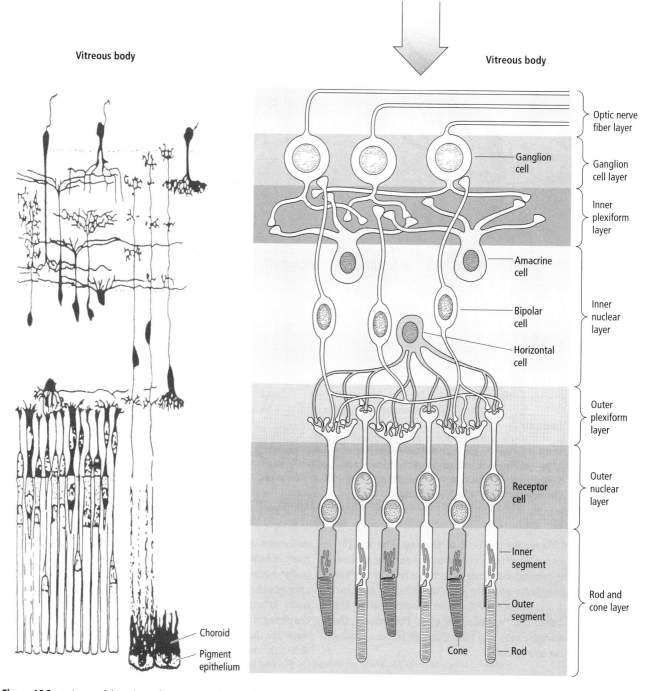

Figure 16.2 ● Layers of the retina and component cells. Note that light has to pass from the front of the eye through the vitreous body and all of the retinal layers to finally reach the receptor cells, rods, and cones.

The visu
sensory (
extraordi
environm

The ey
cial sense
each cons
but also f
retina co
transmit
form refl
sensory i
conveyec
a visual i

the pigment epithelium which underlies the choroid, and an inner layer, the retina proper or neural retina (Fig. 16.2). The **pigment epithelium** consists of a layer of pigmented cells that absorb light that has passed through the retina. The **neural retina** contains the layers of nerve cells responsible for the processing and transmission of visual information. The photosensitive portion of the neural retina extends from the ora serrata to the optic disc. The nonphotosensitive

portion of the retina extends from the ora serrata anteriorly, where it lines the inner surface of the ciliary body and iris.

The elements of the **optic nerve** collect into a bundle at the **optic disc** and pierce all the three layers of the bulb to exit the eye (Fig. 16.1). The optic disc is insensitive to light (since it lacks photoreceptors) resulting in a **blind spot** in the visual field. The **macula lutea** (L., "yellow spot") is a yellow spot of the retina in the back of the eye, whose central pit, the **fovea** centralis, contains only cones and represents the site of maximal visual acuity and color perception.

Retinal layers

The **neural retina** is a multilayered structure. These layers contain supporting glia (**Müller cells**) and astrocytes, as well as six types of neurons that process visual input prior to its transmission to the diencephalon. They are the **photoreceptors** (100–120 million **rods** and 6–7 million **cones**), the **conducting neurons** (**bipolar cells** and **ganglion cells**), and the **association neurons** or **interneurons** (**horizontal cells** and **amacrine cells**), which modulate the activity of the bipolar and ganglion cells.

The retina consists of the following 10 layers (Fig. 16.2).

1 **Pigment epithelium**. The deepest layer of the retina consists of pigmented cells. This is a non-neural layer that absorbs excess light which has passed through the other retinal layers, and is immediately next to the choroid.

2 **Rod and cone layer**. This layer includes the outer and inner segments of the photoreceptor cells (rods and cones). The discs of the photoreceptors contain visual pigments that undergo chemical changes (following absorption of light) leading to the initiation of local receptor potentials.

3 **External (outer) limiting membrane**. Although this appears to be a membrane, actually its not. It is formed by intercellular junctions—the zonulae adherents—binding the apical aspect of the Müller cells.

4 **Outer nuclear layer**. This consists of the cell bodies of the rods and cones.

5 **Outer plexiform layer**. This is a synaptic area that contains the terminals of the rods and cones, as well as those of the retinal interneurons (horizontal cells) and bipolar cells. The rods and cones synapse with the horizontal and bipolar cells. The horizontal cells join the photoreceptor cells laterally.

6 **Inner nuclear layer**. This consists of the somata of the retinal interneurons (horizontal, bipolar, and amacrine cells), which integrate and modulate the activity of the photoreceptors.

7 **Inner plexiform layer**. This is a synaptic area containing the terminals of the bipolar, amacrine, and ganglion cells. Amacrine cells link the ganglion cells laterally.

8 **Ganglion cell layer**. This consists of the somata of the ganglion cells (multipolar neurons).

9 **Optic nerve fiber layer**. This is composed of the axons of the ganglion cells that gather to form a thick bundle, the optic nerve. These axons terminate primarily in the lateral geniculate nucleus (LGN) of the thalamus.

10 **Internal (inner) limiting membrane**. This membrane is composed of a basal lamina interposed between the vitreous body and the Müller cells. The vitreous body is a gelatinous substance filling the vitreous space of the bulb of the eye, posterior to the lens. The internal limiting membrane separates the neural retina from the vitreous body.

Sensory input from the photoreceptors is transmitted to a synaptic zone stimulating bipolar cells, which in turn transmit the information to ganglion cells. Horizontal and amacrine cells link the conducting neurons laterally within the retina. The convergent circuitry of the rods on the bipolar cells results in a decrease in visual acuity. High acuity would result from a 1 : 1 ratio of rods to bipolar cells: one tiny portion of the visual field would be mapped to one bipolar cell. Instead, many rods representing a larger portion of the visual field are mapped to one bipolar cell, so that cell represents a larger portion of the visual field. There is little convergence in the macula lutea of the retina, the site of highest visual acuity.

The supporting **Müller cells** (specialized glia cells) extend the entire thickness of the retina from the internal to the external limiting membrane.

The **cones** (Fig. 16.3B) are activated by *high intensity light* (**photopic vision**). They mediate sharp vision and color vision. They detect fine detail, have the highest acuity, and are more numerous in the central portion of the retina and less concentrated at the periphery. There are three different types of cones in the human retina, the membrane of each cone being associated with a different pigment, and responding to a different wavelength of light (red, blue, or yellow-green sensitive).

Rods are of a single type only (Fig. 16.3A). They are stimulated by *low intensity light*; thus they transmit visual input in dim illumination (**scotopic vision**) but they cannot detect colors. They are more concentrated in peripheral regions of the retina. At night, when looking straight at a light located at a distance, it disappears when projected on the fovea (which contains only color-sensitive cones), but when looking away from it, the image falls on more peripheral regions of the retina, where rods are more numerous, and therefore the image becomes visible.

Molecular biology of the rods and cones

A light-absorbing photopigment is synthesized in the inner segment of both rods and cones; rod membranes are associated with rhodopsin, whereas cone membranes are associated with iodopsin

Rods and cones are composed of an inner segment, a connecting stalk, and an outer segment. The **inner segment** encloses the cellular organelles and is the site of protein synthesis, such as the protein component of the photopigments. The **connecting stalk** is the narrow segment interposed between the inner and outer segments. The photoreceptor cells derive their name from the morphology of their **outer segment**—that of a rod being cylindrical, and that of a cone being conical. The outer segment is the dendritic end of the photoreceptor and is a photosensitive-modified cilium, which is located adjacent to the retinal pigment epithelium. The photoreceptor outer segment consists of a stack of horizontally oriented, membranous, flattened discs derived from the plasma membrane. In rods, the hollow discs located at the apical end of the outer

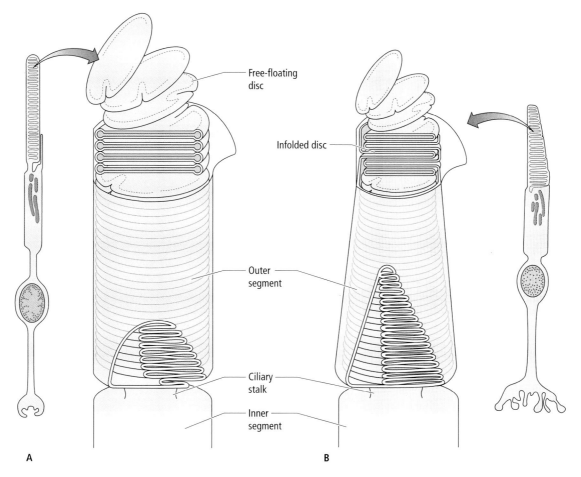

Figure 16.3 ● Schematic representation of the retinal receptor cells outer segment: (A) the outer segment of a rod; and (B) the outer segment of a cone.

segment are intracellular, and are completely separated from the plasma membrane. The discs located closer to the base of the rod outer segment, and the entire outer segment of the cones, consist of shelf-like infoldings of the plasma membrane. They are thus a continuation of the plasma membrane with their interior being continuous with the intercellular space (Fig. 16.3).

A light-absorbing photopigment is synthesized in the inner segments of both rods and cones, and is then transported to their respective outer segments (by passing through the connecting stalk), where it is incorporated into disc membranes as transmembrane proteins. The membrane of rods is associated with the pigment **rhodopsin** (G., "visual purple"), whereas the membrane of cones is associated with a pigment that consists of a component chemical of **iodopsin**. Rhodopsin and iodopsin are almost identical chemically, with the exception of their spectral sensitivity difference (thus, only the photochemistry of rhodopsin is discussed below). Both rhodopsin and iodopsin consist of two components: an **opsin**, which is a protein moiety, and a **chromophore** (G., "bearing color"), which absorbs photons. In rods the opsin is known as **scotopsin** (G. scotos, "darkness"), whereas in cones the opsins are known as **photopsins** (G. photos, "light"). The chromophore associated with rods is

retinal, a substance derived from vitamin A. Normal vision is dependent on a sufficient intake of vitamin A. A severe dietary deficiency of vitamin A results in **night blindness**, a condition characterized by the inability to see in poor illumination.

Rhodopsin is a transmembrane homologue of G-protein-linked receptor molecules that acts by activating a trimeric G-protein (**transducin**, G_t). It is composed of a protein segment, **opsin** (embedded in the membranes of rod discs), to which a vitamin A derivative, **11-*cis*-retinal**, is covalently attached. The plasma membrane of the rod outer segment contains cGMP-gated Na^+ channels to which cGMP is bound in the absence of light. The cGMP–Na^+ channel complex maintains the channel in an open state, so that Na^+ as well Ca^+ can enter the outer segment. The constant flow of Na^+ ions into the outer segment causes a high rate of neurotransmitter release from the synaptic region of the rod, resulting in the inhibition of postsynaptic retinal neurons in the dark.

When a photon hits the 11-*cis*-retinal molecule, it isomerizes to **all-*trans*-retinal**, and this change in molecular configuration causes an alteration in the conformation of the opsin to which it is attached. This conformational change of the opsin moiety results in the binding of rhodopsin to transducin which, in turn, dissociates and its alpha subunit activates the enzyme **cGMP phosphodiesterase**. Since this enzyme functions to hydrolyze cGMP, decreasing its cytosolic concentration, cGMP is released from the Na^+ channels causing the closure of these channels. The lack of Na^+ flow into the outer segment causes a hyperpolarization of the rod with a resultant shutdown of neurotransmitter release from its synaptic region. Since the neurotransmitter substance inhibits the postsynaptic retinal neurons, the absence of the neurotransmitter acts to excite them. Thus a single photon has the capability of eliciting a visual response.

The closed state of the Na^+ channel also shuts off the flow of Ca^+ into the outer segment of the rod. This decrease in cytosolic Ca^+ causes the uncoupling of Ca^+ from the cytosolic protein **recoverin**, resulting in its activation. The activated recoverin stimulates guanylyl cyclase to manufacture cGMP which, by binding to the guanylyl cyclase, opens the Na^+ channels so that the rod can revert to its dark-phase (resting) state.

Lens

The lens is a biconvex, transparent adjustable structure, whose shape can be adjusted in order to focus the corneal image on the retina

The human eye consists of two "lenses," the cornea and the lens (see Fig. 16.1). Light rays entering the eye are actually refracted mostly by the cornea, and not the lens. The lens is a biconvex, transparent adjustable structure, whose shape can be adjusted in order to focus the corneal image on the retina. The lens is suspended posterior to the iris by the **suspensory ligaments of the lens**, which are anchored to the ciliary processes of the ciliary body. The lens inverts and reverses the image and focuses it on the retina. In order for incoming light to reach the retina, it has to pass through the following refractive media of the eye:

1 The **cornea**. This is the chief refracting medium of the eye. It serves to focus a crude image on the retina.
2 The **anterior chamber** of the eye. This is a fluid-filled (aqueous humor) space between the lens and the cornea.
3 The **lens**. The shape (thickness) of the lens can be altered, which can fine focus the corneal image on the retina.
4 The **vitreous body**. This is a transparent gelatinous substance filling the vitreous space of the bulb of the eye, posterior to the lens.
5 Most layers of the **neural retina**. In order for light to reach the photoreceptors (rods and cones), which are located at the "back" of the retina, light has to first go through the overlying retinal layers (layers 3–10, see above) in order to reach them.

CENTRAL VISUAL PATHWAYS

The visual pathway consists of photoreceptors, first order and second order neurons residing in the retina, and third order neurons in the lateral geniculate nucleus of the thalamus

Incoming light rays impinging on the retina pass from its inner layers to its outermost neural layer where they cause the retinal **photorecep-**

tor cells (modified neurons), the **rods** and **cones**, to become *hyperpolarized*. The photoreceptors then stop releasing neurotransmitters and the **bipolar cells (first order neurons)** are no longer inhibited, and fire. The bipolar cells along with the interneurons, the **horizontal** and **amacrine cells**, process, integrate, and modulate visual input. The bipolar cells relay this sensory input to the **ganglion cells (second order neurons)** of the retina. Therefore, stimulation within the retina proceeds from the rod and cone layer to the bipolar cell layer and finally to the ganglion cell layer. Although light travels from the inner to the outer layers of the retina, visual electrical signals are transmitted in the opposite direction from the outer to the inner layers of the retina.

Although light travels from the inner to the outer layers of the retina, visual electrical signals are transmitted in the opposite direction from the outer to the inner layers of the retina

The **ganglion cells** possess nonmyelinated axons (see Fig. 16.2b) that course on the *inner surface* of the retina (separated from the vitreous body only by the internal limiting membrane), converge at the **optic disc**, and cross a sieve-like perforated area of the sclera, the **lamina cribrosa**, to emerge from the back of the bulb of the eye. At this point, the axons become myelinated and they form a large bundle, the **optic nerve (CN II)**. The optic nerve is enveloped in a meningeal cover, exits the bony orbit by passing through the **optic canal**, and enters the middle cranial fossa. The optic nerves of the right and left sides join superior to the body of the sphenoid bone in the middle cranial fossa to form an intersection of fibers, the **optic chiasma** (G., "optic cross") (Fig. 16.4) where partial decussation of the optic nerve fibers (axons) of the two sides occurs. All ganglion cell axons arising from the temporal half of the retina course in the lateral aspect of the optic chiasma without decussating, to join the optic tract of the same side. All ganglion cell axons arising from the nasal half of the retina decussate at the optic chiasma, and enter the optic tract of the opposite side, to join the temporal fibers. Thus, each optic tract consists of ganglion cell axons arising from both eyes (the ipsilateral temporal half and the contralateral nasal half of the retina). The fibers retain a retinotopic organization in the optic tract as it courses around the cerebral peduncle to end and relay visual information primarily in the **lateral geniculate nucleus** (LGN) of the thalamus, which processes visual input. The optic nerve also ends and relays visual information in: (i) the **superior colliculus**, a mesencephalic relay nucleus for vision having an important function in somatic motor reflexes; (ii) the **pretectal area**, which mediates autonomic reflexes such as the control of pupillary constriction and lens accommodation (see discussion on visual reflexes below); and (iii) the **hypothalamus**, which has an important function in circadian rhythms (day–night) and the reproductive cycle (Fig. 16.5).

An overview of the central visual pathway is given in Fig. 16.6.

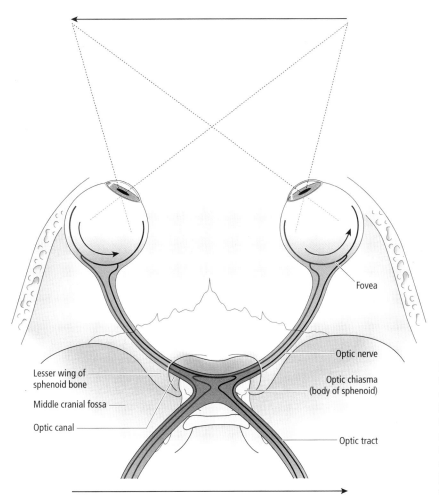

Figure 16.4 ● Schematic diagram of the eyes, optic nerves, optic chiasma, and optic tracts. Each optic nerve contains visual information from the ipsilateral eye. Fibers from the temporal half of each retina course along the lateral aspect of the optic chiasma to join the ipsilateral optic tract. In contrast, fibers from the nasal half of each retina course in the central region of the optic chiasma where they cross to join the contralateral optic tract. Thus each optic tract carries information from both eyes.

Lateral geniculate nucleus

The LGN houses the cell bodies of third order neurons of the visual pathway and serves as a thalamic relay station that processes/regulates the flow of visual information to the primary visual cortex

The **lateral geniculate nucleus** (Fig. 16.7) is a relay station of the dorsal thalamus whose principal function is to process and regulate the flow of visual information and relay it to the **primary visual cortex**. The LGN houses the cell bodies of **third order neurons** of the visual pathway. Their axons form the thalamocortical projection (optic radiation) that relays visual input to the primary visual cortex. The LGN is a laminated structure consisting of six distinct layers that are readily identifiable in a horizontal section. Although each LGN receives information from the contralateral visual hemifield, each of its layers receives input from only one eye. Layers 1, 4, and 6 receive ganglion cell axons arising from the contralateral retina, whereas layers 2, 3, and 5 receive ganglion cell axons arising from the ipsilateral retina. Layers 1 and 2 consist of large neurons and are therefore referred to as the **magnocellular layers**; they receive information from ganglion cells that are sensitive to *movement* and *contrast* but are insensitive to color. Layers 3–6 consist of small neurons and are referred to as the **parvocellular layers**; they receive

information from the ganglion cells responding to *color* and *form*. The macular area of the retina has a greater representation in the LGN than the peripheral (paramacular) areas of the retina. Furthermore, the lateral half of the LGN receives visual information from the lower retinal quadrants (upper visual field quadrants), whereas its medial half receives visual information from the upper retinal quadrants (lower visual field quadrants).

In addition to the retinal ganglion cell axon terminals (second order neurons) arriving at the LGN (**retinogeniculate projections**), the LGN also receives a greater number of afferents from the visual cortical areas (**corticogeniculate projections**). These fibers are associated with stimulating visual attention of the individual, and reciprocally regulating the transmission of sensory input from the LGN to the primary visual cortex.

Superior colliculus

The superior colliculus functions in the control of reflex movements that orient the eyes, head, and neck in response to visual, auditory, and somatic stimuli

The **superior colliculi** (L. colliculus, "little hill") (Fig. 16.5) are two prominent elevations projecting from the posterior surface of the

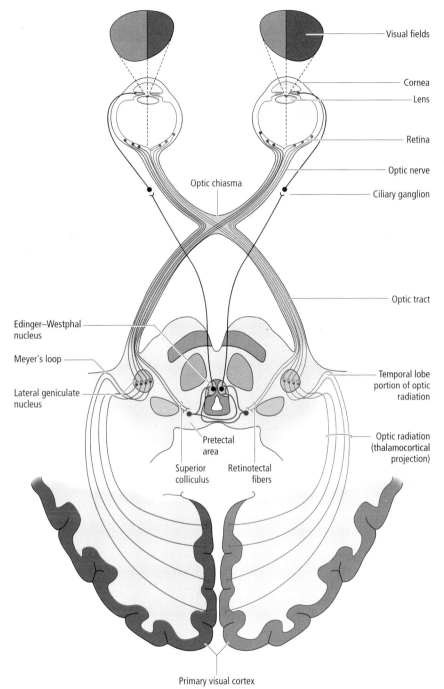

Figure 16.5 ● The visual pathways. Ganglion cell axons (axons of second order neurons) leaving the retina form the optic nerve. The ganglion cell axons arising from the temporal half of each retina pass along the lateral aspect of the optic chiasma to join the ipsilateral optic tract. The ganglion cell axons arising from the nasal half of each retina cross at the optic chiasma to join the contralateral optic tract. Ganglion cell axons terminate in the lateral geniculate nucleus of the thalamus and the superior colliculus and pretectal area of the midbrain. Third order neurons of the lateral geniculate nucleus project via the geniculocalcarine tract (optic radiation, thalamocortical projections) to the primary visual cortex (Brodmann's area 17) located in the banks of the calcarine sulcus on the medial surface of the occipital lobe.

mesencephalon. They are also laminated structures, each consisting of seven layers. The superior colliculus is a relay nucleus of the mesencephalon that receives sensory input (afferents) from:

- the **visual system** to **layers 1–3** (from the retina via retinotectal fibers, and from the visual cortex via corticotectal fibers);
- the **auditory system** to **layers 4–7** (principally from the inferior colliculus); and
- the **somatosensory system** to **layers 4–7** (spinotectal tract).

Following the integration of all the sensory input, appropriate reflex responses are produced by the neurons of the superior colliculi.

The superior colliculus has important functions in the control of **reflex movements** that **orient the eyes, head, and neck** in response to **visual, auditory, and somatic stimuli** (tracking moving objects) via its outputs (efferent projections). Efferents from the superior colliculus include projections to the reticular formation, the inferior colliculus, the LGN and the pulvinar of the thalamus, the oculomotor, trochlear, and abducens nuclei via the medial longitudinal fasciculus (MLF), the pontine nuclei and the cerebellum via

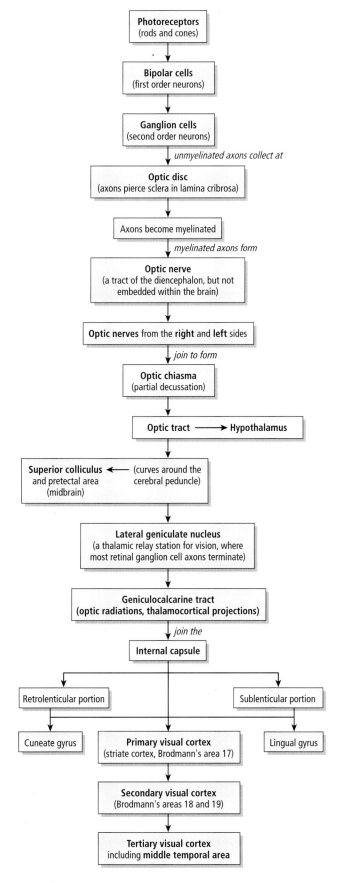

Photoreceptors
(rods and cones)

↓

Bipolar cells
(first order neurons)

↓

Ganglion cells
(second order neurons)

unmyelinated axons collect at

↓

Optic disc
(axons pierce sclera in lamina cribrosa)

↓

Axons become myelinated

myelinated axons form

↓

Optic nerve
(a tract of the diencephalon, but not embedded within the brain)

↓

Optic nerves from the right and left sides

join to form

↓

Optic chiasma
(partial decussation)

↓

Optic tract ⟶ Hypothalamus

↓

Superior colliculus ⟵ (curves around the cerebral peduncle)
and pretectal area
(midbrain)

↓

Lateral geniculate nucleus
(a thalamic relay station for vision, where most retinal ganglion cell axons terminate)

↓

Geniculocalcarine tract
(optic radiations, thalamocortical projections)

join the

↓

Internal capsule

↙   ↘

Retrolenticular portion   Sublenticular portion

↓   ↓

Cuneate gyrus   Primary visual cortex
(striate cortex, Brodmann's area 17)   Lingual gyrus

↓

Secondary visual cortex
(Brodmann's areas 18 and 19)

↓

Tertiary visual cortex
including middle temporal area

Figure 16.6 ● The visual pathway.

the tectopontocerebellar tract, and the cervical levels of the spinal cord via the crossed tectospinal tract.

Geniculocalcarine tract (optic radiations, thalamocortical projections)

Axons of third order neurons originating from the LGN form the geniculocalcarine tract (optic radiations, thalamocortical projections), which terminate in the primary visual cortex

The fibers of the **geniculocalcarine tract** follow the contour of the lateral wall of the lateral ventricle (Fig. 16.8), joining the retrolenticular and sublenticular components of the internal capsule, the **corona radiata**, and then pass posteriorly toward the medial and posterior surface of the **occipital lobe** where the **visual cortex** is located. Each one of the axons of the geniculocalcarine tract carries visual input only from one eye.

The geniculocalcarine tract fibers maintain retinotopic organization and form an upper, an intermediate, and a lower division. The **upper division** consists of fibers conveying information from the **superior retinal quadrants**. This division projects via the retrolenticular portion of the internal capsule to the superior bank of the calcarine fissure of the primary visual cortex. The **lower division** consists of fibers conveying information from the **inferior retinal quadrants**. The lower division fibers collectively form **Meyer's loop** (Fig. 16.8). These fibers loop anteriorly and inferiorly around the anterior horn of the lateral ventricle then posteriorly via the sublenticular part of the internal capsule to the inferior bank of the calcarine fissure of the primary visual cortex. The **intermediate division** of the geniculocalcarine tract consists of fibers relaying visual information to the primary visual cortex from the **macular region of the retina** (Table 16.1).

Visual cortex

The visual cortex is the site where visual information is processed and its significance determined

The neurons of the visual cortex respond to different visual stimuli transmitted by neurons conveying color, motion, three-dimensional vision, or a combination of various visual stimuli. The LGN projects visual information to the **primary visual cortex** (V-1) (Fig. 16.9). The primary visual cortex projects to the **secondary visual cortex** (V-2), where information is processed and subsequently relayed to the **tertiary visual areas** (V-3, V-4, and the middle temporal area) **of the cortex**. The tertiary visual areas function in identifying an object as well as in determining its location and color. Furthermore, the middle temporal area has an important function in detecting moving objects.

The primary visual cortex resides mainly in the medial surfaces of the occipital lobes on the banks of the **calcarine fissure**, although it extends into their posteromedial surface. The primary visual cortex is also referred to as the **striate cortex** due to its striped characteristic exhibiting a noticeable band of myelinated fibers, the "**stripe of Gennari**."

The primary visual cortex receives visual input from the macula of the retina in its caudal third, and from the

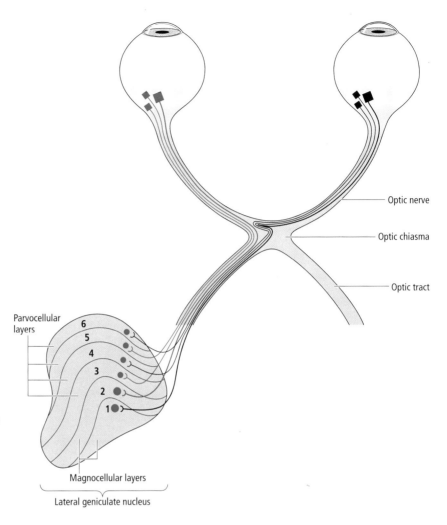

Figure 16.7 ● Retinal ganglion cell projections to the lateral geniculate nucleus of the thalamus. Note that layers 1, 4, and 6 of the lateral geniculate nucleus receive visual information from the contralateral retina, whereas layers 2, 3, and 5 receive visual information from the ipsilateral retina. (Modified from Nolte, J (1999) *The Human Brain, An Introduction to Its Functional Anatomy*, 5th edn. Mosby, St Louis, Missouri; fig. 17.25C.)

Table 16.1 ● Topographic relationships of projections from the retina to the lateral geniculate nucleus (LGN) to the banks of the calcarine sulcus.

Visual field quadrants	Retinal field quadrants	LGN	Optic radiations	Calcarine banks
Upper	Lower	Lateral half	Inferior part	Inferior
Lower	Upper	Medial half	Superior part	Superior

paramacular (and more peripheral) fields of the retina in its rostral portions. The macular representation in the primary visual cortex is much larger than that of other areas of the retina, reflecting the high visual acuity of the macula.

VISUAL REFLEXES

Pupillary light reflex

The pupillary light reflex enables the eye to adapt to varying light intensity, which protects the eye and also facilitates vision

Inherent in the structure of the visual system is its ability to adapt to environmental changes such as varying light intensity, in order to protect the eye and to facilitate vision. The **pupillary light reflex** is an autonomic response; it is mediated independently of cortical input.

The iris contains two smooth muscles, the sphincter pupillae and dilatator pupillae, which control the diameter of the pupil. When the circularly arranged fibers of the sphincter pupillae contract the diameter of the pupil is decreased, therefore reducing the amount of light that falls on the retina. The fibers of the dilatator pupillae muscle are arranged radially, and when they contract the pupillary aperture dilates, allowing more light to enter the eye to reach the retina. The size of the pupillary aperture depends on two factors: (i) the tone of the autonomic nervous system—if the activity of the *sympathetic* nervous system dominates, the pupillary

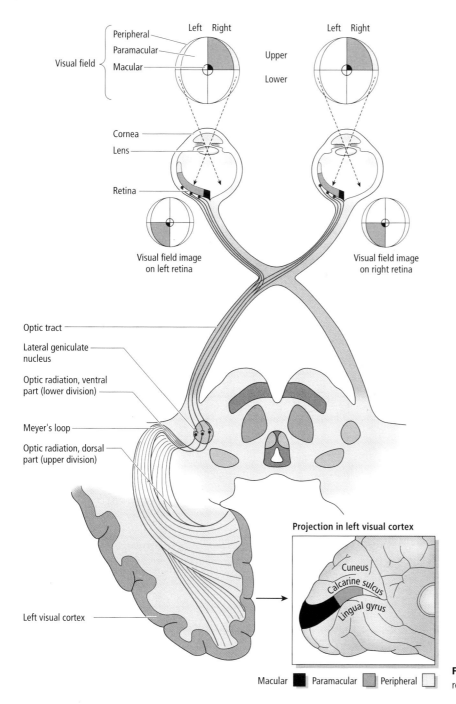

Figure 16.8 ● Visual field representation in the retina and primary visual cortex.

aperture *dilates*; if the activity of the *parasympathetic* nervous system dominates, the pupillary aperture *constricts*; and (ii) the amount of light that reaches the retina—varying the light intensity results in a corresponding alteration of pupillary size. Normally, bright light causes the pupils to constrict, whereas dim light causes the pupils to dilate.

The pupillary light reflex of an individual may be tested by illuminating one eye with a small flashlight and observing that normally, simultaneous pupillary constriction results in both eyes. The reaction in the illuminated eye is the **direct** pupillary light reflex, whereas the reaction in the nonilluminated eye is the **consensual pupillary light reflex**.

The pupillary light reflex pathway is summarized in Fig. 16.10.

Afferent limb of the pupillary light reflex

Bright light stimulating the photosensitive **retina** is transmitted via the **optic nerve**, **optic chiasma**, **optic tract** and

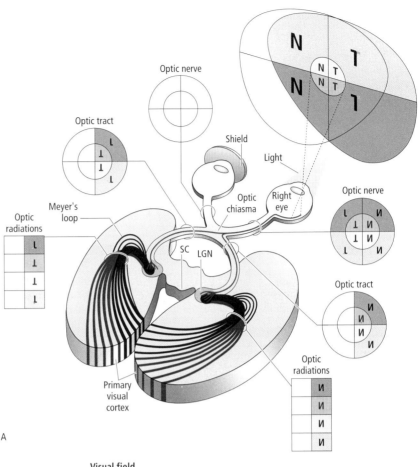

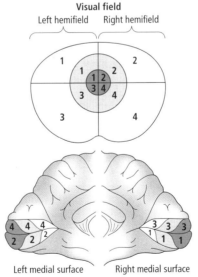

Figure 16.9 ● (A) Visual field representation in the visual pathway: T, temporal half of the visual field; N, nasal half of the visual field; SC, superior colliculus; LGN, lateral geniculate nucleus. In the right retina and right optic nerve, the image from the visual field is backwards and upside down. Note that the left eye has a shield over it, thus no visual information is perceived by that eye. At the level of the optic chiasma, the ganglion cell axons coursing in the medial half of the right optic nerve decussate to the opposite side to course in the medial half of the left optic tract, to terminate in the left lateral geniculate nucleus. In contrast, the ganglion cell axons coursing in the lateral half of the right optic nerve remain ipsilaterally and course in the lateral half of the right optic tract, to terminate in the right lateral geniculate nucleus. Visual information is relayed to the primary visual cortex in a banded pattern. The alternating clear bands represent the areas occupied by the axons of the optic radiations relaying visual information from the left eye. (B) Visual field representation in the primary visual cortex. The peripheral area of the visual field is represented in the anterior region of the primary visual cortex on the medial surface of the occipital lobe. In contrast, the central or macular area of the visual field is represented in the posteriormost region of the primary visual cortex. (Modified from Fitzgerald, MJT, Folan-Curran, J (2002) *Clinical Neuroanatomy and Related Neuroscience*. WB Saunders, New York; fig. 25.10.)

the **brachium of the superior colliculus** (without synapsing at the LGN) to the **pretectal area** located in the cranial aspect of the mesencephalon (Fig. 16.11). The pretectal area sends bilateral projections to the **Edinger–Westphal nuclei** of the oculomotor nuclear complex.

Efferent limb of the pupillary light reflex

Each Edinger–Westphal nucleus (containing preganglionic parasympathetic neurons) (Fig. 16.11) projects via the **oculomotor nerve** to the ipsilateral **ciliary ganglion** (a

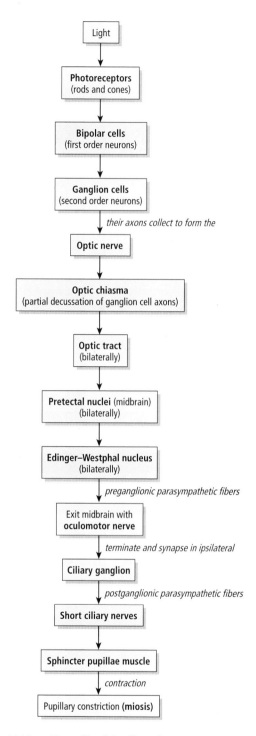

```
Light
   ↓
Photoreceptors
(rods and cones)
   ↓
Bipolar cells
(first order neurons)
   ↓
Ganglion cells
(second order neurons)
   ↓ their axons collect to form the
Optic nerve
   ↓
Optic chiasma
(partial decussation of ganglion cell axons)
   ↓
Optic tract
(bilaterally)
   ↓
Pretectal nuclei (midbrain)
(bilaterally)
   ↓
Edinger–Westphal nucleus
(bilaterally)
   ↓ preganglionic parasympathetic fibers
Exit midbrain with
oculomotor nerve
   ↓ terminate and synapse in ipsilateral
Ciliary ganglion
   ↓ postganglionic parasympathetic fibers
Short ciliary nerves
   ↓
Sphincter pupillae muscle
   ↓ contraction
Pupillary constriction (miosis)
```

Figure 16.10 ● The pupillary light reflex pathway.

parasympathetic ganglion of the oculomotor nerve) synapsing with postganglionic parasympathetic neurons housed in this ganglion. The postganglionic parasympathetic fibers project via the short ciliary branches of the **trigeminal nerve** to the ipsilateral **sphincter pupillae muscle**, causing it to contract. This results in bilateral pupillary constriction, with a consequent reduction in the amount of light reaching the retina of both eyes.

Pupillary dilation reflex

Pupillary dilation occurs when sympathetic activity is dominant, such as when the individual is experiencing pain, fear, or rage

Pupillary dilation is mediated by the sympathetic division of the autonomic nervous system. Pupillary dilation occurs when sympathetic activity is dominant, such as when the individual is experiencing pain, fear, or rage.

Neurons of the posterior aspect of the **hypothalamus** project to the **ciliospinal center** of the spinal cord located in the intermediolateral cell column of cord levels (C8) T1–T2 (Fig. 16.12). Here they synapse with preganglionic sympathetic neurons. Preganglionic sympathetic fibers exit the spinal cord, enter the sympathetic trunk and ascend to the **superior cervical ganglion** where they synapse with postganglionic sympathetic neurons. Postganglionic sympathetic fibers form the internal carotid arterial perivascular plexus and follow vessel branches to the orbit where they join the long and short ciliary branches of the **trigeminal nerve** and terminate in the **dilatator pupillae muscle**. Sympathetic innervation of this muscle causes it to contract, increasing the pupillary diameter, resulting in **mydriasis** (Fig. 16.13).

Convergence accommodation reflex

The convergence accommodation reflex alters the thickness of the lens, which facilitates the projection of a focused image on the retina

As visual attention is consciously switched from a far away object to one near by, the thickness of the lens of each eye changes from a flatter to a more rounded, biconvex shape in order to be able to project a focused image on the retina. This is accomplished by an initial conscious fixation on the near object, followed by the subconscious convergence accommodation reflex, consisting of three reflex changes (Fig. 16.14).

1 **Convergence.** As attention is shifted from a far to a near object, both eyes converge simultaneously. This is mediated by bilateral contraction of the medial recti muscles, which are innervated by the **medial rectus subnucleus** of the oculomotor nerve (CN III). This convergence permits the visual image to be projected and focused on the foveae of both retinas. If this is not accomplished, the individual will experience diplopia (double vision). Unlike other reflexes, this reflex involves the cerebral cortex.

2 **Accommodation.** Parasympathetic stimulation causes contraction of the ciliary muscle of the iris thus releasing the tension it exerts on the suspensory ligaments of the lens. Since the lens is no longer being stretched, it thickens (lens **accommodation**), focusing the image on the retina.

3 **Pupillary constriction.** Pupillary constriction enhances the outline of the image formed on the retina. This is a distinct and independent process from that which occurs in the pupillary light reflex.

Visual input is transmitted from the retina to the primary visual cortex (Brodmann's area 17) via the visual pathway. The

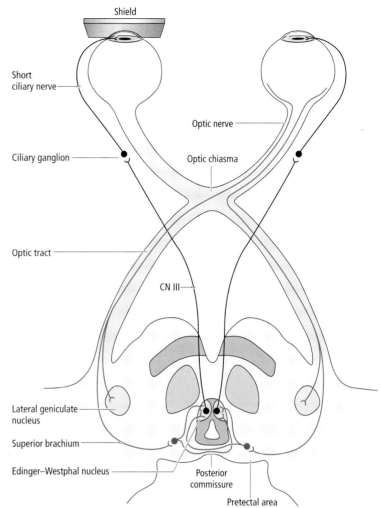

Figure 16.11 ● The pupillary light reflex pathway. When light is flashed into one eye, normally, both pupils constrict simultaneously as follows. The information is transmitted from the illuminated eye via the optic nerve and then the optic tract to the pretectal area in the midbrain. The pretectal area projects to the Edinger–Westphal nucleus bilaterally—connecting it to the parasympathetic neurons of both sides, thus initiating a bilateral pupillary response. The Edinger–Westphal nucleus contains the cell bodies of preganglionic parasympathetic neurons whose axons join the oculomotor nerve of its respective side, to terminate in the ciliary ganglion. In the ciliary ganglion, the preganglionic parasympathetic terminals synapse with the postganglionic parasympathetic neurons whose axons project via the short ciliary nerve of the trigeminal nerve to the sphincter pupillae muscle, causing the pupil to constrict.

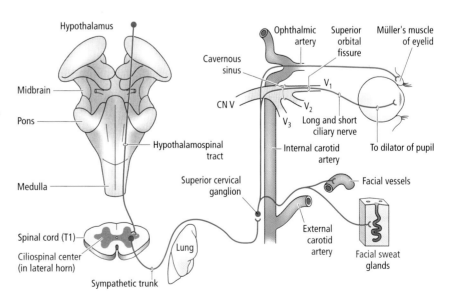

Figure 16.12 ● The pupillary dilation pathway. Axons arising from the hypothalamus form the hypothalamospinal tract, which descends ipsilaterally to terminate in the ciliospinal center of the intermediolateral cell column of the spinal cord at the T1 level. Preganglionic sympathetic neurons project their axons arising from the ciliospinal center to the superior cervical ganglion where they synapse with postganglionic sympathetic neurons. The postganglionic neurons give rise to axons that form a perivascular plexus, following vessels to the orbit where they terminate in the dilator pupillae muscle, causing pupillary dilation. (Modified from Fix, JD (1995) *Neuroanatomy*. Williams & Wilkins, Media; fig. 17.4.)

primary visual cortex transmits the information to the visual association cortex (Brodmann's area 19) where reflex activity is initiated. Fibers from this area form the **corticotectal tract** (the afferent limb of reflex), which projects bilaterally to the superior colliculus and/or the pretectal area. These areas then project to **Perlia's nucleus** of the oculomotor nuclear complex, which in turn project to the Edinger–Westphal nucleus and the medial rectus subnucleus (also of the

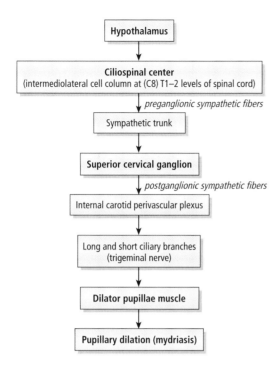

Figure 16.13 ● The pupillary dilation pathway.

oculomotor nuclear complex). Motor fibers from the medial rectus subnucleus and preganglionic parasympathetic fibers from the Edinger–Westphal nucleus join the **oculomotor nerve** (the efferent limb of reflex) to distribute to the medial rectus muscle and the ciliary ganglion, respectively. The medial recti muscles adduct the eyes (convergence). Postganglionic parasympathetic fibers arising from the ciliary ganglion join the short ciliary nerves of the ophthalmic division of the trigeminal nerve to distribute to the sphincter pupillae muscle and to the ciliary muscle. Contraction of the sphincter pupillae muscle results in pupillary constriction (miosis), whereas contraction of the ciliary muscle results in thickening of the lens (accommodation) (Fig. 16.15).

Corneal blink reflex

When a foreign object contacts the eye, the corneal blink reflex elicits a forceful blinking of both eyes to protect them from possible injury

The **corneal blink reflex** consists of (Fig. 16.16):
- **receptors** (at the peripheral terminals of pseudounipolar neurons in the ophthalmic division of the trigeminal nerve);
- an **afferent limb** (peripheral processes of pseudounipolar neurons in the ophthalmic division of the trigeminal nerve);

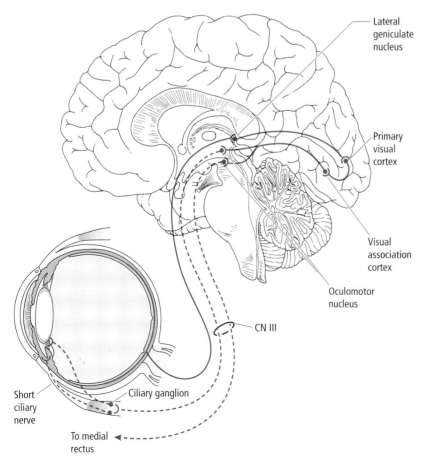

Figure 16.14 ● The convergence accommodation (near) reflex pathway. Visual input passes via the visual pathway to the visual association cortex. It is believed that the visual association cortex projects bilaterally, to the superior colliculus and/or the pretectal area, both of which in turn project to Perlia's nucleus of the oculomotor nuclear complex. Perlia's nucleus of each side projects to the Edinger–Westphal nucleus and the medial rectus subnucleus of the oculomotor nucleus. Each oculomotor nucleus stimulates the contraction of the ipsilateral medial rectus muscle, causing adduction of the eye. The Edinger–Westphal nucleus projects preganglionic parasympathetic fibers to the ciliary ganglion where they synapse with postganglionic parasympathetic neurons that innervate the sphincter pupillae (pupillary constriction) and the ciliary muscle (lens accommodation) causing the lens to thicken for near vision. Note that the accommodation reflex is as described above, and is a bilateral response.

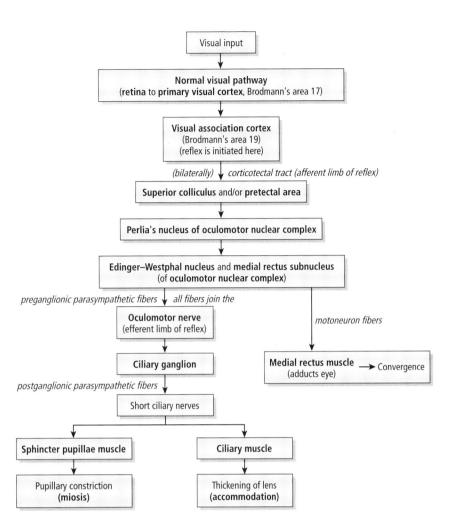

Figure 16.15 ● The convergence accommodation (near) reflex pathway.

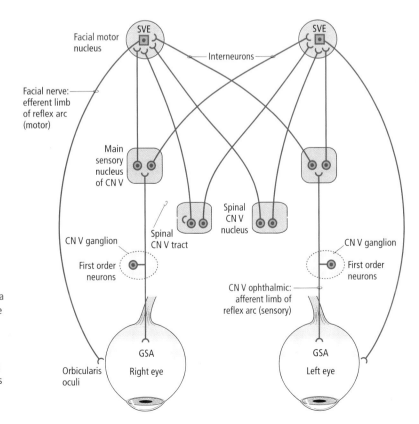

Figure 16.16 ● The corneal blink reflex. When a wisp of cotton is gently brushed against the cornea of one eye, both eyes blink. Touch sensation is transmitted from the cornea via the pseudounipolar neurons of the trigeminal ganglion to the ipsilateral spinal nucleus and main sensory nucleus of the trigeminal nerve. The spinal and main sensory nuclei of the trigeminal nerve both send bilateral projections to the facial motor nuclei where they synapse with the motoneurons that innervate the orbicularis oculi muscles, causing simultaneous blinking of both eyes. GSA, general somatic afferent; SVE, special visceral efferent.

- an **integrator** (spinal nucleus and main sensory nucleus of the trigeminal nerve);
- an **efferent limb** (facial nerve branches to the orbicularis oculi muscle); and
- an **effector** (orbicularis oculi muscle).

When a fine strand of cotton or any other foreign object is brushed against the cornea unilaterally, it evokes an immediate, forceful blinking of both eyes simultaneously. **General somatic afferent** (GSA) sensation from the cornea is transmitted by the receptors at the peripheral processes of **first order pseudounipolar** neurons whose cell bodies are housed in the **trigeminal ganglion**. These peripheral processes course in the ophthalmic division of the trigeminal nerve (afferent limb). The central processes of most of these neurons enter the pons, join the ipsilateral **spinal trigeminal tract** and descend to terminate in the rostral two-thirds of the ipsilateral **spinal trigeminal nucleus** where they synapse with **second order neurons** (interneurons). The remainder of the first order neurons terminate in the ipsilateral main sensory nucleus of the trigeminal nerve. Second order neurons from the spinal trigeminal nucleus as well as from the main sensory nucleus project bilaterally to the **motor nucleus of the facial nerve** where they synapse with motoneurons (**third order neurons**). Fibers of the motoneurons course in the **facial nerve** to terminate in and innervate the orbicularis oculi muscle, causing bilateral blinking (Fig. 16.17).

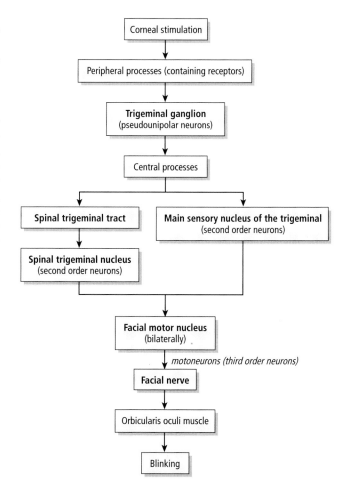

Figure 16.17 ● The corneal blink reflex.

CLINICAL CONSIDERATIONS

Visual deficits

The naming of visual deficits is based on the visual field loss and not the actual impaired or damaged region of the retina or other visual system component

The **visual field**, the region perceived by each eye, is divided by imaginary lines into quadrants (Fig. 16.18). Since light rays travel in straight lines, the temporal half of the visual field is projected onto the nasal half of the retina, whereas the nasal half of the visual field is projected onto the temporal half of the retina. The image within the visual field quadrants is reversed and inverted by the lens when it is projected on the respective retina.

The naming of visual deficits is based on the *visual field loss* and not the actual impaired or damaged region of the retina or other visual system component (Table 16.2).

Anopsia (anopia) (G., "loss of vision") refers to visual field loss. **Hemianopsia** (G. hemi, "half") is the loss of only one-half (temporal or nasal) of the visual field of one or both eyes (Fig. 16.18B). **Quadrantanopsia** (L. quadr, "one-fourth") is the loss of one-fourth (upper temporal or lower temporal; upper nasal or lower nasal) of the visual field of one or both eyes.

A deficit may be homonymous (G. homo, "same") or heteronymous (G. hetero, "different") (Fig. 16.18B). In a **homonymous** deficit, the visual field losses for the two eyes are the same. That is, there is a right or left visual field loss for both eyes. In a **heteronymous** deficit, the visual field losses for the two eyes are not alike. That is, there is a right visual field loss in one eye, and a left visual field loss in the contralateral eye, or vice versa.

A unilateral lesion of the **optic nerve** results in **permanent blindness** in the ipsilateral (corresponding) eye (A in Fig. 16.19).

Unilateral damage to the **temporal (noncrossing) fibers of the optic chiasma** results in an **ipsilateral nasal hemianopsia** (B1 in Fig. 16.19). The noncrossing fibers are often damaged by an aneurysm and/or calcification of the internal carotid artery due to its close proximity to the fibers. Bilateral damage to the **temporal fibers of the optic chiasma** results in a **binasal heteronymous hemianopsia** (B2 in Fig. 16.19).

CLINICAL CONSIDERATIONS (*continued*)

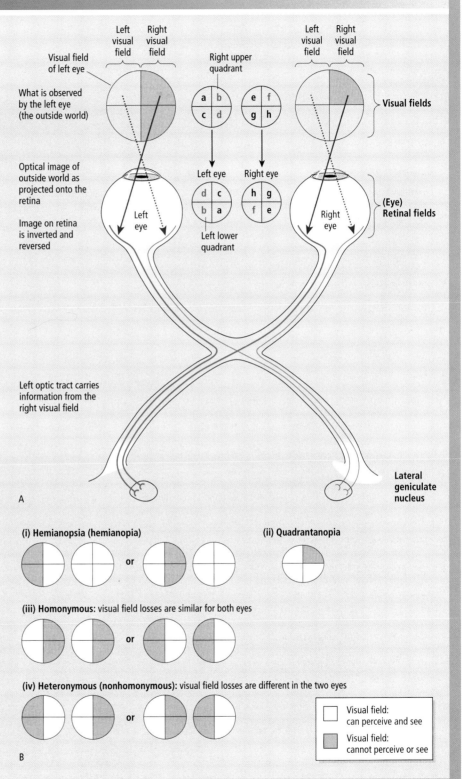

A

(i) Hemianopsia (hemianopia)   **(ii) Quadrantanopia**

(iii) Homonymous: visual field losses are similar for both eyes

(iv) Heteronymous (nonhomonymous): visual field losses are different in the two eyes

| | Visual field: can perceive and see |
| | Visual field: cannot perceive or see |

Figure 16.18 ● (A) The visual fields and their representation on the retina. (B) Visual field loss and the consequent deficits.

B

CLINICAL CONSIDERATIONS (*continued*)

Structure of visual pathway	Lesion	Deficit
Optic nerve	Unilateral	Permanent blindness in ipsilateral eye
Optic chiasma		
Temporal fibers (noncrossing fibers)	Unilateral	Ipsilateral nasal hemianopsia
	Bilateral	Binasal heteronymous hemianopsia
Nasal fibers (crossing fibers)	Bilateral	Bitemporal heteronymous hemianopsia ("tunnel vision")
Optic tract	Unilateral	Contralateral homonymous hemianopsia
Lateral geniculate nucleus	Unilateral	Contralateral homonymous hemianopsia
Lower division of optic radiations (Meyer's loop)	Unilateral	Contralateral upper homonymous quadrantanopsia
Upper division of optic radiations	Unilateral	Contralateral lower homonymous quadrantanopsia
Both upper and lower divisions of optic radiations *or* Ipsilateral primary visual cortex	Unilateral	Contralateral homonymous hemianopsia with macular sparing

Table 16.2 ● Visual deficit(s) resulting following a lesion at various locations in the visual pathway.

A lesion that damages the **crossed fibers** occupying the central region of the **optic chiasma** results in a **bitemporal heteronymous (nonhomonymous) hemianopsia ("tunnel vision")** (C in Fig. 16.19). The central fibers may be damaged due to compression by a tumor of the pituitary gland.

A unilateral lesion caudal to the optic chiasma, affecting the **optic tract** fibers or the **lateral geniculate nucleus**, results in a **contralateral homonymous hemianopsia** (D in Fig. 16.19).

A unilateral lesion affecting **Myer's loop** or the **lower division of the optic radiations**, results in a **contralateral upper homonymous quadrantanopsia** (E in Fig. 16.19). A lesion affecting the fibers of the **upper division of the geniculocalcarine tract (optic radiations)** results in a **contralateral lower homonymous quadrantanopia** (F in Fig. 16.19).

A unilateral lesion that damages the **upper and lower divisions of the geniculocalcarine tract** or produces injury to the ipsilateral **primary visual cortex (area 17)** will result in a **contralateral homonymous hemianopsia with macular sparing** (G in Fig. 16.19). Macular sparing occurs because so much cortex is devoted to the macula that often some central vision is spared.

Lesion in the afferent or efferent limb of the pupillary light reflex pathway

If one of the optic nerves (afferent limb of the pupillary light reflex arc) is damaged, and light is flashed into the eye ipsilateral to the damaged nerve, both direct and consensual pupillary responses will not be present since sensory input is not transmitted centrally. When the light is flashed into the eye on the side of the undamaged optic nerve, both the direct and the consensual pupillary responses will be elicited, if both oculomotor nerves are functional.

If the optic nerve is functional bilaterally, but there is unilateral damage to the oculomotor nerve (efferent limb of the pupillary light reflex arc), light flashed into either eye is perceived by the individual and sensory input is transmitted centrally. When light is flashed into the eye ipsilateral to the oculomotor nerve lesion there is only a consensual pupillary response. When light is flashed into the eye contralateral to the oculomotor nerve lesion, there is only a direct pupillary response. If both oculomotor nerves are damaged and parasympathetic innervation to the sphincter pupillae muscles is interrupted bilaterally, then neither eye will exhibit the direct or consensual responses.

An individual may be blind, but present a normal pupillary light reflex (see Fig. 16.11). This indicates that the site of the lesion producing the blindness involves structures caudal (posterior) to the divergence of the optic tract fibers (destined for the Edinger–Westphal nucleus and/or the pretectal area, which is associated with the pupillary reflex). The lesion may involve the LGN, or the optic radiations, or the primary visual cortex. If the individual is completely blind, a bilateral lesion of the visual cortex is more probable since an extensive, bilateral lesion of the geniculocalcarine tract is incompatible with life.

Lesion in the pupillary dilation pathway

A lesion that damages the sympathetic (preganglionic or postganglionic) fibers of this pathway, results in **Horner's syndrome** ipsilateral to the lesion. One of the characteristics of this syndrome is a persistent **miosis** (pupillary constriction) ipsilateral to the lesion due to the unopposed action of the parasympathetic nervous system. Although an individual with Horner's syndrome exhibits loss of the pupillary dilation reflex, the pupillary constriction reflex is intact, both ipsilateral and contralateral to the lesion.

Lesion in the afferent or efferent limb of the corneal blink reflex pathway

If there is a lesion in the ophthalmic nerve (afferent limb) of the corneal blink reflex arc, corneal sensation is lost on the ipsilateral side, and the corneal blink reflex is not elicited on either side upon stimulation of the cornea ipsilateral to the lesion. If the cornea ipsilateral to the intact ophthalmic nerve is stimulated, it evokes bilateral simultaneous blinking.

If the ophthalmic nerve (afferent limb) of the corneal blink reflex arc is intact bilaterally, but there is a unilateral lesion of the facial nerve (efferent limb), both corneas can sense stimulation when either one is stimulated. However, only the eye ipsilateral to the intact facial nerve will blink.

CLINICAL CONSIDERATIONS (*continued*)

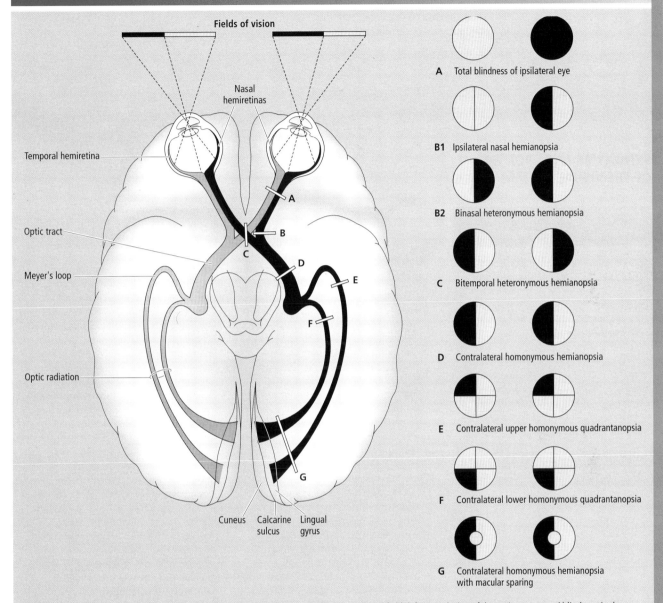

Fields of vision

Nasal hemiretinas

Temporal hemiretina

Optic tract

Meyer's loop

Optic radiation

Cuneus   Calcarine   Lingual
           sulcus   gyrus

A   Total blindness of ipsilateral eye

B1   Ipsilateral nasal hemianopsia

B2   Binasal heteronymous hemianopsia

C   Bitemporal heteronymous hemianopsia

D   Contralateral homonymous hemianopsia

E   Contralateral upper homonymous quadrantanopsia

F   Contralateral lower homonymous quadrantanopsia

G   Contralateral homonymous hemianopsia
     with macular sparing

Figure 16.19 ● Lesions at various points along the visual pathway and consequent visual field deficits: A, lesion of the optic nerve: total blindness in the ipsilateral eye; B1, unilateral lesion of the temporal (noncrossing) fibers of the optic chiasma: ipsilateral nasal hemianopsia; B2, bilateral lesion of the temporal (noncrossing) fibers of the optic chiasma: binasal heteronymous hemianopsia; C, lesion of the crossing fibers of the optic chiasma: bitemporal heteronymous hemianopsia; D, lesion of the optic tract: contralateral homonymous hemianopsia; E, lesion of Meyer's loop (lower division of the optic radiations): contralateral upper homonymous quadrantanopsia; F, lesion of the upper division of the optic radiations: contralateral lower homonymous quadrantanopsia; G, lesion of the upper and lower divisions of the optic radiations or the primary visual cortex: contralateral homonymous hemianopsia with macular sparing.

Note that the clinical case at the beginning of the chapter refers to a patient with visual loss, papilledema of the optic disc, an abnormal pupillary light reflex, and pain in the right eye.

1 What forms the optic disc?

2 At what point do the ganglion cell axons become myelinated?

SYNONYMS AND EPONYMS OF THE VISUAL SYSTEM

Name of structure or term	Synonym(s)/ eponym(s)
Geniculocalcarine tract	Optic radiations
	Thalamocortical projections
Hemianopsia	Hemianopia
Heteronymous	Nonhomonymous
Intermediolateral horn of the spinal cord	Lateral horn of the spinal cord
	Lateral column of the spinal cord
Miosis	Pupillary constriction
Mydriasis	Pupillary dilation
Primary visual cortex	Brodmann's area 17
Sphincter pupillae muscle	Constrictor pupillae muscle
Striate cortex	Band of Genari

FOLLOW-UP TO CLINICAL CASE

This patient has **optic neuritis**. This refers to inflammation of the optic nerve arising from any cause. However, it most commonly occurs in **multiple sclerosis** (MS) or another demyelinating disease. Not all patients with optic neuritis have or will ever develop MS, but most do. Therefore optic neuritis typically refers to demyelination of the optic nerves. MS affects only the central nervous system. Although almost all of the cranial nerves are components of the peripheral nervous system, the optic nerves are unusual since they are actually tracts and thus components of the central nervous system.

This case is a typical presentation of optic neuritis, i.e., visual loss affecting one eye (occasionally both) and sometimes with pain on eye movement and papilledema. Papilledema refers to swelling of the optic disc as seen on ophthalmoscopic exam. This may or may not be present, depending on the part of the optic nerve that is affected. If visual acuity is severely impaired then the pupil of the affected eye will not constrict to light properly, i.e., less than the unaffected eye. This can result in a Marcus Gunn pupil, as determined in the swinging light test. The examiner shines a penlight into each eye in succession. When the light is directed in the normal eye, both pupils constrict. When it is swung to the affected eye, the pupil paradoxically dilates (this is enhanced by the fact that it had been constricted just prior). This is referred to as an afferent pupillary defect in the affected eye.

Optic neuritis is treated by intravenous corticosteroids over 3–5 days. The majority of cases resolve completely or nearly so over the course of weeks or months. An MRI of the optic nerves may reveal the inflammation. However, an MRI is used mainly in the detection of any other brain lesion that may be indicative of MS. Visually evoked potentials can also be used to detect subclinical abnormality of the optic nerves to confirm the presence of MS in suspected cases.

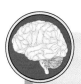

3 What component of the pupillary light reflex arc is affected by the papilledema in this patient?

QUESTIONS TO PONDER

1. What is the pathway of the light entering the eye and that of the visual electrical signals through the layers of the retina?

2. A physician was testing the pupillary light reflex of one of his patients. When he illuminated the right eye, both direct and consensual pupillary light reflexes were elicited. However, when he illuminated the left eye, neither pupil responded. Where might the lesion be?

3. A physician was testing the pupillary light reflex of one of her patients. When she illuminated the right eye, only the consensual pupillary light reflex was elicited. When she illuminated the left eye, only the direct papillary light reflex was elicited. Where might the lesion be?

4. A physician is testing the corneal blink reflex in one of her patients. When brushing a wisp of cotton across the patient's right cornea, only the right eye blinked. When she brushed the cotton across the patient's left cornea, again only the right eye blinked. Where may the lesion be?

5. Following a thorough examination of a patient's visual system, the physician concluded that the patient had a bitemporal heteronymous hemianopsia. Where in the visual pathway is the lesion? What might cause this type of visual disorder?

6. What causes Horner's syndrome?

CHAPTER 17

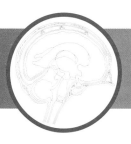
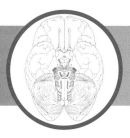
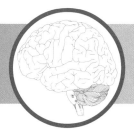

Auditory System

CLINICAL CASE

A 49-year-old woman complains of right-sided hearing loss which began a year ago. This has slowly and progressively become worse. Hearing from the left ear is normal. She first noticed this when it became difficult to hear with the phone held to her right ear. She has also noted vague and persistent imbalance and dizziness over the past couple months. There is some ringing in her right ear. The patient has no other complaints.

Examination reveals mild hearing loss and difficulty distinguishing different sounds on the right. The appearance of the external auditory canal and eardrum is normal. Gait examination reveals mild ataxia when attempting to walk in a straight line. The rest of the neurologic exam is normal.

The special sense of **hearing** is mediated by the **cochlear nerve**, the cochlear division of the vestibulocochlear nerve (CN VIII), that innervates a specialized receptor organ, the **organ of Corti** enclosed in the cochlea (G. cochlos, "snail shell"), a bony structure located in the inner ear within the petrous portion of the temporal bone (Fig. 17.1). Originally, the principal function of the inner ear was the maintenance of equilibrium (balance), but the phylogenetically older vestibular apparatus (for balance) developed a special receptor for sound perception.

EAR

The ear is divisible into three parts: the **outer ear**, the **middle ear**, and the **inner ear**, each performing a necessary function for the perception of sound (Fig. 17.1; Table 17.1).

Outer ear

The components of the outer ear facilitate the reception of sound waves by funneling them toward the tympanic membrane

The **outer ear** is comprised of the cartilaginous **auricle (pinna)** and the **external auditory meatus (canal)**, both of which serve to facilitate the reception of sound waves conducted by the air by funneling them towards the **tympanic membrane (eardrum)** located at the internal extent of the meatus. The contour of the helical-shaped auricle alters the frequency spectrum of sound depending on the position of the listener in reference to the location of the sound source. The tympanic membrane resembles a resilient trampoline that oscillates in response to incoming sound waves. Moreover, it forms a partition and seals off the external auditory meatus from the middle ear cavity.

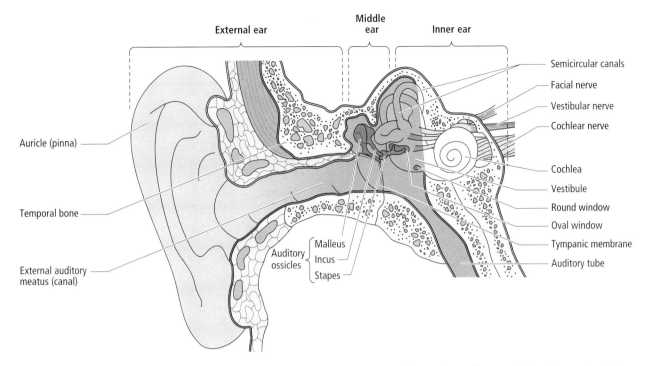

External ear | Middle ear | Inner ear

Semicircular canals
Facial nerve
Vestibular nerve
Cochlear nerve

Auricle (pinna)

Cochlea
Vestibule
Round window
Oval window
Tympanic membrane
Auditory tube

Temporal bone

Auditory ossicles {
Malleus
Incus
Stapes

External auditory meatus (canal)

Figure 17.1 ● The external, middle, and inner ear. (Modified from Canfield Willis, MC (1996) *Medical Terminology*. Williams & Wilkins, Baltimore; plate 26.)

Middle ear

The middle ear functions in the transmission and transduction of tympanic membrane vibrations to the inner ear (from an air to a fluid medium)

The **middle ear**, also referred to as the **tympanic cavity**, consists of an irregular-shaped *air-filled* chamber, embedded in the petrous portion of the temporal bone. It contains several important elements:

1 Three small articulating bones: the auditory ossicles (the **malleus**, the **incus**, and the **stapes**).
2 Two miniature skeletal muscles: the tensor tympani muscle, which attaches to the malleus, and the stapedius muscle, which attaches to the stapes.
3 Two membrane-covered foramina in the bone: the oval window and the round window.
4 Two additional openings: the Eustachian (pharyngeal, auditory) tube, which permits communication between the middle ear and nasopharynx, and the communication to the mastoid air cells.
5 The chorda tympani nerve: a branch of the facial nerve (CN VII), which passes through but has no function in the middle ear.

The middle ear functions in the *transmission* and *transduction* of tympanic membrane vibrations to the inner ear (from an air to a fluid medium) (Fig. 17.2). The **oval window** and the **round window** both serve necessary functions in these processes.

The **ossicles** are linked in series by synovial joints and are suspended within the tympanic cavity. Since they extend from the tympanic membrane to the membrane of the oval window, they conduct oscillations from the tympanic membrane to the membrane of the oval window. The intensity of these vibrations is dampened by the **tensor tympani** and the **stapedius muscles**. When the tensor tympani contracts, it tenses the tympanic membrane by pulling on the malleus, therefore reducing the vibrations transmitted from this membrane to the ossicles. When the stapedius contracts, it pulls on and stabilizes the stapes, therefore reducing the vibrations that are transmitted by the footplate of the stapes to the oval window of the membranous labyrinth of the inner ear, and eventually to the auditory receptors. By dampening vibrations, they serve a protective reflex function for the auditory apparatus.

The **Eustachian tube** (also referred to as the **pharyngeal** or **auditory tube**) serves to equalize the atmospheric pressure between the middle and outer ear. At higher elevations, the atmospheric pressure in the external auditory meatus is lower than that of the middle ear cavity and causes the tympanic membrane to curve outwards (towards the external auditory meatus) stimulating pain receptors of the tympanic membrane. Since the wall of the Eustachian tube is normally collapsed, pressure differences can be relieved by the action of swallowing, chewing, yawning, or coughing, which open the Eustachian tube, allowing equalization of pressure on the two sides of the tympanic membrane.

Part of ear	Components	Function
Outer ear	Auricle	Alters the frequency spectrum of sound
	External auditory meatus	Funnels sound waves toward the tympanic membrane
	Tympanic membrane	Separates external ear from internal ear
		Transmits sound wave vibrations to the ossicles
Middle ear	Ossicles	Amplify sound waves
	Malleus	Conduct oscillations from the tympanic membrane
	Incus	to the membrane of the oval window
	Stapes	
	Muscles	Dampen intensity of tympanic membrane vibrations
	Tensor tympani	Tenses tympanic membrane by pulling on malleus
	Stapedius	Pulls on and stabilizes the stapes
	Windows	
	Oval window	Permit the conversion of air waves into fluid waves
	Round window	of the inner ear
	Openings	
	Eustachian tube	Equalizes atmospheric pressure between middle and outer ear
	Opening to the mastoid air cells	Unknown
	Nerve	
	Chorda tympani	No function in ear, just passes by
Inner ear	Bony labyrinth	Contains perilymph
	Vestibule	Encloses the saccule and the utricle
	Semicircular canals	Enclose the semicircular ducts
	Cochlea	Encloses the cochlear duct
	scala vestibuli	Waves propagated in its perilymph agitate the vestibular membrane
	scala tympani	Its perilymph propagates waves toward the round window
	Membranous labyrinth	Contains endolymph
	Three semicircular ducts	Contains the receptors for head movement
	Saccule	Contains the receptors for head movement
	Utricle	Contains the receptors for head movement
	Endolymphatic sac	Connects the scala vestibuli and scala tympani to
	Endolymphatic duct	the subarachnoid space
	Cochlear duct	Contains endolymph and the organ of Corti (the receptor for hearing)

Table 17.1 ● Components of the outer, middle, and inner ear.

Inner ear

The inner ear encloses the cochlea, which contains the organ of Corti (the receptor for hearing), and the vestibular apparatus, which contains the receptors associated with maintenance of equilibrium

The *fluid-filled* **inner ear** is embedded in the petrous portion of the temporal bone. It consists of a **bony (osseous) labyrinth** (G., "maze") and a **membranous labyrinth** forming an interconnected system of channels and chambers that are filled with fluid. The bony labyrinth is divided into three regions: the **vestibule**, the three **semicircular canals**, and the **cochlea** (Fig. 17.3). The vestibule and the semicircular canals are associated with the maintenance of equilibrium and are discussed in Chapter 18. The membranous labyrinth fits inside and is supported by the bony labyrinth and follows its general contour.

Cochlea

The cochlea's interior is divided into three parallel, fluid-filled, compartments by two membranes, the vestibular (Reissner's) membrane and the basilar membrane

The **cochlea** is a spiral, bony shell, resembling a snail shell (Figs 17.1–17.3), which winds 2.5–2.75 turns about its osseous axis, the **modiolus**. Bubble-like hollow areas dispersed within the modiolus house groups of nerve cell bodies of the

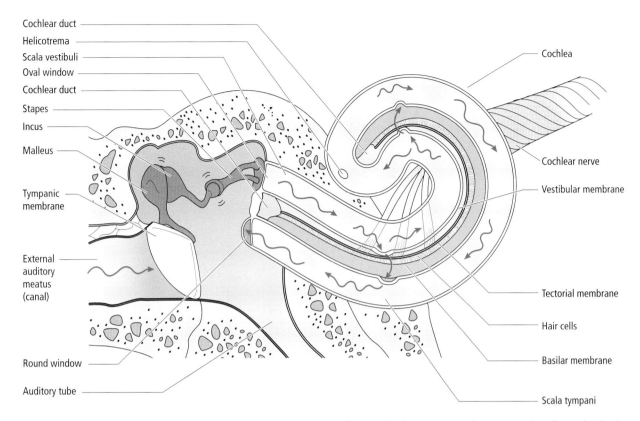

Cochlear duct
Helicotrema
Scala vestibuli
Oval window
Cochlear duct
Stapes
Incus
Malleus
Tympanic membrane
External auditory meatus (canal)
Round window
Auditory tube

Cochlea
Cochlear nerve
Vestibular membrane
Tectorial membrane
Hair cells
Basilar membrane
Scala tympani

Figure 17.2 ● The transmission of sound waves from the outer to the inner ear. Sound waves strike the tympanic membrane, causing it to vibrate. The vibrations of the tympanic membrane are transmitted to the three bones in the middle ear which in turn transmit the vibrations to the oval window. Oscillations of the oval window are then sequentially transmitted to the perilymph of the scala vestibuli and the endolymph of the cochlear duct, and then to the basilar membrane. Sound is detected by the receptor hair cells of the organ of Corti resting on the basilar membrane. Vibrations are conveyed to the perilymph in the scala tympani which cause the elastic membrane covering the round window to release pressure waves into the middle ear cavity.

bipolar sensory neurons that collectively form the **cochlear (spiral) ganglion**. The peripheral processes of these bipolar neurons terminate in the basal aspect of the hair cells of the **organ of Corti**, the cochlear receptor for hearing, whereas the central processes of these neurons form the root of the **cochlear nerve**.

The cochlea's interior is divided into three parallel, fluid-filled, compartments by two membranes, the vestibular (Reissner's) membrane and the basilar membrane. Each compartment is referred to as a scala (L., "staircase") since each spirals about the modiolus like a winding staircase. They are: the (bony) **scala vestibuli** (L., "staircase of the vestibule"); the (membranous) **scala media (cochlear duct)** (L., "staircase of the cochlear duct"), which is wedged between the vestibular and the basilar membranes (as a blind-ending duct ending at the apex of the cochlea); and the (bony) **scala tympani** (L., "stairway of the tympanic cavity") (Fig. 17.3B). The interior of the scala vestibuli and scala tympani is lined by a simple squamous epithelium.

The perilymph-filled, bony, scala vestibuli of the cochlea is in direct communication with the perilymph-filled, bony, vestibule of the vestibular apparatus. The scala vestibuli and scala tympani, both of which are filled with perilymph, are joined at the **helicotrema** (G. helicon, "helix;" trema, "hole"), a small connecting aperture located at the apex of the cochlea,

which permits perilymph from the scala vestibuli to flow into the scala tympani. These canals are connected to the subarachnoid space via the endolymphatic duct, and the perilymph flows into the subarachnoid space thus contributing to the cerebrospinal fluid. It should also be noted that the scala vestibuli communicates with the **oval window** and the scala tympani communicates with the **round window**.

The cochlear duct, also referred to as the scala media, contains endolymph. On cross-section of the cochlea, the triangular-shaped cochlear duct is wedged between the scala vestibuli and the scala tympani with its apex attached to the spiral lamina of the modiolus. The **vestibular (Reissner's) membrane**, the roof of the cochlear duct, serves as a division between the cochlear duct and the scala vestibuli. This membrane consists of squamous epithelium. Its function is unclear; however it is believed to play a role in the transmission of vibrations from the perilymph of the scala vestibuli to the endolymph of the cochlear duct. The floor of the cochlear duct, which separates it from the scala tympani, is the **basilar membrane**. The basilar membrane is an elastic structure exhibiting a gradual increase in width, and a decrease in stiffness from the oval window (at the cochlear base) to the helicotrema (at the cochlear apex). The gradual decrease in stiffness permits this membrane to be sensitive to *high frequency* vibrations near the **cochlear base**, and *low frequency*

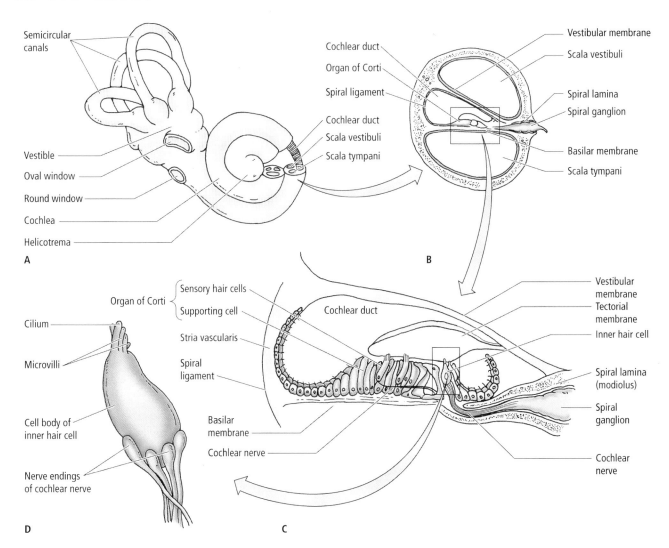

Figure 17.3 ● Components of the inner ear. (A) The vestibulocochlear apparatus. (B) Cross-section through the three scalae of the cochlea: the scala vestibuli, scala media (cochlear duct), and scala tympani. (C) The organ of Corti resting on the basilar membrane. (D) A sensory hair cell.

vibrations near its **apex**, at the helicotrema. Thus, the vestibular membrane is interposed between the scala vestibuli and the cochlear duct, whereas the basilar membrane is interposed between the cochlear duct and the scala tympani. The inner surface of the bony labyrinth bordering the scala media is the stria vascularis, which produces endolymph.

The receptors associated with the sense of hearing form a structure, the (spiral) organ of Corti, which rests like a carpet along the floor of the cochlear duct on the basilar membrane. The organ of Corti consists of **supporting epithelial cells** and neuroepithelial receptor "**hair cells**." Each hair cell displays numerous **stereocilia** (long microvilli) and a single **kinocilium** projecting from its apical cell surface. The free ends of the stereocilia project into the **tectorial membrane**, an acellular, gelatinous substance, joined to the **osseous spiral lamina** (a bony shelf protruding from the modiolus). The hair cells are the receptors of the auditory system that act as transducers, that is, they serve to convert mechanical energy into electrical energy that can be relayed to the brainstem. Hair cells synapse with the peripheral ends (dendritic processes)

of the bipolar neurons whose cell bodies are housed in the spiral ganglion. The central processes of these bipolar neurons form the cochlear nerve, which joins the vestibular nerve to form the vestibulocochlear nerve (CN VIII). This nerve courses through the internal acoustic meatus to enter the cranial vault, and then enters the brainstem at the pontomedullary angle.

AUDITORY TRANSMISSION

As sound wave vibrations are transmitted from the tympanic membrane to the oval window membrane, they are amplified approximately 20-fold

The **auricle** and **external auditory meatus** channel sound waves to the **tympanic membrane**, which cause it to vibrate (see Fig. 17.2). Oscillations of the tympanic membrane cause the three **ossicles** to vibrate in sequence, conducting the vibration to the **oval window**. The articulating ossicles form a lever system, and not only mediate vibrations from the tympanic membrane to the membrane

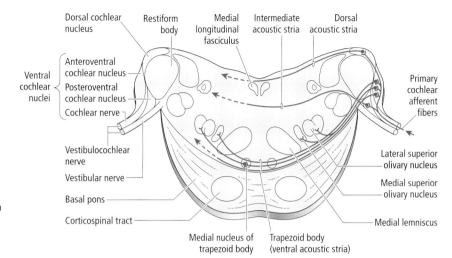

Figure 17.4 ● The main efferent projections from the cochlear nuclei. (Modified from Burt, AM (1993) *Textbook of Neuroanatomy*. WB Saunders, Philadelphia; fig. 12.15.)

of the oval window, but—a fact of paramount importance—*amplify* these vibrations as they are converted from **air waves** of the outer ear into **fluid waves** (perilymph) of the inner ear. Since liquids are more resistant to the conduction of sound waves, the incoming sound waves hitting the tympanic membrane have to be amplified by the ossicles in order to ensure adequate vibration of the perilymph. Since the tympanic membrane is much larger than the oval window membrane, and the sound waves reaching the oval window membrane are amplified by the ossicles, the compound effect is that the vibrations reaching the oval window have been amplified approximately 20-fold from the original vibrations at the tympanic membrane. The rapid oscillations of the **stapes** footplate cause the membrane covering the oval window to vibrate, which in turn agitates the perilymph fluid of the vestibule, causing fluid displacement and the formation of pressure waves. The pressure waves are propagated from the base of the cochlea, through the scala vestibuli, along the helical path to the apex of the cochlea. Although perilymph waves in the **scala vestibuli** also flow via the **helicotrema** to the **scala tympani**, the effect of these waves is probably minor and causes little stimulation of the organ of Corti.

Perilymph waves in the scala vestibuli agitate the **vestibular membrane**, which begins to oscillate. The oscillating vestibular membrane generates waves in the endolymph of the **cochlear duct**, which in turn causes the **basilar membrane** to oscillate. Basilar membrane oscillations are initiated at the base of the cochlea and advance along the basilar membrane as a traveling wave towards the apex of the cochlea. Wave formation in the scala vestibuli and scala tympani is possible only because of the flexibility of the elastic membrane covering the **round window**, which vibrates and allows pressure formed by the waves to be released into the middle ear cavity, as the round window membrane protrudes towards it. Without the round window to compensate for the pressure exerted on the oval window, waves could not be propagated in the scala tympani since fluid completely enclosed in a bony compartment is resistant to compression.

The bases of the hair receptor cells rest on the basilar membrane, whereas the tips of their cilia and stereocilia extend into the overlying tectorial membrane. It is the basilar membrane oscillations that cause a shearing force and deformation of the hair cells' cilia and stereocilia, which are inserted (fixed) in the less mobile overlying tectorial membrane (Fig. 17.3C). This deformation causes depolarization of the cell membrane, and stimulation of the hair cells is transmitted to the dendritic processes of the bipolar sensory neurons. Sensory stimulation is then relayed by the cochlear nerve to the cochlear nuclei in the brainstem (Fig. 17.4).

The pathway of auditory stimulation is summarized in Fig. 17.5.

CENTRAL AUDITORY PATHWAYS

The auditory pathway relays sensory input by projecting bilaterally in the brain, that is, auditory input from each ear ultimately flows to both cerebral hemispheres

Auditory input travels in the **auditory pathway**, which begins with the **first order neurons** housed in the **spiral (cochlear) ganglion** and continues as a chain of multisynaptic relays into the medulla, pons, mesencephalon, diencephalon (thalamus), and finally the cerebral cortex. Due to the complexity of the auditory pathways, only the main pathways are discussed here. The auditory pathway transmits sensory input related to *frequency* (pitch), *amplitude* (loudness), and *location* of the sound.

The auditory pathway relays sensory input by projecting bilaterally in the brain; that is, auditory input from each ear (similar to visual input from each eye) ultimately flows to both cerebral hemispheres. The only site of unilateral (ipsilateral) projection in the auditory pathway is the first relay, since each cochlear nerve projects to its ipsilateral cochlear nuclei. All subsequent relays of the auditory pathway are bilateral.

The spiral (cochlear) ganglion is unusual since its nerve cell bodies are not aggregated into a single ganglion. Instead, the cell bodies form numerous swellings that are embedded

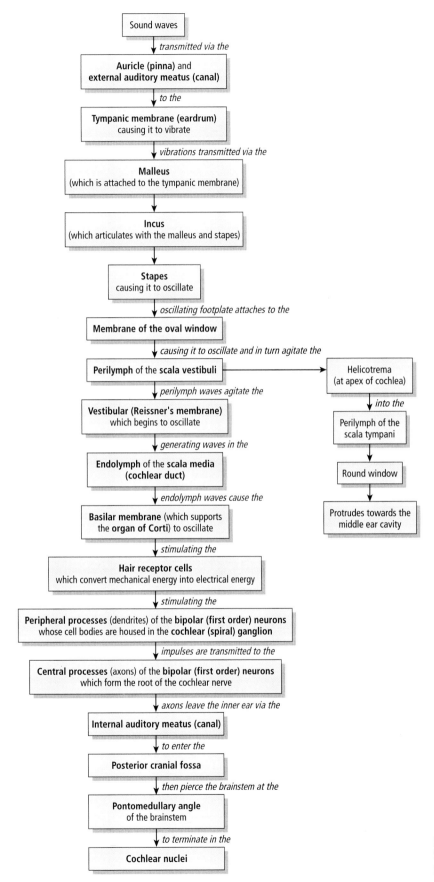

Figure 17.5 ● The pathway of auditory stimulation from the external auditory meatus to the cochlear nuclei in the brainstem.

in hollow bubbles within the modiolus of the cochlea. The dendritic terminals of the peripheral processes of these neurons terminate in the organ of Corti and synapse with its specialized "hair cell" receptors. The central processes of these neurons collect to form the **cochlear nerve** (the cochlear division of the vestibulocochlear nerve, CN VIII). In the inner ear, the cochlear nerve joins the vestibular nerve to form the vestibulocochlear nerve. From the inner ear, the vestibulo-cochlear nerve then passes through the internal acoustic meatus to enter the posterior cranial fossa of the cranial vault. As it enters the brainstem at the pontomedullary angle, the vestibulocochlear nerve again separates into its two components, the vestibular nerve and the cochlear nerve. The vestibular nerve terminates in the vestibular nuclei, whereas the cochlear nerve terminates in the **cochlear nuclei**. The vestibular and cochlear nuclei extend into the pons and the medulla. The central processes of the first order neurons of the cochlear nerve enter the ventral cochlear nucleus where they bifurcate, some branches terminating in the dorsal cochlear nucleus, with others terminating in the ventral cochlear nucleus. Thus, the **ventral cochlear nucleus** as well as the (smaller) **dorsal cochlear nucleus** are the first relay stations of auditory input. The ventral cochlear nucleus is subdivided into a posteroventral cochlear nucleus and an anteroventral cochlear nucleus. The **anteroventral cochlear nucleus** is the major nucleus of termination of cochlear nerve fibers.

Second order fibers arising from the cochlear nuclei either ascend ipsilaterally from the anteroventral cochlear nucleus to the medial and lateral superior olivary nuclei, or decussate forming three different separate pathways: the **dorsal, inter-mediate**, and **ventral acoustic striae** (see Fig. 17.4). Most of the decussating fibers arising from the anteroventral cochlear nucleus form a very noticeable group of fibers, the **trapezoid body**, also known as the ventral acoustic striae in the ventral pontine tegmentum. The fibers in the trapezoid body project to and terminate *contralaterally* either in:

- the **medial nucleus of the trapezoid body**, which in turn projects to the **lateral superior olivary nucleus**;
- the **medial superior olivary nucleus**; or
- the **dorsal nucleus of the lateral lemniscus** and the **inferior colliculus** (by ascending in the contralateral lateral lemniscus) (Fig. 17.6).

Second order fibers arising from the **posteroventral cochlear nucleus** form the intermediate acoustic stria ventral to the medial longitudinal fasciculus. These fibers subsequently join the ipsilateral and contralateral lateral lemniscus to ascend to, and terminate in, the ventral nucleus of the lateral lemniscus and the inferior colliculus, bilaterally (Fig. 17.7).

Second order fibers arising from the dorsal cochlear nucleus form the dorsal acoustic stria, which decussates on the ventral aspect of the floor of the fourth ventricle. These fibers join the contralateral lateral lemniscus to ascend to, and terminate in, the inferior colliculus.

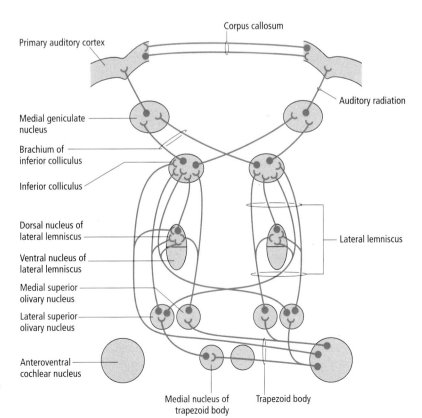

Figure 17.6 ● The principal ascending auditory pathways emerging from the anteroventral cochlear nucleus. (Modified from Burt, AM (1993) *Textbook of Neuroanatomy.* WB Saunders, Philadelphia; fig. 12.16.)

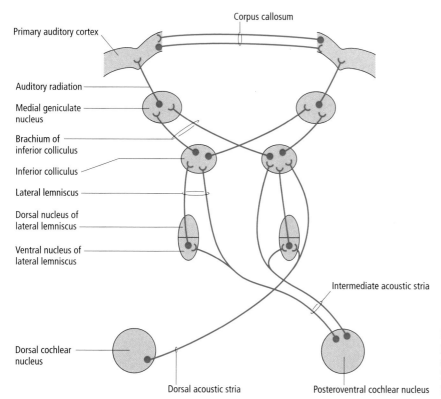

Corpus callosum

Primary auditory cortex

Auditory radiation

Medial geniculate
nucleus

Brachium of
inferior colliculus

Inferior colliculus

Lateral lemniscus

Dorsal nucleus of
lateral lemniscus

Ventral nucleus of
lateral lemniscus

Intermediate acoustic stria

Dorsal cochlear
nucleus

Dorsal acoustic stria

Posteroventral cochlear nucleus

Figure 17.7 ● The principal ascending auditory pathways emerging from the posteroventral and dorsal cochlear nuclei. (Modified from Burt, AM (1993) *Textbook of Neuroanatomy*. WB Saunders, Philadelphia; fig. 12.17.)

Superior olivary nuclei (nuclear complex)

The superior olivary nuclei process auditory information from both ears and determine the direction that a sound is coming from and its intensity

The **superior olivary nuclei** form a nuclear complex housing **third order neurons**, located in the pontine tegmentum at the level of the facial nucleus. The main nuclei of this complex are the **medial superior olivary nucleus** and the **lateral superior olivary nucleus**, both of which receive second order fiber terminals from the cochlear nuclei (as discussed above), and have an important function in *sound localization*. The superior olivary nuclei process auditory information from both ears, and determine the direction and location that a sound is coming from in the following manner. The medial superior olivary nucleus processes auditory input by comparing the amount of *time* it takes for a sound to reach each ear, whereas the lateral superior olivary nucleus processes auditory input by comparing the *intensity* (volume) of a sound arriving at each ear. Thus a sound arising from a source, such as a telephone located to one's right, arrives at the right ear sooner than it does in the left ear, and the sound is slightly louder in the right ear than it is in the left ear. If a sound arises from a source that is located at an equal distance from both ears, then the sound arrives at both ears at the same time. The neurons in the lateral superior olivary nucleus are stimulated by impulses transmitted by second order fibers arising from the ipsilateral anteroventral cochlear nucleus and are inhibited by impulses transmitted by second order fibers arising from the contralateral anteroventral cochlear nucleus.

Lateral lemniscus

The lateral lemniscus is the main ascending pathway of the auditory system in the brainstem, conveying auditory input from both ears

The lateral lemniscus is the main ascending pathway of the auditory system in the brainstem, conveying auditory input from both ears. In summary, the lateral lemniscus (L., "ribbon") contains the following.

1 Second order fibers arising from the contralateral anteroventral cochlear nucleus (which do not synapse in the superior olivary complex) that terminate in the dorsal nucleus of the lateral lemniscus and the inferior colliculus.
2 Second order fibers arising from the ipsilateral and contralateral posteroventral cochlear nucleus that terminate in the ventral nucleus of the lateral lemniscus and in the inferior colliculus.
3 Second order fibers arising from the contralateral dorsal cochlear nucleus that terminate in the ventral nucleus of the lateral lemniscus and in the inferior colliculus.
4 Third order fibers originating from the superior olivary nuclear complex (the fibers arising from the medial superior olivary nucleus join the ipsilateral lateral lemniscus, whereas those that arise from the lateral superior olivary nucleus join the ipsilateral and contralateral lateral lemniscus) that terminate in the dorsal nucleus of the lateral lemniscus and in the superior colliculus.
5 Fibers arising from the dorsal and ventral nuclei of the lateral lemniscus that project to the ipsilateral inferior colliculus.

Nuclei of the lateral lemniscus

The diffuse ventral and dorsal nuclei of the lateral lemniscus are located within the substance of the lateral lemniscus

The **ventral nucleus of the lateral lemniscus** contains neurons that process auditory input from only *one ear*, whereas the **dorsal nucleus of the lateral lemniscus** houses neurons that process auditory input from *both ears*.

Inferior colliculus

The inferior colliculus is associated with sound localization

The **inferior colliculus** (L., "little hill"), located in the roof of the caudal midbrain, is a mesencephalic relay nucleus of the auditory system. It receives afferents ascending in the lateral lemniscus from the cochlear nuclei, the superior olivary nuclear complex, and the nuclei of the lateral lemniscus. The inferior colliculus also receives afferents from the contralateral inferior colliculus and the auditory cortex.

The inferior colliculus gives rise to a prominent bundle, the **brachium of the inferior colliculus** (L. brachium, "arm"), an arm-like structure whose fibers end in the ipsilateral **medial geniculate nucleus**, a thalamic relay station of the auditory system. The inferior colliculus also projects to the contralateral medial geniculate nucleus and the superior colliculus (which is involved in visual reflexes) to mediate audiovisual reflex activity such as turning the head and eyes in the direction of a startling noise. The inferior colliculus is associated with sound localization.

Medial geniculate nucleus

The medial geniculate nucleus processes auditory input related to sound intensity (loudness) and frequency (pitch), and transmits it to the auditory cortex

Fibers arising in the **medial geniculate nucleus** form the **auditory radiations** that join the sublenticular portion of the posterior limb of the internal capsule to terminate in the primary auditory cortex. The medial geniculate nucleus processes auditory input related to *sound intensity* (loudness) and *frequency* (pitch), and transmits it to the auditory cortex.

Auditory cortex

The primary auditory cortex corresponding to Brodmann's areas 41 and 42 is located deep in the lateral fissure of Sylvius, in the transverse temporal gyri of Heschl

The **primary auditory cortex** receives the auditory radiations from the lateral geniculate nucleus. This cortical region has a tonotopic representation of frequencies; that is, neurons responding to low frequencies reside in its rostral extent, whereas neurons responding to high frequencies reside in its caudal extent. The primary auditory cortex is arranged into two-dimensional, alternating, vertically oriented columns of neurons (Fig. 17.8). One dimension of the auditory cortex is composed of **frequency columns**. The cells in each frequency column respond to an auditory stimulus of a particular frequency. As mentioned above, cells responding to low frequencies reside in the frequency columns located in

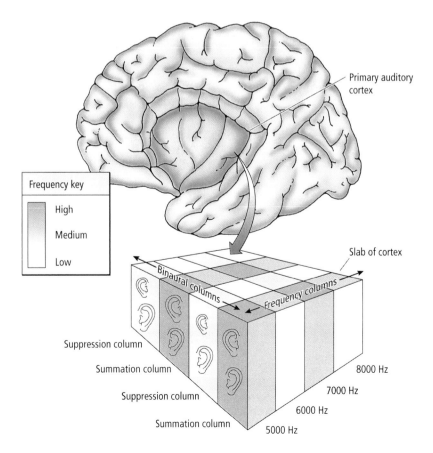

Figure 17.8 ● Lateral view of the cerebral hemisphere showing the location of the primary auditory cortex and an illustration of its organization. (Modified from Matthews, G (2001) *Neurobiology*. Blackwell Publishing, Oxford; fig. 17.14.)

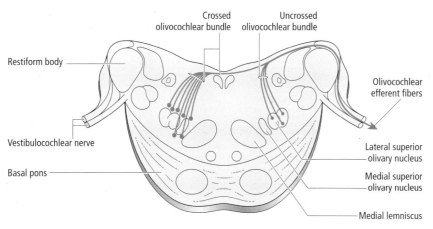

Figure 17.9 ● The olivocochlear pathway arises from the superior olivary nuclei and terminates in the organ of Corti where it inhibits the transmission of auditory information to higher brain centers. (Modified from Burt, AM (1993) *Textbook of Neuroanatomy.* WB Saunders, Philadelphia; fig. 12.18.)

the rostral extent of the transverse temporal gyri of Heschl, whereas frequency columns containing cells responding to gradually higher frequencies are lined up in sequence toward the caudal extent of the primary auditory cortex. The other dimension of the auditory cortex is composed of alternating **binaural columns**. There are two types of binaural columns: summation columns and suppression columns. The neurons residing in the **summation columns** respond to an auditory stimulus that stimulates both ears simultaneously. In contrast, the neurons in the **suppression columns** respond maximally to an auditory stimulus that stimulates only one ear, but respond minimally when the auditory stimulus stimulates both ears.

The primary auditory cortex of each side sends projections to the contralateral side via the corpus callosum. The **primary auditory cortex** plays an important function in the detection of alteration in pattern as well as the localization of a sound.

The **secondary auditory cortical areas**, although numerous, are not well defined. They border the primary auditory cortex and form reciprocal connections with the primary auditory cortex. The secondary auditory cortical areas play an important function in the interpretation of sounds, and via connections with Wernicke's area function in the comprehension of language.

Descending auditory projections

The olivocochlear bundle has an inhibitory effect on cochlear nerve activity, modulating and sharpening auditory transmission

The **superior olivary nucleus**, one of the nuclei of the olivary nuclear complex, gives rise to the **olivo-** **cochlear bundle** (an efferent pathway) whose fibers descend both ipsilaterally and contralaterally to terminate in the spiral organ of Corti, where they synapse with receptor hair cells (Fig. 17.9). This tract has an inhibitory effect on cochlear nerve activity, modulating and sharpening auditory transmission. Thus the cochlea is innervated by the peripheral (afferent) processes of the first order bipolar neurons of the cochlear nerve, as well as the olivocochlear (efferent) fibers arising from the brainstem.

Sound attenuation reflex

A loud noise heard in one ear causes a reflex contraction of both the tensor tympani and stapedius muscles of both ears

A loud noise heard in one ear causes a reflex contraction of both the tensor tympani and the stapedius muscles of both ears, and therefore dampen, bilaterally, the transmission of excessively loud and/or startling sound wave signals from the outer to the inner ear. The sound waves entering one ear follow the normal auditory pathway via the **cochlear nerve** to the ipsilateral **ventral cochlear nucleus**. Each ventral cochlear nucleus projects bilaterally to the **superior olivary nuclei**. They in turn project bilaterally to the **facial motor nuclei** and the **motor nuclei of the trigeminal nerve**. Each facial motor nucleus projects to the ipsilateral stapedius muscle. Each motor nucleus of the trigeminal nerve projects to the ipsilateral tensor tympani muscle (Fig. 17.10).

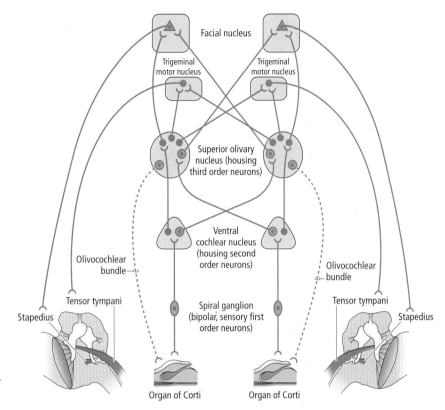

Figure 17.10 ● The sound attenuation reflex. Auditory information is transmitted from the organ of Corti via the central processes of bipolar sensory neurons to the ipsilateral ventral cochlear nucleus. Subsequent connections are bilateral. Information is then transmitted sequentially to the superior olivary nucleus which in turn projects to the trigeminal motor and facial motor nuclei. The trigeminal motor nucleus projects to the tensor tympani and the facial motor nucleus projects to the stapedius muscle, causing their contraction and dampening of auditory input.

CLINICAL CONSIDERATIONS

Hearing defects can result from many causes. A unilateral lesion in the facial nerve (CN VII) proximal to giving rise to the branch to the stapedius muscle results in **hyperacusis**, characterized by abnormally acute hearing in the affected ear. This condition often occurs in individuals with Bell's palsy.

Hearing defects may be categorized into conduction deafness and sensorineural (nerve or perceptive) deafness.

Conduction deafness usually involves the auditory apparatus of the outer and/or middle ear and is caused by a defect in the *mechanical transmission* of sound from the air-filled outer and/or middle ear to the fluid-filled inner ear, which interferes with sound conduction. Conduction deafness may result from:

1 **Cerumen** (wax) **buildup** in the external auditory canal.
2 **Perforation of the tympanic membrane**.
3 **Otitis media**, which is a middle ear inflammation and is accompanied by fluid accumulation in the middle ear chamber (which if not treated may progress to meningitis or brain abscesses).
4 **Otosclerosis** (G. oto, "ear;" sklerosis, "hardening"), which is the most common pathologic condition resulting in conduction deafness in adults. It is a consequence of new bone deposition of the labyrinthine spongy bone bordering the oval window with subsequent fixation of the stapes on the oval window. Otosclerosis can be surgically corrected by releasing the stapes. A hearing aid often improves conduction deafness.

Sensorineural (nerve) deafness results following a lesion involving the cochlea, the cochlear nerve, or the central auditory pathways. A lesion involving the cochlea, the cochlear nerve, or the cochlear nuclei results in an ipsilateral hearing deficit. Injury to the hair receptor cells may be caused from extensive exposure to loud noise, antibiotics, or other drugs such as aspirin, or various prenatal infections, such as rubella, cytomegalovirus, or syphilis.

The most prevalent sensorineural hearing deficit occurring in the elderly is **presbycusis** (G. presbus, "old man;" cusis, "hearing"). This condition results from the gradual degeneration of the spiral organ of Corti.

Acoustic neuroma (schwannoma or neurilemoma) is a tumor arising from the Schwann cells covering the vestibulocochlear nerve (CN VIII). This tumor appears in the internal auditory meatus, or close to the cerebellopontine angle after the nerve leaves the brainstem in the posterior cranial fossa. This tumor causes nerve destruction resulting in **total loss of hearing (deafness)** in the ipsilateral ear and **tinnitus** ("ringing" sensation in the ear) and/or vestibular symptoms.

Lesions involving the central auditory pathways (anywhere rostral to the cochlear nuclei) result in **minor hearing impairments** mainly in the **contralateral** side. This is due to the bilateral projections of the auditory pathway. The individual will have difficulty in localizing sounds in the contralateral side if the lesion involves the ascending auditory pathways rostral to the level of the pons, or if the primary or secondary auditory cortex is involved.

Recent studies support that genetic mutations are the underlying cause of some cases (< 1%) of congenital bilateral deafness. The **Jervell–Lange-Nielsen syndrome** is a recessively inherited genetic disorder associated with bilateral deafness. This syndrome results from the formation of defective ion channel complexes in the stria vascularis lining the lateral wall of the cochlear duct (scala media). The cells of the stria vascularis regulate the ionic composition of endolymph in the cochlear duct, which is an important component in the formation of nerve impulses in the auditory system.

Note that the clinical case at the beginning of the chapter refers to a patient whose symptoms include hearing loss and ringing in the right ear, imbalance, dizziness, and ataxia.

1 What can cause hearing loss?

SYNONYMS AND EPONYMS OF THE AUDITORY SYSTEM

Name of structure or term	Synonym(s)/ eponym(s)
Auricle	Pinna
Bony labyrinth	Osseous labyrinth
Cochlear ganglion	Spiral ganglion
Eustachian tube	Auditory tube
	Pharyngeal tube
External auditory meatus	External auditory canal
Internal auditory meatus	Internal acoustic canal
Lateral fissure	Lateral fissure of Sylvius
Mesencephalon	Midbrain
Primary auditory cortex	Transverse temporal gyri of Heschl
	Brodmann's areas 41 and 42
Scala media	Cochlear duct
Sensorineural deafness	Nerve deafness
	Perceptive deafness
Spiral organ of Corti	Organ of Corti
Superior olivary nuclei	Superior olivary nuclear complex
Trapezoid body	Ventral acoustic striae
Tympanic membrane	Eardrum
Vestibular membrane	Reissner's membrane

FOLLOW-UP TO CLINICAL CASE

Hearing defects may result from conduction deafness or sensorineural deafness. Conduction deafness usually involves the auditory apparatus of the outer and/or middle ear and is caused by a defect in the mechanical transmission of sound from the air-filled outer and/or middle ear to the fluid-filled inner ear, which interferes with sound conduction. Sensorineural (nerve) deafness results following a lesion involving the cochlea, the cochlear nerve, or the central auditory pathways.

This case requires further testing since clinical evaluation alone will not determine the cause of deafness. The other noted symptoms are vague or nonspecific, although the dizziness and imbalance could possibly indicate vestibular or cerebellar dysfunction. This patient should have a full examination by an otolaryngologist and imaging of the base of the skull, mastoid, inner ear, and auditory canals. MRI is best but CT may be adequate. This patient's MRI (with contrast) showed an **acoustic neuroma** of the right eighth cranial nerve, more properly known as a **schwannoma**.

An acoustic neuroma is a fairly common, benign tumor of Schwann cells (which provide myelin for all peripheral nerves, including cranial nerves). Schwannomas commonly arise from cranial nerve VIII although they can affect any nerve, particularly the cranial nerves. Acoustic neuromas are bulbous or fusiform tumors that are seen in the cerebellopontine angle. The most common and initial symptom of an acoustic neuroma is typically unilateral hearing loss. Dizziness (even occasionally vertigo) and ataxia can arise from dysfunction of the vestibular portion of cranial nerve VIII or from cerebellar dysfunction secondary to compression. Other symptoms, such as facial numbness or weakness, can arise from compression of the corresponding cranial nerves.

Acoustic neuromas are unilateral, with one notable exception. Neurofibromatosis type II leads to multiple tumors, including bilateral acoustic neuromas. A cerebellopontine angle meningioma can be confused with an acoustic neuroma. The mainstay of treatment is surgical excision. Hearing can only sometimes be restored.

2 The patient's MRI showed that she has an acoustic neuroma on the right side. How does this tumor cause the patient's symptoms of hearing loss, imbalance, dizziness, and ataxia?

3 What other cranial nerve emerges from the brainstem near cranial nerve VIII that may also be compressed by an acoustic neuroma and cause symptoms?

QUESTIONS TO PONDER

1. What is the function of the middle ear?

2. What is the function of the Eustachian (pharyngeal, auditory) tube?

3. What is the tonotopic organization of the basilar membrane?

4. What structures are involved in the transduction of the sound waves from the outer ear to the inner ear?

5. What is the function of the olivocochlear bundle?

6. Which cranial nerves are involved in the auditory attenuation reflex?

CHAPTER 18

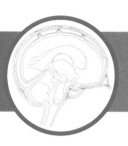
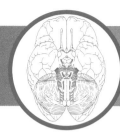
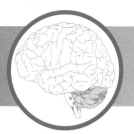

Vestibular System

CLINICAL CASE

A 65-year-old woman presents to the office with 2 weeks of dizziness. She described the dizziness as a whirling sensation that made her feel as though her head was spinning. Each spell lasts for about 10–20 seconds. She has several spells per day, and notes that turning in bed and looking upward exacerbates this condition. Since these spells are so incapacitating, she is afraid to move. She feels normal in between these spells. She does not have any ringing in the ears, or visual, hearing, or speech problems. Walking and balance are normal, except during the dizzy spells. There has not been any trauma, history of similar dizziness, or recent infection.

Kinesthesis (G. kinein, "to move;" esthesis, "sensation") is mediated by a somatosensory system that makes us aware of the relative position and motion of our various body parts with respect to one another, and to objects in our environment that we may come in contact with. The position and motion of different body parts are detected and monitored by special receptors located in the muscles, tendons, and joints. Our kinesthetic sense assists us in the maintenance of our posture and the control of a myriad of voluntary motor activities.

Working with our kinesthetic sense is the sense of equilibrium (balance), mediated by the **vestibular system**. The vestibular system, a proprioceptive (somatosensory) system, mediates the special functions of posture maintenance, muscle tone, equilibrium, and coordination of head and eye movements. Also, it transmits sensory information to the brain regarding the position of the body and spatial orientation.

The vestibular system is equipped with two groups of receptors. One group detects *angular acceleration* (rotational movement) of the head, as in turning the head from side to side. The other group of receptors detects *spatial orientation* of the head in space, relative to gravity and linear acceleration or deceleration forces.

Sensory input from the visual, vestibular, and proprioceptive systems is integrated by the nervous system, especially the cerebellum, to generate motor responses that maintain equilibrium, posture, muscle tone, and reflex movements of the eyes, all of which are carried out at the subconscious level.

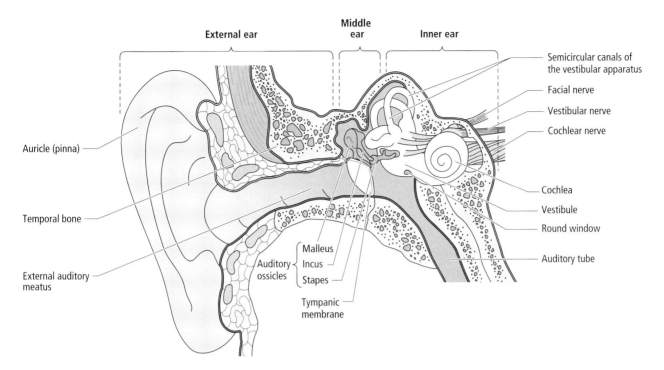

Middle
ear

External ear

Inner ear

Semicircular canals of
the vestibular apparatus

Facial nerve

Vestibular nerve

Cochlear nerve

Auricle (pinna)

Cochlea

Vestibule

Round window

Temporal bone

Auditory tube

External auditory
meatus

Malleus
Auditory
ossicles   Incus

Stapes

Tympanic
membrane

Figure 18.1 ● The external, middle, and inner ear. (Modified from Canfield Willis, MC (1996) *Medical Terminology*. Williams & Wilkins, Baltimore; plate 26.)

VESTIBULAR APPARATUS

The sensory apparatus of the vestibular system resides in the inner ear, housed in the petrous portion of the temporal bone and is composed of a bony (osseous) labyrinth and a membranous labyrinth

The sensory apparatus of the vestibular system resides in the inner ear, housed in the petrous portion of the temporal bone and is composed of a bony (osseous) labyrinth (G., "maze") and a membranous labyrinth. Sensory information about the orientation and motion of the **head** (not the body), is detected by the receptors in the **vestibular (sensory) apparatus** (Figs 18.1, 18.2) and is relayed to the **vestibular nuclei** in the brainstem and the **cerebellum** by the **vestibular nerve** (the vestibular division of the vestibulocochlear nerve, CN VIII). The vestibular system, in concert with the cerebellum, then mediates appropriate postural adjustments.

Bony (osseous) labyrinth associated with equilibrium

The components of the bony labyrinth associated with equilibrium include the three semicircular canals and the vestibule

The **bony labyrinth** of the inner ear (Fig. 18.2) includes the **cochlea**, three bony **semicircular canals**, and the **vestibule**. The cochlea is a special receptor that mediates hearing and has no function in equilibrium (and is discussed in Chapter 17). The semicircular canals and the vestibule, however, are associated with equilibrium.

Semicircular canals

There are three **semicircular canals** in the inner ear. They are the anterior (superior), lateral (horizontal), and posterior (inferior) canals. The semicircular canals are oriented along three planes of angular or rotational movement, at nearly right angles to each other. Both ends of the C-shaped canals attach to and open into the bony vestibule (Fig. 18.2). The **anterior canal** (a vertically oriented semicircular canal) of each side, is positioned *anterolateral* to the median plane (about 45° from the coronal plane). It is oriented parallel to the **posterior canal** (also a vertically oriented semicircular canal), on the contralateral side, which is positioned *posterolateral* to the median plane (about 45° from the coronal plane). These two canals function as a pair. The two **lateral canals** of the right and left sides are oriented in the same (horizontal) plane, and they too function as a pair.

Pilots and astronauts refer to the three planes of rotational movement as pitch, roll, and yaw. **Pitch** refers to forward and backward tilting of the head, as when we nod our head "yes." **Roll** refers to tilting the head sideways from one shoulder to the other shoulder, and **yaw** refers to movement of the head form side to side, as when indicating "no." The lateral semicircular canals are oriented in the horizontal yaw plane, whereas the anterior and posterior semicircular canals are oriented in the half pitch/half roll planes.

When the head is in its normal upright position, the anterior and posterior canals are oriented almost in the vertical plane, whereas the lateral canals are oriented almost in the

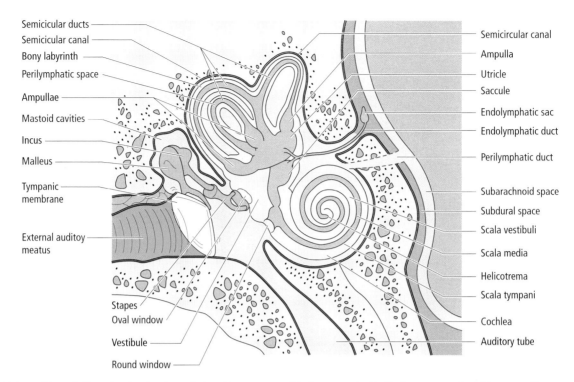

Figure 18.2 • Schematic illustration showing the vestibulocochlear apparatus of the inner ear embedded in the petrous portion of the temporal bone.

horizontal plane. During a certain movement that affects a particular functional pair of canals (i.e., the two lateral canals, or the right anterior and left posterior, or the right posterior and left anterior), the receptors in one canal of the pair are stimulated and excite the afferent axons of the vestibulo-cochlear nerve, whereas the receptors in its complementary canal on the contralateral side, are inhibited and diminish neural activity.

Vestibule

The **vestibule** is a component of the bony labyrinth, receiving the open ends of the three semicircular canals. It is a perilymph-filled space that is continuous with the perilymphatic space of the semicircular canals. The vestibule houses two membranous sacs, the **utricle** and **saccule**. The utricle and saccule each contain an elliptical-shaped sensory receptor, the **macula** (L., "spot") (see below).

Membranous labyrinth associated with equilibrium

The components of the membranous labyrinth associated with equilibrium are the three semicircular ducts, the utricle, and the saccule. They all contain endolymph, and are bathed in perilymph

The **membranous labyrinth** is housed within the bony labyrinth, and reflects its general shape and contour. The space separating the bony labyrinth from the membranous labyrinth is the **perilymphatic space**, filled with a fluid referred to as **perilymph**, which is comparable to extracellular fluid. The membranous labyrinth consists of a series of **membranous sacs** and **ducts** filled with another viscous fluid, referred to as **endolymph**, which is comparable to intracellular fluid. The components of the membranous labyrinth associated with equilibrium are the **three** (membranous) **semicircular ducts** (which are enclosed in the respective three bony semicircular canals) and the (membranous) **utricle** and **saccule**, two sac-like structures that are enclosed within the bony vestibule. The region of the membranous labyrinth containing the receptor for hearing is the cochlear duct, which is enclosed in the bony cochlea (discussed in Chapter 17). Endolymph percolates (flows) in the three membranous semicircular ducts, the utricle, the saccule, and the cochlear duct. The **ductus reuniens** permits communication between the lumen of the cochlear duct with the lumen of the components of the vestibular membranous labyrinth. Both ends of each of the semicircular ducts are attached to, and empty into, the utricle.

Each semicircular duct has a single dilated segment, an **ampulla** (L., "dilation"), near one of its ends. The ampullae of the three semicircular ducts, as well as the utricle and saccule, contain in their interior the **sensory receptors of the vestibular system**. The receptors in the ampullae of the semicircular ducts are the **cristae ampullares**, whereas the receptors in the utricle and the saccule are the **macula utriculi** and the **macula sacculi**, respectively (Figs 18.3, 18.4). Thus there are a total of five receptors (three cristae and two maculae) in each vestibular sensory apparatus. The cristae ampullares of the semicircular canals rest in a patch of neuroepithelium at the base of each ampulla. The macula utriculi rests in a strip of neuro-epithelium on the base of the utricle, whereas the macula sacculi is oriented vertically on the medial wall of the saccule.

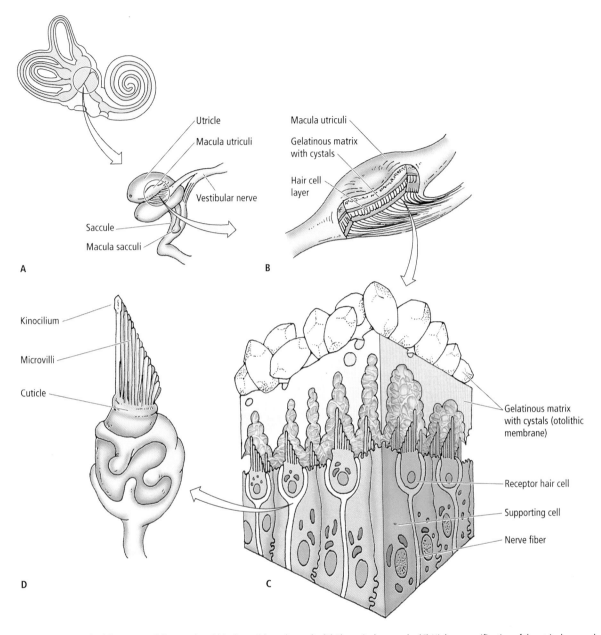

Figure 18.3 ● The macula. (A) Location of the macula within the utricle and saccule. (B) The utricular macula. (C) Higher magnification of the utricular macula illustrating the otoliths on the otolithic membrane, the receptor cells, and the peripheral fiber terminals of the vestibular nerve synapsing with the receptor hair cells. (D) Higher magnification of a receptor hair cell showing its single kinocilium and numerous microvilli.

Note that the clinical case at the beginning of the chapter refers to a patient whose symptoms include intermittent spells of dizziness. The patient was diagnosed with benign positional vertigo that may be caused by free floating debris or particles in the endolymph of the membranous labyrinth in the inner ear.

1 What structures make up the membranous labyrinth?

2 What is the sensory structure that is enclosed within, and is unique to, the utricle and the saccule?

Vestibular receptors

The vestibular receptors (cristae ampullares, macula utriculi, and macula sacculi) consist of a distinct area of neuroepithelium containing mechanoreceptor "hair cells"

The **vestibular receptors** consist of a distinct area of neuroepithelium inside the membranous labyrinth, composed of mechanoreceptor "**hair cells**" and support cells that fill the spaces among the hair cells (see Figs 18.3, 18.4). The hair cells display sensory "hairs," many stiff **stereocilia** (specialized, elongated microvilli, and not true cilia), and a single immotile **kinocilium**. These hair cells, like the

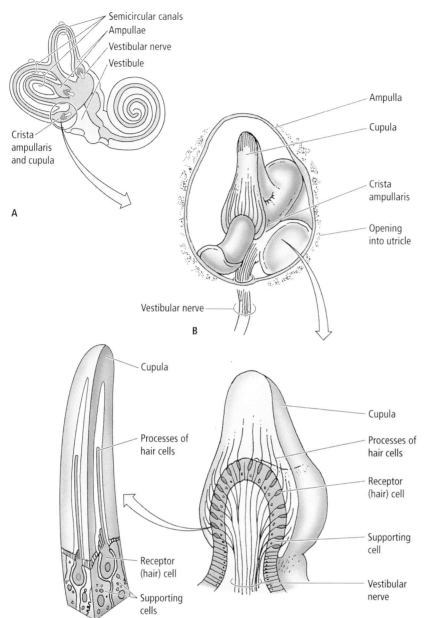

Semicircular canals
Ampullae
Vestibular nerve
Vestibule

Crista
ampullaris
and cupula

A

Ampulla
Cupula
Crista
ampullaris
Opening
into utricle

Vestibular nerve

B

Cupula
Processes of
hair cells
Receptor
(hair) cell
Supporting
cells

D

Cupula
Processes of
hair cells
Receptor
(hair) cell
Supporting
cell
Vestibular
nerve

C

Figure 18.4 ● Three-dimensional view of the semicircular canals. (A) Location of the crista ampullaris within the ampullae of the three semicircular canals. (B) An enlarged crista ampullaris. (C) Higher magnification of a sectioned crista ampullaris showing the cupula, receptor hair cells, and peripheral processes of the vestibular nerve synapsing with the receptor hair cells (D).

hair cells in the cochlea that are involved in hearing, are *transducers* that transform the mechanical stimulation imposed on them, into electrical signals. Electrical signals are transmitted to, and are then conveyed by, the vestibular nerve to the brainstem and cerebellum. Both afferent and efferent nerve endings terminate on the basal and lateral aspects of the hair cells. The neuroepithelia of the **cristae ampullares**, **macula utriculi**, and **macula sacculi** are covered with a **gelatinous glycoprotein membrane**. The stereocilia and kinocilia are embedded in this membrane. Movement of the hair cells with respect to the membrane results in a process by which mechanical deformation of the stereocilia and kinocilia is transformed into an electrical potential.

Otoliths

In the utricle and saccule, the gelatinous glycoprotein membranes overlying their macula have otoconia (or otoliths) on their free surface

In the utricle and the saccule, the gelatinous glycoprotein membranes overlying their macula have, on their free surface, **otoconia** (G., "ear dust") also referred to as **otoliths** (G., "ear stones")—crystals consisting of calcium carbonate (see Fig. 18.3). Since the gelatinous glycoprotein membrane of the utricle and the saccule has otoliths, it is referred to as the **otolithic membrane**, and the utricle and the saccule are referred to as **otolithic organs**. The otoliths have a specific gravity that is greater than that of the endolymph which surrounds them, and they are consequently pulled by gravity. Gravity applies a continuous linear acceleration on the head, and thus deflects the gelatinous membrane, which in turn stimulates the hair cells.

The glycoprotein membrane of the **cristae ampullares** is dome-shaped and is called the **cupula**, which is devoid of crystals (see Fig. 18.4). The cupula increases resistance to the flow of endolymph and unlike the otolithic membranes is *not* influenced by gravitational forces. Instead, it **responds to endolymphatic flow**. The cupula is a mechanical structure that narrows the lumen of the canal and so increases resistance to flow. The three cristae ampullares enclosed in the semicircular duct ampullae (one crista in each ampulla) detect angular acceleration or deceleration (rotational movement) of the head (as in turning or tilting the head). The differing orientation of the three semicircular ducts enable an individual to perceive motion in all planes. Head rotation in a particular plane will result in endolymphatic flow in the functional pair of canals oriented closest to the plane of rotation, and is almost perpendicular to the axis of rotation. Head rotation in a plane that is not parallel to that of any one canal, will activate more than one canal.

The receptors in the utricle and saccule (the macula utriculi and macula sacculi within the utricle and the saccule, respectively) detect spatial orientation of the head in space relative to gravity and linear acceleration or deceleration forces. The receptors in the utricle and in the saccule are oriented *perpendicular* to each other, and therefore can detect motion in two different planes. When the head is upright, the **macula utriculi** is oriented in the *horizontal plane* (on the base of the utricle) and can be stimulated (activated) by linear forces (acceleration or deceleration) in the horizontal plane (as occur in a car, when it increases speed or slows down). The **macula sacculi** is oriented in the *vertical plane* (on the medial wall of the saccule) and can be stimulated (activated) by linear forces (acceleration or deceleration) in the vertical plane (as occur in an ascending or descending elevator). Note that the macula utriculi and the macula sacculi perceive head orientation when the body itself is at rest, but is exposed to external forces.

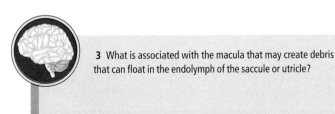

3 What is associated with the macula that may create debris that can float in the endolymph of the saccule or utricle?

Mechanisms of action of the vestibular apparatus

When the body is at rest, and the head is tilted, the otoconia (resting on the gelatinous membrane of the macula utriculi and the macula sacculi) are pulled by gravitational forces, causing the membrane to slant, which in turn deflects the

"hairs" (of the hair cells) embedded in it. The hair deflection stimulates the mechanoreceptor hair cells, which in turn transmit the stimulation to the vestibular nerve dendrites synapsing with them.

In angular (rotational) movement of the head (Fig. 18.5), the bony semicircular canals and the enclosed membranous semicircular ducts rotate at the same velocity as the head. However, the viscous endolymph filling the ducts resists flow initially, and thus "falls behind" due to inertia (that is, the endolymph does not move as fast as the canals). This resistance causes a relative motion difference between the faster moving cupula (which is attached to the interior of the semicircular ducts) and the slower endolymphatic flow. This motion difference results in flow of the endolymph in the direction opposite to that of the crista's cupula, pressing against and tilting the cupula. This action deflects the stereocilia embedded in the cupula. The stereocilia that are deflected away from the kinocilium (caused by the endolymphatic flow away from the kinocilium) elicits hyperpolarization (inhibition) of the hair cell. Whereas the stereocilia that are deflected toward the kinocilium (by endolymphatic flow toward the kinocilium) stretch the hair cell membrane and elicit depolarization (excitation) of the hair cell, and therefore initiate a nerve impulse that is relayed to the vestibular nerve afferent peripheral nerve endings. Flow of endolymph *in the direction of the ampulla* of the horizontal canal results in deflection of the stereocilia toward the kinocilium, which **stimulates the hair cell**. In the anterior and posterior semicircular canals, flow of endolymph in the direction of the ampulla has the opposite effect, that is the **hair cells are inhibited**. If rotation is sustained, the endolymph of the semicircular canals eventually moves at the same rate as the cupula. When this occurs, the cupula is no longer pushed and bent by the endolymph, and the stereocilia and kinocilia are no longer deflected. Since the hair cells are no longer depolarized, the **semicircular canal receptors are not activated by sustained rotation**. Following about 20 seconds of continued rotation, however, the cupula slowly recoils back to its resting position. When the head stops rotating, so do the ducts and the canals. However, the endolymphatic flow persists within the membranous duct due to its momentum, pressing on, and bending the cupula from its resting position in the opposite direction (in the same direction as the head had been rotating), causing the stereocilia to bend away from the kinocilium, thus inhibiting the hair cell from firing completely. A few seconds later, endolymphatic flow ceases and within 20 seconds the cupula once again recoils back to its resting position, permitting the hair cell to emit impulses at a tonic level. Therefore, the semicircular canal conveys a positive signal at the onset of head rotation only if movement is in the correct direction, and conveys a negative signal when head rotation ceases.

It is important to note that the function of the equilibratory senses mediated by the vestibular system is to *perceive differences in the relative movement* between the endolymph and the receptor gelatinous membrane (as occur during the onset and cessation of rotation), rather than to merely detect motion (when sustained rotation is in progress).

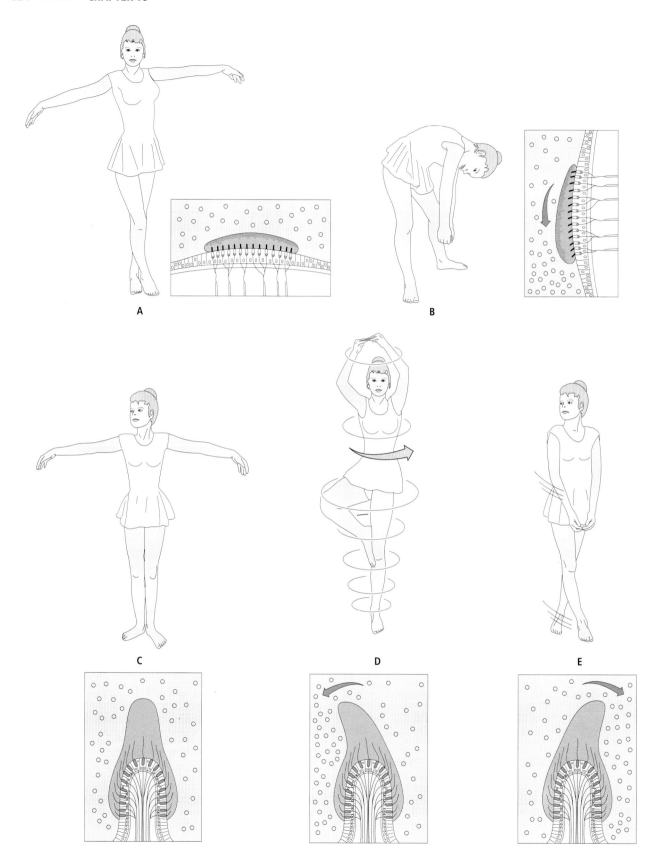

Figure 18.5 • Function of the semicircular canals in balance maintenance. (A, B) The maculae detect spatial orientation of the head relative to gravity and linear acceleration or deceleration forces. (C–E) The cristae respond to endolymphatic flow. They detect angular acceleration or deceleration (rotational movement) of the head (as in turning or tilting the head). As a person at rest (C) begins to rotate (D), the crista ampullaris is tilted by the flow of the endolymph opposite to the direction of the rotation. When the person stops rotating (E), the crista ampullaris is tilted by the flow of the endolymph in the same direction as the rotation.

Slow, slight rotation sends signals to the brain that indicate movement. Fast, intense rotation (as well as motion sickness that occurs in a car or boat) overwhelms the receptors, sending a flood of signals to the brain, with consequent dizziness and/or nausea. When an individual is aboard a ship in a room without a window and cannot see outside, his vestibular system sends information to the brain that he is moving (since the ship is moving), however he cannot "see" that he is actually moving. The inconsistency of the sensory information (or sensory mismatch) that is sent to the brain by the vestibular and visual systems causes him to feel **seasick**. Going out on deck where he can *see* that he is moving, which confirms the vestibular input to the brain, alleviates the symptoms.

When an individual (such as an astronaut) is exposed to an environment with zero gravity, he experiences **space sickness**, an unusual phenomenon affecting his sense of equilibrium. Some scientists believe that in space, the brain receives only slight or no vestibular sensory input due to the lack of gravity, causing space sickness. Others believe that space sickness is similar to car or sea sickness and is caused by a sensory mismatch as described above.

VESTIBULAR NERVE (CN VIII)

The cell bodies of the first order bipolar neurons of the vestibular pathway reside in the vestibular (Scarpa's) ganglion, a sensory ganglion of the vestibular nerve

The cell bodies of the first order **bipolar neurons** of the vestibular pathway reside in the vestibular (Scarpa's) ganglion, a sensory ganglion of the vestibular nerve. The peripheral processes of these bipolar neurons (Fig. 18.6) terminate in the **cristae ampullares** of the semicircular ducts, the **macula utriculi** of the utricle, and the **macula sacculi** of the saccule, where they form synapses with the mechanoreceptor epithelial "**hair cells**." The hair cells are transducers; that is, they transform mechanical stimulation into electrical stimulation (action potentials), which is relayed to the dendritic terminals of the first order bipolar neurons. The central

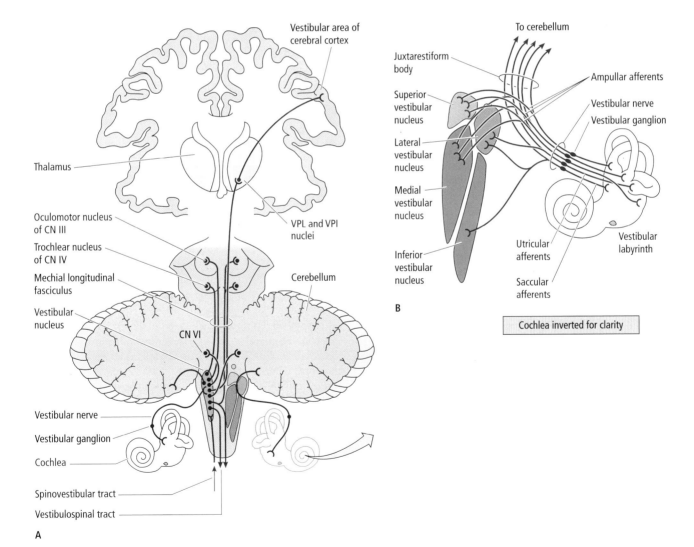

Figure 18.6 ● (A) The vestibulocochlear apparatus, termination of the central processes of the vestibular nerve in the vestibular nuclei, and their projections to the oculomotor, trochlear, and abducens nuclei. VPI, ventral posterior inferior; VPL, ventral posterior lateral. (B) The termination of the central processes of the first order afferent neurons of the vestibular ganglion in the brainstem vestibular nuclei and the cerebellum.

processes of the bipolar neurons gather to form the root of the **vestibular nerve** (the vestibular division of the vestibulo-cochlear nerve, **CN VIII**). In the inner ear, the vestibular nerve joins the cochlear nerve, to form the **vestibulocochlear nerve**. Although the two nerves accompany one another wrapped in a common connective tissue sheath, they are anatomically and functionally two distinct nerves. From the inner ear, the vestibulocochlear nerve passes through the internal auditory meatus to enter the posterior cranial vault. As the vestibulocochlear nerve enters the brainstem at the pontomedullary angle, it separates into its two component nerves. The fibers of the cochlear nerve synapse in the cochlear nuclei in the medulla (as discussed in Chapter 17). The vestibular nerve fibers enter the **vestibular nuclei** located in the pons and upper medulla, where most of the central processes of the vestibular nerve bifurcate into ascending and descending terminals. Some first order vestibular fibers, however, do not terminate in the vestibular nuclei, but take an alternate route by going around them, joining the **juxtarestiform body** in the inferior cerebellar peduncle and terminating *directly* in the **ipsilateral flocculo-nodular lobe of the cerebellum**. This direct termination of the central processes of the first order bipolar neurons in the cerebellum is unique to the vestibular system.

CENTRAL PATHWAYS OF THE VESTIBULAR SYSTEM

Sensory input from the vestibular system is integrated to produce coordinated movement of the head, eyes, and body, and to maintain equilibrium and muscle tone

Unlike other sensory systems, the projections of the vestibular system are mainly reflexive in nature (Fig. 18.7). Sensory input is integrated to produce coordinated movement of the head, eyes, and body, and to maintain equilibrium and muscle tone. The vestibular system mainly projects to the following structures:

1   The **motor nuclei** of the oculomotor, trochlear, and abducens nerves that innervate the extraocular muscles and thus control reflex eye movements.
2   The **cerebellum**, which integrates sensory input from various systems and coordinates head and body movement.
3   The **reticular formation** at the pontine and medullary levels, where reflex motor activity is initiated.
4   The **spinal cord**, where postural adjustments can be made.

Vestibular nuclear complex

The vestibular nuclear complex is composed of four vestibular nuclei, and the central processes of the first order bipolar neurons of the vestibular (Scarpa's) ganglion that terminate there

The **vestibular nuclear complex** is composed of four vestibular nuclei (Fig. 18.6.), and the central processes of the first order bipolar neurons of the vestibular (Scarpa's) ganglion that terminate there. The four vestibular nuclei are:

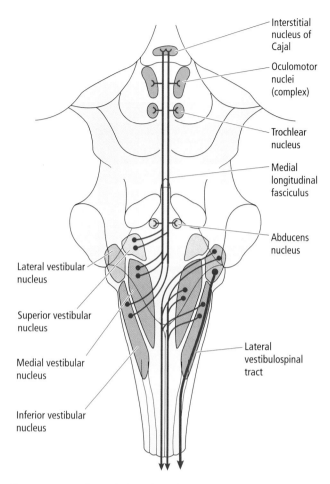

Figure 18.7 ● The vestibular nuclei and their ascending and descending projections.

1   The superior (Bechterew's) vestibular nucleus.
2   The medial (Schwalbe's) vestibular nucleus.
3   The lateral (Deiter's) vestibular nucleus.
4   The inferior (spinal, descending) vestibular nucleus.

The vestibular nuclei are located in the upper medulla and lower pons, lateral to the fourth ventricle, in close proximity to the cerebellum. The superior nucleus is located entirely in the pons, whereas the other three nuclei extend into both the caudal pons and the rostral medulla. These nuclei contain the cell bodies of second order neurons whose fibers carry outflow signals to various destinations.

The **superior** and **medial vestibular nuclei** receive the first order neuron terminals relaying sensory input from the cristae ampullares of the **semicircular canals**. Following the reception of this sensory input, these nuclei then relay it via two structures:

1   The **medial longitudinal fasciculus** (MLF) to the extra-ocular muscle nuclei to elicit compensatory ocular movements triggered by movements of the head.
2   The **medial vestibulospinal tract** to the cervical spinal cord to elicit suitable head movements.

The **lateral vestibular nucleus** receives vestibular sensory input mainly from the maculae of the **utricle**, but may also receive input from the **saccule** and semicircular canals. This nucleus projects via the lateral vestibulospinal tract to motoneurons or interneurons at all spinal cord levels to make postural adjustments.

The **inferior vestibular nucleus** receives vestibular sensory input from the semicircular canals as well as the utricle. Most of the first order vestibular fibers terminate in this nucleus. It projects to the reticular formation and the cerebellum.

Termination of the vestibular nerve first order afferent fibers

The first order afferent fibers of the vestibular nerve project to, and terminate directly in, either the vestibular nuclear complex or the flocculonodular lobe of the cerebellum

The **vestibular nuclei** and the **cerebellum** serve as the **first relay centers of the vestibular pathway**. The vestibular nerve is unique since it is the only cranial nerve that sends some of its first order afferent fibers relaying sensory input *directly* from peripheral receptors to the cerebellar cortex.

Afferent projections (input) to the vestibular nuclei

Most of the afferents arriving at the vestibular nuclei arise from the cerebellum

The vestibular nuclei receive afferent (input) projections from numerous sources. There are a number of input sources to the vestibular nuclei:

1   The central processes of the bipolar first order neurons of the **vestibular nerve**, which transmit sensory input from the vestibular receptor apparatus in the inner ear (as discussed above; see Fig. 18.6).
2   The **vestibulocerebellum** (the flocculus and nodulus) and part of the uvula, which project their fibers to the ipsilateral vestibular nuclei via the juxtarestiform body (Fig. 18.8).
3   The **spinocerebellum** (the vermis of the anterior lobe of the cerebellum), which projects its fibers to the ipsilateral vestibular nuclei via the juxtarestiform body.
4   The **fastigial nucleus** of the cerebellum, which projects bilaterally to the vestibular nuclei via the fastigiovestibular tract.
5   The reciprocal connections from the **contralateral vestibular nuclei**.

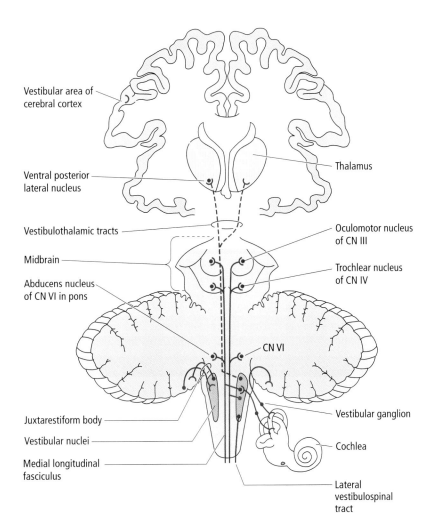

Figure 18.8 ● The main central projections of the vestibular system. Output fibers from the vestibular nuclei join the ascending medial longitudinal fasciculus (MLF) to terminate in the motor nuclei innervating the extraocular muscles where they function in vestibulo-ocular reflexes. Output fibers from the vestibular nuclei joining the descending MLF and the lateral vestibulospinal tracts, terminate in the motor horn of the spinal cord where they function in postural reflexes.

Vestibular area of cerebral cortex

Ventral posterior lateral nucleus

Vestibulothalamic tracts

Midbrain

Abducens nucleus of CN VI in pons

Juxtarestiform body

Vestibular nuclei

Medial longitudinal fasciculus

Thalamus

Oculomotor nucleus of CN III

Trochlear nucleus of CN IV

CN VI

Vestibular ganglion

Cochlea

Lateral vestibulospinal tract

6   The **spinal cord**.
7   The **pretectal nuclei**.

The spinal cord sends proprioceptive information to the vestibular nuclei via the spinovestibular tract regarding the orientation status of the body so that postural adjustments can be made.

Efferent projections (output) from the vestibular nuclei

The vestibular nuclei project **second order fibers** to the following areas (see Fig. 18.7):

1   The **oculomotor**, **trochlear**, and **abducens motor nuclei** as well as the **accessory oculomotor nuclei**: the interstitial nucleus of Cajal, and the nucleus of Darkschewitch via the **medial longitudinal fasciculus (MLF)**.
2   The **contralateral vestibular nuclei**, most of which are reciprocal inhibitory connections.
3   The **inferior olivary nucleus** (via the vestibulo-olivary tract), which in turn projects to the cerebellar vermis via the restiform body.
4   The **ipsilateral flocculus** and **nodulus** (both of which are associated with equilibrium and receive sensory information from the semicircular canals).
5   The **uvula**.
6   The **fastigial nucleus** of the cerebellum (bilaterally), via the juxtarestiform body (note that the juxtarestiform body consists of two-directional traffic; that is, it carries both afferent and efferent fibers connecting the vestibular nuclei and the cerebellum).
7   **Spinal cord** ventral horn alpha and gamma motoneurons and interneurons.
8   The **vestibular labyrinth**, where descending efferent fibers modulate afferent input to the vestibular nuclei.

Ascending projections

The superior and medial vestibular nuclei give rise to fibers that join the MLF and terminate in the cranial nerve nuclei, which innervate the extraocular muscles

The **superior vestibular nucleus** fibers join the ipsilateral and contralateral MLF and project to the oculomotor nuclear complex as well as the trochlear nuclei bilaterally. Some of the fibers arising from the **medial vestibular nucleus** join the ipsilateral and the contralateral MLF to terminate in the oculomotor nuclear complex and the abducens nucleus bilaterally, whereas other medial vestibular nuclear fibers join only the contralateral MLF and terminate in the contralateral trochlear nucleus and inter-stitial nucleus of Cajal.

Fibers arising from the **inferior vestibular nucleus** join the ipsilateral and contralateral MLF to terminate in the oculomotor and trochlear nuclei bilaterally.

All of these ascending (output) connections function in the *coordination of eye movements*. Since the MLF also carries descending fibers from the medial vestibular nucleus to the spinal cord (see below), it functions in the coordination of head, eye, and neck movements.

Descending projections

The vestibular nuclei regulate the activity of spinal cord alpha and gamma motoneurons by their lateral and medial vestibulospinal tracts

The **lateral vestibulospinal tract** originates only from the lateral vestibular nucleus. This tract descends ipsilaterally and terminates at all levels of the spinal cord although it projects more fibers at the cervical and lumbar levels, where it synapses with both interneurons and with alpha and gamma motoneurons in the spinal cord ventral horn. On its way to the spinal cord, the lateral vestibulospinal tract gives rise to collaterals that synapse in the reticular formation of the medulla. Functionally, the lateral vestibulospinal tract regulates the activity of spinal cord motoneurons in order to *maintain posture*. It forms excitatory synapses with the alpha and gamma motoneurons whose fibers innervate extensor (antigravity) muscles in the neck, trunk, and lower limb, as well as inhibitory synapses via interneurons to the alpha and gamma motoneurons that innervate flexor muscles (causing their relaxation).

The **medial vestibulospinal tract** originates primarily from the medial vestibular nucleus. This tract descends bilaterally in the MLF and terminates in the cervical spinal cord where it, too, forms synapses with interneurons and alpha and gamma motoneurons, innervating neck extensors. Functionally, since the medial vestibulospinal tract terminates in the cervical spinal cord, it serves to *coordinate head* and *ocular movements*.

The **inferior vestibular nucleus** gives rise to fibers that terminate in the inferior olivary nucleus, the reticular formation in the medulla, the cerebellum, and the cervical spinal cord via the MLF.

All output vestibular projections distribute collaterals in the medullary, pontine, and mesencephalic reticular formation. These relays play an important function in the reflexive control and coordination of head and eye movements.

Vestibular thalamic and cortical projections

The vestibular nuclei project to the thalamus via the MLF. The thalamus in turn relays vestibular input to the primary vestibular cortex

The **superior** and **lateral vestibular nuclei** give rise to second order fibers that join the MLF bilaterally to ascend to the **ventral posterior lateral** and **ventral posterior inferior nuclei of the thalamus**. The thalamus gives rise to third order fibers that terminate in the **primary vestibular cortex (Brodmann's area 3a)** in the parietal lobe, located next to the primary motor area (Brodmann's area 4). Brodmann's area 3a is believed to be the site of integration of sensory input from the vestibular and other proprioceptive systems (see Fig. 18.8). The associations between Brodmann's areas 3a and 4 serve in the regulation of motor activity.

CONTROL OF OCULAR MOVEMENTS

The majority of eye movements are mediated by reflex activity involving several neural systems that are interconnected by complex pathways

Eye movements are categorized into conjugate eye movements and disconjugate (disjunctive) eye movements. **Conjugate eye movements**, in which both eyes turn toward the same direction simultaneously (i.e., to the right or to the left), include: (i) **smooth pursuit** eye movements, which are involuntary, slow, and smooth, and occur during the tracking of a moving object (note that smooth pursuit can only be elicited if there is an actual moving stimulus to track); (ii) **optokinetic** eye movements, which are tracking eye movements and are triggered by motion of the visual field; (iii) **saccadic** eye movements, which are rapid and abrupt, voluntary or involuntary, and change the point of visual fixation; and (iv) **vestibular** eye movements, which are involuntary eye movements triggered by head movements (i.e., the vestibuloocular reflex). **Disconjugate eye movements** consist of **vergence** eye movements in which both eyes turn in opposite directions simultaneously. Vergence eye movements are involuntary and may be: (i) **convergent** (both eyes are adducted, i.e., rotate toward the midline, when we focus on an object close to our face); or (ii) **divergent** (i.e., eyes rotate away from the midline toward their normal position when we are looking at an object as we move it away from our face).

The motor nuclei (oculomotor, trochlear, and abducens nuclei, containing lower motoneurons) innervating the extraocular muscles receive inputs from various sources, which indirectly control voluntary or involuntary ocular movements. There are four principal projection sources to these nuclei.

1 **Upper motoneurons** from the **frontal eye field** controlling *voluntary eye movements.*
2 The **vestibular system**, which detects head motion and *coordinates head* and *eye movements* via: (i) the pontine reticular formation lateral gaze center (also referred to as the **paramedian pontine reticular formation**) that controls *conjugate horizontal ocular movements*; and (ii) a **center for vertical gaze** in the periaqueductal gray of the mesencephalon, which controls *conjugate vertical ocular movements*, in order to keep the eyes fixed on a stationary object as the head is moving.
3 Projections from the **visual cortex** to the rostral midbrain (vertical gaze center and lateral gaze center), that play a role in the *tracking of a moving object* by moving the eyes in order to maintain the image of a moving object on the retina.
4 Projections from the *auditory system* that play a role in causing a sudden (reflex) turning of the eyes in the direction of a startling sound.

Vestibular control of eye movements

As the head moves, reflex activity mediated by vestibular neural circuits connects the vestibular system with the cranial nerve nuclei to elicit compensatory ocular movements, so that an object can remain in the field of vision

The extraocular muscles that control ocular movements receive innervation from motoneurons whose cell bodies are housed in the oculomotor, trochlear, and abducens nuclei. The superior oblique is innervated by the trochlear nerve, the lateral rectus is innervated by the abducent nerve, whereas the remainder of the extraocular muscles, the superior and inferior rectus, the medial rectus, and the inferior oblique, are innervated by the oculomotor nerve. To produce smooth, coordinated ocular movements as one extraocular muscle contracts, its antagonists relax.

As the head moves, the eyes may gaze at a motionless object by reflex activity mediated by vestibular neural circuits that connect the vestibular system (which detects orientation and movement of the head in space) with the cranial nerve nuclei (innervating the appropriate extraocular muscles). This elicits compensatory ocular movements, so that the object can remain in the field of vision.

Conjugate horizontal ocular movements

Vestibulo-ocular reflex

During movement of the head in the horizontal plane (right to left or vice versa), information is transmitted from the canal-specific vestibular system via reflex circuit connections to the abducens and oculomotor nuclei, which innervate extraocular muscles controlling horizontal eye movement

When the head is turned (e.g., to the right), it induces subtle endolymphatic flow in both horizontal semicircular canals. The endolymph flows to the left since its inertia causes it to "fall behind" relative to the movement of the head. The endolymphatic flow causes deflection of the cupula in the right horizontal canal ampulla, bending the "hair cell" sensory hairs toward the kinocilium, and increasing the neural activity of the crista ampullaris of the right horizontal canal ampulla. There is a simultaneous decrease in neural activity of the crista ampullaris of the left horizontal canal ampulla. The depolarized hair cells (in the right horizontal canal ampulla) transmit sensory information to the peripheral (dendritic) terminals of the first order, vestibular ganglion neurons. The central processes of these neurons terminate in the ipsilateral (in this example, right) vestibular nuclei where they synapse with neurons whose axons join the MLF and terminate in the contralateral (left) **abducens nucleus** (Fig. 18.9). In the abducens nucleus, the axon terminals synapse with and *stimulate* the motoneurons that project directly to, and innervate, the contralateral (left) **lateral rectus muscle** as well as another group of neurons that cross the midline, join the contralateral (right) MLF and terminate in the contralateral (right) **oculomotor nucleus** where they synapse with the motoneurons that innervate the right **medial rectus muscle**. Thus the muscles that would cause

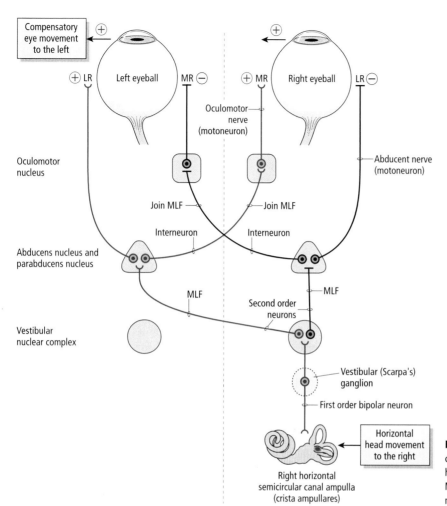

Figure 18.9 ● Central connections mediating compensatory horizontal eye movement in response to horizontal head movement. LR, lateral rectus muscle; MLF, medial longitudinal fasciculus; MR, medial rectus muscle.

conjugate horizontal ocular movement in the opposite direction to that of the head movement are stimulated.

The second order vestibular fibers that terminate in the ipsilateral (right) abducens nucleus *inhibit* the motoneurons that project directly to, and innervate, the ipsilateral (right) lateral rectus muscle as well as another group of neurons that cross the midline, join the contralateral MLF, and terminate in the contralateral (left) oculomotor nucleus where they synapse with the motoneurons that innervate the contralateral (left) medial rectus muscle. Thus, the muscles that would cause conjugate (simultaneous) horizontal ocular movement in the same direction as the head movement are inhibited.

The outcome of this mechanism is the **reflex turning of both eyes to the left** to maintain an image on the retina as the head is turned to the right.

In summary, when an individual fixes his gaze on ("stares at") an object and then begins to turn his head, for example to the right, the eyes will reflexly (via MLF vestibular connections to the extraocular nuclei) "turn" to the left (as the head is moving), which is opposite to the direction of head movement. This turning of the eyes (dictated by vestibular reflex connections) compensates for the shifting of head position in order to *maintain visual fixation* on an object. Otherwise, without this vestibular reflex mechanism coupling head and eye

movements, as the erect head moves from a certain position (to the right or to the left) the eyes would remain still, perceiving a changing visual field in the duration of head movement. The vestibulocerebellum regulates **vestibulo-ocular reflex** activity in order to produce compensatory ocular movement for the head movement and can cancel it so that the eyes can move from a target.

Conjugate vertical ocular movement

During vertical head movement, information is transmitted from the vestibular system to the trochlear and oculomotor nuclei, which innervate extraocular muscles controlling vertical eye movement

During movement of the head in the vertical plane (tilting upward, backward; or downward, forward), information is transmitted from the canal-specific vestibular system via reflex circuit connections to the trochlear and oculomotor nuclei, which innervate extraocular muscles controlling vertical eye movement. If the head is erect and the eyes are fixed ("stare at") on an object, as the head is tilted forward or backward, a reflex will be automatically activated. This causes a "reflex turning" of the eyes upward or downward, respectively, in order to maintain visual fixation on the object.

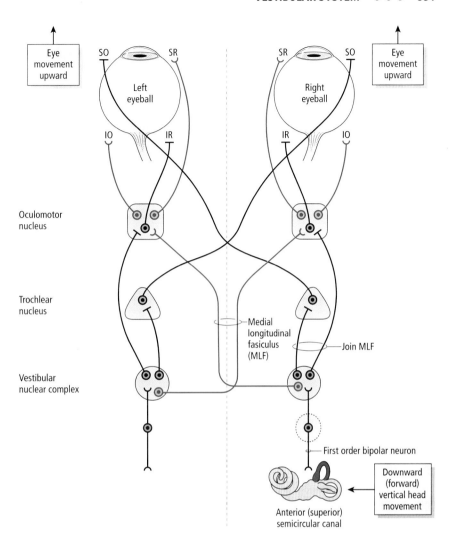

Figure 18.10 ● Central connections mediating compensatory vertical (upward) eye movement in response to downward (forward) movement of the head. IO, inferior oblique muscle; IR, inferior rectus muscle; SO, superior oblique muscle; SR, superior rectus muscle.

Conjugate upward ocular movement

When the head tilts forward, the eyes reflexly turn upward

When tilting the head forward, the eyes will reflexly turn upward. This is caused by endolymphatic flow in the anterior (superior) vertical semicircular canal and the subsequent deflection of its cupula. Deflection of the cupula stimulates the hair cells, which transmit sensory input to the ipsilateral vestibular nuclei. The first order fibers synapse with both inhibitory and excitatory second order vestibular neurons (Fig. 18.10).

Second order inhibitory vestibular neurons join the ipsilateral MLF and ascend to, terminate in, and inhibit: (i) the ipsilateral trochlear nucleus, whose neurons give rise to fibers that decussate and then exit the brainstem to innervate the **contralateral superior oblique muscle**; and (ii) the oculomotor nucleus, which sends fibers to innervate the **ipsilateral inferior rectus muscle**.

Second order excitatory vestibular neurons give rise to fibers that decussate, join the contralateral MLF, and ascend

to terminate in the contralateral oculomotor nucleus where they synapse with neurons that innervate the **contralateral superior rectus** and **inferior oblique muscles**.

In summary, as the head tilts *forward*, the eyes *turn upward* by the simultaneous inhibition of the neurons that innervate the superior oblique and inferior rectus muscles of both eyes, and the stimulation of the neurons that innervate the superior rectus and inferior oblique muscles of both eyes.

Conjugate downward ocular movement

When the head tilts backward, the eyes reflexly turn downward

When tilting the head backward, the eyes will reflexly turn downward. This is caused by endolymphatic flow in the posterior (inferior) vertical semicircular canal and the subsequent deflection of its cupula. Deflection of the cupula stimulates the hair cells, which transmit sensory input to the ipsilateral vestibular nuclei. The first order neurons synapse

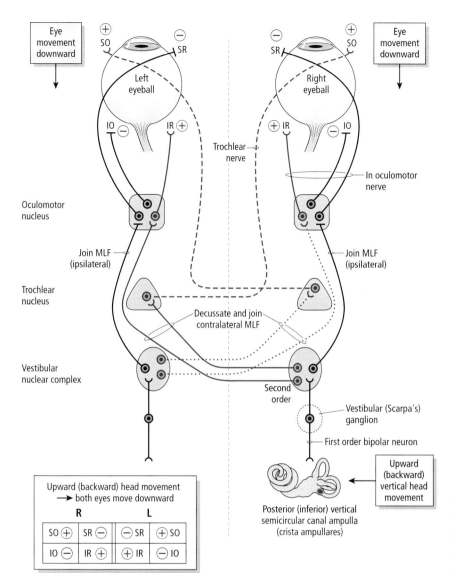

Figure 18.11 ● Central connections mediating compensatory vertical (downward) eye movement in response to upward (backward) movement of the head. IO, inferior oblique muscle; IR, inferior rectus muscle; MLF, medial longitudinal fasciculus; SO, superior oblique muscle; SR, superior rectus muscle.

with both inhibitory and excitatory second order vestibular neurons (Fig. 18.11).

Second order inhibitory vestibular neurons join the ipsilateral MLF and ascend to terminate in the oculomotor nucleus where they synapse with neurons that inhibit the **ipsilateral superior rectus** and **inferior oblique muscles**.

Second order excitatory vestibular neurons give rise to fibers that decussate, join the contralateral MLF, and terminate in: (i) the trochlear nucleus, where they synapse with neurons that give rise to fibers that cross the midline and exit in the trochlear nerve, to innervate the **superior oblique muscle**; and (ii) the oculomotor nucleus, where they synapse with neurons that innervate the **inferior rectus muscle**.

In summary, when the head tilts *backward*, the eyes *turn downward* by the simultaneous inhibition of the superior rectus and inferior oblique muscles of both eyes and the stimulation of the superior oblique and inferior rectus muscles of both eyes.

VESTIBULAR NYSTAGMUS

Horizontal nystagmus is a normal movement of the eyes when it is induced by activation of the vestibular apparatus; spontaneous nystagmus is indicative of a lesion affecting the vestibular nuclei

Horizontal nystagmus is a normal movement of the eyes when it is induced by activation of the vestibular apparatus. The distinguishing characteristic of nystagmus is a rhythmic, back and forth movement of the eyes, with a slow component in one direction, and a fast component (rapid return) in the other direction following asymmetric stimulation of the vestibular sensory apparatus of the two sides.

Spontaneous nystagmus, however, is pathologic, and is indicative of a lesion affecting the vestibular nuclei. A lesion in the vestibular apparatus, nerve, nuclei, or pathways, or the vestibulocerebellum, may produce nystagmus.

In addition to horizontal nystagmus, there are also vertical and rotatory nystagmus. **Vertical nystagmus** may result following damage involving the superior vestibular nucleus in the pons. Extensive damage in the pontomedullary junction affecting the entire vestibular nuclear complex results in **rotatory nystagmus**.

To test the functional integrity of the vestibular system, two clinical tests—the rotation test and the caloric test—may be performed.

In the **rotation test**, the individual sits in a Barany chair with his head upright and tilted at 30° anteriorly. In this position the horizontal semicircular canals are oriented parallel to the plane of rotation. The individual is then rotated about 10 complete rotations to either the right or left, maintaining a continuous angular acceleration of the head. The rotation is then suddenly ceased. If, for example, the individual (with normal vestibular apparatus) is rotated to the right, the rotation will stimulate the right horizontal semicircular canal and then the stimulation will be transmitted to the right vestibular nuclei. The endolymphatic flow will tilt the cupula of the right horizontal semicircular canal to the left, due to the

relative motion difference of the cupula and the endolymph. As rotation continues, the endolymph will "catch up" and flow at the same speed as the canal and head, which will no longer activate the cupula. Sudden stopping of the rotation causes the endolymph, due to its inertia, to continue flowing in the direction of rotation, tilting the cupula to the left, which will inhibit the hair cells. During rotation, the eyes will move slowly to the left (slow component) in order to maintain visual fixation, and then will flick back (fast component) to the center (right) (Fig. 18.12). The nystagmus is in the direction of the spin, to the right. As the rotation is suddenly stopped, the direction of nystagmus is in the opposite direction (to the left), to that which occurs during rotation (which was to the right). This is known as **postrotatory nystagmus**. Normally, postrotatory nystagmus lasts for about half a minute.

In addition to the above reactions, the individual will lean or fall to the right (the same direction as the rotation) and experience vertigo (subjective sensation of rotation) to the left (opposite to the direction of rotation). If the subject is asked to

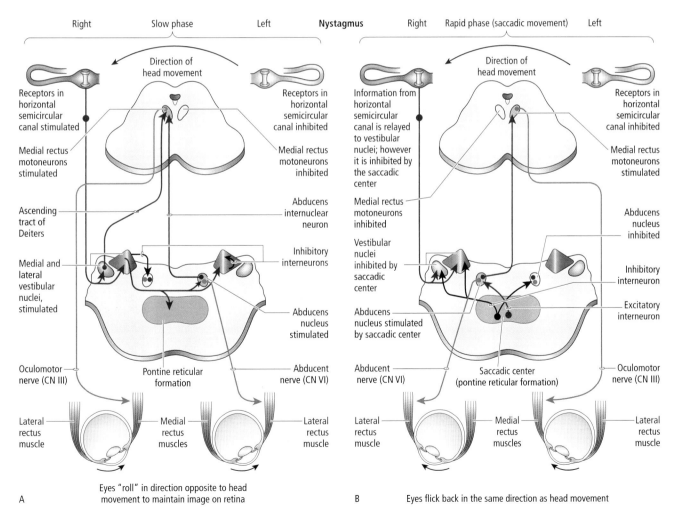

Figure 18.12 ● Vestibular nystagmus: (A) slow phase, and (B) rapid phase. (Modified from Netter, FH (1983) *The Ciba Collection of Medical Illustrations*, Vol. 1 *The Nervous System*, Part I *Anatomy and Physiology*. CIBA, New Jersey; plate 31.)

point at a target, he will exhibit **past pointing**, in which the subject's arm points in the direction of the rotation. Since nystagmus is named after the fast component, in this case it is to the right.

CALORIC NYSTAGMUS

The caloric test may be utilized to stimulate each vestibular apparatus, or specific semicircular canals, in conscious or unconscious individuals

The **caloric test** may be used to stimulate each vestibular apparatus, or specific semi-circular canals, in conscious or unconscious individuals. The caloric test allows for the examination of the vestibular apparatus of only one side at a time. In a rotational test, on the contrary, both sides are stimulated simultaneously.

For the caloric test, the **horizontal canal** has to be oriented in the vertical plane. To stimulate the horizontal canal, the subject sits upright with his head inclined about 60° posteriorly. The external auditory meatus is subsequently irrigated with cold or warm water. The cold or warm temperature of the water produces vestibular apparatus fluid circulation currents. Cold water produces a sinking of the fluid, whereas warm water produces a rising of the fluid.

In a subject with a normal vestibulo-ocular system, when the left ear is irrigated with cold water, flushing causes nystagmus (fast component) toward the opposite side (to the right), with accompanying past pointing and falling on the same side as the stimulation. When the same ear is irrigated with warm water, the nystagmus (fast component) is to the left (that is, the subject exhibits the opposite response).

If the subject is comatose, nystagmus is not observable. If the brainstem is undamaged, cold irrigation will cause both eyes to turn to the side of the cold irrigation. If the subject has a lesion affecting the MLF bilaterally, cold irrigation will cause the eye ipsilateral to the irrigation to turn toward the side of the cold irrigation. If there is a lesion in the caudal brainstem, affecting the vestibular nuclear complex, deviation of the eyes is not present.

SYNONYMS AND EPONYMS OF THE VESTIBULAR SYSTEM

Name of structure or term	Synonym(s)/eponym(s)
Anterior semicircular canal	Superior semicircular canal
Bony labyrinth	Osseous labyrinth
Cranial nerve VIII	Vestibulocochlear nerve
Disjunctive ocular movements	Disconjugate ocular movements
Frontal eye field (FEF)	Brodmann's area 8
Inferior vestibular nucleus	Spinal vestibular nucleus
	Descending vestibular nucleus
Lateral semicircular canal	Horizontal semicircular canal
Lateral vestibular nucleus	Deiter's vestibular nucleus
Medial vestibular nucleus	Schwalbe's vestibular nucleus
Otoconia (G. oto, "ear;" conia, "dust")	Otoliths (G. oto, "ear;" liths, "stones")
Posterior semicircular canal	Inferior semicircular canal
Saccule	Sacculus
Saccule and utricle	Otolithic organs
Superior vestibular nucleus	Bechterew's vestibular nucleus
Utricle	Utriculus
Vestibular ganglion	Scarpa's ganglion
Vestibular nuclei	Vestibular nuclear complex

FOLLOW-UP TO CLINICAL CASE

This patient has **benign positional vertigo**. This is the most common identifiable vertigo and it occurs most frequently in older individuals, although it can occur at any age. It is common and probably underdiagnosed. It is thought to be caused from free floating debris or particles in the endolymph of one of the semicircular canals, most commonly the posterior semicircular canal. Free floating particles are also derived from calcium carbonate crystals or otoliths. These crystals are normally associated with the macula in the utricle or the saccule and can at times become "dislodged and float in the endolymph."[1] The cause of this pathology is unknown, but it is sometimes associated with trauma. This condition most often resolves on its own eventually, but can recur. Medications are often ineffective in the treatment of this condition. For a more complete description, please refer to the article by Furman and Cass.[1]

The evaluation of dizziness requires that the patient describes exactly what he or she mean by dizziness. Dizziness can result from vertigo, which is an illusion of movement when there is actually no movement occurring. This is the same sensation produced when one is spun around and then suddenly stopped. The term dizziness is often used to refer to a vague sensation of imbalance, dysequilibrium, or light-headedness. This is often nonspecific and indeed non-neurologic. In contrast, vertigo is quite specific and usually indicates a problem either in the inner ear, the brainstem (specifically the posterolateral medulla), and/or the cerebellum. If it is an inner ear problem, it is often associated with hearing loss and/or tinnitus.

1 Furman JM, Cass SP (1999) Benign paroxysmal positional vertigo. *New England Journal of Medicine* **341**(21): 1590–96.

QUESTIONS TO PONDER

1. Which sensory systems work with the vestibular system to maintain equilibrium, posture, muscle tone, and reflex movements of the eyes?

2. Give the location of the receptors of the vestibular apparatus.

3. Differentiate between the structure and function of the gelatinous glycoprotein membrane of the macula utriculi, the macula sacculi, and the crista ampullaris.

4. What is the effect of endolymphatic flow in the direction of the ampullae of the horizontal, anterior, and posterior semicircular canals?

5. What is unique about the vestibular first order bipolar neuron central projections?

6. What is the source of most of the afferents arriving at the vestibular nuclei?

7. What is the function of the vestibulo-ocular reflex (VOR)?

CHAPTER 19

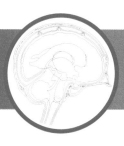
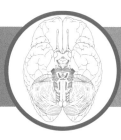
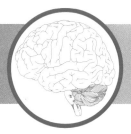

Olfactory System

CLINICAL CASE

A 32-year-old male carpenter fell backwards off a ladder while at work about a month ago. His coworkers said that he hit the back of his head, but the patient does not remember this. He apparently lost consciousness for approximately 10 minutes, and was sent to the emergency room. A head CT performed in the ER was normal, including the sinuses. There was no apparent skull fracture. He recovered alertness and awareness and insisted on going home. Symptoms of headache and dizziness subsided after a few days. However, he has continued to experience a persistent loss of the sense of smell and taste since his accident. Food tastes bland, and he cannot fully sense odors such as coffee, freshly cut lumber, or his wife's perfume.

Examination shows his sense of smell to be greatly diminished when tested with several types of odiferous substances, in both nostrils. Taste sensation was normal for sweet, salty, bitter, and sour. Examination of the nose and sinuses was normal. The remaining general physical and neurologic exam was normal.

The **olfactory system** mediating the special sense of smell is phylogenetically one of the most primitive sensory systems. Although humans do not rely to a great extent on their olfactory sense, the survival of many other animals is greatly dependent on olfaction. This is reflected in the relative size difference of the olfactory systems—that of humans being rather rudimentary compared with that of many other animals. In humans the olfactory epithelium consists of about 10 cm^2, compared to about 170 cm^2 in dogs; dogs also have more than 100 times more receptors in each square centimeter than humans. The olfactory system is not only implicated in the perception and transmission of *olfactory sensation*, but is also believed to affect other neural systems associated with producing or influencing *emotional*, *behavioral*, and *reflex responses* such as reproductive and maternal behaviors, and autonomic visceral functions such as salivation, gastric secretion, and nausea.

The ancestral cerebrum consisted of a pair of swellings, which received olfactory input from the olfactory bulbs and whose principal function was to mediate olfactory sensation. During evolution, the ancestral brain underwent modifications resulting in the enlargement and increased complexity of the cerebrum. These gradual changes were accompanied by the emergence and vast expansion of the neocortex with a consequent movement of the paleocortex to a more internal position at the base of the brain.

OLFACTORY RECEPTOR CELLS

Olfactory receptor cells reside in the olfactory epithelium, and are the only neurons that are in direct contact with the environment

Olfactory receptor cells, the first order bipolar neurons of the olfactory pathway, reside in the olfactory epithelium (and not in a ganglion), and are the only neurons that are in direct contact with the environment.

The nasal cavities are lined by a special membrane, the nasal mucosa, that is modified at the roof and the adjacent superior walls of these cavities into a specialized thick **olfactory epithelium (neuroepithelium)** and underlying connective tissue (Fig. 19.1). This pseudostratified ciliated columnar epithelium includes several cell types, namely basal cells, immature receptor cells, olfactory receptor cells, and supporting cells. The **basal cells** proliferate to form **immature receptor cells** that differentiate to become **olfactory receptor cells**. The **supporting cells** provide both physical and physiological support to all other cells of this epithelium. The olfactory receptor cells are **first order afferent bipolar neurons** that have a lifespan of about 1–2 months. These neurons are unique since they are the only nerve cells that come in direct contact with the environment. It was once thought that the olfactory receptor cells were the only nerve cells to retain the capability to regenerate throughout the lifetime of the organism. However, this is challenged by recent findings that adult neurogenesis also occurs in the dentate gyrus of the limbic system.

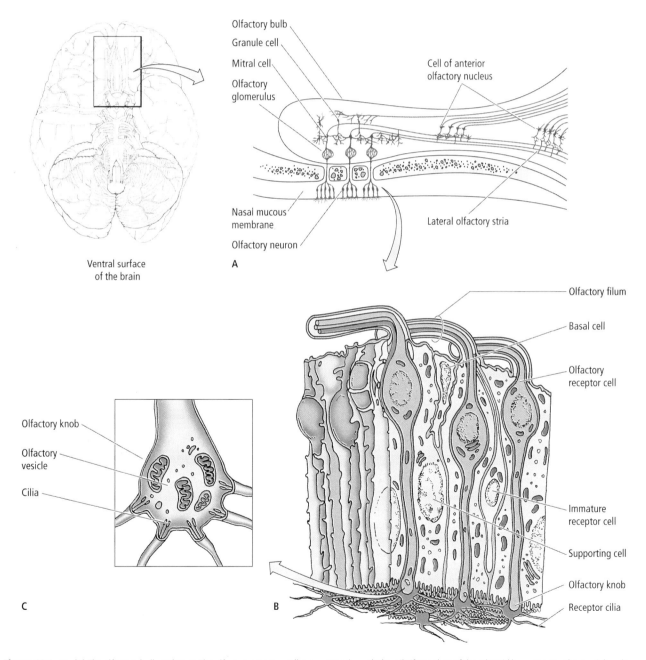

Figure 19.1 ● (A) The olfactory bulb and tract. The olfactory receptor cell axons pass through the cribriform plate of the ethmoid bone to enter the cranial vault where they terminate and synapse in the olfactory bulb. (B) The olfactory epithelium (neuroepithelium). Note the olfactory receptor cells—the first order neurons of the olfactory pathway. (C) Enlargement of an olfactory knob.

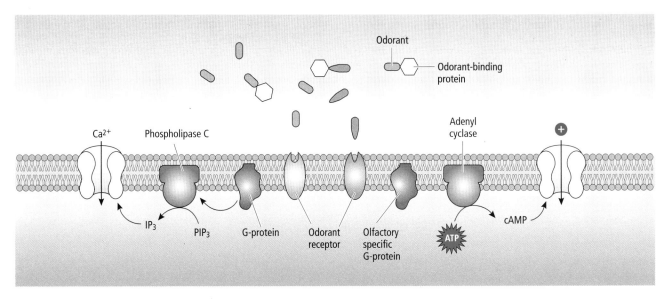

Figure 19.2 ● Olfactory transduction. Odorous substances dissolve in the mucus layer overlying the olfactory neuroepithelium and then bind to odorant-binding proteins that move them through the mucus. The odorous substances subsequently bind to the receptors in the olfactory epithelium, which in turn activates a second messenger pathway.

The connective tissue (lamina propria) underlying the olfactory epithelium contains **Bowman's glands**, whose ducts carry the gland's aqueous secretion that forms a moist blanket on the epithelial surface. The remainder of the nasal mucosa produces a mucus secretion. The apical surface of the olfactory receptor cells possesses modified cilia, which are embedded in the mucus secretions. Odorous substances entering the nasal cavities dissolve in the moist layer of mucus and interact with receptor molecules embedded in the plasmalemma of the ciliary membrane, stimulating the **chemosensitive cilia** of the olfactory receptor cells. Most of the flavor that we "taste" in foods is actually the aroma that passes from the back of the mouth, reaching the superior recesses of the nasal cavity lined with olfactory epithelium.

OLFACTORY TRANSDUCTION

Odorous substances interact with and bind to odorant-receptor protein molecules embedded in the plasmalemma of the ciliary membrane, where transduction takes place

Odorous substances entering the nasal cavities dissolve in the moist mucus layer overlying the olfactory epithelium. These substances then interact with **odorant-binding proteins** immersed in the mucus layer. After diffusing through the mucus layer, the odorous substances interact with and bind to **odorant-receptor protein molecules** (transmembrane G-protein-coupled receptors) embedded in the plasmalemma of the ciliary membrane, where transduction takes place. Each olfactory receptor cell contains about a dozen identical receptors (all of them being identical structurally), all of which are coded by one gene. Each olfactory receptor cell contains only one type of receptor, however this same type of receptor may also be exhibited by thousands of other olfactory receptor cells distributed throughout the olfactory epithelium.

There are about 1,000 distinct olfactory receptors that make up the largest family of G-protein-coupled receptors. These receptors function in the detection of a wide range of odorous molecules. The binding of an odorous substance to the odorant-receptor protein molecules stimulates the initiation of a second messenger pathway associated with an olfactory-specific G-protein, which subsequently stimulates adenyl cyclase, which generates cAMP. The cAMP elevation unlocks a cyclic nucleotide-gated cation channel embedded in the ciliary membrane permitting sodium and calcium cations to pass into the cell (Fig. 19.2). This stimulates the **chemosensitive cilia** of the olfactory receptor cells and a wave of depolarization (generator potential) is propagated from the dendrites to the cell body of the olfactory receptor cell. A high enough depolarization triggers a nerve impulse that is propagated along the axon of the olfactory receptor cell, centrally to the olfactory bulb.

OLFACTORY NERVE (CN I)

Olfactory receptor cells give rise to unmyelinated axons, the slowest impulse-conducting axons of the CNS

Each olfactory receptor cell gives rise to an unmyelinated centrally directed axon. They are the slowest impulse-conducting axons of the central nervous system (CNS). The axons of these bipolar cells converge and assemble to form 15–20 bundles (fascicles)—the **olfactory fila** (L., "threads") (Fig. 19.1B). The olfactory fila course superiorly, traversing the sieve-like perforations of the cribriform plate of the ethmoid bone of the skull to terminate in the ventral surface of the ipsilateral **olfactory bulb**, where they synapse with second order neurons. Collectively, all the olfactory fila from each nasal cavity form the **olfactory nerve (CN I)** on both respective sides. The olfactory nerve fibers carry only **special visceral afferent** (SVA) modality, denoting the special sense of olfaction. The olfactory receptor cells are unique not only because they serve the functions of **sensory receptors** (chemoreceptors that become activated by chemical stimuli in their surroundings), **transducers** (generate graded potentials), and **first order neurons** (relaying olfactory sensation centrally to the olfactory bulbs), but also because they reside in a peripheral structure, the olfactory epithelium, instead of being housed within a sensory ganglion.

In addition to the sympathetic and parasympathetic innervation supplying the glands and blood vessels of the connective tissue, the olfactory mucosa also receives afferent sensory innervation from the trigeminal nerve. The free nerve endings of the peripheral trigeminal afferents ramify in the olfactory epithelium and the underlying lamina propria. Trigeminal fibers not only mediate pain sensations from the nasal mucosa, but are also believed to transmit noxious odor perception to subconscious levels, thus eliciting the autonomic secretomotor reflex in response to the presence of noxious chemicals (such as ammonia).

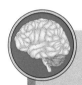

Note that the clinical case at the beginning of the chapter refers to a patient with a persistent loss of the sense of smell and taste following head trauma.

1 Which component of the olfactory system is most susceptible to injury during head trauma such as that sustained by the patient in this case?

CENTRAL CONNECTIONS OF THE OLFACTORY SYSTEM

Olfactory bulb

The olfactory bulbs, outgrowths of the telencephalon, receive the central processes (axon terminals) of the olfactory receptor cells

The **olfactory bulbs** are two oval-shaped, flattened structures located on the basal aspect of the frontal lobes, that are lodged in two fenestrated depressions formed by the cribriform plate of the ethmoid bone in the anterior cranial fossa. The two olfactory bulbs receive the central processes (axon terminals) of the first order olfactory receptor cells (see Fig. 19.1A) whose terminations are organized and mapped in an orderly manner. This is the **first relay station** of the olfactory system where synaptic integration occurs (Fig. 19.3). Since the olfactory bulbs are rostral dilations of the olfactory tracts, which are outgrowths of the telencephalon rather than typical cranial nerves, this first relay station of the olfactory system bypasses the diencephalon and is actually located in the cerebral cortex. (This situation is contrary to other sensory systems that normally project to regions of the diencephalon such as the thalamus, *prior* to the cortical projection.)

The olfactory bulbs are laminated structures consisting of five layers surrounding a center of white matter. The layers are: the **olfactory nerve layer**, which is the most superficial, the **glomerular layer**, the **external plexiform layer**, the **mitral cell layer**, and the deepest layer, the **inner plexiform layer** containing granule cells. This laminated cellular architecture

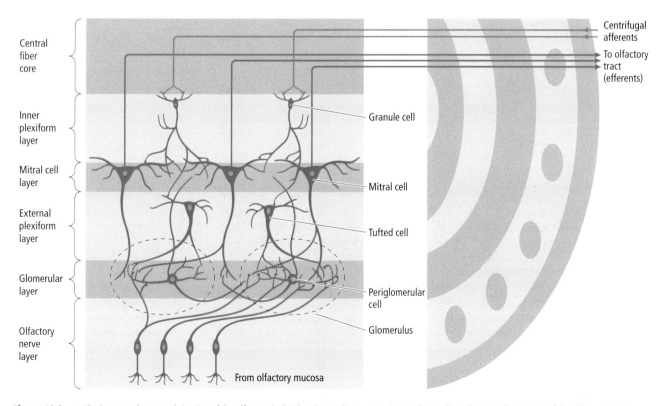

Figure 19.3 ● The layers and neuronal circuitry of the olfactory bulb. The glomeruli are synaptic complexes where the central processes of the olfactory receptor cells synapse with the neurons in the olfactory bulb.

is more clearly defined in animals other than humans, reflecting the exquisite olfactory system that these animals possess. The center of white matter of the olfactory bulb consists of *afferent* fiber terminals (centrifugal afferents), which have reached the bulb from other brain centers to modulate neural activity within the bulb, and *efferent* axons leaving the olfactory bulb via the **olfactory tract** to reach other cortical areas.

Olfactory receptor cell axons are highly convergent as they terminate in the glomeruli of the olfactory bulbs. **Glomeruli** (Fig. 19.3) are spherical synaptic complexes where olfactory receptor cell axons establish synapses with **interneurons** (the **juxtaglomerular, periglomerular cells**) and the **main relay second order neurons** of the bulb, the **mitral** and **tufted cells**. Each olfactory receptor cell has an input to several dendritic processes (residing in a glomerulus) of a single mitral or tufted cell. In the rabbit each glomerulus receives up to a thousand converging olfactory receptor cell axons. Neural activity involving combinations of glomeruli is responsible for the perception of a "single" odor. That is, if several sets of dendrites are stimulated, the "odor" perceived is different than if only one of those sets of dendrites is stimulated. The juxtaglomerular and periglomerular interneurons modulate the transmission of the sensory afferent information from the olfactory receptor cells that is communicated to the mitral and tufted cells. These interneurons also control mitral and tufted cell output by regulating the stream of signals that reach other brain centers from the olfactory bulb. The olfactory bulbs also receive **centrifugal fibers** providing biofeedback input from neurons residing in other sites of the CNS. Centrifugal afferent fibers are projected to the olfactory bulb from the **locus ceruleus**, the **medial** and **dorsal midbrain raphe nuclei**, the **medial septal nucleus**, and the **nuclei of the diagonal band of Broca**. Each olfactory bulb also receives sensory input from the olfactory bulb of the opposite side, which is first processed in the contralateral **anterior olfactory nucleus** (Fig. 19.4). This input is believed to adjust the capacity of the second order neurons and interneurons to respond to incoming signals.

Olfactory tract

The olfactory tract carries afferent fibers to the olfactory bulb and efferent fibers from both the olfactory bulb (mostly axons of the mitral and tufted cells) and the anterior olfactory nucleus

Each olfactory tract arises from the olfactory bulb, courses posteriorly, and diverges to form the **medial** and **lateral olfactory striae (tracts)** (Fig. 19.4). The two striae and a small region rostral to the anterior perforated substance collectively form a triangular-shaped region, the **olfactory trigone**.

The principal fibers carried by the **olfactory tract** are the *efferent* axons of second order output neurons of the bulb —the mitral and tufted cells. Others include the *afferent* centrifugal fibers.

Mitral and tufted cells occupying the olfactory bulb send collaterals to a cortical structure, the ipsilateral **anterior olfactory nucleus** located in the vicinity of the junction between the olfactory bulb and tract (Fig. 19.4). Efferent fibers

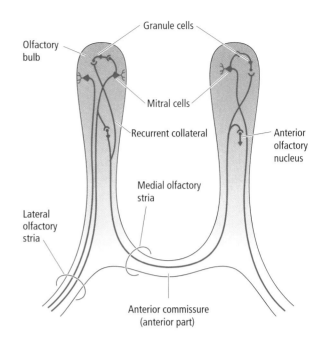

Figure 19.4 ● The olfactory bulb, anterior olfactory nucleus, and olfactory tract, and its division into the medial and lateral olfactory striae.

arising from neurons of this nucleus accompany the efferent axons of the mitral and tufted cells coursing in the olfactory tract. The fibers arising from the anterior olfactory nucleus project to both olfactory bulbs; some of these fibers project to the nearby ipsilateral olfactory bulb, whereas others join the medial olfactory stria and cross via the **anterior commissure** to terminate in the *contralateral* olfactory bulb and anterior olfactory nucleus. The majority of the fibers coursing in the medial olfactory stria are derived from neurons housed in the anterior olfactory nucleus. The medial olfactory stria also carries fibers from mitral and tufted cells, which terminate in the ipsilateral **anterior perforated substance** and the **medial septal nuclei**. These nuclei form connections with the limbic system and are therefore implicated in the *emotional* and *visceral response to odors* (to the great benefit of companies manufacturing perfumes).

The lateral olfactory stria, consisting primarily of mitral cell axons, is the **main central pathway of the olfactory system**. Its second order fibers project mostly to **paleocortical structures**.

Olfactory cortex

The primary olfactory cortex projects to the thalamus, which in turn projects to the orbitofrontal cortex

The **lateral olfactory stria**, consisting of second order fibers, projects mostly to **paleocortical structures** and the amygdala. The paleocortical structures that are targets of the lateral olfactory stria consist of parts of the **primary olfactory cortex** (the lateral olfactory gyrus and anterior half of the uncus, collectively referred to as the "**piriform cortex**") and the **periamygdaloid cortex**, which forms the rest of the olfactory component of the uncus and the **amygdala**

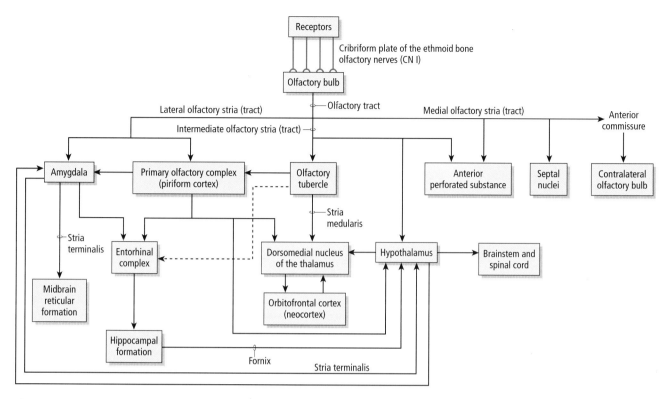

Figure 19.5 ● The connections of the olfactory system. The olfactory receptor cell axons pass through the cribriform plate of the ethmoid bone to terminate in the olfactory bulb. Each olfactory bulb is continuous posteriorly with the olfactory tract, which divides into the medial, intermediate, and lateral olfactory striae. From there, olfactory information is transmitted to the amygdala, the primary olfactory cortex, the olfactory tubercle, the anterior perforated substance, the septal nuclei, and the contralateral olfactory bulb via the anterior commissure. (Modified from Fix, JD (1995) *Neuroanatomy*, 2nd edn. Williams & Wilkins, Baltimore; fig. 20.1; and Burt, AM (1993) *Textbook of Neuroanatomy*. WB Saunders, Philadelphia; fig. 13.13.)

(Fig. 19.5). *Some* fibers terminate in the **lateral olfactory gyrus (nucleus of the lateral olfactory stria)**. However, *most* of the fibers terminate in the anterior half of the **uncus** forming part of the **primary olfactory cortex** located in the ventromedial aspect of the temporal lobe. Still other fibers terminate in the **amygdala** and the **anterior perforated substance**. The lateral olfactory stria also sends collaterals to the anterior olfactory nucleus and to subcortical limbic structures. The primary olfactory cortex (consisting of paleocortex) projects to the **dorsomedial nucleus of the thalamus**, which in turn projects mainly to the orbital gyri of the **orbitofrontal cortex** of the frontal lobe (the **neocortical** region of the olfactory system). However, the primary olfactory cortex also sends *direct* projections to the neocortex and is the only sensory system that *bypasses the thalamus* in projecting to the telencephalon.

The olfactory system neocortical projections terminating in the orbitofrontal cortex have an important function in the *conscious awareness of odors*. The neocortex functions as a correlating and coordinating center for the vast spectrum of sensory and motor input it receives from all sensory and motor systems (Fig. 19.5).

The primary olfactory cortex also projects to the **hypothalamus**, the amygdala, and the **olfactory association cortex (secondary olfactory cortex, entorhinal cortex)** located next to the primary olfactory cortex. The entorhinal cortex also receives *direct* projections from the olfactory tract. Functionally, the entorhinal cortex is closely associated with the hippocampus, affecting memory and emotional behavior. Projections to the hypothalamus are associated with sexual and maternal behavior.

CLINICAL CONSIDERATIONS

Anosmia, the complete loss of the sense of smell, or **hyposmia**, the partial loss of the sense of smell, may result following injury to the olfactory apparatus, ipsilateral to the lesion. These conditions may occur subsequent to head trauma, especially if there is fracture or damage to the cribriform plate of the ethmoid bone. In the event that the olfactory bulb becomes dislodged from its normal position, the delicate first order afferent fibers traversing the fenestrations of the cribriform plate of the ethmoid bone may be injured or torn. However, since these bipolar neurons retain the capacity to regenerate, they may successfully reconnect to the olfactory bulb and restore synaptic contacts in the appropriate layers of the bulb, resulting in the recovery of function and sense of smell.

Other prevalent conditions such as **rhinitis** or **sinusitis**, resulting from irritation and/or swelling of the nasal mucous membrane, may temporarily disrupt olfaction. Moreover, exposure to various contaminants may adversely affect olfaction. Extensive damage may result in permanent loss of the sense of smell. Nasal congestion resulting from a cold or viral infection may also affect the sense of smell. A complete loss of olfaction is usually accompanied by a partial or complete loss of gustation (taste), as commonly experienced during a bad cold when the individual is unable to taste food.

Individuals with lesions in the orbitofrontal cortex—the neocortex necessary for conscious awareness of odors—are able to detect the presence of odors but are unable to distinguish between different odorous substances.

A viral or bacterial infection in the ears, air sinuses, or throat may spread to the upper recesses of the nasal cavities introducing infectious agents into the cranial vault. The meningeal membranes may subsequently become infected spreading the infection to the subarachnoid space and cerebrospinal fluid, resulting in **meningitis**, a serious and life-threatening inflammation of the brain and its surrounding membranes, the meninges. The upper recesses of the nasal cavity communicate with the cranial vault via perforations of the cribriform plate of the ethmoid bone, which can serve as a conduit for the spread of infection, especially following head trauma involving the cribriform plate.

Individuals diagnosed with Alzheimer's disease, Parkinson's disease, or Huntington's disease, also experience a deterioration in olfactory function as a result of degenerating olfactory pathways. Individuals suffering from epilepsy may perceive odors that are not present or experience **parosmia**, a distorted perception of odors.

SYNONYMS AND EPONYMS OF THE OLFACTORY SYSTEM

Name of structure or term	Synonym(s)/eponym(s)
Amygdala	Amygdaloid nucleus
Interneurons	Internuncial neurons
Lateral olfactory gyrus	Nucleus of the lateral olfactory stria
Lateral olfactory stria	Lateral olfactory tract
Medial olfactory stria	Medial olfactory tract
Olfactory association cortex	Secondary olfactory cortex
	Entorhinal cortex
Olfactory epithelium	Olfactory neuroepithelium
Parosmia	Dysosmia
Plasmalemma	Cell membrane

FOLLOW-UP TO CLINICAL CASE

In this case the etiology of the patient's olfactory dysfunction is obvious: **head trauma**, which is a very common cause of olfactory dysfunction. Its cause is rarely of neurologic origin. The most common etiologies include upper respiratory infections, sinus disease, or any other nasal obstruction or congestion. Medications can induce loss of or alteration of the sense of smell. Neurodegenerative diseases such as Alzheimer's disease, Parkinson's disease, or Huntington's disease are also associated with loss of olfactory sensation.

Most cases of olfactory loss caused by head trauma are thought to arise from shearing injury to the olfactory nerve fibers as they pass through the cribriform plate of the ethmoid bone. However, it can also arise from injury to the olfactory bulbs, olfactory tracts, or the frontal or temporal lobes. An individual is often unaware of unilateral loss of olfactory sensation in only one nostril but it becomes noticeable when the lesion is bilateral. Olfactory dysfunction occurs in approximately 5–10% of patients with head trauma.[1] Loss of and/or alteration of the sense of smell can occur. There is some correlation between the severity of head trauma and the presence of, or the degree of, olfactory disturbance.[2]

Patients with a loss of the sense of smell often complain of loss of, or alteration in, taste as well. However, loss of taste sensation to sweet, sour, salty, and bitter is much rarer than olfactory dysfunction. Trigeminal nerve endings in the nasal membranes detect irritants. Therefore, to only test olfactory function, nonirritating substances such as coffee or vanilla should be used. Ammonia or vinegar are irritants and can be detected through the trigeminal nerve endings.

Recovery of normal olfactory function in cases caused by head trauma is rare. There is no effective treatment.

1 Costanzo RM, Zasler ND (1991) Head trauma. In: Getchell TV, ed. *Smell and Taste in Health and Disease*. New York: Raven: 711–30.
2 Doty RL, Yousem DM, Pham LT, Kreshak AA, Geckle R, Lee WW (1997) Olfactory dysfunction in patients with head trauma. *Archives of Neurology* **54**: 1131–40.

2 Besides head trauma what are some other causes that may lead to loss of the sense of smell?

3 What is the likelihood of the recovery of normal olfactory function following head trauma?

QUESTIONS TO PONDER

1. What makes the olfactory receptor cells unique?

2. Where are the odorant-binding proteins located?

3. Where are the odorant-receptor molecules located?

4. How many types of receptors are located in the ciliary membrane of a single olfactory receptor cell?

5. Describe the events following the binding of an odorous substance to an odorant-receptor protein.

CHAPTER 20

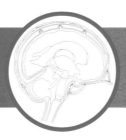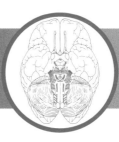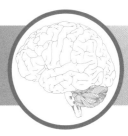

Limbic System

CLINICAL CASE

A 38-year-old woman complained to her primary care physician of two separate attacks during which she experienced fear and anxiety. These occurred suddenly without warning or precipitation by any circumstance. These episodes were brief, lasting a minute or so each. She noted increasing levels of anxiety and irritability even in between these attacks. Friends and family were concerned about her increasingly "odd" behavior and unprovoked outbursts of anger. There were brief episodes during which she became incoherent. There was concern about panic attacks or even a more severe psychiatric condition such as schizophrenia.

The patient had another attack that was witnessed by a friend. There was a sudden feeling of fear and anxiety as in the prior attacks, accompanied by agitation and crude verbalizations. This quickly progressed to loss of responsiveness and convulsive activity that lasted for less than a minute. After this episode she had a neurologic evaluation and testing.

The **limbic system** consists of a diverse group of structures including phylogenetically ancient cortical areas, a group of associated subcortical nuclei, as well as associated pathways that interconnect regions of the telencephalon, diencephalon, and brainstem. A major function of the limbic system is to modulate the hypothalamus.

As a result of its complex nature and widespread connections, the areas considered to constitute the limbic system are sometimes inconsistent among authors; however, the structures most commonly included under the limbic system are the cingulate, subcallosal, parahippocampal, and dentate gyri, the hippocampus proper, the subiculum, the amygdaloid body, the septal area, and some nuclei of the thalamus and hypothalamus (Table 20.1). The two main structures of the limbic system are the **hippocampal formation** (which includes the **hippocampus proper**, the **dentate gyrus**, and the **subiculum**) and the **amygdala**. The hippocampal formation is involved in the consolidation of short-term memory into long-term memory, whereas the amygdala regulates emotional expression via modulation of the hypothalamus. An emotion (L. emovere, "to disturb") is an intense subjective sensation—including anger, distress, excitement, fear, happiness, hate, love, or sadness—that may be felt toward another individual or an object. The behavioral expression of emotions is usually accompanied by physiological (visceral and/or somatic) responses.

Associated pathways such as the alveus, fimbria of the fornix, fornix, perforant pathway, cingulum, septohippocampal tract, ventral amygdalohypothalamic tract, mammillothalamic tract (mammillary fasciculus), mammillointerpeduncular tract, mammillotegmental tract, stria terminalis, and stria medullaris thalami, are also included in the limbic system (Table 20.1).

The limbic system, which is unique to mammals, functions in: (i) *species preservation*, which includes reproduction and associated instinctive behavior; (ii) *self-preservation*,

Table 20.1 ● Components of the limbic system.

Structure	Components
Cortex	Limbic lobe
	Cingulate gyrus
	Subcallosal gyrus
	Parahippocampal gyrus
	Hippocampal formation
	Dentate gyrus
	Hippocampus proper (Ammon's horn, cornu ammonis)
	Subiculum (subicular cortex)
Nuclei	Amygdaloid body (nucleus, complex)
	Septal nuclei (nuclear complex)
	Some thalamic nuclei
	Some hypothalamic nuclei
Pathways	Alveus
	Fimbria
	Fornix
	Perforant pathway
	Cingulum
	Septohippocampal tract
	Ventral amygdalohypothalamic tract
	Mammillothalamic tract (mammillary fasciculus)
	Mammillointerpeduncular tract
	Mammillotegmental tract
	Stria terminalis
	Stria medullaris thalami

which includes feeding behavior and aggression; and (iii) the *expression of fear*, *motivation*, and other emotions, as well as *memory* and *learning*. The limbic system not only exerts its influence on the expression of emotions, but also via its extensive connections with the hypothalamus (which integrates the functions of the endocrine and the autonomic nervous system). This influences the corresponding visceral responses (i.e., increase in heart rate and breathing, sweating, etc.), which supplement the expression of emotion.

The limbic system generates the emotional background for intellect. Furthermore, it serves to balance emotional and cognitive mechanisms. The limbic system, also referred to as the "visceral brain," processes information about a certain situation and then, via its visceral control, produces visceral responses. What a person "knows" or "thinks" is mediated by the neocortex.

Since the limbic system is involved in diverse functions and consists of intricate interconnections, it is often difficult to associate a particular component of the limbic system with a particular function.

LIMBIC LOBE

The limbic lobe consists of the subcallosal, cingulate, and parahippocampal gyri, as well as the hippocampal formation, collectively forming a cortical perimeter around the corpus callosum

The **limbic lobe** (L. limbus, "border") (Fig. 20.1) was characterized by Broca in 1878 as a composite of cortical structures ("le grand lobe limbique") that formed a transitional border intervening between the centrally positioned diencephalon and

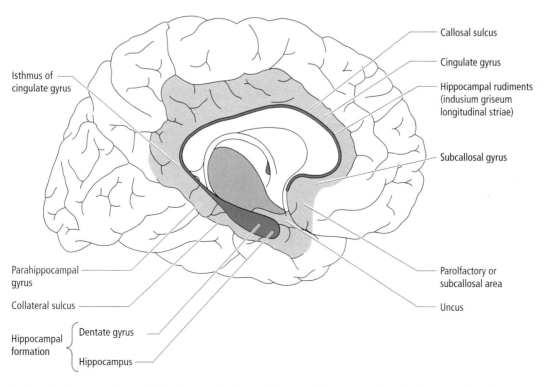

Figure 20.1 ● The cortical structures of the limbic lobe: the subcallosal, cingulate, and parahippocampal gyri and the hippocampal formation.

the overlying telencephalon. The limbic lobe consists of the **subcallosal**, **cingulate**, and **parahippocampal gyri**, as well as the **hippocampal formation**, all of which collectively form a cortical perimeter around the corpus callosum. The subcallosal and parahippocampal gyri consist of **neocortex** (G. neo, "new"); the cingulate gyrus consists of **mesocortex** (G. mesos, "middle," "intermediate"); and the hippocampal formation consists of **archicortex** (G. archein, "beginning," "original," "primitive") (Table 20.2). Neocortex is phylogenetically new, whereas the archicortex consists of ancient cortex. The mesocortex is a transitional cortex positioned between the archicortex and neocortex. The limbic lobe is considered to be a component of the more extensive limbic system.

Table 20.2 • Cortical components of the limbic lobe.

Part of cortex	Components

Allocortex	Archicortex
	    Hippocampal formation
	        hippocampus proper
	        dentate gyrus
	        subiculum
	Paleocortex
	    Piriform cortex of the
	        parahippocampal gyrus

Juxtallocortex	Mesocortex Cingulate gyrus

Isocortex	Neocortex
	    Subcallosal gyrus
	    Parahippocampal gyrus

Subcallosal, cingulate, and parahippocampal gyri

The **subcallosal gyrus** consists of gray matter, which underlies the basal surface of the rostral extent of the corpus callosum (Fig. 20.1). It curves superiorly around the genu of the corpus callosum and then extends posteriorly, superior to the corpus callosum, as the **cingulate gyrus**. At its posterior inferior extent, the cingulate gyrus in turn continues as the **parahippocampal gyrus**.

Hippocampal formation

The hippocampal formation consists of three regions: the hippocampus proper, the dentate gyrus, and the subiculum

The **hippocampal formation** consists of three regions, the **hippocampus proper** (also referred to as the **hippocampus**, **Ammon's horn**, or **cornu ammonis**), the **dentate gyrus**, and the **subiculum (subicular cortex)** (Fig. 20.1; Table 20.3). Structures associated with the hippocampal formation, via neuroanatomical connections, include the **entorhinal cortex**, the **supracallosal gyrus (indusium griseum)**, **fasciola cinerea (gyrus fasciolaris)**, and the **septal area** (a primitive precommissural area). The hippocampal formation extends from the amygdala anteriorly to the splenium of the corpus callosum posteriorly. On cross (coronal) section, its intrinsic structure is most striking in its middle third.

The hippocampal formation consists of archicortex, which during the early stages of its development scrolls inferiorly and medially on the floor of the lateral ventricle (Fig. 20.2). The function of the hippocampal formation in recent memory and learning is well established.

Component	Layers	Cell bodies	Dendrites	Axon terminals
Hippocampus proper	Molecular (deepest)		Pyramidal cell apical dendrites	Granule cells of dentate gyrus ("mossy fibers") Perforant pathway Septohippocampal tract Pyramidal cell axon collateral branches
	Pyramidal (middle) Polymorphic (superficial)	Pyramidal cells Interneurons	Pyramidal cell basal dendrites	Pyramidal cell axon collateral branches
Dentate gyrus	Molecular (outer)	Some	Apical dendrites of granule cells	Perforant pathway Alveus Collateral branches of granule cells
	Granule cell (middle) Polymorphic (deepest)	Granule cells Interneurons		
Subiculum	Three-layered cortex next to hippocampus Six-layered cortex next to parahippocampal gyrus			

Table 20.3 • The hippocampal formation.

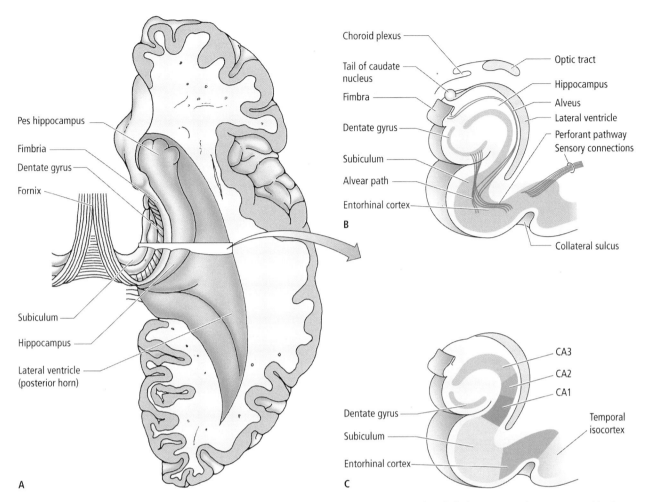

Figure 20.2 ● (A) Dissection of the right cerebral hemisphere illustrating the interior of the lateral ventricle with the hippocampus, dentate gyrus, and fornix. (B) Coronal section exposing the fiber pathways. (C) Coronal section exposing the three sectors of the hippocampus proper.

Hippocampus proper

The hippocampus proper is a phylogenetically ancient cortical structure that forms a comma-shaped prominence on the floor and medial wall of the temporal (inferior) horn of the lateral ventricle

The **hippocampus proper** (G. hippocampus, "seahorse") is a phylogenetically ancient cortical structure that forms a comma-shaped prominence on the floor and medial wall of the temporal (inferior) horn of the lateral ventricle. The hippocampus is an infolding of the cortex of the human brain, embedded within the parahippocampal gyrus of the temporal lobe. The ventricular surface of the hippocampus is coated with an ependymal layer. At its anterior extent, the hippocampus displays a swelling with several grooves resembling a paw, and is thus referred to as the **pes hippocampus** (L. pes, "foot"). The hippocampus extends from the amygdala anteriorly, and then tapers as it courses posteriorly to the inferior surface of the splenium of the corpus callosum.

On coronal section (Fig. 20.3A), the hippocampus appears similar to a seahorse as a result of its arched form, thus its name. Due to its C-shaped outline in coronal section, the hippocampus also resembles a ram's horn, and is called Ammon's horn (cornu ammonis or CA) after an Egyptian deity with a ram's head.

Layers of the hippocampus proper

The hippocampal archicortex consists of three layers

When viewed in transverse (coronal) section, the hippocampus (consisting of archicortex), displays three zones: CA1, CA2, and CA3 (Fig. 20.2C). The hippocampus of the human brain also consists of an additional zone, CA4. Based on their cytoarchitectural characteristics, these zones are of importance to researchers. Area CA1 lies next to the subiculum, whereas CA3 lies close to the dentate gyrus. The hippocampal archicortex consists of three layers: the **molecular**, **pyramidal**, and **polymorphic layers** (Fig. 20.3A; Table 20.3).

Molecular layer

The molecular layer is the deepest layer of the hippocampal archicortex and is located in the core of the hippocampal formation; it merges with the molecular layer of the dentate gyrus and neocortex

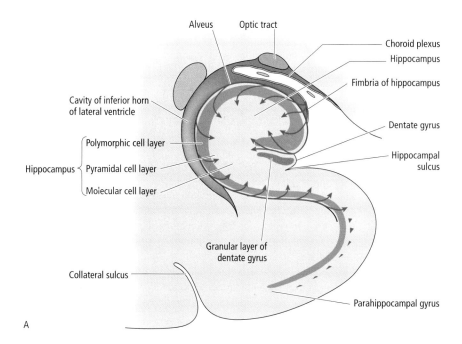

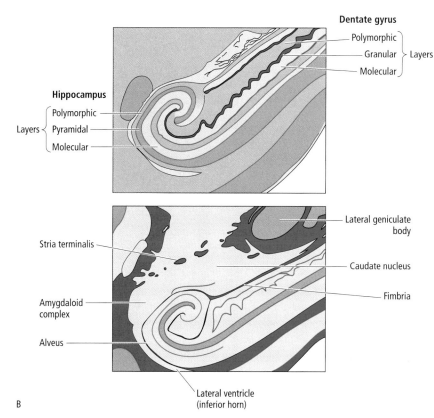

Figure 20.3 ● (A) Coronal section through the hippocampus and its associated structures. (Modified from Snell, RS (1997) *Clinical Neuroanatomy for Medical Students*, 4th edn. Lippincott–Raven, New York; fig. 16.4.) (B) Sagittal sections of the hippocampal formation illustrating the association of the hippocampus and dentate gyrus to the inferior horn of the lateral ventricle, the caudate nucleus, and the amygdala. The respective layers of the hippocampus and the dentate gyrus are illustrated in the top view.

The **molecular layer** (the deepest layer), which is located in the core of the hippocampal formation, consists of apical dendritic trees and axon terminals. The apical dendrites belong to hippocampal pyramidal cells (see below). The axon terminals belong to granule cells whose cell bodies reside in the granule cell layer of the dentate gyrus, the perforant pathway arising in the entorhinal cortex, the septohippocampal tract arising from the septal area, and the pyramidal cell axon collateral branches, arising from the pyramidal cell layer of the hippocampus. This layer merges with the molecular layer of the dentate gyrus and the neocortex.

Pyramidal layer

The pyramidal layer is the middle, most prominent, layer of the hippocampal archicortex; it merges with the internal pyramidal layer of the neocortex

The **pyramidal layer** (the middle layer) is the most prominent layer of the hippocampal formation and consists of **pyramidal cells**. Their dendrites ramify in the molecular layer, whereas their axons pass in the opposite direction, across the polymorphic layer, and then course in the alveus, fimbria, and the fornix. Pyramidal cell axon collateral branches, referred to as **Schaffer collaterals**, cross the polymorphic and pyramidal layers to reach the molecular layer where they form synaptic contacts with the dendrites of other pyramidal neurons. The pyramidal layer of the hippocampal formation merges with the internal pyramidal layer of the neocortex.

Polymorphic layer

> The polymorphic layer of the hippocampal archicortex is the superficial layer, consisting of interneurons

The **polymorphic layer** (the superficial layer) shares structural characteristics with the deepest layer of the neocortex. This layer lies deep to the alveus and consists of interneurons, as well as pyramidal cell dendrites and axon collateral branches.

Dentate gyrus

> The dentate gyrus gets its name from its tooth-like configuration, created by numerous blood vessels that pierce the ventricular surface of the hippocampus and dentate gyrus

The **dentate gyrus** (L. dentate, "tooth-shaped") (see Fig. 20.3; Table 20.3) is a notched band of cortex that is interposed between the upper aspect of the parahippocampal gyrus and the fimbria. This gyrus gets its name from its tooth-like configuration created by numerous blood vessels that pierce the ventricular surface of the hippocampus and then the dentate gyrus, which imparts a notched appearance. Dorsally, the dentate gyrus courses along with the fimbria near the splenium of the corpus callosum where it extends to the indusium griseum. Anteriorly, the dentate gyrus extends to the uncus of the parahippocampal gyrus.

Layers of the dentate gyrus

Similar to the hippocampus, the dentate gyrus also consists of three layers of archicortex. They are an outer **molecular layer**, a middle **granule cell layer** (corresponding to the pyramidal layer of the hippocampus), and a deep **polymorphic layer** (see Fig. 20.3B).

Molecular layer

The **molecular layer** of the dentate gyrus archicortex consists mainly of a small population of nerve cell bodies and granule cell dendrites.

Granule cell layer

> The granule cell layer of the dentate gyrus archicortex contains the cell bodies of granule cells whose axons form the output of the dentate gyrus

The **granule cell layer** consists of the cell bodies of the **granule cells**, the most predominant cell type of the dentate gyrus. The dendritic arborizations of the granule cells ramify in the molecular layer of the dentate gyrus where they form synapses with the terminals of the perforant pathway. The axons of the granule cells (the output neurons of the dentate gyrus), give rise to collateral branches, then exit the dentate gyrus, pass into the molecular layer of the hippocampus as **mossy fibers** and terminate on the dendrites of the pyramidal cells of the hippocampus. *The hippocampus is the only target of the dentate gyrus output.* A large number of the collateral branches project to the molecular layer of the dentate gyrus.

An area of the dentate gyrus known as the **hilus** merges with the polymorphic layer of the CA3 zone of the hippocampus. The hilus consists of interneurons and granule cell axons.

A cross-section of the hippocampal formation exhibits a perceptible double interlocking C. This salient characteristic of the hippocampal formation results from the interlocking of the prominent **pyramidal layer** of the hippocampus proper and the granule cell layer of the dentate gyrus.

Polymorphic layer

The **polymorphic layer** of the dentate gyrus archicortex consists of interneurons.

Subiculum

> The subiculum is a thin band of cortex interposed between the hippocampus proper and the parahippocampal gyrus of the temporal lobe

The **subiculum** is a transitional zone that displays a three-layered archicortex next to the hippocampus, but progressively becomes a more elaborate six-layered neocortex as it approaches the parahippocampal gyrus. The subiculum receives information relayed by the hippocampal pyramidal cells. It gives rise to fibers that join the fornix and terminate in the mammillary nuclei of the hypothalamus, and the anterior nuclear group of the thalamus.

Structures associated with the hippocampal formation

Entorhinal cortex

> The entorhinal cortex gives rise to the most prominent input to the dentate gyrus

The **entorhinal cortex** (Brodmann's area 28) is located ventral to the amygdaloid body and the anterior half of the hippocampal formation. The entorhinal cortex exhibits distinguishing characteristics in two of its layers (layers II and IV) that are visible at light microscopy level. Layer II contains the cell bodies of large multipolar neurons that assemble to form multiple "islands" throughout this layer. Since this layer is close to the cortical surface, the cell islands protrude from the surface of the entorhinal cortex, appearing as tiny swellings, resembling the texture of lemon peel. These swellings are visible grossly. Unlike layer II, layer IV of the entorhinal cortex includes a dense fiber plexus that forms a distinct boundary between layer III, containing small pyramidal cells, and layer V, containing large pyramidal cells.

Widespread areas of the association cortex relay input to the entorhinal cortex and it is via the entorhinal cortex that these cortical association areas have access to the hippocampus and play a role in memory consolidation. The entorhinal cortex gives rise to the most prominent *input* to the **dentate gyrus** of the hippocampal formation via the **perforant pathway** arising from the lateral part of the entorhinal cortex and the **alvear pathway** arising from the medial part of the entorhinal cortex. These pathways are part of the intrinsic circuitry of the hippocampal formation.

Indusium griseum

> The subcallosal gyrus gives way to the indusium griseum, a slender stripe of gray matter that overlies and follows the contour of the superior surface of the corpus callosum in the midline

The **indusium griseum** (supracallosal gyrus) represents a portion of the hippocampal formation that remained attached to the corpus callosum during its development, as the rest of the hippocampal formation moved laterally, inferiorly, and then medially to its final position in the temporal lobe (Fig. 20.4). Dorsally, it curves around the splenium of the corpus callosum and then merges with the dentate and parahippocampal gyri by way of the fasciola cinerea. Two pairs of rudimentary stripes of indusium griseum white matter, the **medial** and **lateral longitudinal striae** arise and terminate in the hippocampal formation, and course bilaterally along the superior surface of the corpus callosum, lateral to the indusium griseum.

Fasciola cinerea

The **fasciola cinerea (gyrus fasciolaris)** (L. fasciola, "band;" cinereus, "ashen-hued") is a transitional zone of intervening cortex that joins the dentate gyrus with the indusium griseum (Fig. 20.5).

Septal area

The **septal area** is located in the telencephalon, in close proximity to the genu of the corpus callosum. This area, which is well developed in humans, includes the **septal nuclear complex** whose nuclei are gathered rostral to the anterior commissure. The septal nuclei are classified into two main groups, the **medial** and **lateral septal nuclei**, which are analogous with the deep telencephalic nuclei rather than the cortex. They are connected with the hippocampal formation via the fornix, and the hypothalamus via the medial forebrain bundle. Furthermore, the septal nuclei send fibers via the stria medullaris thalami to the habenular nucleus.

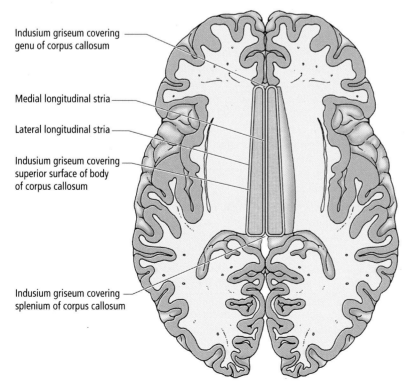

Indusium griseum covering genu of corpus callosum

Medial longitudinal stria

Lateral longitudinal stria

Indusium griseum covering superior surface of body of corpus callosum

Indusium griseum covering splenium of corpus callosum

Figure 20.4 ● Dissection of the superior surface of the cerebrum to reveal the superior surface of the corpus callosum. (Modified from Snell, RS (1997) *Clinical Neuroanatomy for Medical Students*, 4th edn. Lippincott–Raven, New York; fig. 16.4.)

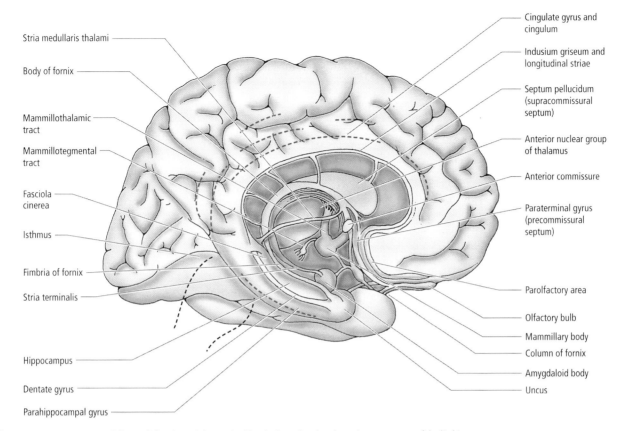

Stria medullaris thalami

Body of fornix

Mammillothalamic tract

Mammillotegmental tract

Fasciola cinerea

Isthmus

Fimbria of fornix

Stria terminalis

Hippocampus

Dentate gyrus

Parahippocampal gyrus

Cingulate gyrus and cingulum

Indusium griseum and longitudinal striae

Septum pellucidum (supracommissural septum)

Anterior nuclear group of thalamus

Anterior commissure

Paraterminal gyrus (precommissural septum)

Parolfactory area

Olfactory bulb

Mammillary body

Column of fornix

Amygdaloid body

Uncus

Figure 20.5 ● Dissection of the medial surface of the cerebral hemisphere showing the main components of the limbic system.

Afferents (input) to the hippocampus proper

Afferent fibers to the hippocampus proper arise from the following sources (Table 20.4): the indusium griseum, cingulate gyrus, septal nuclei, the entorhinal cortex, the dentate gyrus, the parahippocampal gyrus, and the contralateral hippocampus.

Efferents (output) from the hippocampus proper

Efferent fibers of the hippocampus proper arise mostly from the pyramidal cells of the hippocampal pyramidal cell layer

Table 20.4 ● Connections of the hippocampus.

Input sources to the hippocampus	Output targets of the hippocampus
Indusium griseum	Septal nuclei
Cingulate gyrus	Lateral preoptic area of the hypothalamus
Septal nuclei	Anterior part of the hypothalamus
Entorhinal cortex	Mammillary body
Dentate gyrus	Anterior nuclear group of the thalamus
Parahippocampal gyrus	Midbrain tegmentum
Contralateral hippocampus	Habenular nuclei

Efferent fibers of the hippocampus proper (Table 20.4) arise mostly from the pyramidal cells of its pyramidal cell layer. Their axons course in the alveus, fimbria, and fornix, which distributes them to various nuclei. Axons coursing anterior to the anterior commissure terminate in the septal nuclei, the lateral preoptic area of the hypothalamus, and the anterior part of the hypothalamus. Axons coursing posterior to the anterior commissure are distributed to the mammillary body, the anterior nuclear group of the thalamus, and the tegmentum of the mesencephalon. Some hippocampal fibers terminate in the habenular nuclei. A second pathway, the **hippocampo-entorhino-neocortical pathway**, emerges from the hippocampus proper and follows the perforant path back to deeper layers of the entorhinal cortex and from there to the neocortex (Fig. 20.6). This pathway is involved in the consolidation of episodic memories.

Intrinsic circuitry of the hippocampal formation

Widespread areas of the neocortex, particularly the cingulate gyrus, relay signals via the cingulum to the entorhinal cortex

The components of the hippocampal formation (the hippocampus proper, dentate gyrus, and subiculum) serve as successive processing stations in a series of local projections within the hippocampal formation. This local circuit consists of a pathway that arises from the entorhinal cortex.

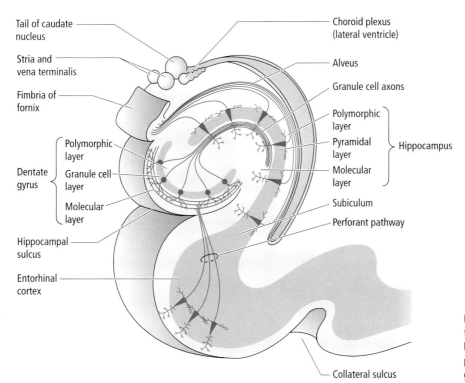

Figure 20.6 ● A transverse section through the temporal lobe at the level of the hippocampus and dentate gyrus. The main pathways connecting the hippocampus, dentate gyrus, and entorhinal cortex are shown.

Although the intrinsic circuitry of the hippocampal formation consists primarily of a closed loop of signal transmission, collateral branches and feedback connections are also present along this pathway, which serve to modify the relay of signals within the hippocampal formation (Figs 20.6, 20.7).

Axons arising from the **entorhinal cortex** (of the parahippocampal gyrus) form the **perforant** and **alvear pathways** (also known as the **lateral** and **medial perforant pathways**, respectively), which end in the molecular layer of the **dentate gyrus**, where their fibers synapse with the dendrites of its **granule cells**. Furthermore, these axons also send collaterals to the **CA1** and **CA3** zones of the hippocampus and the **subiculum**. *The entorhinal cortex provides the major input to the hippocampal formation.*

The granule cells of the dentate gyrus give rise to axons referred to as **mossy fibers**, which project not only to the CA3 zone of the hippocampal formation where they synapse with **pyramidal cells**, but also to its own **polymorphic layer**. The dentate gyrus polymorphic-layer neurons give rise to fibers that synapse with the dendrites and cell bodies of the granule cells, modifying the information relayed by the granule cells. Note that the *dentate gyrus projects only locally*, and does not project outside the hippocampal formation.

The pyramidal cells of the CA3 zone give rise to axons that join the **fimbria**. Prior to joining the fimbria, these axons emit **Schaefer collaterals** that project within CA3, and to the CA1 zone of the hippocampal formation (to synapse with the pyramidal cells there), as well as to the **septal nuclei**.

The pyramidal cells of the CA1 zone send their axons to the subiculum (subicular cortex). The subiculum in turn projects to the deeper layers of the entorhinal cortex, completing a closed circuit. The cells in the deeper layers of the entorhinal

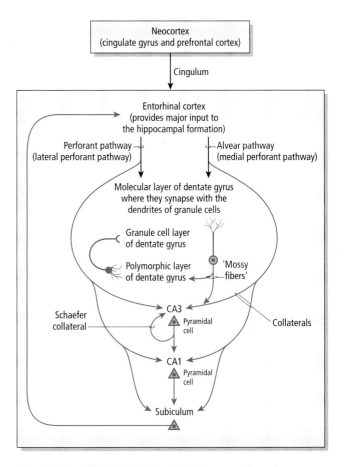

Figure 20.7 ● The intrinsic circuitry of the hippocampal formation.

cortex in turn give rise to axons that project to the superficial layers of the entorhinal cortex. The superficial layers of the entorhinal cortex then give rise to the perforant pathway. The entorhinal cortex also gives rise to a prominent projection to **neocortical association areas**.

Widespread areas of the cerebral cortex project to the entorhinal cortex, which in turn relays this input to specific areas of the hippocampal formation. Association (intrinsic) connections link different areas of the hippocampal formation, whereas commissural fibers link the hippocampal formation of the two sides.

Papez circuit

The **Papez circuit** was proposed by James Papez in the 1930s as the neuroanatomical basis of emotion. Although it is known today that the connections of the limbic system are much more complex, this circuit served as a basis for more modern research. The Papez circuit consists of the following anatomical structures: the hippocampus, fornix, mammillary body, anterior nucleus of the thalamus, mammillothalamic tract, and cingulate gyrus.

The **hippocampal formation** sends fibers via the **fornix** to the **mammillary body**, and other nuclei of the hypothalamus. The mammillary body sends the majority of its output fibers via the **mammillothalamic tract** to the **anterior nuclear group of the thalamus**, which in turn projects to the **cingulate gyrus**. The cingulate gyrus projects back via the **cingulum** to the hippocampal formation, completing the circuit. This circuit, though, is not a closed one, since each relay station has numerous connections with other areas of the nervous system.

Function of the hippocampal formation in memory

Learning is the manner by which knowledge is acquired, and memory is the process by which knowledge is stored and is retrievable in the future. Memory is classified very broadly into **immediate**, **short-term**, and **long-term memory**. Newly learned information is initially stored into immediate or short-term memory, lasting for seconds and minutes, respectively. Recently learned information, if reinforced, may be conveyed and stored into long-term memory for a prolonged period of time, a function which is mediated by the hippocampal formation. Individuals who have lesions in the hippocampal formation are unable to transfer immediate and short-term memory into long-term memory. Learning and memory processes may be interrupted by trauma, cerebral anoxia, Alzheimer's disease, and amnestic confabulatory syndrome (Korsakoff's syndrome) involving the hippocampus.

Recent studies indicate that the mechanism by which short-term memory is assembled/converted into long-term memory may be **long-term potentiation**, a form of neuronal plasticity. Long-term potentiation is a physiological process that occurs at neuronal synaptic contacts, as follows. When a neuron transmits a succession of nerve impulses to another neuron, this persistent/continual stimulation increases the probability that the target neuron will be depolarized by this particular synapse and by additional synaptic contacts established on the target neuron. Depolarization of the target neuron may be due to a higher chance that neurotransmitter will be released by the presynaptic terminal and/or an enhanced response of the postsynaptic terminal. Long-term potentiation in the hippocampal formation has been established at the axon terminals of the perforant pathway (the main cortical input pathway to the hippocampal formation terminating in the **dentate gyrus**), and at the axon terminals of the **CA3 zone** pyramidal cells forming synaptic contacts on **CA1 zone** cells. Recall that the perforant pathway consists of cortical association fibers that emerge from the entorhinal cortex, and migrate to the molecular layers of the hippocampus and the dentate gyrus, where they synapse with pyramidal and granule cells, respectively. Long-term potentiation may be the physiological process via which certain types of memory are formed.

Amygdala (amygdaloid body, complex, nuclei)

The amygdala is divided into three groups of subnuclei, the basolateral (ventrolateral), corticomedial (dorsomedial), and central groups

The **amygdala** (G. amygdalon, "almond") (Fig. 20.8) is an almond-shaped group of nuclei located deep to the uncus of the parahippocampal gyrus anterior to the hippocampus and the temporal horn of the lateral ventricle. The amygdala is divided into three groups of subnuclei (Table 20.5): the large basolateral (ventrolateral) group, and the smaller corticomedial (dorsomedial) and central groups. The basolateral and corticomedial subnuclei receive *afferent* fibers, whereas the central group subnuclei give rise to *efferent* fibers. Each subnucleus has different connections and functions.

The basolateral and corticomedial subnuclei receive afferent fibers, whereas the central group subnuclei give rise to efferent fibers

The amygdala receives sensory input from widespread areas of the nervous system including somatosensory, visual, auditory, and visceral (such as olfactory) stimuli.

The **corticomedial (dorsomedial) nucleus** is the oldest phylogenetically. This nucleus is the termination of olfactory fibers arising from the olfactory bulb via the lateral olfactory stria, and the olfactory cortex. Since this nucleus projects to the ventromedial nucleus of the hypothalamus, it is believed to play a role in eating behaviors.

The **basolateral (ventrolateral) nucleus** is the newest phylogenetically. It is reciprocally connected to the cortical sensory association areas of all four lobes (the visual, auditory, and somatosensory systems) and projects to the medial dorsal nucleus of the thalamus, the basal nucleus (of Meynart), and the ventral striatum. This nucleus influences the various functions of the hypothalamus associated with feeding and drinking behavior, autonomic and somatic reflexes, and responses to stress.

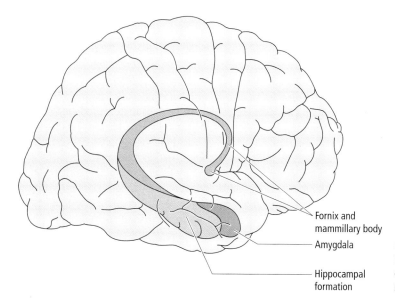

Fornix and
mammillary body

Amygdala

Hippocampal
formation

Figure 20.8 ● The relationship of the amygdala and hippocampal formation. The fornix, the principal efferent pathway of the hippocampal formation, and its termination, the mammillary body, are also shown.

Nucleus	Connections	Functions
Corticomedial (dorsomedial)	Afferents from olfactory bulb and olfactory cortex Efferents to the ventromedial nucleus of the hypothalamus	Behavior associated with hunger and eating
Basolateral (ventrolateral)	Reciprocally connected to the sensory association cortical areas Efferents to the medial dorsal nucleus of the thalamus, basal nucleus (of Meynart), and ventral striatum	Behaviors associated with eating and drinking Autonomic and somatic reflex activity Behavioral reaction to stressful situations
Central	Reciprocally connected to the visceral sensory and autonomic nuclei in the brainstem	Respiratory and cardiovascular responses

Table 20.5 ● Nuclei of the amygdaloid complex.

The basolateral and corticomedial nuclei project to the **central nucleus**. This nucleus has reciprocal connections with the visceral sensory and visceral motor nuclei located in the brainstem. The central nucleus gives rise to the ventral amygdalofugal pathway, which terminates in the autonomic nervous system nuclei of the brainstem. These include the **dorsal motor nucleus of the vagus**, as well as nuclei of the reticular formation involved in respiratory and cardiovascular functions.

Afferent projections to the amygdala

The amygdala receives *afferent* (input) fibers from the following sources (Table 20.6): olfactory bulb, orbitofrontal cortex, cingulate gyrus, basal forebrain, medial thalamus, hypothalamus, and brainstem.

Table 20.6 ● Connections of the amygdala.

Afferent projections to the amygdala	Efferent projections from the amygdala
Olfactory bulb Orbitofrontal cortex Cingulate gyrus Basal forebrain Medial thalamus Hypothalamus Brainstem	Hypothalamus Septal nuclei Ventral striatum Basal nucleus of Meynart

Efferent projections from the amygdala

The principal function of the limbic system is to modulate hypothalamic activity, and it does so via two main pathways, the stria terminalis and the ventral amygdalofugal (amygdaloid) pathway

One of the principal functions of the limbic system is to modulate hypothalamic activity, and this modulation is mediated via two main output pathways arising from the amygdala, which distribute fibers mainly to the hypothalamus, but also to sources of amygdalar input. These *efferent* pathways are: the **stria terminalis** (which conveys fibers primarily from the corticomedial nucleus to the septal nuclei and the hypothalamus) and the **ventral amygdalofugal (amygdaloid) pathway** (which also conveys input fibers to the amygdala) (Table 20.6). The latter pathway is less distinct, and distributes fibers from the central nucleus to the brainstem as well as fibers from the basolateral nucleus that terminate in the thalamus, ventral striatum, and basal nucleus. The signals arising from the striatum are ultimately relayed to the medial dorsal nucleus of the thalamus, which in turn projects to the prefrontal and orbitofrontal cortices. The limbic system projections to the deep cerebral nuclei are associated with underlying emotional aspects that influence movement.

Functions of the amygdala

One of the key roles of the amygdala is the control of ANS function in relation to previous experiences

One of the key roles of the amygdala is the control of autonomic nervous system (ANS) function in relation to previous experiences. ANS modulation is mediated indirectly by reciprocal projections between the amygdala and the hypothalamus (corticomedial nucleus), which in turn coordinates ANS activity, and directly via the descending pathways that arise from the amygdala and terminate in the brainstem autonomic centers (central nucleus).

The mode of amygdaloid control on ANS function differs from that of the hypothalamus (without amygdaloid input). Hypothalamic control of ANS activity is reflex in nature, continuously monitoring the body's internal environment via baroreceptors and osmoreceptors, and making appropriate adjustments, whereas control of ANS activity by the amygdala is mediated by instinct. The amygdala utilizes prior experiences to modulate ANS activity. The basolateral nucleus has abundant reciprocal projections with the sensory association areas of all four lobes and is associated with the processing of input related to past experiences. In contrast, the corticomedial nucleus projects to the hypothalamus, whereas the central nucleus projects to the brainstem. The amygdala, through its connections with the hypothalamus, influences the visceral and somatic aspects that correspond to the behavioral expression of emotion.

Table 20.7 ● Brainstem centers associated with limbic system function.

Structure	Function

Hypothalamic nuclei
    Mammillary nucleus
    Preoptic nucleus
	Control autonomic nervous system responses associated with the expression of emotions

Thalamic nuclei
    Anterior
    Lateral dorsal
    Medial dorsal
	Process information from the hypothalamus and amygdala, and relay information to the limbic lobe, prefrontal, and temporal areas

Habenular nuclei	Serve as relay centers for information arising from the limbic system destined for the midbrain reticular formation
Ventral tegmental area	Regulates processing of memory
Locus ceruleus	Regulates processing of memory
Dorsal raphe	Regulates processing of memory

BRAINSTEM CENTERS ASSOCIATED WITH LIMBIC SYSTEM FUNCTION

Hypothalamus

The hypothalamus mediates ANS (visceral) responses that accompany the expression of emotions

Various emotional states initiate intricate psychological, endocrine, and autonomic responses. The limbic system sends numerous projections to the hypothalamic nuclei, especially the mammillary and preoptic nuclei (Table 20.7). The hypothalamus in turn mediates ANS (visceral) responses that accompany the expression of emotions.

Thalamus

The amygdala and hypothalamus project to the "limbic nuclei" of the thalamus: the anterior nuclear group, and the lateral dorsal and medial dorsal nuclei of the thalamus

The amygdala and hypothalamus project to the "limbic nuclei" of the thalamus, which include the **anterior nuclear group** and the **lateral dorsal** and **medial dorsal nuclei** of the thalamus (Table 20.7). These nuclei then relay this information to the limbic lobe. Furthermore, the hippocampal formation receives *afferent* fibers from the anterior, lateral dorsal, lateral posterior, and intralaminar nuclei of the thalamus.

Habenular nuclei

The limbic system projects to the reticular formation of the mesencephalon via a relay in the habenular nuclei

The limbic system projects to the reticular formation of the mesencephalon via a relay in the **habenular nuclei**. These nuclei project to the **interpeduncular** and **raphe nuclei** of the mesencephalon via the **habenulointerpeduncular tract**. Other habenular efferent fibers terminate in the **hypothalamus**, the **ventral tegmental area**, and the **substantia nigra**.

Ventral tegmental area

The **ventral tegmental area** of the midbrain modulates the processing of memory via *dopaminergic* fibers that terminate in cortical areas related to the limbic system.

Locus ceruleus and dorsal raphe

The **locus ceruleus** sends *noradrenergic* fibers whereas the **dorsal raphe** sends *serotonergic* fibers to the hippocampal formation, limbic lobe, and amygdala, where they modulate the processing of memory.

PATHWAYS OF THE LIMBIC SYSTEM

A number of pathways connect the various components of, and areas associated with, the limbic system (Tables 20.1, 20.8). They are the alveus, fimbria, fornix, perforant pathway, cingulum, septohippocampal tract, ventral amygdalohypothalamic tract, mammillothalamic tract (mammillary fasciculus), mammillointerpeduncular tract, mammillotegmental tract, stria terminalis, stria medullaris (thalami), anterior commissure, diagonal band of Broca, and habenulointerpeduncular tract.

Alveus, fimbria, and fornix

The fornix is the main output pathway of the hippocampal formation relaying information to the hypothalamus and the septal nuclei

Deep to the ependymal layer overlying the ventricular surface of the hippocampal formation, there is a fine layer of white matter, the **alveus** (L., "trough," "canal"). The alveus is composed of a two-way bundle of myelinated axons, most of which belong to the pyramidal cells of the hippocampal formation. These axons gather to become the **fimbria** (L., "fringe"), which extends to the subsplenial area inferior to the corpus callosum. At the subsplenial area each hippocampus (right and left) proceeds as the **crus of the fornix** (L. crus, "leg;" fornix, "arch") (Fig. 20.9). The fornix consists of two crura, one on each side, which are joined by commissural fibers forming the **commissure of the fornix (hippocampal commissure)**. Anterior to the commissure of the fornix, the two crura approach one another and unite in the midline to become the

Pathway	Origin	Termination
Alveus	Pyramidal cells of the hippocampal formation	
Fimbria	Continuation of the alveus	
Fornix	Continuation of the fimbria	Hypothalamus Septal area
Perforant	Entorhinal cortex	Hippocampus proper Dentate gyrus
Cingulum	Cingulate gyrus	Neocortex
Septohippocampal tract	Medial septal nucleus Nuclei of the diagonal band of Broca	Hippocampus proper Dentate gyrus Subiculum Entorhinal cortex
Ventral amygdalohypothalamic tract	Amygdala	Hypothalamus
Mammillothalamic tract (mammillary fasciculus)	Mammillary body	Anterior nuclear group of the thalamus
Mammillointerpeduncular tract	Mammillary body	Interpeduncular nucleus
Mammillotegmental tract	Mammillary body	Midbrain tegmentum
Stria terminalis	Amygdala	Septal area Preoptic area of the hypothalamus Bed nucleus of the stria terminalis
Stria medullaris (thalami)	Habenular nuclei	Septal nuclei Anterior hypothalamus
Anterior commissure	Olfactory bulb Parahippocampal gyrus	Contralateral olfactory bulb and parahippocampal gyrus
Diagonal band of Broca	Parolfactory area	Periamygdaloid area
Habenulointerpeduncular tract	Habenular nucleus	Interpeduncular nucleus of the midbrain

Table 20.8 ● Pathways of the limbic system.

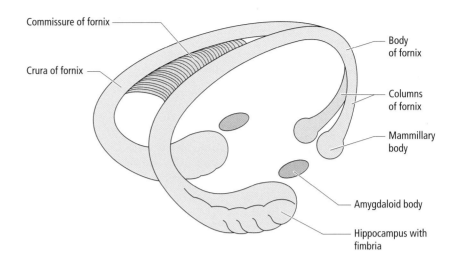

Commissure of fornix

Crura of fornix

Body of fornix

Columns of fornix

Mammillary body

Amygdaloid body

Hippocampus with fimbria

Figure 20.9 ● Three-dimensional view of the relationships between the hippocampus, the fornix, and the mammillary bodies.

body of the fornix. The body of the fornix courses anteriorly following the inferior edge of the septum pellucidum. At the level of the interventricular foramen (of Monro) and the anterior commissure, the fornix becomes arched, proceeding inferiorly and posteriorly diverging again into the **columns of the fornix**. As each column turns inferiorly on each side, it dives into the lateral wall of the third ventricle and then enters the mammillary body of the hypothalamus.

At the level of the anterior commissure, the fornix separates into a precommissural part that lies anterior to the anterior commissure, and a postcommissural part that lies posterior to the anterior commissure. The **precommissural fibers** take their origin primarily from the pyramidal cells of the hippocampus (although some fibers originate from the subiculum and entorhinal cortex) and project to the septal area and basal forebrain. The **postcommissural fibers** emerge from the subiculum, and then enter the hypothalamus where the majority of the fibers project primarily in the mammillary nucleus. Some fibers also terminate in the thalamus and other nuclei of the hypothalamus.

The **fornix** is the *main output* pathway of the hippocampal formation relaying information to the hypothalamus and the septal nuclei. Although most of the axons in the fornix are *efferents* to the ipsilateral hypothalamus and the septal area, some of the fibers are *afferents* to the hippocampus from various brain centers. In addition, the fornix carries commissural fibers to the habenular nuclei, and others connecting the hippocampal formation of the two sides.

Through its connections with the hypothalamus (which coordinates visceral and endocrine functions) and with the temporal lobe, the hippocampus can influence emotional behavior and memory, respectively.

Perforant pathway

The perforant pathway is the main cortical input pathway to the hippocampal formation

The **perforant pathway** (see Figs 20.6, 20.7) is the main cortical input pathway to the hippocampal formation. It consists of cortical association fibers that emerge from the entorhinal cortex, and migrate to the molecular layers of the

hippocampus and the dentate gyrus, where they synapse with pyramidal and granule cells, respectively.

Cingulum

The **cingulum** consists of cortical association fibers located on the deep aspect of the cingulate gyrus. It transmits information that interconnects the surrounding neocortex.

Septohippocampal tract

The **septohippocampal tract** carries fibers that arise from the medial septal nucleus and the nuclei of the diagonal band of Broca. These fibers join the fornix to terminate in the hippocampus, dentate gyrus, subiculum, and entorhinal cortex next to the hippocampal formation.

Ventral amygdalohypothalamic tract

The **ventral amygdalohypothalamic tract** is the main projection pathway from the amygdala to the hypothalamus, which it reaches by traversing the internal capsule.

Mammillothalamic tract (mammillary fasciculus)

The **mammillothalamic tract** is the principal output pathway arising from the hypothalamic mammillary nucleus. It consists of heavily myelinated axons that terminate in the anterior nuclear group of the thalamus.

Mammillointerpeduncular tract

The **mammillointerpeduncular tract** arises from the mammillary body and terminates in the interpeduncular nucleus.

Mammillotegmental tract

The **mammillotegmental tract** arises from the mammillary body and terminates in the midbrain tegmentum.

Stria terminalis

Fibers of the **stria terminalis** take their origin mainly from the amygdaloid body and terminate in the septal area, the medial preoptic area of the hypothalamus, and the bed nucleus of the stria terminalis.

Stria medullaris (thalami)

The **stria medullaris (thalami)** consists of fibers that interconnect the habenular nucleus with the septal nuclei and the anterior hypothalamus.

Anterior commissure

The **anterior commissure** carries decussating fibers transmitting olfactory information between the olfactory bulbs, as well as information between the parahippocampal gyri.

Diagonal band of Broca

The **diagonal band of Broca** consists of fibers that arise from the parolfactory area and terminate in the periamygdaloid area in the temporal lobe.

Habenulointerpeduncular tract (tractus retroflexus)

The **habenulointerpeduncular tract** arises from the habenular nucleus and terminates in the interpeduncular nucleus of the mesencephalon.

CLINICAL CONSIDERATIONS

Injury to the temporal lobes results in the inability to form new memories

Bilateral lesions of the hippocampus may be produced during a forceful impact of the anterior poles of the temporal lobes on the greater wings of the sphenoid bone. Injury to the temporal lobes results in the inability to form new memories.

Studies have shown that the pyramidal neurons in area CA1 of the hippocampal formation (referred to as **Sommer's sector**) are particularly susceptible to cell injury and death if blood oxygen concentration drops to low levels. Cell degeneration within CA1 occurs within 3–4 minutes as a consequence of the decrease in oxygen supply that occurs following a cardiac arrest to individuals who are resuscitated. Injury to the pyramidal cells of the hippocampal formation results in memory loss.

Bilateral lesion or removal of the medial temporal lobe including the amygdala and most of the hippocampal formation, has been performed in the past on individuals who have epileptic seizures. The hippocampus has an exceptionally low threshold for epileptic seizures, which may be transmitted to other parts of the limbic lobe and to the neocortex. Although this surgical treatment reduces the occurrence of seizures in these individuals, they are unable to learn anything or to form new memories, a condition referred to as **anterograde amnesia**. In addition, removal of the hippocampi results in **retrograde amnesia**, a condition in which there is a deficit in more recent memories, but not of those in the distant past. These findings have led to the conclusion that the hippocampal formation is necessary in the formation of long-term memories. It is believed that the hippocampus generates the drive and mediates the translation of short-term into long-term memories, which are stored in the neocortical association areas (visual association cortex, auditory association cortex, somatosensory association cortex, etc.).

Limbic system syndromes

Alzheimer's disease

Alzheimer's disease is a degenerative disorder of the brain and is the most common form of progressive dementia in the elderly

Alzheimer's disease is a degenerative disorder of the brain and is the most common form of progressive dementia in the elderly. Individuals with this disease are unable to form new memories.

This disease is caused by pathologic alterations, including neurofibrillary tangles, neuritic plaques, and neuronal degeneration, which appear initially in the pyramidal cell islands (of layer II) of the entorhinal cortex. From there, degeneration spreads to the CA1 zone of the hippocampus proper, and then back to the deeper layers of the entorhinal cortex. Consequently, this neuronal degeneration hinders the normal flow of information through the hippocampal formation. Confusion and deficits in executive function occur following further spread of neurofibrillary tangles to the temporal pole and prefrontal cortex. Subicular pathology occurs roughly at the same time that neurofibrillary tangles invade the temporal neocortex.

Amnestic confabulatory syndrome (Korsakoff's syndrome)

Amnestic confabulatory syndrome is a disorder that most often results from thiamin nutritional deficiency in chronic alcoholism

Amnestic confabulatory syndrome is a disorder that most often results from thiamin (vitamin B_1) nutritional deficiency in chronic alcoholism. Affected individuals have loss of recent memory, and to compensate for this when they converse, they make up fictitious information or events to fill in the gaps of memory loss. Morphological changes are reported in the hippocampal formation, the columns of the fornix, and the mammillary bodies of the hypothalamus. However, the area that exhibits the most drastic modification is the medial dorsal nucleus of the thalamus.

Klüver Bucy syndrome

Experiments performed on monkeys with bilateral temporal lobe lesions, which included the amygdala as well as the surrounding cortical areas that project to the amygdala, produced what is referred to as the **Klüver Bucy syndrome**. This syndrome, however, is rare in humans, and the following description refers to the original experimental findings. The most striking behavioral characteristics of this syndrome are: lack of fear and anger in previously wild animals, docility, changes in feeding behavior, sexual abnormalities, excessive oral curiosity in examining objects, and visual agnosia (the inability to recognize objects).

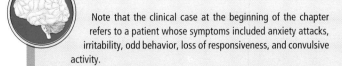

Note that the clinical case at the beginning of the chapter refers to a patient whose symptoms included anxiety attacks, irritability, odd behavior, loss of responsiveness, and convulsive activity.

1 Which part of the brain has a low threshold for epileptic seizures?

SYNONYMS AND EPONYMS OF THE LIMBIC SYSTEM

Name of structure or term	Synonym(s)/ eponym(s)
Amnestic confabulatory syndrome	Korsakoff's syndrome
	Korsakoff's psychosis
Amygdalofugal pathway	Amygdaloid pathway
Amygdaloid body	Amygdaloid nuclear complex
Archicortex	Archipallium
	Allocortex
Basolateral nuclear group of the amygdala	Ventrolateral nuclear group of the amygdala
Commissure of the fornix	Hippocampal commissure
Corticomedial nuclear group of the amygdala	Dorsomedial nuclear group of the amygdala
Fasciola cinera	Gyrus fasciolaris
Habenulointerpeduncular tract	Tractus retroflexus
Hippocampus proper	Hippocampus
	Ammon's horn
	Cornu ammonis
Mammillothalamic tract	Mammillary fasciculus
Mesocortex	Juxtallocortex
Neocortex	Neopallium
	Isocortex
	Homogenetic cortex
Paleocortex	Paleopallium
	Periallocortex
Stria medullaris	Stria medullaris thalami
Subiculum	Subicular cortex
Supracallosal gyrus	Indusium griseum
Telencephalon	Forebrain

FOLLOW-UP TO CLINICAL CASE

This patient initially had symptoms of a psychiatric disturbance and seemed to display some elements of psychosis. However, she then had another episode that began like the previous attacks but then clearly became a seizure. The knowledge that she had a seizure shifts the whole scheme of diagnostic possibilities. A seizure work-up was performed, including an electroencephalogram (EEG) and magnetic resonance imaging (MRI) of the brain.

The EEG showed epileptiform activity coming from the left anterior temporal region. The MRI revealed an astrocytoma in the left anteromedial temporal lobe. The patient underwent resection of the tumor. There were subsequently no more seizures and many, but not all, of her other psychological symptoms improved.

Psychological symptoms are very common in **epilepsy**. They often occur as an aura preceding the onset of more characteristic manifestations of seizure. However, the aura in this case is actually the beginning of the seizure. Fear, anxiety, anger, disorientation, bizarre behavior, altered perception, a feeling of *déjà vu*, and agitation are some of the more common manifestations. Psychological or emotional symptoms are associated with temporal lobe seizures, especially involving the anteromedial temporal lobe, and sometimes frontal lobe seizures. In fact, the most epileptogenic regions of the brain are the temporal and frontal lobes, especially the limbic regions. Thus epilepsy with emotional or psychological manifestations is occasionally confused with psychiatric disease.

Patients with epilepsy, especially temporal lobe epilepsy, sometimes display bizarre behaviors or personality or have psychological disturbances even between the seizures. This can occur in patients with lesions, such as tumors, in specific regions of the brain or even in patients without such lesions. This leads to the hypothesis that the temporal lobe, specifically the medial temporal lobe, may be structurally or physiologically abnormal even if no lesion is detected there.

Very fine resolution MRI imaging of the temporal lobes, using coronal images, often shows medial temporal sclerosis in those with chronic temporal lobe epilepsy. This shows up as subtle scarring and loss of volume of the parahippocampal gyri. There is a loss of neurons and gliosis in the hippocampus and to a variable degree in the surrounding structures.

2 Why are psychological symptoms common in epilepsy?

3 What does fine resolution MRI imaging of the temporal lobe of patients with chronic temporal lobe epilepsy show?

QUESTIONS TO PONDER

1. Distinguish between the limbic lobe and the limbic system.

2. What are the components of the hippocampal formation?

3. What causes the dentate gyrus to appear "tooth-shaped"?

4. Where do the cell bodies of the output neurons of the dentate gyrus reside?

5. What is the source of the most prominent input to the dentate gyrus?

6. What is the source of the efferent fibers of the hippocampus proper?

7. What is the function of the hypothalamus in the expression of emotions?

8. What is the main output pathway of the hippocampal formation?

9. What is the main cortical input pathway to the hippocampal formation?

10. Describe the cause and symptoms of Alzheimer's disease.

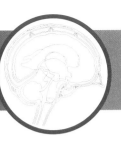
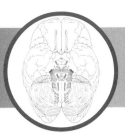
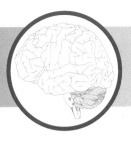

CHAPTER 21

Hypothalamus

CLINICAL CASE

A 23-year-old woman complains of daytime sleepiness and poor sleep at night. Sometimes she has an uncontrollable urge to sleep during the daytime. When she feels sleepy, she takes 5–15-minute naps and feels somewhat refreshed upon awakening. These episodes occur a few times per week. She has also noticed that occasionally her body feels somewhat limp and her head drops. These episodes last only a few seconds and seem to be prompted by laughing, getting very angry, or excited. A few times she has noticed brief episodes of complete paralysis while lying in bed at night prior to falling sleep. Sometimes she has strange and occasionally frightening visual hallucinations before she drifts off to sleep at night. She usually wakes up a few times each night. Her most disabling symptom is the daytime sleepiness, which interferes with her ability to concentrate. These symptoms began several years ago. Family history is negative. She is not taking any medications or drugs.

The general physical and neurologic exam is normal. MRI of the brain is normal.

The **hypothalamus**, a subdivision of the diencephalon, weighs approximately 4 g, and forms less than 1% of the brain's total weight. Although this small region of the brain may seem trivial, it is, on the contrary, the center of numerous, and various, very important functions associated with the survival of the organism, and continuation of the species.

The hypothalamic functions that are crucial to the survival of the organism include the control of appetite, fluid balance, electrolyte balance, glucose concentration, metabolism, sleeping, and body temperature regulation. In addition, hypothalamic function is associated with the continuation of the species, since it plays a role in sexual behavior. The hypothalamus mediates these functions by integrating the functions of the endocrine, autonomic (visceral motor), somatic motor, and limbic systems.

The hypothalamus maintains **homeostasis**, a state of constant internal environment (physiological equilibrium), and responds to both neural and non-neural stimulation. The hypothalamus consists of a group of nuclei each playing a role in one or more of the above functions. Some nuclei consist of neurons that receive and respond to neural input from widespread areas of the nervous system. Other nuclei consist of neurons that respond to non-neural input, such as fluctuations in the temperature, osmotic pressure, and hormone levels of the circulating blood. During stressful situations, however, this state of equilibrium may be disturbed. The body is equipped with receptors that detect changes in various physiological systems. The hypothalamus in turn, through its connections with the endocrine, autonomic, and limbic systems, mediates corrective mechanisms that compensate for the imbalance, and aid the body in restoring physiological equilibrium. Furthermore, through its extensive interconnections with the limbic system, the hypothalamus plays an important role in memory and emotional behavior, and mediates the appropriate visceral responses, such as changes in heart rate and blood pressure, accompanying behavioral expression. For example, an individual who is feeling anxious, experiences an increase in heart rate and breathing.

iorly, the interpeduncular fossa; *superiorly*, the hypothalamic sulcus; *inferiorly*, the tuber cinereum (L., "gray swelling"), *medially*, the third ventricle, and *laterally*, the substantia innominata, subthalamic nucleus, and internal capsule.

HYPOTHALAMIC ZONES AND COMPONENT NUCLEI

The hypothalamus is divided sagittally from medial to lateral into **periventricular**, **medial**, and **lateral zones** for descriptive purposes (Table 21.1). Two prominent, heavily myelinated fiber bundles associated with the hypothalamus—the **mammillothalamic tract** and the column of the **fornix**—form a conspicuous boundary between its medial and lateral zones (Fig. 21.3).

BORDERS

The hypothalamus is located anterior and inferior to the thalamus, surrounding the narrow anterior ventral portion of the third ventricle

The following structures form the borders of the hypothalamus (Figs 21.1, 21.2): *anteriorly*, from superior to inferior, the anterior commissure, lamina terminalis, and optic chiasma; *poster-*

Periventricular zone

The periventricular zone is located next to the midline and consists of numerous small nuclei

The **periventricular zone** is located next to the midline, and consists of numerous, rather small, and difficult to delineate nuclei that line the wall of the third ventricle along

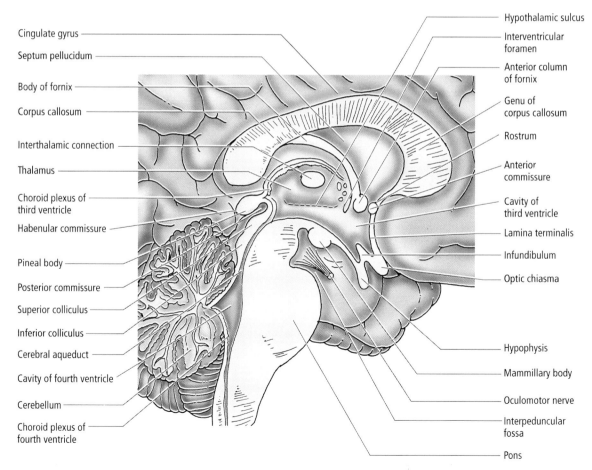

Figure 21.1 ● Sagittal section through the brainstem and part of the cerebral hemispheres illustrating the hypothalamus and its neighboring structures, the diencephalon and midbrain.

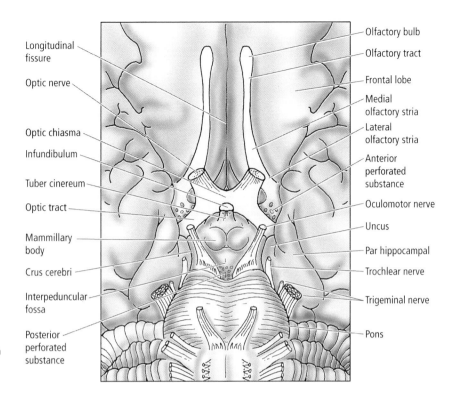

Labels (clockwise from top left and right):
- Longitudinal fissure
- Optic nerve
- Optic chiasma
- Infundibulum
- Tuber cinereum
- Optic tract
- Mammillary body
- Crus cerebri
- Interpeduncular fossa
- Posterior perforated substance
- Olfactory bulb
- Olfactory tract
- Frontal lobe
- Medial olfactory stria
- Lateral olfactory stria
- Anterior perforated substance
- Oculomotor nerve
- Uncus
- Par hippocampal
- Trochlear nerve
- Trigeminal nerve
- Pons

Figure 21.2 ● Schematic ventral view of the brain illustrating the hypothalamus and surrounding structures.

Table 21.1 ● Hypothalamic zones, regions, and component nuclei.

| Zone | Anterior region | | Middle region | Posterior region |
	Preoptic region	Supraoptic (chiasmatic) region	Infundibular (tuberal) region	Mammillary region
Periventricular	Preoptic nucleus Periventricular nuclei	Suprachiasmatic nucleus Periventricular nuclei	Arcuate nucleus	
Medial	Medial preoptic nucleus	Anterior hypothalamic nucleus Paraventricular nucleus Supraoptic nucleus	Dorsomedial nucleus Ventromedial nucleus	Mammillary nuclei Posterior hypothalamic nuclei
Lateral	Lateral preoptic nucleus	Lateral hypothalamic nucleus	Lateral tuberal nuclei Lateral hypothalamic nucleus	Lateral hypothalamic nucleus

the anterior–posterior extent of the hypothalamus. The nuclei of this zone are the **periventricular, suprachiasmatic,** and **arcuate nuclei** (Figs 21.4B, 21.5). The periventricular and arcuate nuclei control the functions of the **anterior pituitary gland** (adenohypophysis), which synthesizes and releases various endocrine hormones into the bloodstream.

The suprachiasmatic nucleus functions in the control of circadian rhythms, and is referred to as the "master clock" of the body.

Medial zone

The medial zone is the intermediate zone, and includes numerous, well-defined nuclei that are involved in various functions

The nuclei located in this zone are in an approximate anterior to posterior sequence, the **medial preoptic, anterior hypothalamic,**

paraventricular, supraoptic, dorsomedial, ventromedial, mammillary, and **posterior hypothalamic nuclei** (Figs 21.4–21.7). The nuclei in this zone control the functions of the autonomic nervous system and the secretory activity of the posterior pituitary gland (neurohypophysis).

Lateral zone

The lateral zone receives input from the limbic system and plays an important role in the behavioral expression of emotions

The lateral zone contains the **lateral preoptic nucleus** anteriorly, the **lateral tuberal nuclei** in the tuberal region, and the **lateral hypothalamic nucleus**, which extends throughout the anterioposterior extent of the lateral zone (Figs 21.4–21.7). In addition, this area also contains the longitudinally oriented fibers of the medial forebrain bundle. This zone contains nuclei that

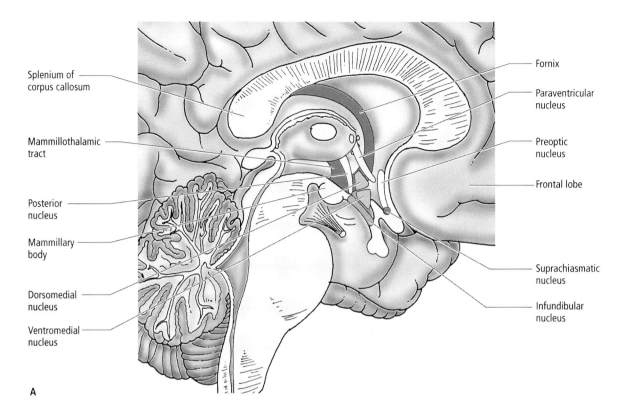

Splenium of corpus callosum

Mammillothalamic tract

Posterior nucleus

Mammillary body

Dorsomedial nucleus

Ventromedial nucleus

Fornix

Paraventricular nucleus

Preoptic nucleus

Frontal lobe

Suprachiasmatic nucleus

Infundibular nucleus

A

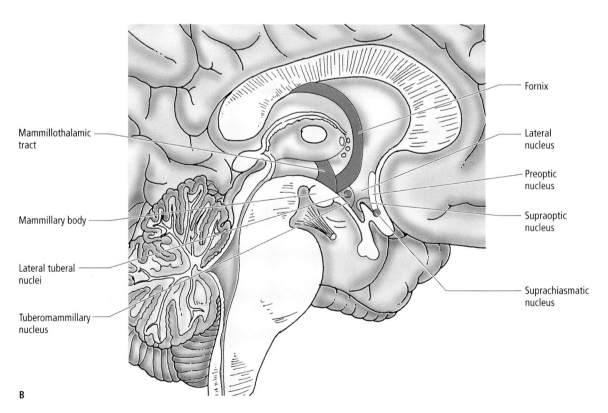

Mammillothalamic tract

Mammillary body

Lateral tuberal nuclei

Tuberomammillary nucleus

Fornix

Lateral nucleus

Preoptic nucleus

Supraoptic nucleus

Suprachiasmatic nucleus

B

Figure 21.3 ● Schematic sagittal section of the brainstem illustrating the hypothalamic nuclei. (A) Nuclei of the medial zone of the hypothalamus positioned medial to the fornix and mammillothalamic tract. (B) Nuclei of the lateral zone of the hypothalamus positioned lateral to the fornix and the mammillothalamic tract.

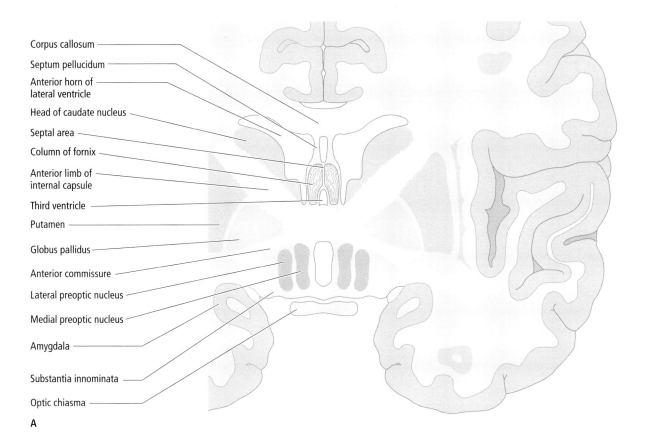

Corpus callosum
Septum pellucidum
Anterior horn of lateral ventricle
Head of caudate nucleus
Septal area
Column of fornix
Anterior limb of internal capsule
Third ventricle
Putamen
Globus pallidus
Anterior commissure
Lateral preoptic nucleus
Medial preoptic nucleus
Amygdala
Substantia innominata
Optic chiasma

A

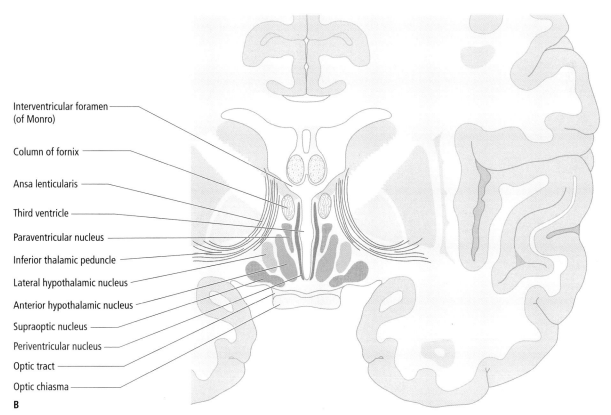

Interventricular foramen (of Monro)
Column of fornix
Ansa lenticularis
Third ventricle
Paraventricular nucleus
Inferior thalamic peduncle
Lateral hypothalamic nucleus
Anterior hypothalamic nucleus
Supraoptic nucleus
Periventricular nucleus
Optic tract
Optic chiasma

B

Figure 21.4 ● Coronal sections through the hypothalamus at the level of: (A) the preoptic region, and (B) the supraoptic region.

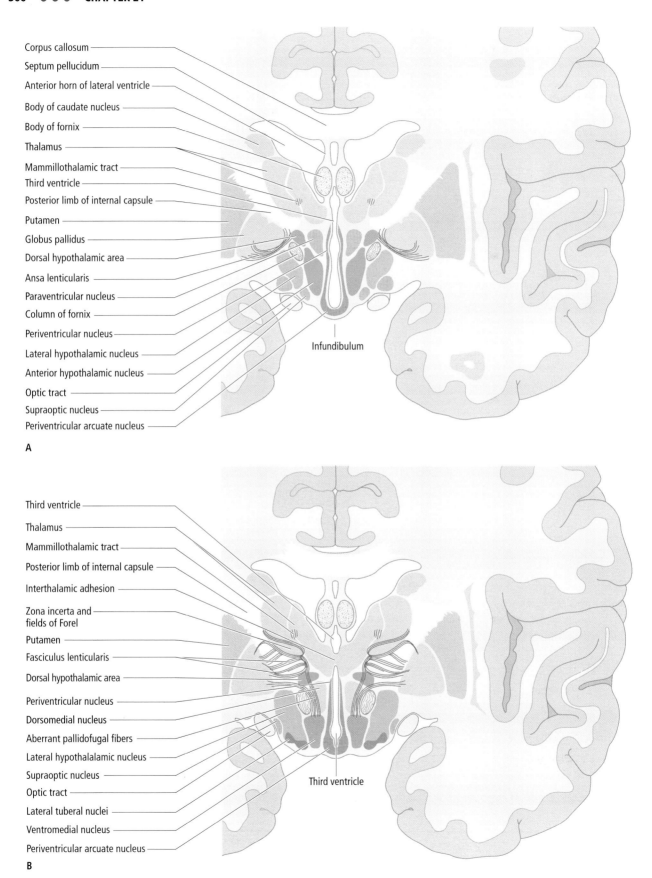

Corpus callosum

Septum pellucidum

Anterior horn of lateral ventricle

Body of caudate nucleus

Body of fornix

Thalamus

Mammillothalamic tract

Third ventricle

Posterior limb of internal capsule

Putamen

Globus pallidus

Dorsal hypothalamic area

Ansa lenticularis

Paraventricular nucleus

Column of fornix

Periventricular nucleus

Lateral hypothalamic nucleus

Anterior hypothalamic nucleus

Optic tract

Supraoptic nucleus

Periventricular arcuate nucleus

Infundibulum

A

Third ventricle

Thalamus

Mammillothalamic tract

Posterior limb of internal capsule

Interthalamic adhesion

Zona incerta and fields of Forel

Putamen

Fasciculus lenticularis

Dorsal hypothalamic area

Periventricular nucleus

Dorsomedial nucleus

Aberrant pallidofugal fibers

Lateral hypothalamic nucleus

Supraoptic nucleus

Optic tract

Lateral tuberal nuclei

Ventromedial nucleus

Periventricular arcuate nucleus

Third ventricle

B

Figure 21.5 ● Coronal sections through the hypothalamus at the level of: (A) the supraoptic region, and (B) the tuberal region.

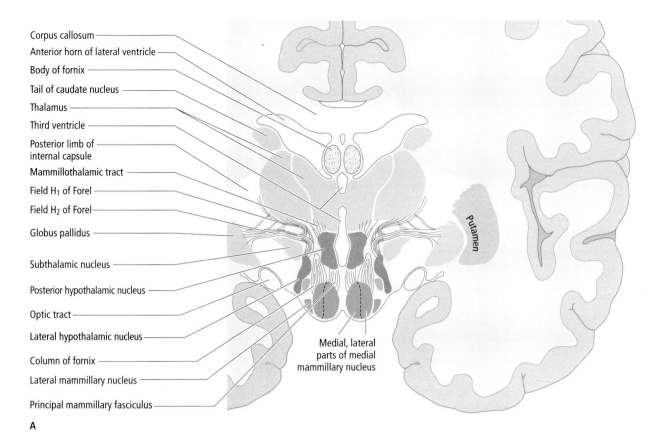

Corpus callosum
Anterior horn of lateral ventricle
Body of fornix
Tail of caudate nucleus
Thalamus
Third ventricle
Posterior limb of internal capsule
Mammillothalamic tract
Field H₁ of Forel
Field H₂ of Forel
Globus pallidus
Subthalamic nucleus
Posterior hypothalamic nucleus
Optic tract
Lateral hypothalamic nucleus
Column of fornix
Lateral mammillary nucleus
Principal mammillary fasciculus

putamen

Medial, lateral parts of medial mammillary nucleus

A

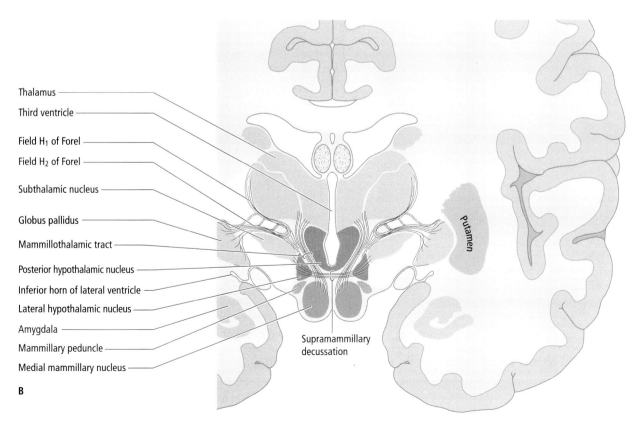

Thalamus
Third ventricle
Field H₁ of Forel
Field H₂ of Forel
Subthalamic nucleus
Globus pallidus
Mammillothalamic tract
Posterior hypothalamic nucleus
Inferior horn of lateral ventricle
Lateral hypothalamic nucleus
Amygdala
Mammillary peduncle
Medial mammillary nucleus

putamen

Supramammillary decussation

B

Figure 21.6 ● Coronal sections through the hypothalamus at the level of: (A) the anterior mammillary region, and (B) the posterior mammillary region.

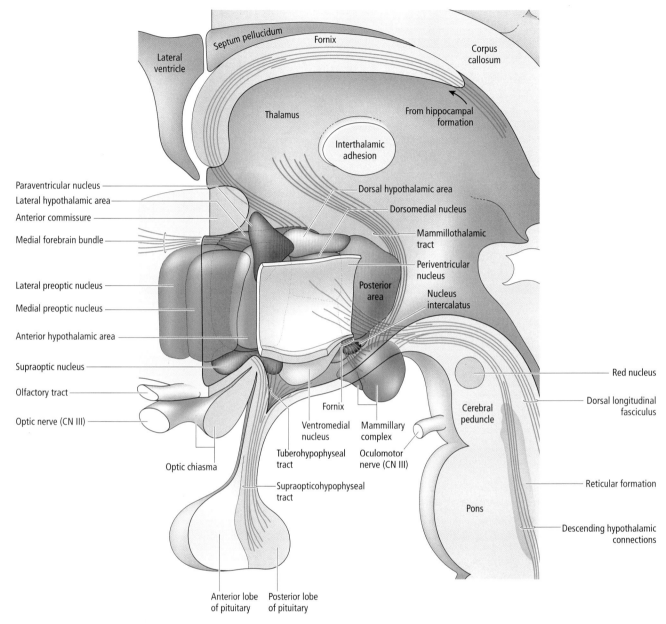

Figure 21.7 ● Schematic diagram of the hypothalamus illustrating its component nuclei. (Modified from Netter, NH (1983) *The CIBA Collection of Medical Illustrations*. Vol. 1, part 1. CIBA, New Jersey; p. 207, plate 55.)

receive information from the limbic system and mammillary bodies and then relay this input to other hypothalamic nuclei and the brainstem. This zone plays an important role in the behavioral expression of emotions.

HYPOTHALAMIC REGIONS (AREAS) AND COMPONENT NUCLEI

The hypothalamus is divided by the optic chiasma, tuber cinereum, and mammillary bodies into four regions in a rostrocaudal sequence

In general, the hypothalamic nuclei are often difficult to identify since their boundaries are not sharply delineated from adjacent nuclei, as they are in other parts of the central nervous system (CNS). In order to define their location more precisely, the hypothalamus is, in addition to being divided sagittally into three mediolateral zones, further divided coronally into four regions in a rostrocaudal sequence. These four regions, which are located near three prominent anatomical structures visible on the ventral surface of the brain (the optic chiasma, tuber cinereum, and mammillary bodies), are the **preoptic region**, **supraoptic (chiasmatic or anterior) region**, **tuberal (infundibular or middle) region**, and **mammillary (posterior) region**. Each of these regions contains nuclei as described below; however, some nuclei may extend into the adjacent zones and regions (see Table 21.1).

Preoptic region

The preoptic region controls the release of reproductive hormones from the adenohypophysis

The **preoptic region**, although located at least in part anterior to the lamina terminalis in the telencephalon, has been accepted in recent years as the anterior telencephalic portion of the hypothalamus (which is a diencephalic structure). It consists of gray matter located in the anteriormost extent of the third ventricle, both anterior and posterior to the plane of the lamina terminalis. Due to the similarities of its connections and functions to those of the anterior part of the medial region of the hypothalamus, the preoptic area is grouped with the anterior hypothalamus.

The preoptic area extends into the periventricular, medial, and lateral zones. It contains the **preoptic** and **periventricular nuclei** in the periventricular zone, the **medial preoptic nucleus** in the medial zone, and the **lateral preoptic nucleus** in the lateral zone.

The preoptic region controls the release of reproductive hormones from the adenohypophysis. There is sexual dimorphism evident in this region, reflecting the different function it has in the male and female. In the female, the anterior pituitary gland releases gonadotropin hormones that ultimately regulate the menstrual cycle, whereas in the male, the pituitary releases gonadotropins continually.

Supraoptic region

The supraoptic region contains nuclei that function in the control of circadian rhythms, temperature regulation, and control of water balance

The **supraoptic region** is located dorsal to the optic chiasma, is continuous rostrally with the preoptic area, and contains six nuclei. They are, from medial to lateral, the suprachiasmatic and periventricular nuclei in the periventricular zone, the anterior hypothalamic, paraventricular, and supraoptic nuclei in the medial zone, and the lateral hypothalamic nucleus in the lateral zone.

The **suprachiasmatic nucleus** is a small nucleus located next to the midline, dorsal to the optic chiasma, adjacent to the third ventricle. This nucleus receives visual information via axons arising from the retina (retinohypothalamic fibers) as they course through the optic chiasma, and functions in the *control of circadian rhythms*. This nucleus is referred to as the "master clock" of the body.

The **anterior hypothalamic nucleus** (see Fig. 21.4B) is located dorsal to the supraoptic nucleus, and is involved in *temperature regulation.*

The **paraventricular** and **supraoptic nuclei** (see Figs 21.4B, 21.5A) have the most abundant blood supply in the brain. The neurons of these two conspicuous nuclei synthesize the neurohypophyseal hormones, antidiuretic hormone (ADH) and oxytocin. These hormones are transported via axons arising from neurons housed in these nuclei to the posterior lobe (neurohypophysis) of the pituitary gland. These unmyelinated axons gather to form the **supraopticohypophyseal (hypothalamohypophyseal) tract**, which courses in the infundibular stalk, and then terminate in the neurohypophysis. The paraventricular nucleus *controls water balance* by functioning in the conservation of water.

In addition to the magnocellular cell group, which projects to the neurohypophysis, the paraventricular nucleus also houses other groups of neurons. One of these groups of cells, the parvocellular group, projects to the median eminence, whereas another group of cells projects to the reticular formation and the autonomic centers of the brainstem and spinal cord.

Tuberal region

The tuberal region contains nuclei that are involved in the control of anterior pituitary gland (adenohypophyseal) hormone release, caloric intake, and appetite

The **tuberal region** is located dorsal to the tuber cinereum and contains the following main nuclei. They are the arcuate (infundibular) nucleus in the periventricular zone, the dorsomedial and ventromedial nuclei in the medial zone, and the lateral hypothalamic nucleus in the lateral zone.

The **arcuate (infundibular) nucleus** is located in the periventricular zone, in the tuber cinereum, arching under the ventral aspect of the third ventricle. The cells of this nucleus produce *hypothalamic-releasing hormones*, and their axons form the **tuberohypophyseal tract** that caries these hormones to the **infundibulum**, where they pass into the **hypophyseal portal system**. The hypophyseal portal system in turn controls anterior pituitary gland (adenohypophyseal) hormone release into the general circulation.

The **dorsomedial nucleus**, when stimulated, produces aggressive behavior in animals. The **ventromedial nucleus** is a "satiety center," which upon stimulation results in satiety. This nucleus contains cells that are sensitive to blood glucose levels, and which are believed to monitor *caloric intake.*

The **lateral hypothalamic nucleus** is involved in the *control of appetite*. When stimulated, it induces eating.

Mammillary region

The mammillary nuclei are associated with emotions, whereas the posterior hypothalamic nucleus serves as a "thermostat" and regulates body temperature

The **mammillary region** includes the prominent mammillary nuclei and the posterior hypothalamic nucleus.

Three to four **mammillary nuclei** collectively form each **mammillary body**. The mammillary bodies appear as two conspicuous elevations on the ventral surface of the hypothalamus. Unlike the other hypothalamic nuclei, which are associated with functions of the endocrine and/or autonomic nervous systems, the mammillary nuclei are a major target projection area of the hippocampal formation via the **fornix**, relaying input related to *emotions*. In addition, information is relayed to the mammillary nuclei via the **mammillary peduncle** from the dorsal and ventral tegmental nuclei as well as from the raphe nuclei. The mammillary nucleus relays input to the anterior nucleus of the thalamus via the prominent **mammillothalamic tract**.

The **posterior hypothalamic nucleus** contains cells that are sensitive to a decrease in the temperature of the blood. This nucleus serves as a "thermostat" and *regulates body temperature* by conserving heat and stimulating heat production. Heat is conserved by vasoconstriction of cutaneous vessels, whereas heat is produced by an increase in thyroid activity and shivering.

CONNECTIONS OF THE HYPOTHALAMUS

The hypothalamus is connected with widespread regions of the nervous system. It receives input related to emotion from the limbic system, as well as input from sensory and motor nuclei from the brainstem and spinal cord. The hypothalamus exerts its influence via its outputs on the endocrine and autonomic nervous systems.

Afferents (input) to the hypothalamus

Most neural input to the hypothalamus arises from the limbic system. Non-neural input is carried to the hypothalamus via the vascular system

The hypothalamus receives **afferent fibers** (neural input) from various structures, however most neural input arises from the limbic system. Other fibers arise from visceral structures and the brainstem. Fibers arise from the following sources: the orbitofrontal cortex, basal forebrain, septal area and septal nuclei, ventral striatum, midline and medial dorsal nucleus of the thalamus, hippocampus, amygdaloid nuclear complex, retina, dorsal and ventral tegmental nuclei, raphe nuclei, locus ceruleus, spinal cord, and reticular formation.

In addition to the neural input, the hypothalamus also receives non-neural input from the vascular system. Hypothalamic neurons serve as receptors that are sensitive to rapid changes in the temperature, osmotic pressure, and hormone levels of the circulating blood. These receptors are referred to as circumventricular organs (CVOs). Although there are six circumventricular organs, only two are associated with the hypothalamus. They consist of hypothalamic neurons that are embedded in the wall of the third ventricle, and are sensitive to alterations in the chemical composition of the cerebrospinal fluid. One of these structures is associated with the lamina terminalis, and is referred to as the organum vasculosum of the lamina terminalis (OVLT). The OVLT is a chemosensory structure that detects and responds to peptides and macromolecules present in the bloodstream. The other CVO is the subfornical organ located inferior to the fornix, near the interventricular foramen. The subfornical organ serves in the regulation of body fluids. The fenestrated capillaries supplying these receptors do not have a blood–brain barrier, thus they permit substances present in the bloodstream to pass through and enter the extracellular space surrounding the receptor cells.

Efferents (output) from the hypothalamus

In addition to the neural output, the hypothalamus also provides output to the adenohypophysis and neurohypophysis

Most hypothalamic output projections terminate in the sources of hypothalamic input. The hypothalamus projects **efferent fibers** (neural output) to the following structures: the septal area and septal nuclei, medial dorsal nucleus of the thalamus, anterior nucleus of the thalamus, hippocampus, amygdaloid nuclear complex, midbrain reticular formation, and brainstem and spinal cord autonomic nuclei.

In addition to the neural output, the hypothalamus also provides output to the adenohypophysis and neurohypophysis. The hypothalamus exerts its influence on the endocrine system via these two projections.

Hypothalamic influence is exerted on the endocrine system directly, via the fibers of the **supraopticohypophyseal tract**, which terminates in the posterior lobe of the hypophysis (neurohypophysis). There these neurons release hormones that pass into the capillaries of the neurohypophysis and then enter the bloodstream.

The hypothalamus also exerts its influence on the endocrine system indirectly, via the local capillary networks of the **hypophyseal portal system**, which carries hormones synthesized by the hypothalamus to the adenohypophysis (anterior pituitary gland).

PATHWAYS OF THE HYPOTHALAMUS

The pathways connecting the hypothalamus with other regions of the nervous system are categorized into afferent or efferent pathways based on the direction of most of the information that they carry. However, none of them carry exclusively afferent or efferent fibers since they all carry information that is bidirectional (Tables 21.2–21.4).

Afferent pathways to the hypothalamus
(Table 21.2)

Fornix

The fornix is the most prominent neural input to the hypothalamus

The **fornix** is a myelinated tract that arises from the hippocampal formation of the limbic system and conveys the most prominent neural input to the hypothalamus. It distributes fibers to the preoptic and anterior areas of the hypothalamus, and then proceeds through the hypothalamus to terminate mostly in the medial nucleus of the mammillary body posteriorly.

Mammillary peduncle

The **mammillary peduncle** carries prominent sensory input from the dorsal and ventral tegmental nuclei of the

Table 21.2 ● Afferent pathways to the hypothalamus.

Tract/pathway	Origin	Termination	Function
Fornix	Hippocampal formation	Preoptic and anterior areas of the hypothalamus Medial mammillary nucleus	
Mammillary peduncle	Dorsal and ventral tegmental nuclei Raphe nuclei	Lateral mammillary nucleus	Relays sensory input from sensory pathways
Stria terminalis (amygdalohypothalamic tract)	Amygdaloid nuclear complex	Medial preoptic area Anterior hypothalamic nucleus	Olfactory information, which influences reproductive behavior
Thalamohypothalamic tract	Medial dorsal and midline nuclei of the thalamus	Lateral preoptic area of the hypothalamus	
Ventral amygdalohypothalamic (amygdalofugal) tract	Basolateral nucleus of the amygdaloid nuclear complex	Lateral hypothalamic nucleus	Influences autonomic nervous system activities
Retinosuprachiasmatic tract	Retina	Suprachiasmatic nucleus	Control of circadian rhythms
Spinohypothalamic tract	Spinal cord	Autonomic control centers of the hypothalamus	Neuroendocrine and cardiovascular responses
Fibers from the reticular formation	Reticular formation	Autonomic control centers of the hypothalamus	Relay nociceptive input to the hypothalamus

mesencephalon as well as from the raphe nuclei to the lateral mammillary nucleus.

Stria terminalis

The **stria terminalis** (amygdalohypothalamic fibers) transmits information from the amygdaloid nuclear complex to the medial preoptic area and the anterior nucleus of the hypothalamus. This pathway transmits olfactory information, which is believed to affect reproductive behavior.

Thalamohypothalamic tract

The **thalamohypothalamic tract** carries fibers from the medial dorsal and midline nuclei of the thalamus to the lateral preoptic area of the hypothalamus.

Ventral amygdalohypothalamic (amygdalofugal) tract

The **ventral amygdalohypothalamic tract** relays amygdaloid signals from the basolateral nucleus to the lateral hypothalamic nucleus where they influence autonomic nervous system activities.

Retinosuprachiasmatic tract

The **retinosuprachiasmatic tract** consists of a bundle of fibers arising from the retina that terminates in the suprachiasmatic

nucleus of the hypothalamus. It is involved in the control of circadian rhythms.

Spinohypothalamic fibers

The spinohypothalamic fibers relay nociceptive input from the spinal cord to the autonomic control centers of the hypothalamus

The **spinohypothalamic fibers**, a component of the anterolateral system of the ascending sensory pathways, consist of axons arising from the spinal cord that relay nociceptive input to the autonomic control centers of the hypothalamus. There they synapse with neurons that give rise to the **hypothalamospinal tract**, which is associated with the autonomic and reflex responses (i.e., endocrine and cardiovascular responses) to nociception.

Fibers from the reticular formation

The ARAS relays nociceptive input to the hypothalamus, which mediates the autonomic and reflex responses to nociception

Most of the nociceptive fibers from the spinal cord ascending in the anterolateral system of the ascending sensory pathways, and the fibers of the trigeminothalamic tract, send collateral branches to the reticular formation as they ascend through the brainstem. There these collateral branches activate the ascending reticular activating system (ARAS), which relays information to the cerebral cortex alerting the individual, but also relays information to the hypothalamus,

Table 21.3 ● Efferent pathways of the hypothalamus.

Tract/pathway	Origin	Termination	Function
Fasciculus mammillaris princeps	Mammillary nuclei		
Mammillothalamic tract	Medial and lateral mammillary nuclei	Anterior nucleus of the thalamus	
Mammillotegmental tract	Lateral mammillary nuclei	Dorsal and ventral tegmental nuclei	
Mammillointerpeduncular tract	Mammillary nucleus	Interpeduncular nucleus	
Supraopticohypophyseal (hypothalamohypophyseal) tract	Supraoptic and paraventricular nuclei	Posterior lobe of the pituitary gland (neurohypophysis)	Releases hormones that pass into the capillaries of the neurohypophysis and then enter the bloodstream
Periventricular bundle	Periventricular zone nuclei	Frontal cortex Medulla Spinal cord	Stimulate ANS responses
Tuberohypophyseal (tuberoinfundibular, infundibular) tract	Arcuate and periventricular nuclei	Infundibular stalk	Regulates the synthesis and release of anterior pituitary hormones
Dorsal longitudinal fasciculus (DLF)	Hypothalamus	Brainstem and spinal cord ANS nuclei and reticular formation	Control of skeletal muscles involved in chewing, swallowing, and shivering
Hypothalamospinal tract	Paraventricular, dorsomedial, ventromedial, and posterior nuclei	Brainstem Spinal cord lateral cell column Sympathetic and parasympathetic (sacral) nuclei	Influences ANS activity

ANS, autonomic nervous system.

limbic system, and serotonergic raphe nucleus magnus. The hypothalamus mediates the autonomic and reflex responses to nociception, the limbic system mediates the emotional/behavioral responses to nociception, and the raphe nucleus is involved in descending control of pain.

Efferent pathways from the hypothalamus
(Table 21.3)

Fasciculus mammillaris princeps

The **fasciculus mammillaris princeps** arises from the mammillary body and then quickly bifurcates to give rise to the **mammillothalamic** and **mammillotegmental tracts**.

Mammillothalamic tract (mammillary fasciculus, tract of Vicq d'Azyr)

The mammillothalamic tract is a myelinated bundle of fibers that arises from the medial and lateral mammillary nuclei and terminates in the anterior nucleus of the thalamus.

Mammillotegmental tract (fasciculus)

The mammillotegmental tract is a component of the medial forebrain bundle. It carries mammillothalamic tract axon collaterals from the lateral mammillary nuclei to the midbrain dorsal and ventral tegmental nuclei in the reticular formation.

Mammillointerpeduncular tract

The **mammillointerpeduncular tract** carries fibers from the mammillary nucleus that terminate in the interpeduncular nucleus. The interpeduncular nucleus plays a role in the sleep–wake cycle.

Supraopticohypophyseal (hypothalamohypophyseal) tract

The supraopticohypophyseal tract carries oxytocin or vasopressin to the posterior lobe of the pituitary

The **supraopticohypophyseal tract** is a short tract consisting of axons that carry oxytocin or vasopressin, synthesized in the cell bodies of hypothalamic neurons residing in the supraoptic and paraventricular nuclei, to the posterior lobe of the pituitary.

Oxytocin and vasopressin are synthesized in different populations of hypothalamic neurosecretory neurons. The secretory substances are transported via these axons to the posterior lobe of the pituitary gland (neurohypophysis). Upon stimulation, the hypothalamic neurosecretory cells transmit impulses to their terminals, which results in the release of the hormones into the general circulation.

Periventricular bundle

The **periventricular bundle** consists of fibers that connect the periventricular zone nuclei with the frontal cortex, the dorsal motor nucleus of the vagus in the medulla, the lateral cell column at T1 to L2, and the sacral parasympathetic nucleus of the spinal cord. The functions of the projections to the brainstem and spinal cord are autonomic system responses.

Tuberohypophyseal (tuberoinfundibular, infundibular) tract

> The tuberohypophyseal tract carries fibers from the arcuate and periventricular nuclei to the infundibular stalk and the anterior pituitary

The tuberohypophyseal tract carries fibers from the arcuate and periventricular nuclei to the infundibular stalk and the anterior pituitary. The axon terminals of the **tuberohypophyseal tract** release "**releasing hormones**" or "**release-inhibiting hormones**" in the hypophyseal portal system, which carries them to the anterior lobe of the pituitary gland where they regulate the synthesis and release of anterior pituitary hormones. The tuberohypophyseal tract and the hypophyseal portal system serve as a connection between the hypothalamus and anterior pituitary gland.

Dorsal longitudinal fasciculus

> The dorsolateral fasciculus carries fibers from the hypothalamus to the brainstem and spinal cord autonomic nuclei and to the reticular formation

The **dorsal longitudinal fasciculus** carries fibers that connect various regions of the CNS. Among these fibers are some that arise from the hypothalamus and descend to terminate in the brainstem and spinal cord autonomic nuclei. In addition, this pathway carries signals from the hypothalamus to the reticular formation. These signals are then relayed via the reticulobulbar tract to the brainstem lower motoneurons, and via the reticulospinal tract to the spinal cord lower motoneurons. By way of the dorsal longitudinal fasciculus, the hypothalamus ultimately influences chewing, swallowing, and shivering.

Hypothalamospinal tract

> The hypothalamospinal tract is a direct route via which the hypothalamus influences preganglionic sympathetic and parasympathetic neurons residing in the spinal cord

The **hypothalamospinal tract** carries fibers arising mainly from the paraventricular nucleus of the hypothalamus. Additional fibers originate from the dorsomedial, ventromedial, and posterior nuclei. These fibers descend to terminate in the brainstem and spinal cord to synapse directly with preganglionic sympathetic (lateral cell column) and parasympathetic (sacral) nuclei neurons. These direct projections to the spinal cord are small in number; the majority of the descending fibers from the hypothalamus that are destined to influence the autonomic centers are believed to synapse at multiple relay centers.

Bidirectional pathways (Table 21.4)

Medial forebrain bundle

> The medial forebrain bundle contains fibers that are believed to play a role in motivation and sense of smell

Tract/pathway	Origin	Termination	Function
Medial forebrain bundle (MFB)	Afferents	Hypothalamus	Motivation and sense of smell
	Septal area		
	Basal forebrain		
	Primary olfactory cortex		
	Brainstem raphe nuclei		
	Ventral tegmental area		
	Locus ceruleus		
	Efferents	Septal area	
	Hypothalamus	Septal nuclei	
		Brainstem reticular formation	
		Autonomic nervous system nuclei	
Stria medullaris thalami	Afferents		
	Habenula	Hypothalamus	
		Supraoptic nucleus	
		Preoptic area	
	Efferents		
	Hypothalamus	Habenula	
	Supraoptic nucleus		
	Preoptic area		

Table 21.4 ● Bidirectional pathways of the hypothalamus.

The **medial forebrain bundle** is not really a distinct bundle as its name implies, but instead consists of a vast array of axons with various origins and terminations. It includes both afferent and efferent fibers to and from the hypothalamus. The afferent fibers to the hypothalamus arise primarily from the septal area. Other fibers arise from the basal forebrain and primary olfactory cortex, as well as from the brainstem raphe nuclei, ventral tegmental area, and locus ceruleus. Efferent fibers arising from the hypothalamus and running in the medial forebrain bundle terminate in the septal area, septal nuclei, and brainstem reticular formation and autonomic nuclei, as well as in the autonomic nuclei of the spinal cord. These fibers are believed to play a role in motivation and sense of smell. The medial forebrain bundle is more prominent in other animals with a keen sense of smell.

Stria medullaris thalami

The **stria medullaris thalami** carries afferent and efferent fibers to and from the hypothalamus, connecting its supraoptic nucleus and preoptic area with the habenula. The habenula is visible in a midsagittal section of the brain, in the medial surface of the thalamus near its caudal end. It appears as a small swelling rostral to the pineal gland, above the posterior commissure. It contains the habenular nuclei and its function is not known.

FUNCTIONS OF THE HYPOTHALAMUS

The hypothalamus functions in the regulation of body temperature, food intake, fluid intake, and control of the autonomic nervous system (Table 21.5). It also plays a role in emotional expression, memory, and aggression.

Regulation of body temperature

The hypothalamus serves as a "thermostat" and plays a central and vital role in body temperature regulation

Temperature-sensitive receptors (thermosensitive free nerve endings) located in the skin detect information about the environmental temperature. Other peripheral temperature-sensitive receptors (similar to those in the skin but located deep in the body) detect information about the body's core temperature. Both environmental and body core (visceral) temperature input is relayed to higher brain centers, including the hypothalamus, via the ascending sensory pathways.

In addition to the peripheral temperature-sensitive receptors, the **preoptic region** and **anterior hypothalamic nuclei** house two types of temperature-sensitive (thermosensitive) neurons that respond to very slight temperature changes (less than 0.1°C) of the blood. One group of these neurons becomes stimulated by increases in blood temperature, whereas another group of neurons becomes stimulated by decreases in blood temperature.

Nucleus	Function(s)
Preoptic	Controls the release of reproductive hormones from the adenohypophysis
Suprachiasmatic	Regulates circadian rhythms; "master clock"
Arcuate	Produces hypothalamic releasing and inhibiting hormones
Periventricular	Produces hypothalamic releasing and inhibiting hormones
Medial preoptic	Regulates the release of reproductive hormones from the adenohypophysis
Anterior	Regulates parasympathetic nervous system activity Regulates body temperature; involved in body heat loss
Dorsomedial	Stimulation of this nucleus causes savage behavior in animals
Ventromedial	Involved in eating behavior; "satiety center"
Mammillary	Processes information related to emotional expression
Posterior	Regulates sympathetic nervous system activity Regulates body temperature Involved in heat conservation and heat production; "thermostat"
Lateral preoptic	Unknown
Lateral	Regulates sympathetic nervous system Involved in eating behavior; "feeding center"
Paraventricular	Produces ADH and oxytocin
Supraoptic	Produces ADH and oxytocin

ADH, antidiuretic hormone.

Table 21.5 ● Hypothalamic nuclei and their functions.

The hypothalamus is a well vascularized brain center. As the circulating blood percolates in the capillary bed surrounding the thermosensitive preoptic and anterior hypothalamic neurons, these neurons become stimulated by warming or cooling of the blood. It is believed that the preoptic and anterior hypothalamic nuclei initiate *heat loss* mechanisms, whereas the **posterior hypothalamic nuclei** activate *heat conservation* and *heat production* mechanisms (Table 21.5). Thus the hypothalamus serves as a "thermostat" that mediates mechanisms that enable the body to return to, and maintain, a normal body temperature.

Temperature regulation involves hypothalamic integration of autonomic, endocrine, somatic motor, and limbic system activities. For example, in response to an increase in body temperature, the **anterior hypothalamus** triggers the appropriate body responses that will result in a decrease in body temperature. These responses include autonomic activities such as sweating and cutaneous vasodilation, and a decrease in somatic motor function. Furthermore, behavioral changes such as seeking a cooler environment or taking off a sweater to reduce body temperature may be appropriate. The neurons that control the parasympathetic nervous system are located in the anterior nucleus of the hypothalamus to mediate the parasympathetic responses associated with decreasing body temperature.

In response to a decrease in body temperature, the **posterior hypothalamus** triggers the appropriate body responses that will produce an increase in body temperature. These responses include: (i) piloerection (formation of goose bumps) and the vasoconstriction of cutaneous vessels, both of which are mediated by the autonomic nervous system to conserve body heat; (ii) an increase in metabolism (via the release of thyroid-stimulating hormone (TSH) by the anterior lobe of the pituitary), mediated by the endocrine system to increase body heat; (iii) shivering, mediated by the somatic motor system to produce heat; and (iv) behavioral (motivational) responses, such as turning the heat on, putting on warmer clothes, and drinking something warm, mediated by the limbic system to increase body temperature. Frontal lobe connections to the limbic system mediate behavioral changes to optimize conditions for homeostasis. The neurons that control the sympathetic nervous system are located in the posterior hypothalamic nucleus. These neurons send their axons to the lateral horn of the spinal cord to mediate the sympathetic responses associated with increasing body temperature.

While body temperature may be regulated by the hypothalamus and associated physiological processes, the temperature range in which these processes are effective is rather slight. For example, the hypothalamus cannot keep the body at a normal temperature range in an extremely cold environment.

Regulation of food intake and the sleep–wake cycle

The hypothalamus contains a "feeding center" and a "satiety center" and has a very important function in food intake regulation

In the past, the **lateral** and **ventromedial nuclei** of the hypothalamus were believed to be associated with eating behavior. Stimulation of the lateral hypothalamic nucleus in experimental animals induced eating, and it was referred to as a "hunger" or "feeding center." Stimulation of the ventromedial nucleus inhibited eating, and was referred to as a "satiety center." It is now known that things are not as simple as were once believed. In addition to the lateral and ventromedial nuclei, the **paraventricular nucleus** also plays a role in the regulation of food intake (Table 21.5), possibly through its projections to the brainstem reticular formation, as well as to the brainstem and spinal cord autonomic nuclei. However, the precise mechanism of food intake regulation is unknown.

The lateral hypothalamic nucleus contains a group of neurons that synthesize **orexins** (G. orexis, "appetite") (also referred to as hypocretins), which are hypothalamic neuropeptides that not only regulate food intake but also the sleep–wake cycle. Fasting causes an increase in orexin synthesis, whereas administration of exogenous orexin induces eating. Orexin is also involved in waking and keeping an individual awake throughout the day. At night, hypothalamic orexin production decreases, causing an individual to fall asleep.

Note that the clinical case at the beginning of the chapter refers to a patient whose symptoms include daytime sleepiness, an occasional limp feeling, complete paralysis, and visual hallucinations prior to falling asleep.

1 What is the neuropeptide synthesized by the hypothalamus that not only regulates food intake but also the sleep–wake cycle?

2 What effect do orexins have on food intake and the sleep–wake cycle?

Regulation of fluid intake

The hypothalamus contains neurons that play a role in water intake

A group of cells located lateral to the lateral nucleus of the hypothalamus, known as the **zona incerta**, are believed to play a role in water intake. Stimulation of the zona incerta results in the drinking of large amounts of water.

Control of the autonomic nervous system

The hypothalamus is the master controller of autonomic functions

The hypothalamus receives visceral input via the ascending sensory system and input related to emotions from the limbic system. The hypothalamus in turn exerts its influence on both the sympathetic and parasympathetic nervous systems, coordinating their functions in order to maintain homeostasis or to produce the appropriate visceral responses that accompany behavioral expression.

Stimulation of the **anterior** (**preoptic** and **anterior nucleus**) and **medial hypothalamus** controls the activities of the **parasympathetic nervous system** (see Table 21.5). Parasympathetic responses include: pupillary constriction, increase in salivary secretion, decrease in heart rate and blood pressure, increase in intestinal peristaltic waves, vasodilation, sweating, piloerection, and urinary bladder contraction.

Stimulation of the **posterior** and **lateral hypothalamus** controls the activities of the **sympathetic nervous system**. Sympathetic responses include: pupillary dilation, decrease in salivary secretion, increase in heart rate and blood pressure, decrease of peristaltic waves, vasoconstriction of cutaneous blood vessels, and urinary bladder relaxation.

Although fibers destined for the control of autonomic centers (sympathetic and parasympathetic) of the brainstem and spinal cord arise from various hypothalamic nuclei, the principal source of these hypothalamic descending fibers is the parvocellular part of the **paraventricular nucleus**. Interestingly, some of the paraventricular neurons project to both parasympathetic and sympathetic centers.

It is important to realize that fibers arising from the anterior and medial hypothalamic nuclei pass posteriorly and laterally on their way to the brainstem and spinal cord. Thus stimulation of the posterior and lateral hypothalamus may not only stimulate the local neurons that project to the sympathetic centers, but also those fibers arising from the anterior and medial hypothalamus that pass by the posterior and lateral hypothalamus, which are destined for the parasympathetic centers.

Fibers arising from the posterior and lateral hypothalamus synapse with the preganglionic sympathetic neurons at the T1 to L2 levels of the spinal cord to elicit the appropriate sympathetic responses. Fibers arising from the anterior and lateral hypothalamus synapse with the parasympathetic neurons at the Edinger–Westphal nucleus, the superior and inferior salivatory nuclei, the dorsal motor nucleus of the vagus, and the S2–S4 parasympathetic nucleus to elicit the appropriate parasympathetic responses.

Role in emotion, memory, and aggression

Through its extensive interconnections with the limbic system, which processes emotions, the hypothalamus plays an important role in emotional behavior

Emotions trigger the relay of a heavy input from the limbic system to the hypothalamus. The hypothalamus in turn, via its connections with the autonomic nervous system, mediates the appropriate visceral responses (such as changes in heart rate, blood pressure, breathing rate, and sweating) accompanying behavioral expression. For example, a student who is feeling anxious before an examination, may experience an increase in heart rate, breathing rate, have sweaty palms, and a dry mouth, all of which are responses mediated by the sympathetic nervous system. The magnitude of the visceromotor responses to emotions depends on the individual, his prior experiences, and his ability to control his emotions and the consequent visceral responses at the neocortical level.

The hippocampus, a region involved in learning and *memory*, gives rise to a prominent fiber bundle, the **fornix**, which among other targets, projects to the mammillary bodies of the hypothalamus. Hippocampal input to the hypothalamus is involved in the influence of memories on emotion.

Stimulation of the **lateral hypothalamus** not only induces eating and drinking behaviors in animals, but also causes the animal to become more active, and even exhibit **aggressive behavior** or rage. Stimulation of the **ventromedial nuclei** of the hypothalamus and surrounding areas produces satiety and tranquility.

HYPOTHALAMOHYPOPHYSEAL CONNECTIONS

The hypothalamus regulates pituitary gland functions

The hypothalamus regulates pituitary gland functions. Hypothalamic influence on the pituitary gland, and ultimately on the endocrine system, travels via two paths: a neural path and a non-neural (vascular) path. The **pituitary gland** (also known as the **hypophysis**), consists of two lobes, the anterior and posterior lobes. The **anterior lobe** is also referred to as the **adenohypophysis** (G. adena, "gland") due to its glandular properties, whereas the **posterior lobe** is also referred to as the **neurohypophysis** due to its neural properties.

Hypothalamic influence on the pituitary gland, and ultimately on the endocrine system, travels via two paths: a neural path and a non-neural vascular path.

In the **neural path**, hypothalamic control is exerted on the neurohypophysis via a neural pathway, the **hypothalamohypophyseal** (supraopticohypophyseal, neurohypophyseal) **tract**. The axon terminals of this pathway release hormones in the extracellular space, which then pass directly into fenestrated capillaries of the posterior pituitary, which in turn empty into the general circulation (Fig. 21.8).

In the **non-neural path**, hypothalamic control is exerted on the adenohypophysis via a vascular network, the **hypothalamic portal system**. This path involves the release of hypothalamic hormones into the hypophyseal portal system, a vascular network confined to the hypothalamopituitary region, which connects the hypothalamic and pituitary vascular beds, and which carries these hormones to the anterior pituitary. The appropriate cells of the anterior pituitary then release hormones into the general circulation (Fig. 21.9).

Neurohypophysis

The hypothalamus contains the cell bodies of neurosecretory cells that display the morphological characteristics of neurons, transmit nerve impulses down their axons, and have endocrine properties

The **supraoptic** and **paraventricular nuclei** of the medial zone of the hypothalamus house the large cell bodies of hypothalamic **neurosecretory cells** (Fig. 21.10). These cells are **neurons** since they have both the morphological characteristics of neurons and upon stimulation transmit nerve impulses down their axons. In addition, these cells also have endocrine properties since they produce hormones (not neurotransmitters) that

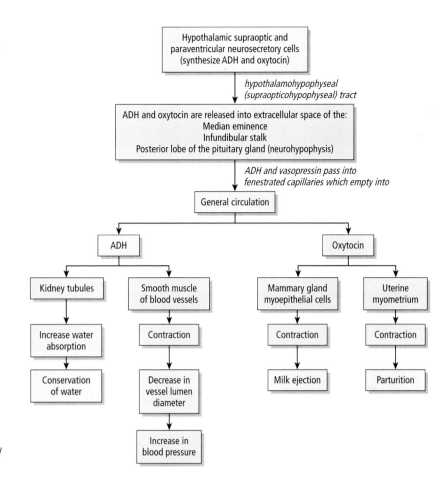

Figure 21.8 ● Hypothalamic control of the pituitary gland (neural path). ADH, antidiuretic hormone.

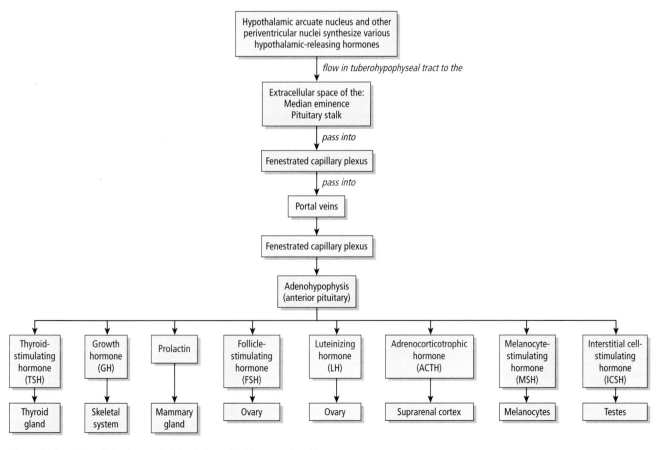

Figure 21.9 ● Hypothalamic control of the pituitary gland (non-neural path).

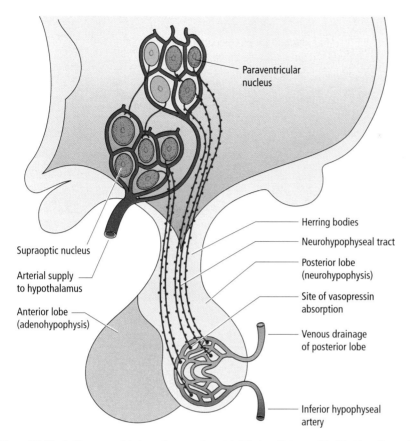

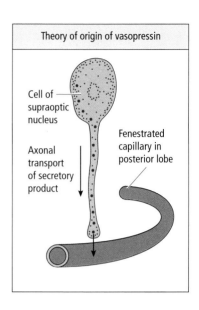

Theory of origin of vasopressin

Cell of supraoptic nucleus

Fenestrated capillary in posterior lobe

Axonal transport of secretory product

Paraventricular nucleus

Herring bodies

Neurohypophyseal tract

Posterior lobe (neurohypophysis)

Site of vasopressin absorption

Venous drainage of posterior lobe

Supraoptic nucleus

Arterial supply to hypothalamus

Anterior lobe (adenohypophysis)

Inferior hypophyseal artery

Figure 21.10 ● The paraventricular and supraoptic nuclei of the hypothalamus. (Modified from Netter, NH (1983) *The CIBA Collection of Medical Illustrations*. Vol. 1, part 1. CIBA, New Jersey; p. 211, plate 59.)

are released into the bloodstream. Thus they are considered to be specialized neurons.

The profuse vascularization of the hypothalamus enables the neurosecretory cells of the supraoptic and paraventricular nuclei to sample the osmolarity of the blood flowing through the hypothalamus. The neurosecretory cells are stimulated even by a slight increase of osmotic pressure in the blood, which triggers the relay of nerve impulses down their axons.

The neurosecretory cells synthesize two peptide hormones, **antidiuretic hormone** (**ADH**, also known as **vasopressin**) and **oxytocin**. Only one of these hormones is synthesized by any one (large) cell, and both hormones are synthesized by the (large) cells of both nuclei. Each of these hormones is synthesized as a prohormone in the cell body of the neurosecretory cells. Each of these hormones then becomes bound to a carrier protein known as a **neurophysin** and is then transported within vesicles (membrane-bound saccules), down the axons of these neurosecretory cells, which gather to form the **supraopticohypophyseal tract**. Although these axons arise from both the supraoptic and paraventricular nuclei, most arise from the supraoptic nucleus and thus the tract is named the supraopticohypophyseal tract. This tract descends only a short distance to terminate in the median eminence, infundibular stalk, and posterior lobe of the pituitary gland. These hormones are either stored in

the axon terminals or are released and then pass into the blood circulation. Hormone release is triggered when nerve impulses are transmitted to the axon terminals of the neurosecretory cells of the supraopticohypophyseal tract. The axon terminals are expanded and form a direct contact with the fenestrated capillary wall. These terminals then liberate ADH, which passes into the fenestrated capillaries and then flows into the general circulation. Unlike other nerve cells, those residing in the supraoptic and paraventricular nuclei do not establish synaptic contacts with other nerve cells. Instead, their function is to detect alterations in the chemical composition of the blood. When these cells are stimulated, they liberate their hormones into the bloodstream.

The ADH released by these nerve terminals passes into the capillary bed of the median eminence, infundibular stalk, and posterior lobe of the pituitary to gain entrance into the general circulation. When the water content of the body is low, the amount of ADH released into the bloodstream is increased. ADH acts on the kidney's distal and collecting tubules causing them to reabsorb water from the tubule lumen, until the water content of the body is restored to normal, resulting in minimal water loss in the urine. When the body's water content is high, only small amounts of ADH are released into the bloodstream. In response to the decreased ADH blood levels, the kidney reabsorbs less water, resulting a dilute urine and water loss. By altering the volume of water lost in the urine, the kidney controls the osmotic pressure in the blood. Thus this hormone enables the body to conserve water and regulate body fluid content. The ADH also acts on the smooth muscle of the vessel wall. It causes contraction of the smooth muscle, which results in a decrease in lumen diameter and a consequent elevation in blood pressure.

In addition, ADH is also released in response to a decrease in blood volume as would result following hemorrhage. Pressure receptors are located in the carotid artery and aortic arch, while stretch receptors are located in the walls of the left atrium and pulmonary veins. These receptors relay this sensory input to the brainstem medulla via the glossopharyngeal and vagus nerves. From there, input is relayed via ascending fibers to the supraoptic nucleus.

The oxytocin released by the nerve terminals, like ADH, also passes into the capillary bed of the median eminence, infundibular stalk, and posterior lobe of the pituitary, to gain entrance into the general circulation. Oxytocin (G. oxy, "rapid;" tokos, "birth;" thus "rapid labor") has two functions. It causes contraction of the uterine myometrium during the final stages of pregnancy, which facilitates parturition, and contraction of the mammary gland myoepithelial cells, resulting in milk ejection of the active mammary gland.

Adenohypophysis

The hypothalamus communicates with the adenohypophysis via the hypophyseal portal system

Small cells located in the **arcuate nucleus** and other **periventricular zone nuclei** of the hypothalamus synthesize various releasing hormones (factors) and release-inhibiting hormones (factors) (Figs 21.9, 21.11). The releasing hormones produced by the hypothalamus are:

- **somatotropin-releasing hormone** (SRH), which stimulates the release of somatotropin (growth hormone);
- **prolactin-releasing hormone** (PRH), which stimulates the release of prolactin;
- **corticotropin-releasing hormone** (CRH), which stimulates the release of adrenocorticotropin;
- **gonadotropin-releasing hormone** (GnRH), which stimulates the release of luteinizing hormone (LH) and follicle-stimulating hormone (FSH);
- **thyroid-stimulating hormone-releasing hormone** (thyrotropin-releasing hormone, TRH), which stimulates the release of TSH; and
- **melanocyte-stimulating hormone-releasing hormone**, which releases melanocyte-stimulating hormone (MSH).

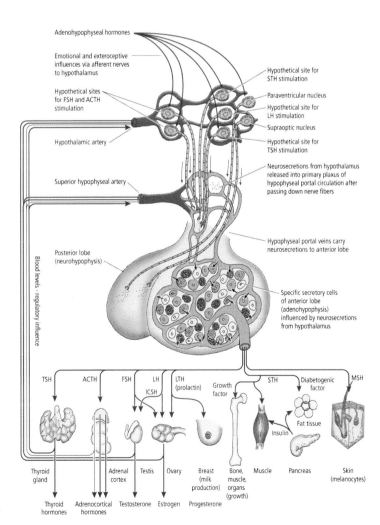

Figure 21.11 ● The interaction between the hypothalamus and anterior pituitary gland. LRH, lutein-releasing hormone; SRH, somatotropin-releasing hormone; for other abbreviations see Fig. 21.9. (Modified from Netter, FH (1983) *The CIBA Collection of Medical Illustrations*. Vol. 1, part 1. CIBA, New Jersey; p. 210, plate 58.)

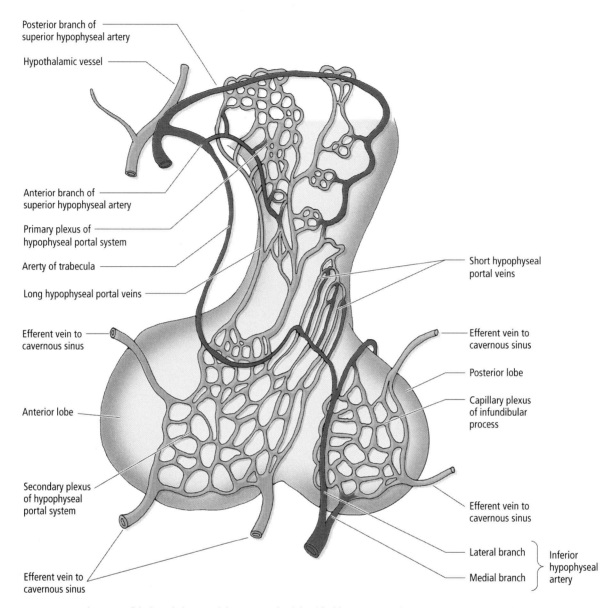

Posterior branch of
superior hypophyseal artery

Hypothalamic vessel

Anterior branch of
superior hypophyseal artery

Primary plexus of
hypophyseal portal system

Arerty of trabecula

Long hypophyseal portal veins

Efferent vein to
cavernous sinus

Anterior lobe

Secondary plexus
of hypophyseal
portal system

Efferent vein to
cavernous sinus

Short hypophyseal
portal veins

Efferent vein to
cavernous sinus

Posterior lobe

Capillary plexus
of infundibular
process

Efferent vein to
cavernous sinus

Lateral branch ⎫ Inferior
             ⎬ hypophyseal
Medial branch ⎭ artery

Figure 21.12 ● Vascularization of the hypothalamus and the pituitary gland. (Modified from Netter, FH (1983) *The CIBA Collection of Medical Illustrations.* Vol. 1, part 1. CIBA, New Jersey; p. 209, plate 57.)

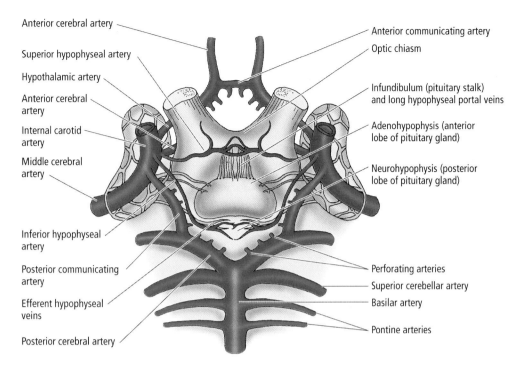

Figure 21.12 ● (*continued*)

The release-inhibiting hormones produced by the hypothalamus are:

- **somatostatin**, which inhibits growth hormone (GH) and TSH release;
- **prolactin-inhibitory factor** (PIF, dopamine), which inhibits the release of prolactin; and
- **melanocyte-stimulating hormone inhibitory factor** (IMIF), which inhibits melanocyte-stimulating hormone (MSH) release.

These releasing or inhibiting hormones are packaged into vesicles that flow down the axons of these neurons, which collectively form the **tuberohypophyseal (tuberoinfundibular) tract**, and are released in the median eminence and the pituitary stalk. There they pass into a capillary plexus that gives rise to portal veins that carry these releasing or inhibiting hormones to the anterior pituitary gland. The adenohypophysis contains cells that synthesize and, when appropriately stimulated, release into the general circulation the following trophic hormones: GH (somatotropin), prolactin, adrenocorticotropic hormone (ACTH, corticotropin), FSH, LH, interstitial cell-stimulating hormone (ICSH) in males, TSH (thyrotropin), and MSH. These hormones are released into the bloodstream and are carried to their target organs (endocrine glands) where they bind to receptors on cells and stimulate (or inhibit) the release of hormones produced by the respective organs.

The pituitary gland receives its blood supply mainly from two vessels; the superior and inferior hypophyseal arteries (Fig. 21.12). The **superior hypophyseal artery** is a branch of the internal carotid or the posterior communicating artery, and supplies the hypophyseal stalk and the anterior lobe of the pituitary gland. The **inferior hypophyseal artery** is a branch of the internal carotid artery, and supplies the posterior lobe of the pituitary gland.

Branches of the superior hypophyseal artery drain into a **capillary plexus** in the median eminence and upper part of the infundibular stalk. This plexus in turn drains into venules, which drain into long portal veins that descend in the infundibular stalk to the adenohypophysis where they branch into another capillary plexus. Both of these plexuses consist of fenestrated capillaries. These capillaries then drain into the nearby cavernous sinus.

A hypothalamic lesion usually extends into a number of its nuclei, affecting their function and resulting in more than one symptom

The hypothalamus is a small region of the brain and a lesion confined to only a single nucleus is uncommon. Instead, a hypothalamic lesion usually extends into a number of nuclei, affecting their function and resulting in more than one symptom. Hypothalamic lesions may result following skull fractures involving the sphenoid bone, cerebrovascular accidents, or most commonly, pituitary tumors. Depending on the nucleus or nuclei damaged, symptoms result from the dysfunction of the autonomic nervous system, water intake, food intake, temperature regulation, and sexual behavior.

Damage to nuclei that control body temperature

Bilateral destruction involving the preoptic and anterior hypothalamic nuclei results in hyperthermia (an elevation in body temperature)

The **preoptic** and **anterior hypothalamic nuclei** are involved in the control of body temperature. In the event that body temperature rises above normal limits, these nuclei initiate heat loss mechanisms in order to restore normal body temperature. Bilateral destruction involving these nuclei results in **hyperthermia**, an elevation in body temperature.

The presence of infectious agents in the body results in the production of pyrogens which may enter the bloodstream and eventually reach the hypothalamus. The pyrogens pass through the fenestrated capillaries of the anterior hypothalamus and contact the hypothalamic receptor cells of the circumventricular organs. In response to this contact, the body's thermostat is changed to a higher temperature point, thus the body's temperature becomes elevated above normal. This is accomplished by inhibition of heat loss mechanisms, cutaneous vasoconstriction, and shivering. Cutaneous vasoconstriction results in the lowering of the body's surface temperature, which is perceived as a cold sensation, usually accompanying a fever.

Bilateral destruction involving the posterior hypothalamic nuclei results in poikilothermia (the inability to regulate body temperature), regardless of environmental temperature

The **posterior hypothalamic nuclei** are also involved in the control of body temperature. In the event that body temperature drops, they initiate mechanisms that will conserve and produce heat to restore body temperature. Bilateral destruction involving the posterior hypothalamic nuclei results in the inability to regulate body temperature (**poikilothermia**) regardless of the environmental temperature. The reason for this phenomenon is that when the cells of the posterior nuclei are damaged, the fibers arising from the anterior hypothalamic nuclei are also damaged as they course through the posterior hypothalamic nuclei on their way to their destination.

Damage to nuclei that regulate food intake

A lesion in the lateral nucleus results in aphagia and a drastic drop in body weight. A bilateral lesion in the ventromedial nucleus results in hyperphagia and excess body weight

The **lateral** and **ventromedial nuclei** of the hypothalamus are involved in eating behavior. The lateral hypothalamic nucleus contains a group of neurons that synthesize **orexins** (G. orexis, "appetite") (also referred to as hypocretins), which are hypothalamic neuropeptides that regulate food intake and the sleep–wake cycle. Stimulation of the lateral nucleus ("feeding center") induces eating, whereas stimulation of the ventromedial nucleus ("satiety center") inhibits eating. Fasting causes an increase in orexin synthesis, whereas administration of exogenous orexin induces eating. A lesion in the lateral nucleus results in **aphagia** (G., "no eating") and a drastic drop in body weight. A bilateral lesion in the ventromedial nucleus results in **hyperphagia** (G., "overeating") and excess body weight.

Undetectable or low levels of orexin (hypocretin) production is associated with **narcolepsy**, a disorder in which an individual falls asleep suddenly, sev-

eral times during the day and at inopportune times. Studies show that the hypothalamus of an individual suffering from narcolepsy contains only one-tenth of the normal number of neurons that produce hypocretin. It is believed that narcolepsy may be caused by deficient hypocretin neurotransmission in some individuals.

3 What is believed to be the cause of narcolepsy?

Damage to the area that controls water intake

A lesion involving the cell group lateral to the lateral hypothalamic nucleus, known as the **zona incerta**, results in a lack of interest in water intake. This may result in severe dehydration and death.

Damage to nuclei that control the autonomic nervous system

A lesion involving the anterior hypothalamic nucleus will result in the disruption of parasympathetic activities, whereas a lesion involving the posterior hypothalamic nucleus will result in the disruption of both sympathetic and parasympathetic activities

The anterior and posterior hypothalamic areas are associated with the control of the autonomic nervous system. A lesion involving the **anterior hypothalamic nucleus** will result in the disruption of parasympathetic activities, whereas a lesion involving the **posterior hypothalamic nucleus** will result in the disruption of both sympathetic and parasympathetic activities. The reason for this is that although the posterior hypothalamic nucleus is involved in the control of the sympathetic nervous system, fibers arising from the anterior nucleus course through the posterior nucleus on their way to their destination. Thus a lesion in the posterior nucleus will damage local hypothalamic neurons controlling sympathetic activities and fibers passing through the nucleus controlling parasympathetic activities.

Damage to hypothalamic nuclei involved in aggression

Stimulation of the **lateral hypothalamus** not only induces eating and drinking behaviors in animals, but also causes animals to become more active, and even exhibit **aggressive behavior** or rage. Bilateral lesions in the lateral hypothalamus cause a lack of interest in eating, drinking, and extreme passivity of the animal. Stimulation of the **ventromedial nuclei** of the hypothalamus and surrounding areas produces satiety and tranquility. Bilateral lesions of the ventromedial areas of the hypothalamus induce excessive eating, drinking, excitability, and aggression.

Diabetes insipidus

Diabetes insipidus is a condition that results following anterior hypothalamic damage of the paraventricular and supraoptic nuclei (but primarily the supraoptic nucleus)

Damage to the anterior hypothalamus may result following the compression of the paraventricular and supraoptic nuclei by a growing tumor at the ventral aspect of the brain. The cells of this nucleus produce ADH (vasopressin), which acts on the kidney tubules to conserve water. As a result of nuclear damage, an inadequate amount of ADH results in **diabetes insipidus**. This condition is characterized by **polydipsia** (excess thirst, with the drinking of large volumes of water) and **polyuria** (the production of large volumes of dilute urine). Diabetes insipidus may also result following damage of the tuberoinfundibular tract. This is a hormonal-type diabetes insipidus, as opposed to the renal type where the renal tubules are incapable of responding to plentiful circulating ADH.

SYNONYMS AND EPONYMS OF THE HYPOTHALAMUS

Name of structure or term	Synonym(s)/ eponym(s)
Adrenocorticotropic hormone (ACTH)	Corticotropin
Amygdaloid nuclear complex	Amygdala Amygdaloid nucleus
Anterior pituitary gland	Adenohypophysis Anterior lobe of the pituitary gland
Antidiuretic hormone (ADH)	Vasopressin
Arcuate nucleus	Infundibular nucleus
Growth hormone (GH)	Somatotropin
Hypophyseal	Hypophysial
Hypothalamic release-inhibiting hormones	Hypothalamic release-inhibiting factors
Hypothalamic-releasing hormones (HRH)	Hypothalamic-releasing factors
Mammillary region of the pituitary gland	Posterior region of the pituitary gland
Mammillotegmental tract	Mammillotegmental fasciculus
Mammillothalamic tract	Mammillary fasciculus Tract of Vicq d'Azyr
Posterior pituitary gland	Neurohypophysis Posterior lobe of the pituitary gland
Prolactin inhibitory factor (PIF)	Dopamine
Stria terminalis	Amygdalohypothalamic fibers
Supraoptic region of the pituitary gland	Chiasmatic region of the pituitary gland Anterior region of the pituitary gland
Supraopticohypophyseal tract	Hypothalamohypophyseal tract Neurohypophyseal tract
Thyroid-stimulating hormone (TSH)	Thyrotropin
Thyroid-stimulating hormone-releasing hormone	Thyrotropin-releasing hormone (TRH)
Trigeminothalamic tract	Trigeminal lemniscus
Tuberal region of the pituitary gland	Infundibular region of the pituitary gland Middle region of the pituitary gland
Tuberohypophyseal tract	Tuberoinfundibular tract Infundibular tract
Ventral amygdalohypothalamic tract	Amygdalofugal tract

FOLLOW-UP TO CLINICAL CASE

This patient has **narcolepsy**. Narcolepsy is a condition which causes abnormal sleep patterns. It is almost always an acquired disease and symptoms typically begin in older childhood or young adulthood. The most common symptom is daytime sleepiness, which often leads to "sleep attacks." Nighttime sleep is often of poor quality, so the total sleep time during a 24-hour period is often normal. Some of the most characteristic and notable symptoms arise secondary to the intrusion of REM (rapid eye movement) states into waking hours. REM is a stage of normal sleep in which there is paralysis of all the muscles except those controlling eye movements and respiration. Dreams often occur in REM sleep. This intrusion of REM into waking hours accounts for episodes of cataplexy, sleep paralysis, and hypnagogic hallucinations.

Cataplexy refers to brief episodes of loss of muscle tone, which is brought about by intense emotions such as laughing or anger. This can cause falls or, in cases where it is just partial, a head drop or jaw drop. It can cause extreme social embarrassment. **Sleep paralysis** refers to brief episodes of complete paralysis, which can occur just before sleep onset or upon waking from sleep. **Hypnagogic hallucinations** are hallucinations, commonly visual and sometimes frightening, which occur before the onset of sleep (hypnagogic) or upon waking from sleep (hypnopompic).

Narcolepsy can be confirmed by a multiple sleep latency test (MSLT). An abnormally short onset of sleep (within 5 minutes) and an abnormally quick onset of the REM stage of sleep confirm the diagnosis of narcolepsy. A regular sleep study should be performed to look for other causes of excessive daytime sleepiness, such as obstructive sleep apnea.

The cause of narcolepsy has recently been determined. The posterior hypothalamus contains neurons that contain orexin (hypocretin). These neurons project widely, including to the cerebral cortex and brainstem. Orexin mediates wakefulness and alertness, and it has been demonstrated that a lack of orexin in animals, or an alteration of the orexin receptors, leads to symptoms reminiscent of narcolepsy. It is thought that there is a selective absence of these orexin-containing neurons in the posterior hypothalamus in narcolepsy.[1] The etiology of this condition is unclear.

The sleepiness and sleep attacks are treated with stimulants such as amphetamines or methylphenidate. A new medication for this, which has less abuse potential and side effects, is modafinil. Cataplexy can be treated with tricyclic antidepressants or similar medicines, which promote the effects of amines such as norepinephrine, dopamine, or serotonin. These medications inhibit REM sleep.[1]

1 Scammell TE (2003) The neurobiology, diagnosis, and treatment of narcolepsy. *Annals of Neurology* **53** (2): 154–66.

QUESTIONS TO PONDER

1. What are the functions of the periventricular zone nuclei of the hypothalamus?

2. What are the functions of the medial zone nuclei of the hypothalamus?

3. What are the functions of the lateral zone nuclei of the hypothalamus?

4. What is the function of the nuclei in the preoptic region of the hypothalamus?

5. What are the functions of the supraoptic region of the hypothalamus?

6. What are the functions of the tuberal region of the hypothalamus?

7. What are the functions of the mammillary region of the hypothalamus?

8. What is the most prominent source of input to the hypothalamus?

9. What is the function of the circumventricular organs?

10. In addition to neural output, what other structure does the hypothalamus influence?

11. What is the most prominent neural input to the hypothalamus?

12. What is the function of the spinohypothalamic fibers?

13. What is the function of the reticular formation fibers terminating in the hypothalamus?

14. What is the function of the supraopticohypophyseal (hypothalamohypophyseal) tract?

15. What is the function of the tuberohypophyseal tract?

16. Summarize the functions of the hypothalamus.

17. A young woman is brought to the doctor because, although she is 18 years old, she has failed to menstruate. Blood tests confirm that she has almost no follicle-stimulating hormone or luteinizing hormone in her circulation. Name the possible problems that could cause this condition.

CHAPTER 22

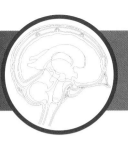
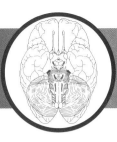
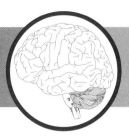

Thalamus

CLINICAL CASE

A 68-year-old hypertensive male had sudden onset of headache and complete loss of sensation of his left face, arm, and leg. This began 10 hours before admission to the emergency room. He had no other complaint.

His blood pressure in the ER was 230/120. Other vital signs were relatively normal. Brief examination in the ER confirmed sensory loss on the left side of his body, with normal strength. Movements on the left were not well coordinated. He was able to ambulate quite well. An urgent head CT was performed, which was diagnostic.

Information arising from the **basal ganglia**, **cerebellum**, **limbic system** and **sensory systems** (with the exception of the sense of olfaction) is relayed to the **thalamus**, a subcortical relay station. Here, this information is processed and integrated and is then transmitted to specific areas of the ipsilateral cerebral cortex. These cortical areas are in turn connected via reciprocal feedback projections to the thalamic subnuclei, making the cerebral cortex the most prominent input source to the thalamus.

The thalamus not only functions in the further processing and integration of *sensory* and *motor* information, but also serves as the main entrance, via which this and additional information reaches the cerebral cortex. Therefore, the thalamus not only controls the flow of numerous streams of information to the cerebral cortex for additional processing but, ultimately, regulates cortical activity.

Although the thalamus projects mainly to the cerebral cortex, it also provides input to the basal ganglia and the hypothalamus.

BORDERS

The thalamus has an anterior and posterior pole, and four surfaces. Its boundaries are: *anteriorly*, the interventricular foramen (of Monro); *posteriorly*, the posterior extent of the pulvinar; *medially*, the third ventricle; *laterally*, the posterior limb of the internal capsule; *dorsally*, its free surface, which contributes to the floor of the lateral ventricle; and *ventrally*, the hypothalamic sulcus on the lateral wall of the third ventricle, separating it from the hypothalamus (Figs 22.1, 22.2).

ANATOMY

The thalamus is the largest subcortical gray mass of the CNS and is the main constituent of the diencephalon

The **thalamus** (G., "inner chamber") (Fig. 22.2) is an oval-shaped mass of gray matter, embedded deep within the white matter of each cerebral hemisphere. Although the right and left thalami are separated along most

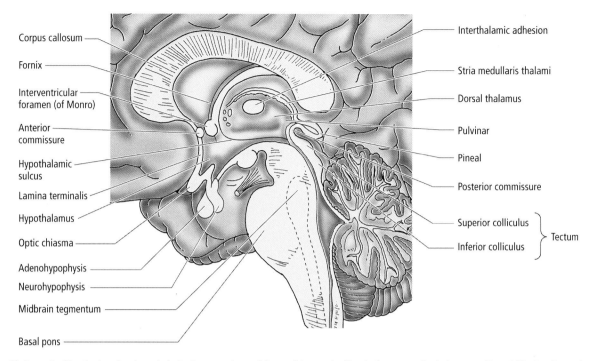

Corpus callosum

Fornix

Interventricular
foramen (of Monro)

Anterior
commissure

Hypothalamic
sulcus

Lamina terminalis

Hypothalamus

Optic chiasma

Adenohypophysis

Neurohypophysis

Midbrain tegmentum

Basal pons

Interthalamic adhesion

Stria medullaris thalami

Dorsal thalamus

Pulvinar

Pineal

Posterior commissure

Superior colliculus

Inferior colliculus

Tectum

Figure 22.1 ● A midsagittal section through the brainstem and part of the overlying cerebral hemisphere. Note the thalamus and its neighboring diencephalic structures and midbrain.

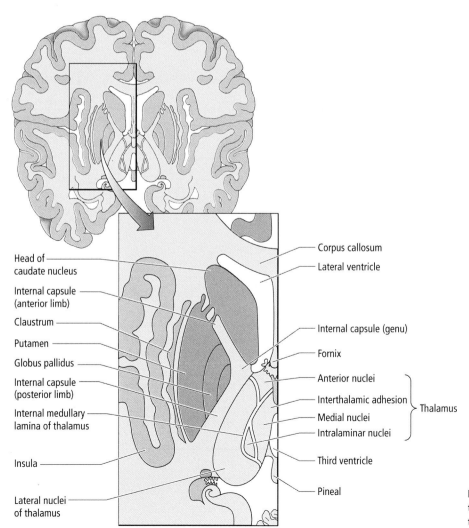

Head of
caudate nucleus

Internal capsule
(anterior limb)

Claustrum

Putamen

Globus pallidus

Internal capsule
(posterior limb)

Internal medullary
lamina of thalamus

Insula

Lateral nuclei
of thalamus

Corpus callosum

Lateral ventricle

Internal capsule (genu)

Fornix

Anterior nuclei

Interthalamic adhesion

Medial nuclei

Intralaminar nuclei

Thalamus

Third ventricle

Pineal

Figure 22.2 ● A horizontal section through the cerebral hemispheres showing the dorsal thalamus, basal ganglia, and internal capsule.

of their medial surface by the narrow, vertically oriented third ventricle, a short, narrow, cylindrical structure—the **interthalamic adhesion (massa intermedia)**, which traverses the third ventricle—forms a bridge between them.

Although the interthalamic adhesion connects the right and left sides of the brain, it is not considered to be a true "commissure" since this structure consists of gray matter only, and has no decussating fibers. The interthalamic adhesion is present in the majority of brains; however, its function is unknown.

The **stria medullaris thalami** and the **stria terminalis**, two thin strands of white matter, lie on the superior surface of the thalamus (Fig. 22.3). The stria medullaris thalami courses on the superomedial margin of the thalamus, separating its superior from its medial surface. It is a slender bundle of two-way fibers connecting the septal nuclei and hypothalamus with the habenular nucleus of the epithalamus. The stria

terminalis carries fibers primarily from the amygdala, which terminate in the hypothalamus, septal area, and bed nucleus of the stria terminalis. It courses on the superolateral surface of the thalamus, separating its superior surface from its lateral surface and from the body of the caudate nucleus.

The lateral aspect of the superior surface of the thalamus contributes to the floor of the lateral ventricle and the medial aspect of the superior surface of the thalamus displays a groove formed by the fornix.

The thalamus rests on the mesencephalon, thus its inferior surface forms a ceiling over the mesencephalic tectum (Fig. 22.1). Numerous tracts such as the medial lemniscus and the trigeminothalamic, rubrothalamic, reticulothalamic, and dentatothalamic (cerebellothalamic) tracts, ascend through the brainstem and pass into the thalamus from its inferior surface. In addition, the brainstem reticular formation extends superiorly into the thalamus through this surface.

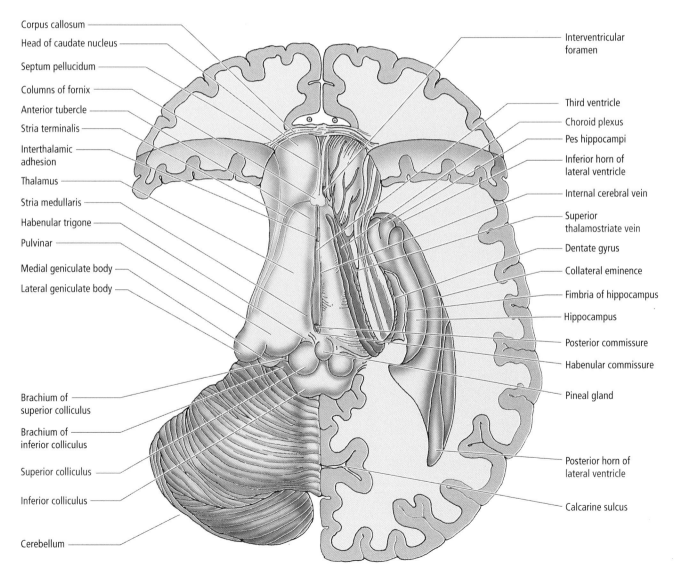

Figure 22.3 ● Schematic representation of the dorsal surface of the thalamus on a horizontally sectioned brain. Part of the cerebral hemisphere has been removed to expose deeper structures such as the thalamus, third ventricle, caudate nucleus, and hippocampus.

INTERNAL AND EXTERNAL MEDULLARY LAMINAE

The thalamus is closely associated with two nearly vertical layers of myelinated fibers, the internal and external medullary laminae

The **internal medullary lamina**, a Y-shaped layer of white matter, partitions the thalamus into three main groups of nuclei, the **anterior**, **medial**, and **lateral groups**, based on their relative position (Figs 22.2, 22.4). The posterior portion of this lamina, the leg of the Y, separates the medial from the lateral thalamic nuclear groups. Its anterior portion, which is divided into two limbs, partially surrounds the anterior nuclear group, and separates it from the neighboring medial and lateral nuclear groups. The internal medullary lamina contains afferent and efferent thalamic fibers that enter or leave the thalamic subnuclei.

The **external medullary lamina** is a curved layer of white matter that follows the contour and covers mostly the anterior and lateral surfaces of the thalamus. It is composed of myelinated **thalamocortical fibers** that originate in the thalamus and terminate in the cerebral cortex, and of reciprocal feedback **corticothalamic fibers** that originate in the cerebral cortex and terminate in the thalamus. The external medullary lamina is covered by a slender layer of gray matter, the **thalamic reticular nucleus**, which is the most lateral (and outermost) nucleus of the thalamus (Fig. 22.4B).

The myelinated thalamocortical fibers arising from the thalamus pass through the external medullary lamina, and radiate from the lateral surface of the thalamus, collectively forming the **thalamic radiations**. These fibers become incorporated in the various parts of the internal capsule and the corona radiata as they ascend to terminate in the cerebral cortex. Corticothalamic fibers also course through the corona radiata and the internal capsule, and when they approach the thalamus they converge to pass through the external medullary lamina to terminate in the various thalamic subnuclei.

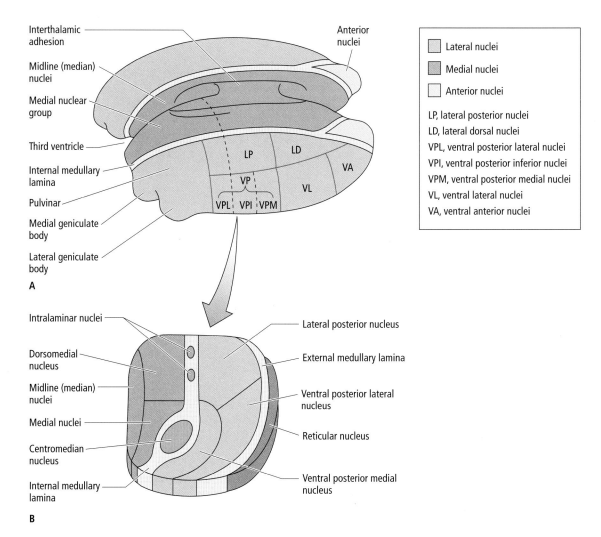

Figure 22.4 ● (A) Schematic representation of the thalamus showing its dorsal and lateral surfaces. (B) Cross-section through the thalamus showing the midline, medial, intralaminar, and lateral groups of nuclei.

Nuclear group	Component subnuclei	Functional group
Anterior	Anteroventral (AV)	Specific relay
	Anteromedial (AM)	Specific relay
	Anterodorsal (AD)	Specific relay
Medial	Dorsomedial (DM)	Association (multimodal)
	Midline (median, periventricular)	Nonspecific
Lateral	Dorsal tier	
	Lateral dorsal (LD)	Association (multimodal)
	Lateral posterior (LP)	Association (multimodal)
	Pulvinar (P)	Association (multimodal)
	Ventral tier	
	Ventral anterior (VA)	Motor relay
	Ventral lateral (VL)	Motor relay
	Ventral posterior (VP)	
	Ventral posterior medial (VPM)	Sensory relay
	Ventral posterior lateral (VPL)	Sensory relay
	Ventral posterior inferior (VPI)	
	Metathalamic nuclei	
	Medial geniculate nucleus	Sensory relay
	Lateral geniculate nucleus	Sensory relay
Intralaminar	Centromedian (CM)	Nonspecific
	Parafascicular (PF)	Nonspecific
Reticular		Nonspecific

Table 22.1 ● Anatomical and functional classification of the thalamic nuclei.

THALAMIC NUCLEI

Anatomical classification

The thalamus is partitioned by the internal medullary lamina into the anterior, medial, and lateral nuclear groups (subdivisions)

Based on their afferent and efferent connections, each thalamic nuclear group functions as an independent unit and serves a particular function (Figs 22.2, 22.4; Table 22.1). The nuclear groups are further divided into **subnuclei**, and the role of each thalamic subnucleus is associated with the source(s) of incoming afferents, and the cortical target areas of its efferents (Table 22.2).

With the exception of the thalamic reticular nucleus, all thalamic subnuclei possess thalamic **projection neurons** that relay processed information to the cerebral cortex. In addition, the thalamic subnuclei also have inhibitory gamma aminobutyric acid (GABA)-ergic **interneurons** whose cell bodies and processes are confined to a single subnucleus.

Although a number of classifications exist, this textbook uses the most common of these and subdivides the subnuclei into anterior, medial, and lateral nuclear groups. The **anterior** and **medial nuclear groups** are phylogenetically the older thalamic nuclei and are collectively referred to as the **paleothalamus**. The subnuclei of the **lateral nuclear group** are newer, and are referred to as the **neothalamus**. Additionally, because of their unique characteristics, two of the thalamic nuclei—the **intralaminar** and **reticular nuclei**—are usually not included in any of the three thalamic nuclear groups listed above, but instead are grouped separately.

Anterior nuclear group

The anterior nuclear group consists of a composite of three subnuclei: the AV, AM, and AD subnuclei

The anterior nuclear group consists of a composite of three subnuclei: the **anteroventral** (AV), **anteromedial** (AM), and **anterodorsal** (AD) **subnuclei**. The subnuclei of the anterior group are wedged in the anterior tubercle of the thalamus, which forms an elevation on the anterior part of the lateral wall of the third ventricle. This is the smallest thalamic nuclear group, and due to the comparable connections and roles of its three subnuclei, they are collectively referred to as the **anterior nuclei of the thalamus**.

The anterior nuclear group, a relay nucleus of the Papez circuit of emotion, has a significant number of connections with the limbic system. It receives afferent fibers relaying information from the mammillary body of the hypothalamus via the mammillothalamic tract, and the hippocampal formation via the fornix. It in turn projects to the cingulate gyrus of the limbic association cortex. Due to its limbic connections, the anterior nuclear group functions in the expression of emotions, and due to its considerable connections with the hippocampal formation, this group of nuclei is also believed

Table 22.2 ● Connections of the thalamic subnuclei.

Nucleus/subnucleus	Afferents (input)	Efferents (output)	Function(s)
Anterior (A)	Mammillary body via mammillothalamic tract Hippocampal formation via fornix	Cingulate gyrus	Expression of emotions Learning, memory
Dorsomedial (DM)			
Parvocellular	Prefrontal association cortex	Prefrontal association cortex	Integration of sensory information
Magnocellular	Amygdala Orbitofrontal cortex Olfactory system Hypothalamus Intralaminar, midline, and lateral posterior thalamic nuclei	Prefrontal association cortex	Expression of emotions
Midline			
Dorsal midline	Striatum, limbic cortex	Striatum, limbic cortex	Modulation of cortical excitability
Ventral midline	Hippocampus	Hippocampus	
Lateral dorsal (LD)	Mammillary body via mammillothalamic tract	Cingulate gyrus Parahippocampal gyrus	Expression of emotions
Lateral posterior (LP)	Superior parietal lobule Precuneus Superior colliculus Pretectal area Occipital lobe	Superior parietal lobule Precuneus	Sensory integration

Pulvinar (P)	Association areas of parietal, temporal, and
	    occipital lobes
	
	Retina, superior colliculus, lateral geniculate
	    nucleus, medial geniculate nucleus,
	    cerebellum
		Association areas of
		    parietal, temporal, and
		    occipital lobes
			Integration of visual, auditory, and
			    somatosensory information

Ventral anterior (VA)			

Magnocellular	Substantia nigra (pars reticulata) via
	    nigrothalamic pathway
	Intralaminar and midline nuclei of the thalamus
	Reticular formation
		Frontal eye field	Control of eye, face, and head
			    movements

Parvocellular	Globus pallidus (internal segment) via pallidothalamic pathway Intralaminar and midline nuclei of the thalamus Reticular formation	Premotor cortex Supplementary motor area	 Control of limb movement
Ventral lateral (VL)			Control of movement
VLa			
Magnocellular	Substantia nigra (pars reticulata)	Supplementary motor area	
Parvocellular	Globus pallidus (internal segment)		
VLp	Contralateral cerebellar nuclei via dentatothalamic tract	Premotor cortex Primary motor cortex	

Ventral posterior medial (VPM)	Orofacial region via trigeminothalamic tracts
	
	Solitary nucleus
		Primary somatosensory
		    cortex in postcentral
		    gyrus
			Processes touch, pressure, pain,
			    and temperature sensation, and
			    proprioception
			Taste

Ventral posterior lateral (VPL) and
ventral posterior inferior (VPI)
	Lateral spinothalamic tract
	
	Medial lemniscus
	
	Anterior spinothalamic tract
		Primary somatosensory
		    cortex in the postcentral
		    gyrus
		Primary somatosensory
		    cortex in the postcentral
		    gyrus
		Primary somatosensory
		    cortex in the postcentral
		    gyrus
			Processes pain and temperature
			    sensation from the body
			
			Processes touch, pressure, joint
			    movement, and vibratory sense
			    from the body
			Processes light touch sensation
			    from the body

Table 22.2 ● *Continued*.

Nucleus/subnucleus	Afferents (input)	Efferents (output)	Function(s)
Ventral posterior inferior (VPI)	Vestibulothalamic fibers	Vestibular area of the somatosensory cortex	
Medial geniculate body (MGB)	Inferior colliculus Other auditory nuclei via brachium of inferior colliculus Lateral lemniscus Primary auditory cortex	Auditory radiation to the primary auditory cortex	Hearing
Lateral geniculate body (LGB)	Retina via optic tract Primary visual cortex Pulvinar Other thalamic nuclei	Optic radiation to the primary visual cortex Pulvinar Other thalamic nuclei	Vision
Intralaminar 　Centromedian	Globus pallidus Premotor cortex Primary motor cortex Ascending sensory systems Reticular formation	Striatum (caudate nucleus and putamen) Other intralaminar nuclei	Sensorimotor integration Maintenance of arousal Pain perception Control of cortical activity
Parafascicular	Striatum Supplementary motor area Ascending sensory systems Reticular formation Striatum	Widespread areas of the cerebral cortex	
Reticular	Corticothalamic, thalamocortical, thalamostriatal, and pallidothalamic collaterals	Other thalamic nuclei Reticular formation	Integrates and controls thalamic activity

to be associated with learning and memory processes. The anterior nuclei are also associated with attention.

Medial nuclear group

The medial nuclear group resides medial to the internal medullary lamina, which separates it from the anterior and lateral nuclear groups

The **medial nuclear group** includes the more prominent **dorsomedial nucleus** (DM; also referred to as the **medial dorsal nucleus**, MD), as well as the diffuse **midline nuclei** (also referred to as the **median** or **periventricular nuclei**) that are located on the most medial surface of the thalamus (adjoining the third ventricle) and within the interthalamic adhesion. It should be noted that some authors classify the midline nuclei as a separate group of nuclei (and not part of the medial group).

The DM nucleus functions in the processing of information related to emotion. It is subdivided into the parvocellular and magnocellular divisions. The **parvocellular** division has reciprocal connections with the prefrontal association cortex, which functions in the integration of sensory information associated with higher order cognitive function. As part of the association loop of the basal ganglia, the globus pallidus and the substantia nigra project to the ventral anterior and

the DM nuclei of the thalamus. These nuclei in turn project via thalamocortical fibers to the prefrontal cortex. The **magnocellular** division is associated with limbic system components such as the amygdala and the orbitofrontal cortex. Additionally, the DM nucleus has extensive connections with the olfactory system, the hypothalamus, and the intralaminar, midline, and lateral posterior subnuclei of the thalamus.

The **midline nuclei** function in the modulation of cortical excitability. They include the **dorsal midline nuclei**, which are associated with the striatum and the limbic cortex, and the **ventral midline nuclei**, which are associated with the hippocampus.

Lateral nuclear group

The lateral nuclear group is interposed between the internal and external medullary laminae, and consists of numerous subnuclei that collectively form the largest nuclear group of the thalamus

The **lateral nuclear group** is interposed between the internal and external medullary laminae, and consists of numerous subnuclei that collectively form the largest nuclear group of the thalamus. The subnuclei of this nuclear group are arranged into two step-like rows, the **dorsal** and **ventral tiers of nuclei** (subnuclei).

Dorsal tier of the thalamic nuclei

> These nuclei are associated with the association areas of the cerebral cortex, and function in the integration of sensory input

The **dorsal tier of the thalamic nuclei** is composed of the lateral dorsal nucleus, lateral posterior nucleus, and the pulvinar nucleus. With the exception of the lateral dorsal nucleus, these nuclei are connected with the *association areas of the cerebral cortex*, and function in the integration of sensory input.

The **lateral dorsal (LD) nucleus** is the caudal continuation of the anterior thalamic nuclear group and may play a role in the expression of emotions. Like the anterior thalamic nuclear group, it receives inputs from the mammillary body via the mammillothalamic tract, and in turn projects to the cingulate and parahippocampal gyri of the limbic system.

The **lateral posterior (LP) nucleus** is the rostral continuation of the pulvinar nucleus and is believed to play a role in sensory integration. Since these nuclei have comparable connections, they are also called the **pulvinar–LP complex**. The LP nucleus is interconnected with the superior parietal lobule (Brodmann's areas 5 and 7) and the precuneus. It also receives afferent terminals from components of the visual system: the superior colliculus, the pretectal area, and the occipital lobe.

The **pulvinar nucleus** (L., "cushion") is the most prominent nucleus of the thalamus and functions in the integration of visual, auditory, and somatosensory information. It has reciprocal projections with the association areas of the parietal, temporal, and occipital lobes. It also receives sensory information from components of the visual system, the medial geniculate nucleus, and the cerebellum.

Ventral tier of the thalamic nuclei

The **ventral tier of the thalamic nuclei** includes the **ventral anterior (VA) nucleus**, **ventral lateral (VL) nucleus**, and **ventral posterior (VP) nucleus** (also referred to as the **ventrobasal complex**). The latter is further subdivided into the ventral posterior medial (VPM) nucleus, the ventral posterior lateral (VPL) nucleus, and the ventral posterior inferior (VPI) nucleus. The ventral tier also includes the **metathalamic nuclei**, including the **medial** and **lateral geniculate nuclei** (MGN and LGN, respectively) or **bodies**.

> The nuclei residing in the anterior aspect of the ventral tier of the system serve as relay stations for the somatic motor system and the brainstem reticular formation

The nuclei residing in the *anterior aspect* of the ventral tier of nuclei (VA and VL), serve as relay stations for the somatic motor system including the basal ganglia and the cerebellum. They also process inputs from the brainstem reticular formation.

> The nuclei residing in the posterior aspect of the ventral tier of the thalamic nuclei serve as relay stations for all of the sensory systems

The nuclei residing in the *posterior aspect* of the ventral tier of nuclei (VPM, VPL, VPI, MGN, and LGN) serve as relay stations for all of the sensory systems (the somatosensory, visual, auditory, and gustatory systems, but excluding the olfactory system).

Ventral anterior nucleus

> The VA nucleus plays a role in the control of the movement of the eyes, face, head, and limbs

The **ventral anterior (VA) nucleus** consists of magnocellular and parvocellular components. The **magnocellular** component is the site of termination of the nigrothalamic pathway, which conveys information from the ipsilateral pars reticulata of the substantia nigra. The **parvocellular** component is the site of termination of the pallidothalamic pathway, which transmits information from the medial (internal) segment of the globus pallidus. In addition, fibers from the intralaminar and midline nuclei of the thalamus, as well as from the brainstem reticular formation, terminate in the VA nucleus. This nucleus sends a spray of fibers throughout the frontal lobe. The magnocellular component of this nucleus is interconnected with the frontal eye fields (Brodmann's area 8). The parvocellular component of this nucleus is interconnected with the premotor cortex and supplementary motor area (Brodmann's area 6). The VA nucleus plays a role in the control of movement. The information arising from the substantia nigra pars reticulata is involved in movements of the eyes, face, and head, whereas that arising from the medial segment of the globus pallidus is associated with movement of the limbs.

Ventral lateral nucleus

> The VL nucleus exerts its influence on somatic motor activity via the cerebral nuclei and the cerebellum

The **ventral lateral (VL) nucleus** is further subdivided anatomically into an anterior (VLa) portion and a posterior (VLp) portion. This nucleus, like the VA nucleus, consists of magnocellular and parvocellular components.

The **VLa** receives afferent fibers from the basal ganglia. Its magnocellular component receives projections from the substantia nigra pars reticulata, and its parvocellular component receives projections from the medial segment of the globus pallidus. The VLa in turn sends efferents to the supplementary motor area (Brodmann's area 6) of the cerebral cortex.

The **VLp** receives prominent projections arising from the deep cerebellar nuclei (mainly from the dentate nucleus) of the opposite side, via the dentatothalamic tract. The VLp then relays the information to the premotor and primary motor cortex (Brodmann's areas 6 and 4, respectively).

It is important to note that there is no overlap in the specific target site of termination of the afferent fibers arising from the substantia nigra, the globus pallidus, and the cerebellum. In addition, fibers from other thalamic nuclei and the reticular formation terminate in the VL nucleus. The VL nucleus exerts its influence on somatic motor activity via the basal ganglia and the cerebellum.

Ventral posterior nucleus
> The VP nucleus relays processed sensory information to the primary somesthetic cortex located in the postcentral gyrus of the parietal lobe (Brodmann's areas 3, 1, and 2)

The **ventral posterior** (VP) **nucleus**, also known as the **ventrobasal complex**, is subdivided into the VPM nucleus, VPL nucleus, and the smaller VPI nucleus, which is interposed between the latter two nuclei. The VP nucleus relays processed sensory information to the primary somesthetic cortex located in the postcentral gyrus of the parietal lobe (Brodmann's areas 3, 1, and 2). These cortical areas send corticothalamic fibers back to the VP nucleus.

The **VPM nucleus** receives the terminals of the trigeminothalmic tracts (the ventral and dorsal trigeminal lemnisci) relaying general somatic afferent information (touch, pressure, pain and temperature sensation, and proprioception) from the orofacial region, and special visceral afferent sensation (taste) from the solitary nucleus.

The **VPL and VPI nuclei** receive terminals of the lateral spinothalamic tract relaying pain and temperature sensation from the body, terminals of the medial lemniscus transmitting discriminatory (fine) touch, pressure, joint movement, and vibratory sensation from the body, and terminals from the anterior spinothalamic tract relaying light (crude) touch sensation from the body.

Additionally, the VPI nucleus receives fibers from the vestibular nuclei (vestibulothalamic fibers) and projects to the vestibular area of the somatosensory cortex.

> Note that the clinical case at the beginning of the chapter refers to a patient whose symptoms include headache and complete unilateral loss of sensation on the left side of the face, arm, and leg. A CT scan is diagnostic of a right thalamic hemorrhage.
>
> **1** Which thalamic nuclei have been damaged by this cerebral hemorrhage, which caused a complete unilateral sensory loss from the face and upper and lower limbs in this patient?
>
> **2** Which ascending sensory tracts terminate in these thalamic nuclei?

Metathalamic nuclei
> The MGN processes auditory input from both ears, whereas the LGN processes visual input from both eyes

The **metathalamic nuclei** include the medial and lateral geniculate nuclei (bodies). They are two oval-shaped elevations located inferior to the pulvinar of the right and left sides.

The **medial geniculate nucleus** or **body** (MGN or MGB) is located on the posterior aspect of the thalamus, inferior to the pulvinar, and lateral to the superior colliculus. This nucleus receives afferent fibers relaying auditory input (from both ears) from the inferior colliculus, as well as some projections from other nuclei of the auditory system via the brachium of the inferior colliculus, and directly via the lateral lemniscus (the principal pathway of the auditory system). The MGN gives rise to the auditory radiation that terminates in the primary auditory cortex residing in the superior transverse temporal gyrus of Heschl (Brodmann's areas 41 and 42). Brodmann's areas 41 and 42 are reciprocally connected with the MGN.

The **lateral geniculate nucleus** or **body** (LGN or LGB), a thalamic relay nucleus for vision, is larger than its medial counterpart. The majority of fibers of the optic tract, bringing information from both eyes, terminate here. This nucleus projects via the geniculocalcarine tract (optic radiation) to the primary visual cortex (Brodmann's area 17) on the banks of the calcarine fissure of the occipital lobe. The LGN is reciprocally connected with the primary visual cortex; additionally, it is interconnected with the pulvinar and other subnuclei of the thalamus. The thalamocortical projections may play a role in arousal of the organism, the control of visual attention, and the regulation of visual input transmission to the primary visual cortex.

Intralaminar nuclei

> The intralaminar nuclei mark the rostral continuation of the ARAS into the thalamus

The **intralaminar nuclei** mark the rostral continuation of the ascending reticular activating system (ARAS) into the thalamus. They consist of multiple, diffuse aggregations of nerve cell bodies embedded within the *internal medullary lamina* and the *interthalamic adhesion* of the thalamus. These nuclei receive sensory information from the spinothalamic tract, the ventral trigeminothalamic tract (ventral trigeminal lemniscus), and the multisynaptic ascending pathways of the reticular formation that relay pain sensation, pain perception, and arousal of the organism. Two of these intralaminar nuclei, the centromedian nucleus and parafascicular nucleus are readily perceptible in the posterior part of the internal medullary lamina. The centromedian nucleus is the most prominent, and is located medial to the VPM and VPL nuclei. The parafascicular nucleus is located medial to the centromedian nucleus.

The prominent **centromedian nucleus** is the site of termination of the fibers arising from the globus pallidus and the premotor (part of Brodmann's area 6) and primary motor cortical areas (Brodmann's area 4), whereas the **parafascicular nucleus** is the site of termination of fibers arising from the supplementary motor area (part of Brodmann's area 6). Both of these nuclei send prominent projections to the basal ganglia (caudate nucleus and putamen). Their projections to the somatosensory areas of the cerebral cortex suggest that they function in sensorimotor integration. Furthermore, as a result of their widespread cortical connections they are believed to play a role in the control of cortical activity.

The intralaminar nuclei are not interconnected with other thalamic nuclei; they only project to each other.

Thalamic reticular nucleus

The thalamic reticular nucleus receives collaterals of the thalamocortical, corticothalamic, thalamostriatal, and pallidothalamic fibers

The **thalamic reticular nucleus** was named for its reticular (mesh-like) appearance, and is not considered part of the brainstem reticular formation. It consists of a thin layer of nerve cell bodies that covers the external medullary lamina on the lateral surface of the thalamus. This is the lateral-most nucleus of the thalamus that is in direct contact with the posterior limb of the internal capsule, laterally.

Almost all of the **thalamocortical fibers** destined for the cerebral cortex give rise to collaterals that end in the thalamic reticular nucleus. In addition, almost all of the **corticothalamic fibers**, on their way to the thalamic subnuclei, course through the thalamic reticular nucleus where they send collaterals to synapse there. The **thalamostriatal** and reciprocal **pallidothalamic fibers** also give rise to collaterals that synapse in the thalamic reticular nucleus.

Unlike the other thalamic nuclei, which project to the cerebral cortex, the thalamic reticular nucleus has no known direct cortical connections. Instead, it relays sensory input locally within the reticular nucleus, to the other thalamic nuclei, and to the reticular formation.

The thalamic reticular nucleus resides in a location where it not only receives a copy of, but can also monitor, thalamic communication with the cortex and the basal ganglia. This nucleus may play a role in the control of thalamic function.

Functional organization of the thalamic nuclei (subnuclei)

Functional organization of the thalamic subnuclei is based on projections between the thalamic nuclei and the cerebral cortex

In addition to the anatomical classification of the thalamic nuclei that was discussed in the previous sections, these nuclei are also categorized according to their function. Functional organization of the thalamic subnuclei is based on projections between the thalamic nuclei and the cerebral cortex (see Table 22.2). The thalamic nuclei have been classified into specific relay (sensory relay and motor relay) nuclei, association (multimodal) nuclei, and nonspecific nuclear functional groups.

The **specific relay nuclei** have reciprocal feedback connections with particular, well-defined, sensory or motor areas of the cerebral cortex (Fig. 22.5). All of the specific relay nuclei rest in the ventral tier of the lateral nuclear group.

The **sensory relay nuclei** of the thalamus include the VPM and VPL nuclei, the MGN, and the LGN. The VPM and VPL nuclei function in the processing and integration of somatosensory information arising from the orofacial region and body, respectively. The MGN and LGN function in the processing of special sensory information related to hearing and vision, respectively.

The **motor relay nuclei** of the thalamus include the VA and VL nuclei. These nuclei relay motor information arising from the somatic motor system—including the basal ganglia and the cerebellum—to the motor cortical areas.

In addition to the nuclei mentioned above, the anterior nuclear group, the smallest collection of thalamic nuclei, is also included in the specific relay nuclei group. Via its connections to the limbic system, the anterior nuclear group plays a role in the processing of emotions, learning, and memory processes.

The **association (multimodal) nuclei**, unlike the specific relay nuclei, receive sensory and motor information from the sensory and motor systems *indirectly* via a relay in other thalamic nuclei, and from many different parts of the brain.

The thalamic association (multimodal) nuclei include the DM, LD, LP, and pulvinar nuclei. These nuclei are referred to as association nuclei because they have widespread connections with the cortical association areas of the frontal, parietal, and temporal lobes. These nuclei are also referred to as multimodal nuclei because they process various modalities. They are involved in the processing of information related to memory and emotional expression, and also consolidate various types of sensory information.

The **nonspecific nuclei** of the thalamus include the intralaminar nucleus and reticular thalamic nucleus. These nuclei receive terminals arising from the caudate nucleus, putamen, cerebellum, and motor cortex. They are involved in the control of arousal and consciousness. Some authors also include the **midline nuclei** in this functional group. The midline nuclei are associated with the striatum and limbic structures, and are believed to function in the modulation of cortical excitability.

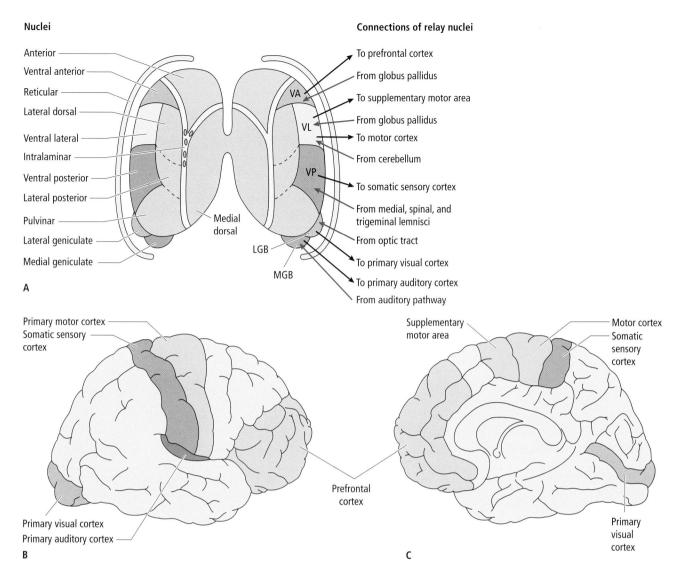

Nuclei

- Anterior
- Ventral anterior
- Reticular
- Lateral dorsal
- Ventral lateral
- Intralaminar
- Ventral posterior
- Lateral posterior
- Pulvinar
- Lateral geniculate
- Medial geniculate

VA
VL
VP
Medial dorsal
LGB
MGB

A

Connections of relay nuclei

- To prefrontal cortex
- From globus pallidus
- To supplementary motor area
- From globus pallidus
- To motor cortex
- From cerebellum
- To somatic sensory cortex
- From medial, spinal, and trigeminal lemnisci
- From optic tract
- To primary visual cortex
- To primary auditory cortex
- From auditory pathway

Primary motor cortex
Somatic sensory cortex

Primary visual cortex
Primary auditory cortex

B

Supplementary motor area

Prefrontal cortex

Motor cortex
Somatic sensory cortex

Primary visual cortex

C

Figure 22.5 ● Schematic representation of the dorsal surface of the thalamus. (A) Thalamic nuclei and connections of the component nuclei of the thalamus. LGB, lateral geniculate body; MGB, medial geniculate body. (B) Lateral surface of the right cerebral hemisphere. (C) Medial surface of the right cerebral hemisphere illustrating the cortical areas where the thalamic nuclei project. (Modified from Fitzgerald, MJT, Folan-Curran, J (2002) *Clinical Neuroanatomy and Related Neuroscience*. WB Saunders, New York; fig. 22.1.)

CLINICAL CONSIDERATIONS

A tumor or stroke that results in thalamic damage and affects the VPM or VPL nuclei, may at first result in diminished or complete loss of touch, pressure, pain or temperature sensation, or proprioception from the *contralateral* orofacial region or body, respectively. Recall that the VPM nucleus of the thalamus receives projections from the main sensory nucleus of the trigeminal (relaying discriminatory touch and pressure sensation) via the dorsal trigeminal lemniscus, and the spinal nucleus of the trigeminal (relaying nondiscriminatory touch and nociceptive and temperature sensation) via the ventral trigeminal lemnisci from the orofacial region. The VPL nucleus receives projections from the dorsal horn of the spinal cord relaying nondiscriminatory touch, pressure, and nociceptive and temperature sensation from the contralateral side of the body via the anterolateral system.

Subsequent to the loss of sensation caused by a thalamic lesion, the individual experiences **paresthesias** (abnormal sensations such as tingling, pinching, or burning, in the absence of an actual stimulus), which may progress to agonizing pain in the parts of the body where loss of sensation has occurred.

This condition is referred to as the **thalamic pain syndrome (Déjérine–Roussy syndrome)**. In many cases, even nonpainful, innocuous stimuli such as a light touch or the contact of clothing on the skin, may trigger a painful sensation. This hypersensitivity is referred to as **allodynia** (a painful sensation elicited from an innocuous stimulus on normal skin), **hyperpathia** (an unusual and intense response to nociceptive stimuli), or **dysesthesia** (an abnormal sensation triggered by the sense of touch). The pain may originate in the thalamus but the individual perceives the pain sensation as if it arises in the part(s) of the body where loss of sensation has occurred.

A lesion damaging the ascending sensory pathways to the thalamus (deafferentation), or the absence of sensory input to the thalamus from a certain part of the body (as occurs following amputation of a limb), may result in neural plasticity within the thalamus. Alterations in neural tissue may produce changes in neural circuitry within the thalamus, causing excruciating chronic pain.

SYNONYMS AND EPONYMS OF THE THALAMUS

Name of structure or term	Synonym(s)/ eponym(s)
Association nuclei of the thalamus	Multimodal nuclei of the thalamus
Auditory radiations	Thalamocortical projections of the auditory system
Basal ganglia	Basal nuclei
	Deep cerebral nuclei
Dentatothalamic tract	Cerebellothalamic tract
Dorsomedial (DM) nucleus of the thalamus	Medial dorsal (MD) nucleus of the thalamus
Frontal eye field	Brodmann's area 8
Geniculocalcarine tract	Optic radiations
	Thalamocortical projections of the visual system
Interthalamic adhesion	Massa intermedia
Lateral geniculate nucleus (LGN)	Lateral geniculate body (LGB)
Medial geniculate nucleus (MGN)	Medial geniculate body (MGB)
Medial segment of the globus pallidus	Internal segment of the globus pallidus
Midline nuclei of the thalamus	Median nuclei of the thalamus
	Periventricular nuclei of the thalamus
Nondiscriminatory touch sensation	Crude touch sensation
Premotor cortex	Part of Brodmann's area 6
Primary auditory cortex	Transverse temporal gyri of Heschl
	Brodmann's areas 41 and 42
Primary motor cortex	Precentral gyrus
	Brodmann's area 4
Primary visual cortex	Brodmann's area 17
	Striate cortex
Somesthetic cortex	Somatosensory cortex
Supplementary motor area (SMA)	Part of Brodmann's area 6
Thalamic radiations	Thalamocortical projections of the thalamus
Trigeminothalamic tracts	Dorsal and ventral trigeminal lemnisci
Ventral posterior nucleus of the thalamus	Ventrobasal complex

FOLLOW-UP TO CLINICAL CASE

A sensory deficit with sudden onset and focal symptoms may be caused by ischemic stroke or hemorrhage of a cerebral vessel affecting one or more of the sensory pathways on the right side of the brain. Headache is a non-specific symptom and may be seen in either ischemic stroke (nonhemorrhagic) or in cerebral hemorrhage, though it may favor the latter. Even a very small hemorrhage is easily detectible on head CT and it becomes evident immediately. The CT in this case showed a moderately sized **right thalamic hemorrhage**. If this were a nonhemorrhagic stroke the CT would have been normal or may have revealed only very subtle changes. With time the stroke would have become apparent on CT (within 48 hours).

The main priority in the treatment of this patient is to stabilize his vital signs. The location of this hemorrhage and the high blood pressure indicate that the probable cause of the hemorrhage was hypertension. However, the patient's blood pressure should not be abruptly lowered to "normal" levels. Intracerebral pressure increases following an ischemic stroke or hemorrhage and it is essential that brain perfusion is maintained. This is accomplished by a modest reduction of the patient's blood pressure.

A lesion affecting the thalamus is usually easily diagnosed since it causes a pure or relatively pure contralateral sensory loss or alteration of sensation. Ischemic strokes and hemorrhages are the most common causes of thalamic lesions. Sometimes a thalamic lesion can cause severe, excruciating pain (referred to as thalamic pain) that is difficult to treat.

In contrast to a stroke that affects the thalamus, a stroke that produces a lesion involving a particular cortical area will produce symptoms such as aphasia (language dysfunction) if the language-dominant hemisphere (usually the left) is affected, or contralateral neglect if the nondominant hemisphere (usually the right) is affected. These symptoms are "cortical" symptoms, and usually are indicative of a lesion (most often a stroke) affecting a particular area of the cerebral cortex.

Hypertension is one of the most common causes of intracerebral hemorrhages. It usually affects the basal ganglia, thalamus, brainstem, or cerebellum. Other causes of intracranial hemorrhage include anticoagulant medication, trauma, aneurysm, or vascular malformation. Blood will resolve spontaneously with time. Depending on the size of the thalamic lesion, symptoms may resolve completely, improve partially, or remain the same over time. A very small thalamic stroke is sometimes clinically "silent" and is only noted incidentally and after the fact on a CT or MRI done for some other reason. Most hemorrhages require a neurosurgical consultation. Large size hemorrhages sometimes need to be removed.

3 Why is it crucial not to lower this patient's blood pressure to normal levels?

QUESTIONS TO PONDER

1. Which group of thalamic nuclei has extensive connections with the limbic system?

2. Which thalamic nuclei are included in the specific relay nuclear group?

3. Which thalamic nuclei receive projections from the cerebellum?

4. Which thalamic nuclei receive sensory information from the orofacial structures and body?

5. Which thalamic nuclei are involved in the control of arousal and consciousness?

CHAPTER 23

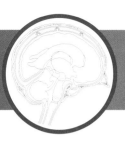
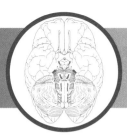
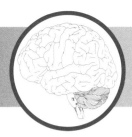

Cerebral Cortex

CLINICAL CASE

A 45-year-old woman, who was previously in perfect health, had two seizures in the past week. Both occurred suddenly and each lasted less than a minute. The first seizure started as twitching of the right side of the face, which progressed to twitching of her right hand and then her right leg. She felt some perioral numbness as well. There was no loss of consciousness or other symptoms, and she was aware of what had occurred. This happened while in bed. The second seizure, as described by her husband, started with facial twitching but she rapidly lost consciousness and then had a generalized convulsion. She bit her tongue and had blood in her mouth. She also had urinary incontinence. She began responding a few minutes after the convulsion, but she was still confused and somewhat agitated for about 30 minutes after that. She had never had a seizure before. In between these spells she had been normal, and examination was normal.

The **cerebral cortex** is the most complex component of the human brain, as a result of its complex and widespread connections. It functions in the planning and initiation of motor activity, perception and conscious awareness of sensory information, learning, cognition, comprehension, memory, conceptual thinking, and awareness of emotions.

The cerebral cortex (L. cortex, "bark") is a multilayered sheet of nerve cell bodies and associated cell processes that covers the paired and prominent cerebral hemispheres of the cerebrum, forming an outer layer much like bark covers a tree. The majority of the cerebral cortex consists of phylogenetically the most highly evolved and complex neural tissue of the human brain.

The central nervous system (CNS) is comprised of white and gray matter. **White matter** consists mostly of nerve cell *axons*, whereas **gray matter** consists mostly of nerve cell *bodies*. Gray matter is arranged into nuclei or cortex. **Nuclei** are aggregations of nerve cell bodies embedded deep within the cerebrum or in the spinal cord. The cerebral cortex consists of 50–100 billion nerve cell bodies arranged into a three to six layered sheet that laminates the brain surface.

The cerebral cortex overlies the subcortical white matter of the cerebral hemispheres. In other animals, the brain's cortical surface appears smooth, whereas in humans the brain surface is convoluted displaying prominent, alternating grooves and elevations as a result of the folding of the cerebral cortex, which occurs during development. The elevations are referred to as gyri, whereas the grooves are referred to as sulci or fissures (Fig. 23.1). **Sulci** are shallow, short grooves, whereas **fissures** are deeper and more constant grooves, with a consistent location on the brain surface. The cortex forming the **gyri** dips down into the pit of the adjacent sulci or fissures to line them. Certain gyri, grooves, and fissures are similar in all normal human brains. Others, however, may vary in different brains and in the two cerebral hemispheres of the same brain. The gyri and sulci greatly increase the total surface area of the cerebral cortex. If the cerebral cortex of a normal human brain were spread out (that is, if the pleats formed by the sulci and fissures were stretched out), the cortex would extend over 0.23 m^2 (2.5 ft^2). In the course of evolution, the cerebral cortex became increasingly folded into alternating gyri and sulci or fissures to facilitate its accommodation in the limited space available in the cranial vault.

The cerebral cortex covering the cerebral hemispheres is divided into the **frontal**, **parietal**, **temporal**, **occipital**, and **limbic lobes**. All of these lobes, with the exception of the limbic lobe, are visible on the lateral aspect of the brain. The limbic lobe is only visible on the medial surface of a midsagittally sectioned brain. In addition to the limbic lobe, the medial surface of the other lobes can also be seen on a midsagittal section of the brain.

The cerebral cortex is classified phylogenetically into the allocortex (heterogenetic cortex), mesocortex (juxtallocortex), and isocortex (homogenetic cortex). The **allocortex** (G. allo, "other") consists of the most primitive **archicortex (archipallium)** (G. archaios, "ancient") of the hippocampal formation and the more recent **paleocortex (paleopallium** or **periallocortex)** (G. palaios, "old") of the parahippocampal gyrus (entorhinal cortex), uncus (piriform cortex), and lateral olfactory gyrus of the olfactory system. The **mesocortex (juxtallocortex)** is a transitional cortex between the allocortex and isocortex, found in the cingulate gyrus and the insula. The **isocortex** is the most recent cortex, also referred to as the **neocortex (neopallium)**, making up the four lobes, the frontal, parietal, temporal, and occipital lobes. The neocortex makes up over 90% of the human cerebral cortex. The remainder is allocortex and mesocortex.

The archicortex consists of three cell layers, the paleocortex from three to five cell layers, and the mesocortex from three to six cell layers, while the neocortex has six distinct cell layers.

The thickness of the cortex also varies from 1.5 mm in the primary sensory areas (being thinnest in the calcarine sulcus of the visual cortex) to 4.5 mm in the motor and association cortical areas. In general, the cortex is usually thickest at the peak of each gyrus and thinnest at the pit of each sulci. The thickness reflects the different cytoarchitectonic arrangements of the various cortical areas. These include cell density,

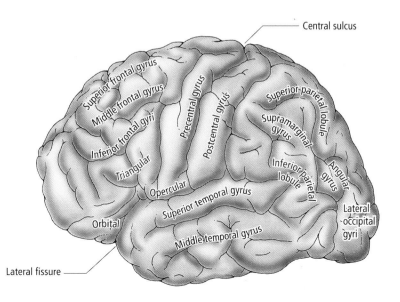

Figure 23.1 ● Lateral view of the cerebral hemisphere showing the principal gyri and sulci of the cerebral cortex.

the types of cells present, fiber density, and the arrangement of the cells and fibers in each of the layers.

The neocortex of the frontal, parietal, temporal, and occipital lobes is anatomically divided into the **primary cortical areas** and **association cortical areas**. The primary cortical areas are subdivided into a primary motor area and the primary sensory areas:

1 The **primary motor area** located in the precentral gyrus of the frontal lobe (corresponding to Brodmann's area 4) contains about one-third of the cell bodies of the upper motoneurons whose axons form the corticospinal tract.
2 The **primary sensory areas** receive sensory information from specific **thalamic nuclei**, including the following four nuclei:

   • The ventral posterior medial (VPM) nucleus of the thalamus, which relays sensory information (touch, pressure, pain, temperature, and proprioception) from the orofacial region to the corresponding head region mapped in the **primary somatosensory cortex** in the postcentral gyrus of the parietal lobe (Brodmann's areas 3, 1, and 2). It also relays input about head movement and orientation to the **primary vestibular area**, the inferior parietal lobule.
   • The ventral posterior lateral (VPL) nucleus of the thalamus, which relays sensory information (touch, pressure, pain, temperature, and proprioception) from various parts of the body to the corresponding body part region mapped in the primary somatosensory cortex.
   • The lateral geniculate nucleus (LGN) of the thalamus, which relays a single modality—visual input from the contralateral visual field to the **primary visual cortex** located in the banks of the calcarine sulcus of the occipital lobe (Brodmann's area 17).
   • The medial geniculate nucleus (MGN) of the thalamus, which relays a single modality—auditory information from both ears to the **primary auditory cortex** in the transverse temporal gyri of Heschl in the lateral fissure of Sylvius (Brodmann's areas 41 and 42).

Most of the cerebral cortex consists of association cortex, which is classified into **unimodal association cortex** and **multimodal (heteromodal) association cortex**. Unimodal association areas are located next to, near, or around the primary sensory cortices and expand on the functions of the respective primary areas. As an example, the primary visual cortex (Brodmann's area 17) projects to the visual association cortex (Brodmann's areas 18, 19, 20, 21, and 37), which processes only a *single modality*, in this case vision, and is thus referred to as unimodal association cortex. In contrast, the multimodal association cortical areas receive inputs from *multiple sensory modalities*; they integrate the information and formulate a composite experience via their higher order cognitive functions. The multimodal association cortex is associated with imagination, judgement, decision making, and making long-term plans.

CELLS OF THE CEREBRAL CORTEX

The multilayered cerebral cortex, which contains an estimated 50–100 billion neurons, is surprisingly populated by only three kinds of neurons: **pyramidal cells**, **fusiform cells**, and **stellate (granule) cells** (Fig. 23.2). Cells of the cerebral cortex have also been classified to include other cells; however these other cells are really variations of the pyramidal, fusiform, and stellate cells.

Pyramidal cells

Pyramidal cells are the most abundant cortical cells and make up about 75% of the cells of the cerebral cortex

Pyramidal cells may be small to giant-sized. They all have a pyramid-shaped cell body, with a dendrite emerging from its apex (Fig. 23.2). This **apical dendrite** is oriented perpendicular to, and courses toward, the cortical surface. Additional dendrites, **basal dendrites** arising from the basal aspect of the cell body, run horizontally and parallel to the cortical surface. A single axon emerges from the base of the pyramidal cell body. Some pyramidal cells have a short axon that courses away from the cortical surface and terminates locally in other cortical layers. The majority of pyramidal cell axons, however, are long, give rise to a recurrent collateral branch prior to leaving the cortex, and then enter the subcortical white matter. These long axons are destined to either serve as commissural, association, or projection fibers. **Commissural fibers** form most of the corpus callosum and cross to the opposite cerebral hemisphere to synapse in the cerebral cortex. **Association fibers** project to cortical association areas in the ipsilateral hemisphere, whereas **projection fibers** leave the cortex, and project to other regions of the CNS, such as the thalamus, striatum, brainstem, or spinal cord.

Pyramidal cells are the main output neurons of the cerebral cortex

The majority of the pyramidal cells serve in the transmission of information away from the cerebral cortex. Pyramidal cells liberate glutamate or aspartate neurotransmitters and form excitatory synapses at their termination. Pyramidal cells of various sizes are the most abundant cortical cells and make up about 75% of the cells of the cerebral cortex. They are also the main output neurons of the cerebral cortex.

Fusiform cells

The projection fibers arising from fusiform cells project mainly to the thalamus

Fusiform cells reside in the deepest cortical layer, and their dendrites project toward the cortical surface (Fig. 23.2). These cells, like the pyramidal cells, project via association, commissural, or projection fibers. The projection fibers arising from fusiform cells project mainly to the thalamus.

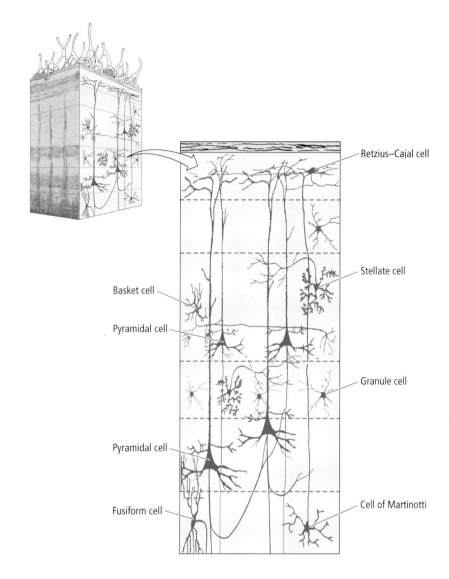

Figure 23.2 ● The different types of neurons of the cerebral cortex.

Labels on figure: Retzius–Cajal cell; Stellate cell; Granule cell; Cell of Martinotti; Basket cell; Pyramidal cell; Pyramidal cell; Fusiform cell

Stellate cells

Stellate cells have a short axon and project locally in the cerebral cortex

Stellate cells are small cells and are also referred to as **granule cells**. Since the dendrites of these cells radiate from their cell body in all planes, these cells have a star-shaped appearance (Fig. 23.2). A short axon emerges from the cell body, which projects locally, in the cerebral cortex.

There are two types of stellate cells based on their morphological and functional characteristics: one type are referred to as **aspiny cells** since they do not have spines on their dendrites. These neurons are believed to be inhibitory interneurons since they utilize gamma aminobutyric acid (GABA), an inhibitory neurotransmitter. The other type located mostly in layer IV of the cerebral cortex, are referred to as **spiny cells** since they have spines on their dendrites. They are believed to be excitatory interneurons, which release glutamate, an excitatory neurotransmitter. Spiny and aspiny cells are located in all cortical layers with the exception of the most superficial layer.

Horizontal cells of Cajal

The cell body and processes of horizontal cells are confined to the superficial layer of the cerebral cortex

The **horizontal cells of Cajal**, also referred to as **horizontal cells**, are spindle-shaped cells, located only in the superficial layer of the cerebral cortex (Fig. 23.2). They give rise to a dendrite and an axon, both of which remain in the superficial layer of the cortex. The axons of these cells run horizontally, that is, they are oriented parallel to the cortical surface and synapse with the pyramidal cell dendrites ramifying in this layer. This type of cell, though, is seldom seen or is completely lacking in adult brains.

Cells of Martinotti

The cells of Martinotti are located throughout the cerebral cortex, and are most populous in the deepest cortical layer

The **cells of Martinotti** are multipolar interneurons displaying short dendrites (Fig. 23.2). Although they are located throughout the cerebral cortex, they are most populous in the deepest cortical layer. Their axons, which give rise to several collateral branches, course toward the surface of the cortex.

TYPES OF CORTEX

Allocortex

The **allocortex** consists of **archicortex** and **paleocortex**.

Archicortex

> The archicortex consists of phylogenetically the most ancient cerebral cortex

The **archicortex** consists of phylogenetically the most ancient cerebral cortex. It consists of only three cell layers: a polymorphic layer, a pyramidal layer, and a molecular layer. The archicortex is located only in the hippocampal formation. This type of cortex is associated with the limbic system, which is involved in memory processes and the expression of emotions.

Paleocortex

> Phylogenetically, the paleocortex formed after the archicortex

Phylogenetically, the **paleocortex** formed after the archicortex, and consists of three to five cell layers. It is found in the primary olfactory cortex (the piriform cortex, consisting of the lateral olfactory gyrus, anterior half of the uncus, and periamygdaloid cortex) and the secondary olfactory cortex, which includes the entorhinal cortex of the parahippocampal gyrus. It mediates the sense of smell, and may also be involved in the processing of emotions.

Mesocortex

> The mesocortex is a transitional cortex between the older allocortex and newer isocortex

The **mesocortex (juxtallocortex)** is a transitional cortex between the allocortex and isocortex. It consists of three to six layers, and is found in the cingulate gyrus and the insula.

Isocortex (neocortex)

> In general, the first four layers (I–IV) of the cerebral cortex serve as input stations (receiving corticopetal fibers), whereas the remaining layers (V and VI) are a major source of output (corticofugal) projection fibers

The **neocortex** consists of six cell layers. In addition to being named, its cell layers are numbered sequentially with Roman numerals (I–VI) in the order which they appear from superficial to deep, that is, from immediately deep to the pia mater to the subcortical white matter (Fig. 23.3).

Although the neocortex consists of six layers, each of these layers is not easily distinguishable in all cortical areas. In the **motor cortex**, layers II–V contain a vast number of large pyramidal cells whose axons leave the cortex, and in their descent to lower centers course in the corona radiata, internal capsule, cerebral peduncle, basis pontis, and pyramids of the medulla to terminate in the brainstem and spinal cord. Nonpyramidal (granule) cells, on the other hand, are not as numerous in these layers of the motor cortex. Due to this morphological characteristic, the motor cortex is referred to as **agranular cortex**. Agranular cortex is typical of the cortical motor areas that are heavily populated by pyramidal cells.

Unlike the motor cortex, the primary **sensory cortex** contains small pyramidal cells, and is heavily populated by nonpyramidal (granule) cells. These cells give the cortex of the primary sensory areas a granular appearance, so it is referred to as **granular cortex**.

In general, the first four layers (I–IV) of the cerebral cortex serve as input stations, receiving **corticopetal fibers**, whereas the remaining layers (V and VI) are a major source of output **corticofugal projection fibers**.

CELL LAYERS OF THE NEOCORTEX

Layer I: molecular (plexiform) layer

> The molecular (plexiform) layer is the most superficial layer of the cerebral cortex, underlying the pia mater

The **molecular (plexiform) layer** is the most superficial layer of the cerebral cortex, underlying the pia mater (Fig. 23.3). As its name implies, the molecular layer consists mainly of interlacing nerve cell processes. Although some cells are present, they are sparse. The most numerous cells in this layer are the horizontal cells of Cajal, which are dispersed throughout this layer. This type of cell, though, is seldom seen or is completely lacking in adult brains.

The interlacing fibers present in this layer consist of both dendrites and axons from various cells. The dendrites arise from the apices of pyramidal and fusiform cells whose cell bodies lie in other (deeper) cortical layers. The axons consist of afferent (thalamocortical) axon terminals arising from the nonspecific, intralaminar, and midline nuclei of the thalamus. These thalamocortical fibers also send collaterals to layers V and VI of the cerebral cortex. In addition, other axons arise from stellate cells and the cells of Martinotti (both of which are interneurons). Overall, this layer contains a myriad of synaptic contacts.

Layer II: external granular layer

> The external granular layer consists mainly of small granule (stellate) cells that give this layer a granular, stippled appearance

The **external granular layer** (Fig. 23.3) consists mainly of small granule (stellate) cells that give this layer a granular, stippled appearance. Other cells include small pyramidal cells. The dendritic trees emerging from these cells extend superficially to the

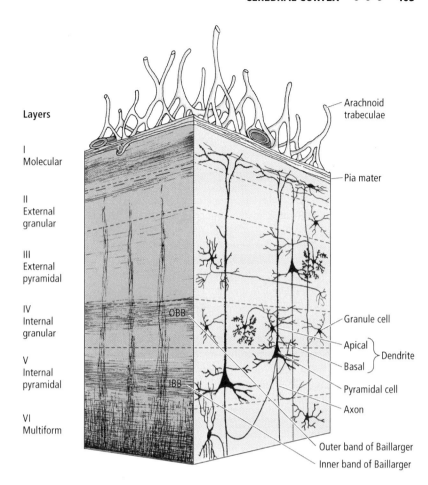

Layers

I
Molecular

II
External
granular

III
External
pyramidal

IV
Internal
granular

V
Internal
pyramidal

VI
Multiform

OBB

IBB

Arachnoid
trabeculae

Pia mater

Granule cell

Apical
Basal } Dendrite

Pyramidal cell

Axon

Outer band of Baillarger

Inner band of Baillarger

Figure 23.3 ● The histology of the cerebral cortex, illustrating the layers and cell types in each of the layers.

molecular layer. Their axons course in the opposite direction to either synapse locally in other cortical layers, or to join the axons of the subcortical white matter, and project to other cortical areas as association fibers.

Layer III: external pyramidal layer

The pyramidal cell axons of this layer are the principal source of corticocortical fibers (association or commissural fibers)

The **external pyramidal layer** (Fig. 23.3) consists predominantly of pyramidal cells. Those pyramidal cells that lie more superficially are medium sized, whereas those lying deeper within this layer, are large-sized cells. Some granule and Martinotti cells are also present. The apical dendrites of the pyramidal cells extend through the external granular layer to reach the molecular layer, whereas their axons join the subcortical white matter to project to other parts of the cerebral cortex mostly as association or commissural fibers. The pyramidal cell axons of this layer are the principal source of corticocortical fibers. In addition, some pyramidal cell axons referred to as projection fibers leave the cortex to terminate in other parts of the CNS. Some thalamocortical fibers from the specific relay thalamic nuclei terminate in this layer of the primary motor cortex. These thalamocortical fibers also send collaterals to layers V and VI.

Layer IV: internal granular layer

Layer IV is the main afferent (input) station of the cerebral cortex and is thicker in the primary sensory areas

The **internal granular layer** (Fig. 23.3) consists mostly of granule (stellate) cells, although some pyramidal cells are also present. The axons of the stellate cells remain in the cerebral cortex. The axons of pyramidal cells course through the deeper cortical layers to either synapse there, or join the axons of the subcortical white matter. The stellate cells receive synapses from fibers arising in the thalamic nuclei. The stellate cells of the **primary somatosensory cortex** receive **thalamocortical fibers** from the VPL and VPM nuclei of the thalamus; those in the **primary visual cortex** receive afferent fibers from the LGN; whereas those of the **primary auditory cortex** receive afferents from the MGN. As the myelinated thalamocortical fibers enter the internal granular layer, they become oriented horizontally to form a layer of white matter, the **outer band (line or stripe) of Baillarger**. This layer of white matter (consisting of thalamocortical fibers from the LGN) is very prominent grossly in the primary visual cortex, and is referred to as the **stripe of Gennari**. Due to the striped appearance of the primary visual cortex, it is also referred to as the **striate cortex**. The thalamocortical fibers also send collaterals to layers V and VI. Layer IV is the main **afferent (input) station** of the cerebral cortex and is especially thicker in the primary sensory areas.

Layer V: internal pyramidal layer

The internal pyramidal layer is the source of the majority of corticofugal (output) fibers of the cerebral cortex

The **internal pyramidal layer** (Fig. 23.3) is thickest in the motor areas of the cerebral cortex since it is a major source of efferent (output) fibers contributing to the corticonuclear and corticospinal tracts. This layer is the source of the majority of corticofugal (output) fibers of the cerebral cortex.

The internal pyramidal layer consists primarily of large and medium-sized pyramidal cells. Stellate and Martinotti cells are also present in this layer. The **primary motor cortex** (Brodmann's area 4) located in the precentral gyrus of the frontal cortex contains a group of giant pyramidal cells, the **cells of Betz**, which are unique to layer V of this cortical area. This layer is the source of the majority of **corticofugal (output) fibers** of the cerebral cortex. The pyramidal cells of this layer give rise to axons that form the corticotectal, corticorubral, corticoreticular, corticopontine, corticonuclear, and corticospinal tracts. All of these tracts terminate at various levels of the brainstem, except for the corticospinal tracts that terminate in the spinal cord. In addition, corticostriate fibers arising from pyramidal cells of this layer descend to terminate in the striatum (caudate nucleus and putamen) of the basal ganglia. Layer V gives rise to fibers that function in *motor* activity.

In addition to the neurons and their processes, this layer also contains a group of horizontally oriented myelinated fibers collectively forming a prominent stripe of white matter, the **inner band (line or stripe) of Baillarger**, located in the deep aspect of this layer. This stripe of white matter consists of collateral branches arising from the axons of cortical association neurons that are destined for layers II and III of the cerebral cortex, as well as collateral branches arising from the pyramidal cells residing in this layer. Layer V is thickest in the motor areas of the cerebral cortex since it is a major source of efferent fibers contributing to the corticonuclear and corticospinal tracts.

In addition to the prominent horizontally oriented outer and inner bands of Baillarger present in layers IV and V, respectively, there are also vertically oriented, but less prominent, groups of afferent and efferent axons that run through the cortical layers.

Layer VI: multiform (fusiform) layer

The multiform (fusiform) layer is the deepest layer of the cerebral cortex and lies immediately next to the white matter underlying the cortex

The **multiform (fusiform) layer** is the deepest layer of the cerebral cortex and lies immediately next to the white matter underlying the cortex (Fig. 23.3). The multiform layer consists mostly of fusiform cells, although pyramidal cells and interneurons are also present. The axons of the fusiform and pyramidal cells course in the underlying white matter as association and commissural fibers that terminate in the cerebral cortex, or as corticothalamic projection fibers that terminate in the thalamus.

VERTICAL COLUMNAR ORGANIZATION OF THE CEREBRAL CORTEX

The cerebral cortex is not only organized into six cell layers that run parallel to the cortical surface, but it is also organized into cell **columns**, which are aligned perpendicular to the cortical surface. The cortical columns are believed to hold the key to cortical function, and represent specific functional units. As an example, within the somesthetic cortex, the cells of certain specific columns are stimulated by impulses related to touch, other columns respond to nociception, whereas others respond to proprioceptive input.

AFFERENTS (INPUT) TO THE CEREBRAL CORTEX

The cerebral cortex receives the following **afferent (input) fibers**: corticocortical (association and commissural) excitatory fibers (which release glutamate or aspartate) from ipsilateral and contralateral cortical areas, thalamocortical excitatory fibers from thalamic nuclei, cholinergic excitatory fibers from the basal forebrain nuclei, noradrenergic inhibitory fibers from the brainstem locus ceruleus, and serotonergic inhibitory fibers from the brainstem raphe nuclei.

The afferent fibers arising from the VPL, VPM, ventral lateral (VL), and ventral anterior (VA) nuclei and the MGN and LGN of the thalamus establish synaptic contacts with the **stellate cells** residing in **layer IV** of the cerebral cortex. Fibers arising from other thalamic nuclei and the remaining cortical input sources establish synaptic contacts in layers I–IV of the cerebral cortex.

The cholinergic and serotonergic afferents to the cerebral cortex function in the control of sleep and arousal.

EFFERENTS (OUTPUT) FROM THE CEREBRAL CORTEX

The cerebral cortex gives rise to efferent fibers that are grouped as association, commissural, or projection fibers

Cortical **efferent fibers** arise from the **output neurons** of the cerebral cortex: the **pyramidal** and **fusiform cells**. Their myelinated axons course deep, pass into the subcortical white matter, and then are distributed to widespread regions of the CNS. Thus the subcortical white matter consists of these three main types of fibers: **association**, **commissural**, and **projection fibers**.

Association fibers

The association cortex of the parietal, occipital, and temporal lobes is connected with the frontal lobe via prominent fasciculi composed of association fibers spanning the four lobes

Association fibers consist of axons arising from small pyramidal cells, primarily from cortical layers II and III. These fibers vary in length from short to long, and project in the ipsilateral hemisphere. Association fibers that connect various cortical areas make up most of the subcortical white matter. These fibers gather to form fasciculi that connect different lobes, but, like a two-way highway, fibers merge into and exit these fasciculi all along their course.

The **short association fibers** connect adjacent gyri. These fibers leave the cortex of one gyrus, enter the underlying white matter, and then loop around the pit of a sulcus and project into the cortex of an adjacent gyrus. Consequently these fibers are also referred to as **U-fibers** or **arcuate fibers** (Fig. 23.4A). These fibers bridge the primary sensory areas with the adjacent cortical association areas.

The **long association fibers** connect different lobes of the same hemisphere. These fibers leave the cortex of one lobe, enter the underlying white matter, gather to form a bundle, and then project to the cortex of a different lobe of the same hemisphere.

Bundles of long association fibers form the following fasciculi: the superior and inferior longitudinal fasciculi, the superior and inferior occipitofrontal fasciculi, and the cingulum (Fig.23.4).

The **superior longitudinal fasciculus** interconnects the frontal lobe with the parietal, temporal, and occipital lobes. As these fibers link these lobes they form a dome over the insula and radiate within the parietal, temporal, and occipital lobes.

The superior longitudinal fasciculus contains a group of fibers, the **arcuate fasciculus**, that forms a distinct arch posterior to the insula. This fasciculus links Broca's area (the frontal lobe motor area for speech) with Wernicke's area (the temporal lobe area for language comprehension).

The **inferior longitudinal fasciculus** (temporo-occipital bundle) connects the temoporal and occcipital lobes.

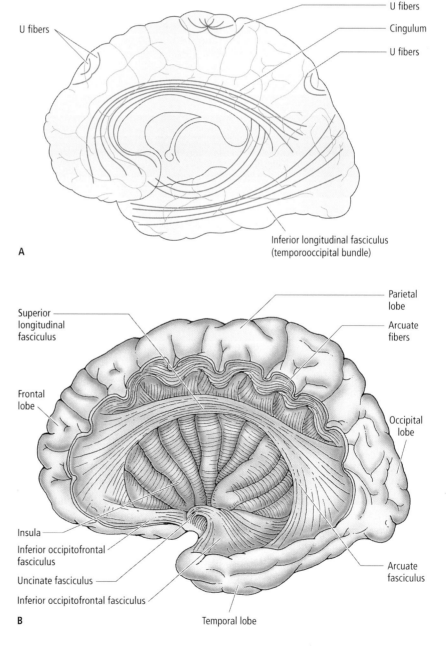

Figure 23.4 ● (A) Schematic representation of the major association fiber system (lateral view). (B) Three-dimensional schematic representation of the major association fiber systems (lateral view).

The **superior occipitofrontal fasciculus (subcallosal bundle)** interconnects the frontal lobe with the occipital lobe. The fibers of the **inferior occipitofrontal fasciculus**, which like their superior counterpart also interconnect the frontal and occipital lobes, radiate in the frontal lobe, pass through the temporal lobe inferior to the insula, to also radiate in the occipital lobe. Some of its fibers curve around on the deep aspect of the lateral sulcus, interconnecting the frontal and temporal lobes, and as a result of their hook-like path are referred to as the **uncinate fasciculus** (L. uncus, "hook").

The **cingulum** is embedded in the cingulate gyrus, and its fibers form a connection between the anterior perforated substance and the parahippocampal gyrus.

Commissural fibers

Commissural fibers arise in one cerebral hemisphere and cross the midline to terminate in the corresponding cortical area of the contralateral hemisphere

Commissural fibers arise in one cerebral hemisphere, and cross the midline to terminate in the corresponding cortical area of the contralateral hemisphere (Fig. 23.5A). These fibers provide an avenue of communication between the corresponding cortical areas of the two hemispheres.

Commissural fibers consist of the myelinated axons of medium-sized pyramidal neurons residing in various layers of the cerebral cortex.

The **corpus callosum** is the most massive commissure in the entire nervous system, linking mainly *corresponding* areas of the neocortex of the two cerebral hemispheres. The corpus callosum, however, also contains commissural fibers that arise in certain cortical areas of one cerebral hemisphere and cross to the opposite side to terminate in *noncorresponding* areas of the contralateral hemisphere. This is true for fibers arising in the **primary visual cortex** of one cerebral hemisphere that cross to the opposite side to terminate in the **visual association cortex** of the contralateral hemisphere. Similarly, parts of the **motor** and **somesthetic cortical areas** where the hand is represented, do not receive commissural fibers from the corresponding motor and sensory cortical areas of the contralateral hemisphere. However, the somesthetic association areas receive commissural fibers that connect the two cerebral hemispheres, thus each hemisphere samples information available to the contralateral hemisphere.

The corpus callosum consists of the following component parts: the rostrum and genu anteriorly, the body forming the roof of the lateral ventricles, and the splenium posteriorly. The **rostrum** and **genu** consist of commissural fibers connecting the anterior cortical areas of the frontal lobe. The **body** consists of most of the commissural fibers that connect the remaining frontal lobe, parietal lobe, and part of the temporal lobe. Posteriorly, the **splenium** consists of commissural fibers that connect the occipital lobes. Cortical commissural fibers emerge mainly from the pyramidal cells residing in the cortical superficial layers and the external granular (layer II) and external pyramidal (layer III) layers.

Other commissures of the brain include the **anterior** (Fig. 23.5B) and **posterior commissures** that bridge the temporal lobes, and the **hippocampal commissure (commissure of the fornix)** connecting the hippocampal formation of the two hemispheres.

Commissural fibers form an anatomical bridge connecting the two cerebral hemispheres, which is essential in the integration of information in the two sides of the brain.

Projection fibers

Projection fibers consist of both afferent and efferent fibers to and from the cerebral cortex, that connect it to the thalamus, basal ganglia, brainstem, and spinal cord

The **afferent fibers** to the cerebral cortex are also referred to as **corticopetal fibers**. They include: (i) **thalamocortical fibers** arising from the **VPL** and **VPM** nuclei of the thalamus relaying sensory information such as touch, pressure, conscious proprioception, two-point tactile sensation, as well as pain and temperature sensation from the body and head to the **sensory cortex**; (ii) the **MGN of the thalamus** relaying auditory information via the auditory radiation to the **auditory cortex**; and (iii) the **LGN of the thalamus** relaying visual information via the optic radiation to the **visual cortex**. Although these afferent fibers terminate in layers I–IV of the cerebral cortex, most terminate in layer IV.

The **efferent fibers** from the cerebral cortex are referred to as **corticofugal fibers**. These fibers consist of axons arising from large pyramidal cells that course in the corona radiata and internal capsule to terminate in the basal ganglia, the brainstem, and the spinal cord. Corticofugal fibers include fibers of the corticoreticular, corticorubral, corticonuclear, corticopontine, corticotegmental, and corticospinal tracts.

INTERNAL CAPSULE AND CORONA RADIATA

The internal capsule is a massive, fan-shaped collection of fibers (white matter) that connect the thalamus to the cerebral cortex

The **internal capsule** is a massive, fan-shaped collection of fibers (white matter) that connect the thalamus to the cerebral cortex. On horizontal section, it appears as a wide letter "L" with its apex directed toward the midline of the cerebrum. It is divided into an **anterior limb**, a **genu** (L., "knee"), and a **posterior limb**. The two limbs converge toward the genu, the angle between the anterior and posterior limbs. The anterior limb is interposed between the head of the caudate nucleus and the lenticular nucleus. The posterior limb is interposed between the thalamus and the globus pallidus. The majority of the internal capsule fibers traversing the cerebrum connect the thalamus to the cerebral cortex. Descending motor fibers arising from the motor cortex destined for the brainstem and the spinal cord also descend in the internal capsule. In addition to the above components, the internal capsule also has a **sublenticular limb** whose fibers run ventral to the lenticular nucleus and a **retrolenticular limb** whose fibers run caudal to the lenticular nucleus.

The anterior limb of the internal capsule includes the anterior thalamic radiations (corticothalamic and thalamocortical

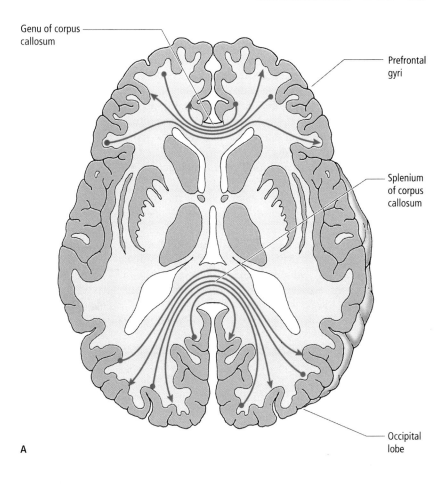

A

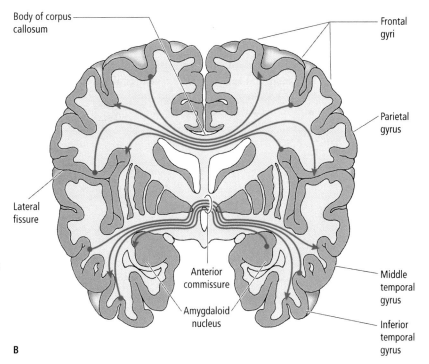

B

Figure 23.5 ● (A) Horizontal schematic representation of the brain showing the fiber connections of the genu and splenium of the corpus callosum. (B) Coronal schematic representation of the brain showing the fibers of the anterior commissure and the body of the corpus callosum. (Modified from Young, PA & Young, PH (1997) *Basic Clinical Neuroanatomy*. Williams & Wilkins, Baltimore; fig. 15.4.)

fibers) serving as a channel between the thalamus and the cerebral cortex. Frontopontine fibers also pass through the anterior limb of the internal capsule. The genu of the internal capsule transmits corticonuclear (corticobulbar) fibers arising from the frontal and motor cortex and descend to terminate in the cranial nerve motor nuclei in the brainstem.

The posterior limb accommodates the corticospinal tract in its posterior third or half and the central thalamic radiations (corticothalamic and thalamocortical fibers). The sublenticular limb carries the auditory radiations arising from the MGN to terminate in the transverse temporal gyri of Heschl. The retrolenticular limb carries visual information from the LGN to the visual cortex via the geniculocalcarine radiations (optic radiations).

As the fibers of the internal capsule emerge from between the caudate nucleus and the lenticular nucleus, they spread out forming a curved radiating crown, the **corona radiata**, containing afferent and efferent fibers to and from the cerebral cortex.

LOBES OF THE CEREBRAL CORTEX

The cerebral cortex of each cerebral hemisphere is divided anatomically into five lobes: the frontal, parietal, temporal, occipital, and limbic lobes

The cerebral cortex of each cerebral hemisphere is divided anatomically into five lobes: the frontal, parietal, temporal, occipital, and limbic lobes (Fig. 23.6). All of the lobes are visible on the lateral aspect of the brain, with the exception of the limbic lobe, which is visible only from the medial surface of the brain.

The **frontal lobe** is involved in motor control, cognitive functions, the processing of emotions, and the motor aspects of language. The **parietal lobe** functions in sensation; it processes touch, pressure, pain and temperature sensation, and proprioception. The **temporal lobe** contains the cortical areas that process hearing, memory, emotions, and the sensory aspects of speech. The **occipital lobe** has the exclusive

function of processing visual information, and the **limbic lobe** functions in the processing of emotions.

Borders

The **frontal lobe** extends from the rostral pole of the cerebral hemisphere, caudally to the central sulcus (of Rolando) and inferiorly to the lateral fissure (of Sylvius) (see Fig. 23.5).

The **parietal lobe** extends from the central sulcus anteriorly, to the parieto-occipital sulcus posteriorly, and the lateral fissure inferiorly.

The **temporal lobe** extends from the lateral fissure superiorly, to its free inferior border, and posteriorly to an imaginary line extending from the posterior extent of the lateral fissure inferior–posteriorly, separating it from the occipital lobe.

The **occipital lobe** extends from the parieto-occipital sulcus to the preoccipital notch, which accommodates the lateral pole of the cerebellar hemisphere. It consists of the cortex covering the caudal pole of the cerebral hemisphere.

The **limbic lobe** is not visible laterally. Unlike the other lobes, which consist of only neocortex, it is composed of archicortex, mesocortex, and some neocortex.

FUNCTIONAL AREAS OF THE CEREBRAL CORTEX

The cerebral cortex was originally classified by Brodmann into 52 different cytoarchitectural areas

The cerebral cortex consists of certain cell types arranged into three to six layers, as described above. The thickness of these layers, and the number and type of cells within each layer, however, varies in different regions of the cortex.

The cerebral cortex was originally classified by Brodmann into 52 different cytoarchitectural areas, but he did not assign a function to each area at that time. He numbered them 1 to 52, which reflected the order in which he examined and mapped them (Fig. 23.7). Additional studies have provided

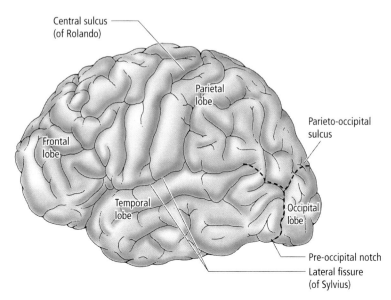

Figure 23.6 ● Lateral view of the brain showing four of the five lobes of the cerebrum.

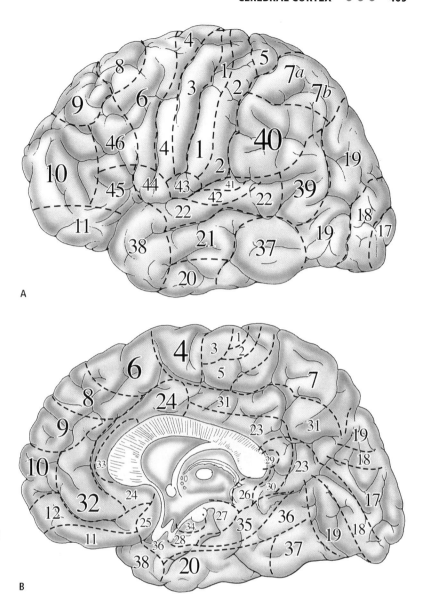

A

B

Figure 23.7 ● Views of the cerebral hemisphere showing the cytoarchitectural map of the cerebral cortex: (A) lateral view, and (B) medial view. Numbers represent Brodmann's areas. (Modified from Noback, CR et al. (1996) *The Human Nervous System*. Williams & Wilkins, Media; figs 25.5, 25.6)

information correlating a function to many of these areas, referred to as **Brodmann's areas**. The anatomical/functional correlation, however, is not as accurate as was thought in the past. Some of these areas are so commonly referred to that both name, and number, should be known by the student. These areas are: the primary somatosensory cortex (Brodmann's areas 3, 1, and 2), motor cortex (Brodmann's areas 4, 6, and 8), secondary sensory cortex (Brodmann's areas 5 and 7), visual cortex (Brodmann's areas 17, 18, and 19), and auditory cortex (Brodmann's areas 41 and 42).

The functional areas of the cerebral cortex are shown in Fig. 23.8.

Cortical areas controlling motor activity

The motor areas of the cerebral cortex located anterior to the central sulcus control the motor activity of the entire opposite side of the body

The *motor activity* of the entire opposite side of the body is controlled by the **motor areas** of the cerebral cortex that are located an-terior to the central sulcus. Fibers arise from the primary motor cortex (M-I), the secondary motor cortex (M-II), and the primary somatosensory (somesthetic) cortex (S-I) of the frontal and parietal lobes to terminate in the motor nuclei of the brainstem and spinal cord.

Primary motor cortex

The precentral gyrus of the cerebral hemisphere controls movement of the contralateral head and body

The **primary motor cortex** resides in the precentral gyrus of the frontal lobe, and corresponds to Brodmann's area 4. It plays an important role in the execution of distinct, well defined, *voluntary* movement (Fig. 23.8). The precentral gyrus of the right cerebral hemisphere controls movement of the left side of the head and body, whereas that of the left cerebral hemisphere controls the right side of the head and body. The body is mapped on the primary motor cortex somatotopically

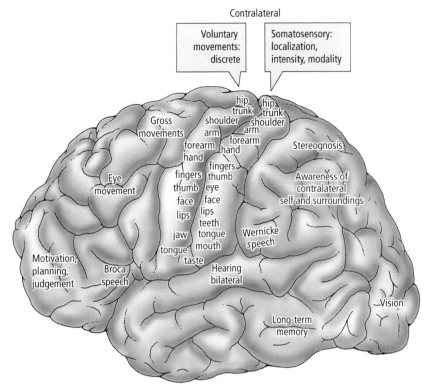

Figure 23.8 ● Lateral view of the cerebral hemisphere showing the functional areas of the cerebral cortex. (Modified from Young, PA, Young, PH (1997) *Basic Clinical Neuroanatomy*. Williams & Wilkins, Baltimore; fig. 15.6c.)

as an upside down homonculus (L., "little person") (Fig. 23.9). The part of the precentral gyrus controlling movement of the toes is located near its superior aspect, whereas the part of the precentral gyrus controlling movement of the tongue, mouth, and larynx is located near its inferior aspect (bordering the lateral fissure). A noticeable characteristic of the primary motor cortex in humans is that more than half of it is associated with the motor activity of the hands, tongue, lips, and larynx—reflecting the manual dexterity and ability for speech that humans possess. It also contributes to the motor control of the limb musculature, specifically to the control of the distal muscles of the extremities (i.e., the muscles controlling movements of the hands and feet). Nerve cells in the primary motor cortex are organized into groups, each group sending its axons to the cranial nerve motor nuclei, or the reticular formation, or the spinal cord gray matter, where they control the motor activity of a single muscle. The total cortical area that mediates motor activity of a particular body region is proportional to the complexity of the movements produced in that region.

Prior to the onset of movement, the primary motor cortex receives instructions and information about the pattern of the intended movement from the other motor areas of the cortex.

Secondary motor cortex

The principal function of the secondary motor cortex is the programing of complex motor activity, which is then relayed to the primary motor cortex, where the execution of motor activity is initiated

The **secondary motor cortex** consists of four regions: the supplementary motor area, the premotor cortex, the frontal eye field, and the posterior parietal motor area. The first three of these motor cortical areas reside in the frontal lobe (rostral to the central sulcus); the posterior parietal motor area is located in the parietal lobe. The principal function of the secondary motor cortex is the programing of complex motor activity, which is then relayed to the primary motor cortex where the execution of motor activity is initiated. The primary motor cortex then translates this information into the execution of movement, and relays it mainly to the brainstem or spinal cord. Most of the nerve signals that arise in the secondary motor cortex mediate complex movements produced by groups of muscles performing a particular task, unlike the discrete muscle contractions elicited by stimulation of the primary motor cortex.

The **supplementary motor area** (SMA) corresponds to the medial and superolateral aspect of Brodmann's area 6. This area receives axon terminals from the basal ganglia (the globus pallidus and the pars reticulata of the substantia nigra) via a relay in the ventral lateral (VLa) nucleus of the thalamus. Input from the basal ganglia assists the SMA in its role in the programing phase of the patterns and sequences of complex movements, and the coordination of bilateral movements. The SMA mediates muscle contractions of the axial (trunk) and proximal limb (girdle) musculature (i.e., the muscles controlling movements of the arm and thigh).

The **premotor cortex** (PMC) corresponds to most of Brodmann's area 6 on the lateral aspect of the frontal lobe.

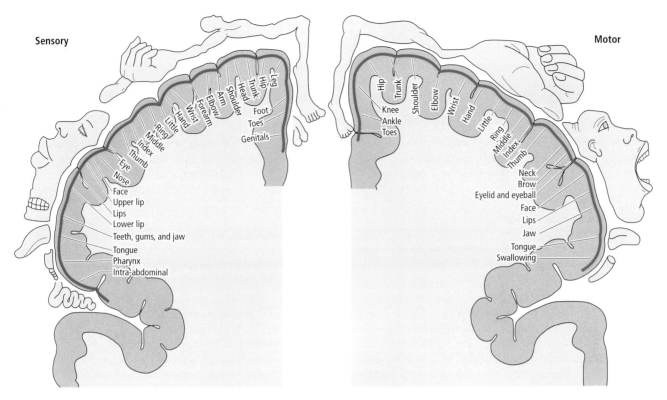

Sensory

Motor

Figure 23.9 ● Coronal section through the cerebral hemisphere showing homunculi of the primary somatosensory cortex (left) and the primary motor cortex (right).

The PMC receives axon terminals from the cerebellum via a relay in the ventral lateral (VLp) nucleus of the thalamus, and fibers from the cortical association areas. Input from the cerebellum assists the PMC in its role in movement. The main function of this area is the motor control of axial and proximal limb musculature. It also plays a role in orienting the body and upper limbs in the direction of a target. Once a motor task has been initiated, activity in the PMC diminishes, reflecting its key function in the planning phase of motor activity.

The **frontal eye field** (FEF) corresponds to Brodmann's area 8. This cortical area is located rostral to the premotor area, on the lateral aspect of the frontal lobe. This area contains nerve cell bodies whose axons join the corticonuclear tract and descend to terminate in the eye movement control centers located in the midbrain reticular formation and the paramedian pontine reticular formation. They in turn transmit information to the motor nuclei of cranial nerves III, IV, and VI, which control voluntary eye movements. The FEF plays a role in the coordination of eye movements, particularly those mediating voluntary visual tracking of a moving object via conjugate deviation of the eyes.

The **posterior parietal motor area** (PMA) corresponds to Brodmann's areas 5 and 7. Area 5 is associated with tactile discrimination and stereognosis, as well as statognosis in relation to reaching and guiding movements (Fig. 23.8). Area 7 (the posterior parietal visual area) is involved with movements that require visual guidance.

Primary sensory areas of the cerebral cortex

The **primary sensory areas** are involved in distinguishing and integrating sensory input relayed there primarily by the thalamic nuclei.

Primary somatosensory (somesthetic) cortex (S-I)

The primary somatosensory cortical area receives sensory information arising from the contralateral half of the head and body

The **primary somatosensory cortex** is located in the postcentral gyrus on the lateral surface of the parietal lobe, and corresponds to Brodmann's areas 3, 1, and 2 (see Fig. 23.1A). The primary somatosensory cortex also comprises the dorsal part of the paracentral lobule, which resides and is visible only on the medial surface of the cerebral hemisphere. This cortical region is the site of termination of the thalamocortical fibers arising from the VPL and VPM nuclei of the thalamus. These fibers relay sensory information from the contralateral half of the body and head, respectively. The body is represented on the somatosensory cortex by an upside-down homunculus (Fig. 23.9). The foot is represented on the superior medial surface of the hemisphere, the leg, thigh, trunk, shoulder, arm, and forearm on the superior surface of the postcentral gyrus, whereas the hand, head, teeth, tongue, larynx, and pharynx are on the lateral surface of the postcentral gyrus. The total cortical area representing a body part is proportional to the discriminative capability of the body part.

The primary sensory cortex also includes Brodmann's area 3a, which is buried in the central sulcus. This area receives sensory input from muscle receptors.

Some of the cells residing in the primary somatosensory cortex give rise to fibers that descend to terminate in the brainstem and spinal cord gray matter. There they influence motor activity, not by synapsing with motoneurons, but instead by modulating the transmission of sensory input from peripheral structures into the brainstem and spinal cord.

Primary visual cortex (V-I)

The primary visual cortex receives visual input from the LGN, which relays visual information arising from the contralateral visual field

The neurons residing in the visual cortex respond to different visual stimuli relayed by neurons conveying color, motion, three-dimensional vision, or a combination of various visual stimuli.

The **primary visual cortex** is located mainly in the medial surface of the occipital lobes on the banks of the **calcarine fissure**, although it extends into their posterolateral surface. The primary visual cortex is the thinnest cortex of the entire brain. Layer IV of this cortex is prominent due to a thick layer of myelinated fibers, the **external band of Baillarger**. This band is characteristically so thick in this cortex that it gives the primary visual cortex a grossly visible striped appearance, and is referred to as the **stripe of Gennari**. The primary visual cortex thus is also referred to as the **striate cortex**.

The LGN projects visual information to the primary visual cortex (V-I) (Brodmann's area 17). This cortical area receives visual input arising from the contralateral visual field: the temporal half of the ipsilateral retina and the nasal half of the contralateral retina.

The primary visual cortex receives fibers of the geniculocalcarine tract (optic radiation) arising from the LGN of the thalamus. Table 23.1 lists the topographic relationships of fibers from the retina to the LGN, and then to the banks of the calcarine sulcus.

The primary visual cortex receives visual input from the macula of the retina in its caudal third, and from the paramacular (and more peripheral) fields of the retina in its rostral portions. The macular representation in the primary visual cortex is much larger than that of other areas of the retina, reflecting the high visual acuity of the macula.

The primary visual cortex is arranged into columns oriented perpendicular to the cortical surface, extending from the cortical surface (under the pia mater) to the subcortical white matter. Nerve cells in a particular cortical column are functionally similar. Columns in the primary visual cortex include the **ocular dominance columns**, the site where fibers relaying information from the ipsilateral or the contralateral eye terminate, and the **orientation columns**, where nerve cells are responsive to visual stimuli that have a comparable spatial orientation. Layers II and III of the primary visual cortex also contain vertically oriented aggregates of nerve cells that are responsive to color.

Primary auditory cortex (A-I)

The primary auditory cortex resides deep in the lateral fissure (of Sylvius) in the hidden superior surface of the superior temporal gyrus

The **primary auditory cortex** (Brodmann's areas 41 and 42) resides deep in the lateral fissure (of Sylvius), in the hidden superior surface of the superior temporal gyrus, containing the transverse temporal gyri of Heschl, and in the floor of the lateral fissure. The primary auditory cortex of each side receives information from both ears by way of the medial geniculate body of the thalamus, and then sends projections to the contralateral side via the corpus callosum. The primary auditory cortex plays an important function in the detection of pattern alteration as well as in the location of the sound.

The primary auditory cortex receives the **auditory radiations** from the **lateral geniculate nucleus**. This cortical region has a tonotopic representation of frequencies, that is, neurons responding to low frequencies reside in its rostral extent, whereas neurons responding to high frequencies reside in its caudal extent. The primary auditory cortex is arranged into two-dimensional, alternating, vertically oriented columns of neurons. One dimension of the auditory cortex is composed of **frequency columns**. The cells in each frequency column respond to an auditory stimulus of a particular frequency. As mentioned above, cells responding to low frequencies reside in the frequency columns located in the rostral extent of the transverse temporal gyri of Heschl, whereas frequency columns containing cells responding to gradually higher frequencies are lined up in sequence toward the caudal extent of the primary auditory cortex.

The other dimension of the auditory cortex is composed of alternating **binaural columns**. There are two types of

Visual field quadrants	Retinal field quadrants	LGN	Optic radiations	Calcarine banks
Upper	Lower	Lateral half	Inferior part	Inferior
Lower	Upper	Medial half	Superior part	Superior

Table 23.1 ● The topographic relationships of fibers from the retina to the lateral geniculate nucleus (LGN) and the banks of the calcarine sulcus.

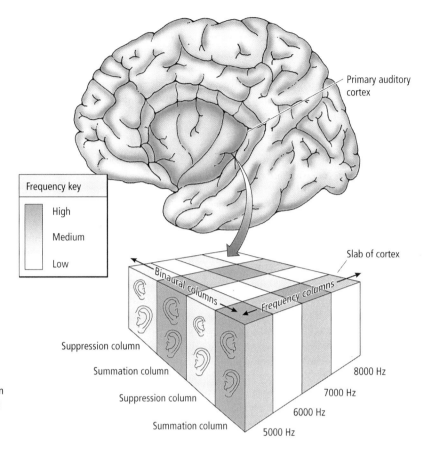

Figure 23.10 ● The location and functional organization of the primary auditory cortex. (Modified from Matthews, G (2001) *Neurobiology*. Blackwell Publishing, Oxford; fig. 17.14.)

binaural columns: summation columns and suppression columns. The neurons residing in the **summation columns** respond to an auditory stimulus that stimulates both ears simultaneously. In contrast, the neurons in the **suppression columns** respond maximally to an auditory stimulus that stimulates only one ear, but respond minimally when the auditory stimulus stimulates both ears (Fig. 23.10).

Primary vestibular area

The primary vestibular area receives input related to the orientation and movement of the head

The cortical area that receives vestibular information is ambiguous. However, it is believed that the vestibular nuclei project primarily crossed fibers to the contralateral VPM nucleus of the thalamus, which in turn relays this input to the **inferior parietal lobule**, the **primary vestibular area**, and the **superior temporal gyrus** next to the primary auditory cortex. This area receives input related to head movement and position.

Taste area

The cortical area where taste information is relayed resides next to the area where general sensory input from the tongue is transmitted

Taste receptors relay gustatory information to the **solitary nucleus** in the brainstem. The solitary nucleus then transmits the information via the ipsilateral central tegmental tract to the VPM nucleus of the thalamus. The thalamus then projects this input to the inferior extent of the **postcentral gyrus** (Brodmann's area 43). The cortical area where taste information is relayed resides next to the area where the general sensory input from the tongue is transmitted.

Olfactory area

The **primary olfactory area** is located in the **prepiriform** and **periamygdaloid regions** of the cerebral cortex. These regions, however, unlike other cortical areas, have not been assigned a Brodmann's area number.

Sensory association areas of the cerebral cortex

The sensory association areas receive inputs from the primary sensory areas and further process, integrate, and interpret the incoming sensory input

Sensory association areas are also referred to as **secondary sensory areas**, and usually surround the primary sensory areas. They receive input from the primary sensory areas and further process, integrate, and interpret the incoming sensory input. The cerebral cortex of the human brain is classified into **sensory**, **motor** and **association cortex**. The human brain contains more association cortex than the brain of any other animal, and thus is the principal component of the human cerebral cortex.

The sophisticated functions of the human association cortex is what distinguishes us from other animals. Our ability to learn, reason, and plan our daily activities and lives, and our language skills, are some examples of association cortical functions.

Somesthetic association area

The somesthetic association area functions primarily in the integration of sensory input from various sensory systems

A **somesthetic association area** is located in the cortex of the **superior parietal lobule** (Brodmann's areas 5, 7, and 40). This cortex receives input mainly from the primary somesthetic cortex; however fibers arising from the VPL and VPM nuclei of the thalamus also terminate here. This cortex functions primarily in the integration of sensory input from various sensory systems. One way of testing the function of the somesthetic association cortex of a patient is by placing an object (e.g., a spoon) in his hand, and while his eyes are closed ask him to identify the object by using his other senses (e.g., touch). In order to identify the object, an individual needs to feel the size, shape, texture, and weight of the object, but in addition, to recognize it by associating it with previous sensory experiences linked to it. This should enable the individual to recognize and identify the object without looking.

Visual association areas

The secondary visual areas function in identifying an object, determining its location and color, comparing it to prior visual experiences, and determining its significance

The primary visual cortex projects to the surrounding **visual association cortex** (extrastriate cortex; Brodmann's areas 18 and 19), which consists of the secondary and tertiary visual cortical areas. The primary visual cortex projects to the **visual association areas** where information is processed and subsequently relayed to the **tertiary visual areas** (**V-3**, **V-4**, and the **middle temporal area**) of the cortex. The secondary visual areas function in identifying an object, determining its location and color, comparing it to prior visual experiences, and determining its significance. Furthermore, the middle temporal area has an important function in detecting moving objects.

Auditory association areas

The secondary auditory cortical areas function in the interpretation of sounds and the comprehension of language

The **secondary auditory cortical areas**, although numerous, are not well defined, and include Brodmann's area 22 and part of area 42. They surround the primary auditory cortex and form reciprocal connections with the primary auditory cortex. The secondary auditory cortical areas function in the interpretation of sounds and, via their connections with Wernicke's area, function in the comprehension of language.

Language areas

There are two cortical areas that function in the processing of language: Wernicke's area and Broca's area

There are two cortical areas that function in the processing of language: Wernicke's area and Broca's area. The left cerebral hemisphere is the dominant hemisphere in language functions in the majority of individuals.

Wernicke's area (see Fig. 23.8) consists of auditory association cortex (part of Brodmann's area 22), as well as parts of the supramarginal and angular gyri (Brodmann's areas 37, 39, and 40, usually in the left, dominant hemisphere). Wernicke's area is also referred to as the receptive (sensory) language area, general interpretative area, or the gnostic area. It plays an important role in the comprehension and formulation of language. In the right cerebral hemisphere this cortical area is an auditory association area that serves to determine the emotional undertones of language. When we hear someone speak, the person's voice often reveals if he/she is happy, upset, angry, etc.

Broca's area (see Fig. 23.8), the motor speech area (Brodmann's areas 44 and 45), is located in the opercular and triangular portions of the inferior frontal gyrus. This area not only functions in the initiation of a sequence of complex movements (via its connections with the primary motor cortex), which are essential in the production of speech (a motor function), but also has expressive language capacities (e.g., grammar). The supplementary motor area is also necessary in the production of language.

Wernicke's and Broca's areas of speech are interconnected via the **arcuate fasciculus** (Fig. 23.11), which is necessary for language and the ability to communicate.

The following is a general description of how a word that is heard is repeated (Fig. 23.12A). Auditory sensory input (a word) reaching the ear is relayed via the auditory pathway to the primary auditory cortex where it is "heard." The primary auditory cortex transmits the input to the auditory association cortex, which functions in the interpretation of sound. This sound is comprehended in Wernicke's area, which projects the information by way of cortical association fibers (the arcuate fasciculus) to Broca's area. Broca's area is involved in the planning of the motor activity that is necessary for the word to be produced. Broca's area projects this information to the premotor cortex where motor activity is planned and relayed to the primary motor cortex, which initiates the movements necessary to produce speech. When an individual reads and says the words (Fig. 23.12B), the visual pathway relays the sensory visual input to the primary visual cortex where the words are "seen." The primary visual cortex transmits this input to the association visual cortex

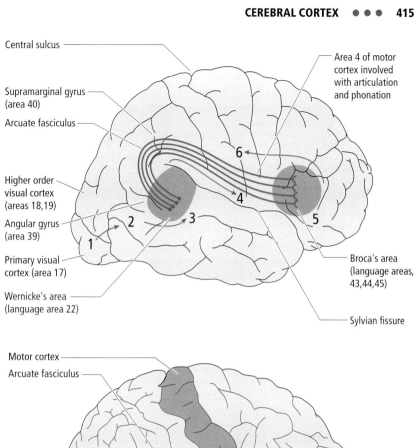

Figure 23.11 ● Diagram showing the possible progression of neural transmission from the visual cortex through the cortical areas associated with speech to the primary motor cortex in the production of speech. For example, when an individual sees an object and is asked to name it, information is relayed from (1) the visual cortex (Brodmann's areas 17, 18, and 19) to (2) the angular gyrus (Brodmann's area 39), to (3) Wernicke's area (Brodmann's area 22), by way of (4) the arcuate fasciculus, to (5) Broca's area of speech (Brodmann's areas 43, 44, and 45), and finally to (6) the primary motor cortex (Brodmann's area 4) which gives rise to the corticonuclear tract that terminates in the brainstem motor nuclei of the cranial nerves associated with vocalization. (Modified from Noback, CR et al. (1996) *The Human Nervous System*. Williams & Wilkins, Media; fig. 25.7.)

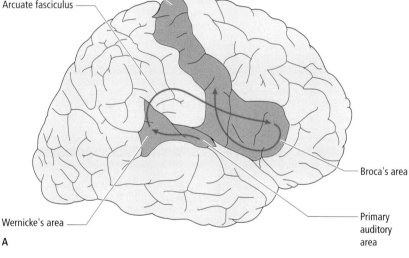

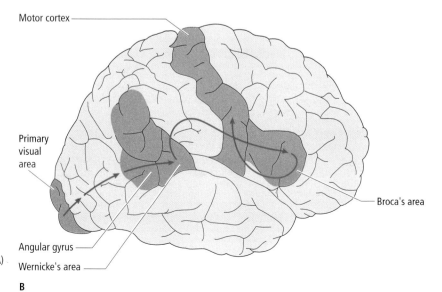

Figure 23.12 ● Neural pathways associated with: (A) hearing a word that is then spoken, and (B) reading a word that is then spoken.

where the significance of the words is determined. The visual information is then relayed to Wernicke's area where the words are comprehended, and the creation of the words takes place. Wernicke's area then projects to Broca's area, which, as described above, dictates the motor activity necessary to produce the words.

Prefrontal association cortex

The prefrontal cortex is associated with the thalamus, limbic system, and basal ganglia

The **prefrontal cortex** is located in the frontal lobe, anterior to the motor cortex, and consists of multimodal association cortex. It has extensive reciprocal connections with the dorso-

medial, ventral anterior, and intralaminar thalamic nuclei via corticothalamic and thalamocortical projection fibers. In addition, its orbital region is associated with the limbic system, whereas its dorsolateral region is interconnected with the association areas of the parietal, temporal, and occipital lobes via long association bundles. Furthermore, both of these cortical regions are a source of fibers that terminate in the caudate nucleus and putamen of the basal ganglia. Commissural fibers arising from the prefrontal cortex pass via the corpus callosum to the opposite hemisphere to terminate not only in the cortex of the prefrontal area, but also in that of the other lobes.

The dorsolateral region of the prefrontal cortex functions in *working memory*. Observing a laboratory demonstration at school and then being able to repeat the task soon afterwards, is an example of working memory. Individuals with lesions

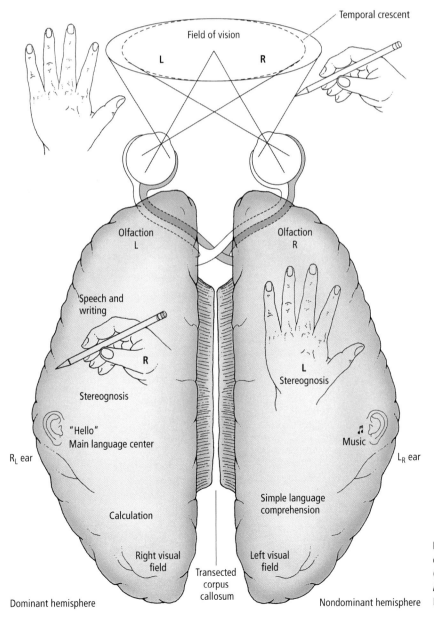

Figure 23.13 ● Functions associated with the dominant and nondominant cerebral hemispheres. (Modified from Noback, CR *et al*. (1996) *The Human Nervous System*, 5th edn. Williams & Wilkins, Baltimore; fig. 25.9.)

to the dorsolateral region have difficulty in problem solving and in paying attention. The main function of the **orbital region** is the expression of an appropriate behavioral response in a particular situation. Individuals with lesions in the orbital region are impulsive and exhibit an inappropriate behavioral response for a given circumstance.

The prefrontal cortex may play a role in the individual's level of intelligence, education, as well as psychological state. It is believed that the prefrontal cortex may correspond to the neocortical area of the limbic system.

CEREBRAL DOMINANCE

In the human brain, the left cerebral hemisphere is usually the dominant hemisphere (in about 95% of the population), whereas the right hemisphere is the nondominant hemisphere (Fig. 23.13). The dominant hemisphere mediates processes related to language, speech, problem solving, and mathematical skills. The nondominant hemisphere mediates spatial perception, recognition of faces, as well as music and poetry skills.

CLINICAL CONSIDERATIONS

Although the brain processes pain sensation arising from other injured body tissues, the brain itself has no pain sensation

Over the years, clinical information has been derived from studying patients treated for various cortical lesions resulting from trauma, cerebral vascular accident (stroke), or tumors. In addition, cortical function has also been studied by observations made on conscious patients (under local anesthesia) while undergoing brain surgery. Interestingly, although the brain processes pain sensation arising from other injured body tissues, the brain itself has no pain sensation; thus recordings and observations can be made during brain surgery while the patient is awake. The cerebral cortex is an extraordinary structure since, following a cerebral lesion, some cortical functional reorganization can result to some degree in restored cortical function.

Sectioning of the corpus callosum

The corpus callosum forms an anatomical bridge connecting the two cerebral hemispheres, which is essential for the integration of information in the two sides of the brain

Historically, surgical sectioning of the corpus callosum has been performed to alleviate symptoms of epilepsy. This surgical procedure has proved to be effective in preventing seizures from being transferred from one cerebral hemisphere to the other. Although individuals seem normal following this surgery, postoperative studies have revealed some interesting findings. When patients were asked to read words that were presented in their right visual field, they were able to see and to read the words. However, when words were presented in their left visual field, they could not read them as they were not even aware that the words were there. One explanation is as follows: visual information from the right visual field is relayed to the left cerebral hemisphere (via the visual pathway, which was not affected when the corpus callosum was sectioned), which is the dominant hemisphere in the processing of language in most individuals. Thus the patients were able to see and read the words. In contrast, visual input from the left visual field is relayed to the right cerebral hemisphere (again, via the visual pathway, which was not affected when the corpus callosum was sectioned), the nondominant hemisphere for language. As a result of the bisection of the corpus callosum the visual input relayed to the right cerebral hemisphere has no way of *also* reaching the left hemisphere containing the language areas. Consequently, patients could not see or read the words, as if they had a left homonymous hemianopia. These individuals are *not* blind. When they were asked to select with their hand an object that corresponds to the object that was presented in their left visual field, they selected the matching object. This showed that the visual system is functioning prop-

erly, and that it is the language function that is not. Although the above studies support the finding that the left cerebral hemisphere is the "dominant" hemisphere in the processing of language, other studies indicate that the right hemisphere may also be involved to some extent in language comprehension.

Lesions involving the corpus callosum

Lesions involving the corpus callosum, which unites the two cerebral hemispheres, results in disconnection syndromes

The corpus callosum receives its blood supply from the anterior and posterior cerebral arteries. Its genu and body are supplied by the anterior cerebral artery and the splenium is supplied by both the anterior and posterior cerebral arteries. A stroke involving the **anterior cerebral artery** may affect the **anterior corpus callosum** and result in **apraxia** (impairment of the capacity to execute various movements) of the left arm as a consequence of the isolation/disconnection of the language-dominant (left) hemisphere from the right motor cortex.

A stroke involving the **posterior cerebral artery** or a lesion involving the **posterior corpus callosum** on the left side, may result in **alexia** (the inability to recognize words or to read). Visual input from the left visual field is relayed to the right, intact visual cortex, which is isolated/disconnected from the language-dominant (left) hemisphere. If the basilar artery is affected, which gives rise to both the posterior cerebral arteries, infarction of the visual cortex will be bilateral and will cause cortical blindness; however, the affected individual is unaware that he cannot see.

Lesions in the motor cortex

A unilateral lesion in the primary motor cortex will affect mainly the fine movements of the contralateral distal limbs (hand and foot)

A unilateral lesion in the primary motor cortex (Brodmann's area 4) (see Fig. 23.7A) results in paralysis of the upper and lower limbs contralateral to the lesion. Initially, a **contralateral flaccid paralysis** occurs. About 2 weeks following the lesion, the individual will regain function of the proximal limb musculature. Lesions confined to the primary motor cortex are rare. If the lesion also involves area 6, the paralysis will persist and **spasticity** (increased muscle tone and exaggerated tendon reflexes) will appear in the distal limb muscles. With this type of lesion, fine movements of the distal limbs (hand and foot) will be affected most.

The **corticonuclear** and **corticospinal tracts** arising from the primary motor cortex synapse with interneurons and lower motoneurons of the brainstem and spinal cord, respectively, which normally cause an increase in

CLINICAL CONSIDERATIONS (*continued*)

muscle tone. The fibers arising from the secondary motor cortex that relay motor input to the basal ganglia and reticular formation exert an inhibitory influence diminishing muscle tone. A lesion in the secondary motor cortex will eliminate this inhibitory effect, and will ultimately result in **muscle spasticity**.

A unilateral lesion in the secondary motor cortex (Brodmann's areas 6 and 8) (see Fig. 23.7A) results in the inability to coordinate hand movements bilaterally. The individual will have no difficulty in coordinating the same movement with both hands concurrently. However, when attempting to perform different movements with each hand concurrently, it will be difficult or impossible to execute.

A unilateral lesion of both the primary and secondary motor cortical areas will produce a more severe form of **contralateral paralysis**.

Following trauma to the head involving the brain, scar tissue formation in the brain often results in epileptic seizures. A lesion of the primary motor cortex, with subsequent scar tissue formation, results in **Jacksonian epileptic seizures**. In this type of seizure convulsions may occur only in a certain part of the body, or additional parts of the body may be involved as well, depending on the site of the primary motor cortex that is affected by the lesion.

Note that the clinical case at the beginning of the chapter refers to a patient who had two seizures. Each started with twitching of the right side of the face, the right hand, and the right leg, and then progressed to loss of consciousness and generalized convulsions.

1 Based on the twitching of the right face, hand, and leg, which part of the cerebral cortex do you suspect was the focus of the seizure?

2 What is the name of the seizures resulting from a lesion (and subsequent scar tissue formation) in the primary motor cortex?

3 This patient did not have any prior history of seizures. What could cause the onset of seizures in an adult?

Lesions in the frontal eye field

Normally, stimulation of the frontal eye field results in deviation of both eyes toward the contralateral side. A unilateral lesion in the frontal eye field (Brodmann's area 8) results in both eyes deviating to the side ipsilateral to the lesion. In addition, the affected individual will be unable to turn the eyes contralateral to the lesion. The effects of frontal eye field lesions are not permanent.

Lesions in Broca's area

A unilateral lesion in Broca's area of speech in the dominant cerebral hemisphere results in Broca's aphasia

A unilateral lesion in Broca's area (Brodmann's areas 44 and 45) (see Fig. 23.11) of speech in the dominant cerebral hemisphere results in **Broca's** (motor, expressive, nonfluent) **aphasia** (G. a, "absence;" phasis, "speech"). An individual with this condition has difficulty expressing a thought, is nonfluent, and speaks slowly and with difficulty, although he does not have a lower motoneuron lesion innervating the muscles used in phonation, and these muscles are normal. In addition, his use of words is distorted. He only uses the main or necessary words of a sentence (this is referred to as **telegraphic**

speech). An individual who has a severe form of Broca's aphasia is incapable of speaking. This is known as **mutism**. Although spoken and written language comprehension in Broca's aphasia is a relatively preserved skill, it is still affected by the lesion. Interestingly, the individual is aware that what he is saying makes no sense. As mentioned earlier, Broca's area is involved in the planning of motor activity that is necessary for words to be produced. Broca's area projects this information to the premotor cortex where motor activity is planned and relayed to the primary motor cortex, which initiates the movements necessary to produce speech. A lesion in Broca's area will disrupt the Broca's area input to the premotor cortex. Broca's aphasia also impairs an individual's ability to express a thought or concept by writing it down. This is known as **agraphia** (G. a, "absence;" graphein, "to write").

Lesions in Wernicke's area

A unilateral lesion in Wernicke's area in the dominant hemisphere results in Wernicke's aphasia

A unilateral lesion in Wernicke's area in the dominant hemisphere (usually the left hemisphere), involving Brodmann's areas 22, 37, 39, and 40 (see Fig. 23.11), results in **Wernicke's** (sensory, receptive, fluent) **aphasia**. Since this area plays a role in the comprehension and formulation of language, an individual with a severe form of this condition has difficulty comprehending the spoken word and is unable to read (**alexia**: G. a, "absence;" lexis, "word") or write in understandable language (**agraphia**), even though the visual and auditory systems are normal. Even if speech is fluent, and the patient can speak with ease, the combination and order of the words selected is meaningless and makes no sense to him or others. This is referred to as **fluent paraphasic speech** ("word salad"). Interestingly, this individual is unaware of his deficiencies. In milder forms of Wernicke's aphasia, an individual may use the wrong word (e.g., "airplane" for "bird") or use a word that sounds like the word he intended to say in a sentence (such as "cook" instead of "book").

Lesions in Wernicke's and Broca's areas

A lesion affecting both Wernicke's and Broca's areas in the dominant hemisphere, results in a severe condition referred to as **global aphasia**. An affected individual is unable to comprehend what he hears or reads, cannot write, and in addition is unable to formulate normal language.

Lesions in the superior longitudinal fasciculus

A lesion in the arcuate fasciculus component of the superior longitudinal fasciculus results in conduction aphasia

A lesion in the arcuate fasciculus component of the superior longitudinal fasciculus will interrupt the connection between Brocas's and Wernicke's areas (see Fig. 23.11), the two language areas, and will result in **conduction aphasia**. An individual with this type of lesion is able to comprehend what he hears (since Wernicke's area is intact) and his language expression is fluent; however, he has difficulty processing what he hears and then formulating a proper response.

Lesions in other afferent fibers terminating in Broca's or Wernicke's areas

Lesions involving other afferent fibers from various cortical areas terminating in Broca's or Wernicke's areas produce aphasic syndromes referred to as transcortical aphasias

Lesions involving other afferent fibers from various cortical areas terminating in Broca's or Wernicke's areas also produce aphasic syndromes, referred to as **transcortical aphasias**. The lesions are extrinsic and do not involve Broca's or Wernicke's language areas. However, affected individuals present symptoms characteristic of Broca's or Wernicke's aphasia as a consequence of the lack of input to the language areas, which is essential for normal linguistic function and capacity.

Lesions in the primary somesthetic area

A unilateral lesion in the primary somesthetic area results in contralateral loss of two-point discrimination, graphesthesia, stereognosis, and vibratory and position sense

A unilateral lesion in the primary somesthetic area (Brodmann's areas 3, 1, and 2) (see Fig. 23.7A) results in **contralateral loss** of **two-point discrimination**, **graphesthesia** (the ability to recognize letters or numbers as they are stroked on the skin), and **stereognosis** (the ability to determine the size, shape, and texture of an object following tactile examination), as well as the loss of **vibratory** and **position sense**. In addition, the significance of the qualitative and quantitative perception of the stimulus is diminished or absent. Usually, pain, temperature, and light touch sensation are only minimally impaired; however, the individual is unable to localize the stimulus.

Lesions in the secondary somesthetic area

A lesion in the secondary somesthetic area results in agnosia

A lesion in the secondary somesthetic area results in minimal sensory loss (provided that the primary somesthetic cortex is intact). However, since the secondary somesthetic area plays an important role in the memory of somatosensory information and sensory integration, the individual has a condition referred to as **agnosia** (G. a, "absence;" gnosis, "knowing"). Agnosias are classified according to the particular secondary (association) cortex affected.

If there is a lesion in the secondary somesthetic cortex the deficits resulting from the lesion are referred to as **astereognosis** and **tactile agnosia**. An individual with this type of lesion (which involves the secondary sensory cortex representing the contralateral hand) is unable to identify a familiar object such as a spoon placed in his palm while his eyes are closed. Although he can feel the object in his palm, and information about it (such as its size, shape, weight, and texture) *is* transmitted to the primary sensory cortex, he is unable to identify it as the sensory association cortex (which stores tactile sensory information based on prior experiences, with a spoon in this case) is not functioning. Thus, this new information cannot be assembled and compared to stored information and matched, which is necessary for the identification of the object.

Astereognosis does not only affect an individual's ability to recognize objects without looking at them, but also results in him experiencing a loss of awareness of the position of parts of his body contralateral to the lesion. A condition, referred to as **cortical neglect**, is a severe form of astereognosis, in which the affected individual ignores or denies the presence of one side of his body. This condition most frequently results from an extensive lesion in the superior aspect of the nondominant parietal lobule (the posterior parietal association cortex: Brodmann's areas 5, 7, 39, and 40). Since the individual does not recognize certain parts of his body as being his, he will not wash his left hand, or shave the left side of his face, etc.

Lesions in the primary visual area

A unilateral lesion in the primary visual area results in blindness of the contralateral visual field

A unilateral lesion in the primary visual area (Brodmann's area 17) (see Fig. 23.7A) results in blindness of the contralateral visual field, referred to as a **contralateral homonymous hemianopsia**. If destruction of the primary visual cortex is the result of a vascular lesion, **macular sparing** may occur, that is, central vision is unaffected. It is believed that this is due to the presence

of collateral anastomotic channels between the middle and posterior cerebral arteries.

A bilateral lesion in the primary visual area results in complete blindness, also referred to as **cortical blindness**.

Lesions in the association visual areas

A lesion in the association visual areas results in visual agnosia

A lesion in the association visual areas (Brodmann's areas 18 and 19) (see Fig. 23.7A) (usually bilaterally) results in **visual agnosia**. Since the visual pathways and primary visual cortex are intact, the individual is able to "see" an object or person. However, although he may be looking at a familiar object (such as a toaster) or person, he is unable to identify them, or describe the function of the toaster. An individual with visual agnosia may recognize an object one day but not the next. Also, he may recognize certain familiar objects but not others. Interestingly, an object may be identified by other senses, such as touch.

Dyslexia is a type of visual agnosia. Individuals with this disorder are unable to read and write words, although they can see and recognize letters.

Lesions in the primary auditory area

A unilateral lesion in the primary auditory area results in partial deafness

A unilateral lesion in the primary auditory area results in **partial deafness**. This is due to a bilateral deficit in hearing since auditory information arising in each ear is relayed to the cortical primary auditory area *bilaterally*. Usually, individuals with this type of lesion experience a greater loss of hearing in the ear contralateral to the cortical lesion. Recall that a greater number of fibers relaying auditory input to the cortex decussate, whereas a lesser number of fibers project ipsilaterally. An individual with this lesion has difficulty in localizing sounds on the opposite side.

A bilateral lesion of the primary auditory area results in **total deafness**.

Lesions in the auditory association area

A unilateral lesion in the auditory association areas results in different agnosias

A unilateral lesion in the auditory association area of the dominant (left) hemisphere results in **receptive aphasia**. A unilateral lesion in the nondominant (right) hemisphere results in **amusia**, a condition in which the individual is unable to recognize familiar voices or music.

A bilateral lesion of the auditory association area results in **auditory agnosia** in which the individual does not recognize complex sounds.

Lesions in the cortical vestibular area

A lesion in the cortical vestibular area results in vertigo

A unilateral lesion in the superior temporal gyrus (see Fig. 23.1) results in **subjective vertigo**, in which the individual has the strange experience of feeling as though he is spinning around his environment.

In contrast, a unilateral lesion in the parietal lobe in the lower margin of the intraparietal sulcus results in **objective vertigo**, in which the individual feels as though the environment is revolving around him.

Lesions in the prefrontal association cortex

An individual with a lesion in the prefrontal association cortex displays changes in various personality traits as well as in higher order functions and/or executive functions

An individual with a lesion in the prefrontal association cortex displays changes in various personality traits as well as changes in higher order func-

CLINICAL CONSIDERATIONS (*continued*)

tions and/or executive functions such as judgement, creativity, analytic think-ing, responsibility, etc. These are more pronounced if the lesion is *bilateral*. In addition, the individual behaves in a manner that is socially inappropriate. His behavior is characterized by a lack of self-respect or concern for others, he loses the social skills necessary to interact with others, is easily distracted, and is emotionally unstable.

Dorsolateral convexity lesions result in apathetic, lifeless behavior; orbitofrontal lesions result in disinhibited behavior and poor judgement; left frontal lesions result in depressed behavior; and right frontal lesions result in manic behavior.

Lesions in the supramarginal gyrus

A unilateral lesion in the parietal lobe of the dominant hemisphere results in various conditions collectively known as apraxias

A unilateral lesion in the parietal lobe of the dominant hemisphere results in various conditions collectively known as apraxias (G. a, "absence;" praxia, "action"). **Apraxia** is a condition in which an individual's ability to perform certain skilled movements that are normally triggered by a stimulus is impaired, although the individual does not have any sensory or motor deficits.

A unilateral lesion in the supramarginal gyrus (Brodmann's area 40) (see Fig. 23.1) of the parietal lobe results in an **ideomotor apraxia**, in which the individual's ability to perform a desired activity is impaired. For example, although the individual can perform certain motor activities, his impairment prevents him from doing them on command. **Ideational apraxia** is a condition in which the individual is able to perform certain activities separately, for example picking up a glass, filling it with water, and drinking it; however, when asked to perform these activities in that sequence, he is unable to do them.

Lesions in the supramarginal and angular gyri of the dominant hemisphere

Lesions in the supramarginal and angular gyri of the dominant hemisphere may result in dysgraphia, dyscalculia, or dyslexia

Lesions in the supramarginal and angular gyri (see Fig. 23.1) of the dom-inant hemisphere result in one or more of the following clinical symptoms of Gerstmann's syndrome: (i) **dysgraphia** (G. dys, "faulty;" graphein, "to write"), a condition in which the affected individual has difficulty writing although the sensory and motor systems are intact; (ii) **dyscalculia**, a con-dition in which the individual has difficulty making calculations, right–left confusion, and finger agnosia (in which the individual does not know one finger from another); and (iii) **dyslexia**, in which the lesion interferes with the ability to read.

Lesions in the parietal association area of the nondominant hemisphere

Lesions in the parietal association area that involve the inferior parietal lobule result in the following deficits: (i) distorted concepts of body image, in which the individual is not aware of the left side of his body (e.g., does not shave the left side of his face, does not wash the left side of his body, etc.); (ii) a lack of awareness that he is ill; (iii) disorientation, for example he does not know where objects are located in his house, or where locations are on a map; and (iv) an inability to draw simple figures.

SYNONYMS AND EPONYMS OF THE CEREBRAL CORTEX

Name of structure or term	Synonym(s)/eponym(s)	Name of structure or term	Synonym(s)/eponym(s)
Allocortex	Heterogenetic cortex	Multimodal association areas of	Heteromodal association areas of
Archicortex	Archipallium	the cerebral cortex	the cerebral cortex
Astereognosis	Stereoanesthesia	Outer band of Baillarger	Outer line of Baillarger
Auditory radiations	Geniculotemporal radiations		Outer stripe of Baillarger
Broca's area	Brodmann's areas 44 and 45	Paleocortex	Paleopallium
Cental sulcus	Central sulcus of Rolando	Parietal motor area (PMA)	Brodmann's areas 5 and 7
Corticofugal fibers	Output projection fibers from the	Posterior limb of the internal capsule	Thalamolenticular part (older term)
	cerebral cortex	Prefrontal cortex	Brodmann's areas 9–12 and 45–47
Corticonuclear fibers	Corticobulbar fibers (older term)	Premotor cortex (PMC)	Premotor area
Corticopetal fibers	Afferent fibers to the cerebral		Part of Brodmann's area 6
	cortex	Primary auditory cortex	Brodmann's areas 41 and 42
Frontal eye field (FEF)	Brodmann's area 8		Transverse temporal gyri of Heschl
Geniculocalcarine radiations	Optic radiations	Primary motor cortex	Precentral gyrus
	Geniculocalcarine tract		Brodmann's area 4
Girdle musculature	Proximal limb musculature	Primary somatosensory cortex	Primary somesthetic cortex
Hippocampal commissure	Commissure of the fornix		Brodmann's areas 3, 1, and 2
Horizontal cells	Horizontal cells of Cajal	Primary visual cortex	Brodmann's area 17
Inner band of Baillarger	Inner line of Baillarger		Striate cortex
	Inner stripe of Baillarger	Retrolenticular part of the internal	Retrolenticular limb of the internal
Isocortex	Neocortex	capsule	capsule
	Neopallium	Secondary auditory cortical areas	Brodmann's areas 22 and 42
	Homogenetic cortex	Secondary somatosensory cortex	Secondary somesthetic cortex
Jacksonian seizure	Jacksonian march		Brodmann's areas 5 and 7
Lateral fissure	Lateral fissure of Sylvius	Short association fibers (of the	Arcuate fibers
Layer I of the cerebral cortex	Molecular layer	cerebral cortex)	U-fibers
	Plexiform layer	Somesthetic association area	Superior parietal lobule
Layer II of the cerebral cortex	External granular layer		Brodmann's areas 5, 7, and 40
Layer III of the cerebral cortex	External pyramidal layer	Stellate cells of the cerebral cortex	Granule cells of the cerebral cortex
Layer IV of the cerebral cortex	Internal granular layer	Sublenticular limb of the internal	Sublenticular part of the internal
Layer V of the cerebral cortex	Internal pyramidal layer	capsule	capsule
Layer VI of the cerebral cortex	Multiform layer	Superior occipitofrontal fasciculus	Subcallosal bundle
	Fusiform layer	Supplementary motor area (SMA)	Part of Brodmann's area 6
Medial geniculate nucleus (MGN)	Medial geniculate body (MGB)	Trunk musculature	Axial musculature
Mesocortex	Periallocortex	Visual association cortex	Extrastriate cortex
	Juxtallocortex		Brodmann's areas 18 and 19
		Wernicke's area	Brodmann's area 22

FOLLOW-UP TO CLINICAL CASE

The onset of seizures in a previously healthy individual without a history of seizure mandates careful evaluation. Brain imaging is required, preferably with MRI (a CT is done in the emergency room setting to look for a cerebral hemorrhage). MRI in the patient discussed revealed a **meningioma** over the midlateral aspect of the left hemisphere, in the vicinity of the primary motor cortical area.

The first seizure experienced by this patient was a focal motor, or simple partial, seizure. Normal consciousness was maintained and motor manifestations occured only on the contralateral side to where the brain focus of the seizure was. In this case, the seizure focus began in or around the facial part of the left primary motor cortex and spread progressively to involve the upper extremity and then the lower extremity part of the primary motor cortex (refer to the somatotopic representation of the face and upper and lower limbs on the motor homunculus; see Fig. 23.9). This is referred to as a **Jacksonian march** or **Jacksonian seizure**. It is rare to see the full march of clonic activity, but it is historically and conceptually important to know about it.

The second seizure almost certainly had its onset in the same spot as the first one, except that this one spread rapidly and became generalized, i.e., involving both hemispheres. This generalization results in loss of consciousness and often generalized convulsions (generalized tonic-clonic seizures). Tongue biting and/or urinary incontinence is also often associated with generalized tonic-clonic seizures. When there is alteration of consciousness with a seizure but it is not generalized, it is called complex partial.

Seizures are a cortical phenomenon. A seizure indicates an abnormality of the electrophysiology of the cortical neurons. The full electrophysiology of seizure initiation and progression is beyond the scope of this discussion. The cortical neurons become hyperexcitable and typically produce "positive" symptoms rather than symptoms indicating loss of function. The manifestations of seizures are widely varied, and depend on which part of the cerebral cortex is affected. The most "epileptogenic" regions, in descending order, are the temporal lobes, frontal lobes, parietal lobes, and occipital lobes.

Seizures are either primary or secondary. A secondary etiology is more common with new-onset seizures in adults, and can be caused by strokes, tumors, vascular malformations, hemorrhage, and any other lesion causing cortical irritation. Subcortical lesions do not cause seizures. Primary seizures are more common in children, who often "outgrow" them, and there is no identifiable lesion on brain imaging. There is often a hereditary component. However, seizures in children can certainly be secondary and new-onset seizures in adults can be primary (or at least show no identifiable lesion).

4 Which lobe of the cerebral cortex is the most epileptogenic lobe?

QUESTIONS TO PONDER

1. Distinguish between unimodal and multimodal association cortices.

2. Which cells are the most common cell type and the main output neurons of the cerebral cortex?

3. Why is it that patients who have their corpus callosum sectioned to relieve symptoms of epilepsy can see and read words presented in their right visual field, but cannot see or read words presented in their left visual field?

4. Describe what is likely to happen following a stroke involving one or more of the blood vessels that supply the corpus callosum?

5. Name the artery that supplies Broca's and Wernicke's areas, and the symptoms that may occur following the occlusion of the vessel's branches that supply the above language areas?

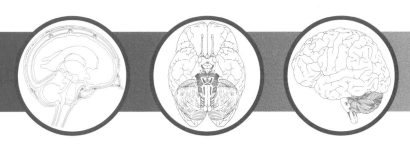

Questions to ponder: answers to odd questions

CHAPTER 1

Question 1: Although these two anatomical components of the nervous system are treated as if they were separate entities, they are in fact intimately related to one another. Although the central nervous system is housed in the skull and spinal column, many of its neurons, whose cell bodies are located in the brain and in the spinal cord, have processes that leave the confines of their bony housing and enter other regions of the body. Here they are referred to as nerve fibers of the peripheral nervous system. Therefore, in many instances, the peripheral nervous system is an extension of the central nervous system.

Question 3: Oligodendroglia are one of the types of neuroglia located in the central nervous system. These cells act as "insulators," protecting neurons from coming into contact with extraneous cells and/or elements located in the central nervous system. Since most neurons have numerous processes, many of which may be quite long, each neuron requires a large number of oligodendroglia to form that physical barrier.

Question 5: There is little voluntary control over a two neuron reflex arc. As an example, the patellar reflex, which is a two neuron reflex arc, cannot be suppressed by an individual. However, due to the presence of the interneuron in a three neuron reflex arc, the motor action of the three neuron reflex arc can be suppressed. As an example, the normal reflex in response to a needle prick to the finger tip is to withdraw the finger from harm's way; however, if the finger is being pricked in a physician's office for the purposes of a blood test, the patient, although aware of the pain, will (usually) suppress the withdrawal component of the reflex.

CHAPTER 2

Question 1: The process of transforming the embryoblast to a trilaminar germ disc is known as gastrulation. This process establishes the presence of the three germ layers—the ectoderm, mesoderm, and endoderm—each of which will be responsible for the development of specific structures of the body. As an example, the ectoderm gives rise to the central nervous system, the mesoderm to the development of the vertebral column, and the endoderm to the epithelium of the gut.

Question 3: Genes code for the synthesis of specific proteins, many of which are enzymes that are responsible for the occurrence of specific events. Certain genes have been conserved through evolution and their study in lower organisms, such as the fruitfly, has provided information that is directly applicable to the developmental processes of higher organisms, including humans. A family of genes, known as the homeobox genes, code for the synthesis of transcription factors, proteins that bind to and regulate the expression of other genes.

The time sequence of the events controlled by products of these homeobox genes and by growth factors are essential for normal development because certain genes can be switched on only if some other genes have already been activated and if still other genes have not as yet been switched on. In other words, there are "windows of opportunity" for the occurrence of certain events and if that timeframe is missed then development will not proceed normally. Therefore, these homeobox genes become activated in a specific order, and their sequential expression establishes a pattern of developmental events. In order for development to progress in a normal manner, cells must interact with each other. These interactions may involve the physical contact of two cells or the release of a particular substance by one cell, referred to as the signaling cell, to act as a message for the other cell, known as the target cell.

Question 5: Both develop as an outgrowth of the forming brain and an invagination of the ectoderm.

The pituitary: The infundibulum of the diencephalon is a downward evagination of the floor of the third ventricle. As the infundibulum grows down, it meets an ectodermal diverticulum of the oral cavity, known as Rathke's pouch. These two structures fuse with each other to form the pituitary gland (hypohysis). The neurohypophysis (median eminence, stalk, and pars nervosa) arises from the infundibulum, whereas the adenohypophysis (pars tuberalis, pars distalis, and pars intermedia) derives from Rathke's pouch. A small colloid-filled cleft frequently remains as a vestige of the lumen of Rathke's pouch, in the pars intermedia.

The eye: During the third week of gestation, the ventrolateral wall on each side of the future diencephalon gives rise to an optic vesicle. These hollow vesicles grow in a lateral direction; they reach and induce the ectoderm to form the lens placode, the precursor of the lens of the eye. The optic vesicle invaginates to form a two-layered structure, known as the optic cup, which gives rise to the nervous and pigmented layers of the retina; the connection between the optic cup and the forming brain becomes known as the optic stalk, the future optic nerve. The rim of the optic cup encircles the prospective lens to form the iris.

CHAPTER 3

Question 1: Although the soma of a neuron is relatively large, the axon and dendrites of many neurons possess a lot more cytoplasm than does the cell body. Therefore, the soma is responsible for the formation of much of the protein, macromolecules, and neurotransmitter material that the entire cell requires. Because of this high biosynthetic demand, the neuron must be equipped with the biosynthetic machinery to manufacture these substances. Since the soma is the only expanded portion of the neuron, its organelles must be localized at that site.

Question 3: Since the intracellular concentration of K^+ is greater than the extracellular concentration, potassium is driven by a concentration gradient from the cell into the extracellular space. Potassium ions travel through ion channels that are not gated and are known as K^+ leak channels. Because only K^+ ions are permitted through these channels an electrical imbalance is established (more positive ions are present on the extracellular aspect of the membrane than on the intracellular aspect). At the point where the concentration gradient's "desire" to push potassium out of the cell and the electrical imbalance's "desire" to return potassium into the cell equal each other, the net flow of K^+ ions becomes zero. This does not mean that there is no flow of K^+ ions across the membrane, it simply means that the same number of K^+ ions flow into the cell as out of the cell. The establishment of this equilibrium potential (modified for K^+ ions) is described by the Nernst equation. This equation can be applied for all ions, and is solved for the most common ions. However, the Nernst equation assumes that only the particular ion in question is permitted to traverse the cell membrane. However, this is not a true situation as ion channels of the plasma membrane are open simultaneously, thus permitting several ions to cross the plasmalemma. The Goldman equation describes the membrane potential as a function of the relative permeability of the cell membrane to more than a single species of ions. Since the neuron membrane is influenced by at least three ions—Na^+, K^+, and Cl^-—all three are considered in the

Goldman equation. The Goldman equation is very similar to the Nernst equation, but it considers more than just a single ion type. It is interesting to note that the two equations would be identical if the permeability of two of the three ions were zero. Therefore, the Goldman equation describes the complexity of the existing situation better than does the Nernst equation and provides a more realistic prediction of resting membrane potential for neurons.

Question 5: An increase in the number of postsynaptic potentials (e.g., by the rapid release of multiple quanta of chemical messengers from a single axon terminal or from many axon terminals on the same neuron), results in their summation. Hence, hundreds of nearly simultaneous, small postsynaptic potentials may be necessary to achieve the threshold required for the formation of an action potential when those currents arrive at the initial segment of the axon. Generally, inhibitory synapses are closer to the initial segment of the axon than are excitatory synapses. Since inhibitory synapses function to hyperpolarize the postsynaptic membrane, they tend to diminish the flow of currents formed at the excitatory potential making it more difficult to reach threshold levels at the initial segment of the axon. This sequence of events is referred to as the summation of inhibitory postsynaptic potentials and excitatory postsynaptic potentials.

CHAPTER 4

Question 1: The neurotransmitter substances that bind specifically to ligand-gated ion channels cause those channels to open directly, thus the target neuron responds immediately, resulting in an ionotropic effect. Those neurotransmitter substances that bind to G-protein-coupled receptors exert an indirect effect on ion channels. Since the G-proteins act as intermediaries, the effect on the target neuron is slower than in the previous instance. Thus, these neurotransmitter substances are known as neuromodulators, and they are said to exert a metabotropic effect.

Question 3: Biogenic amines are derived from amino acids and exert a metabotropic effect. They bind to G-protein-coupled receptors and activate the second messenger system within the target neuron, which in turn will open ion channels. These substances include the catecholamines dopamine, norepinephrine, and epinephrine as well as histamine and serotonin. Upon release from the presynaptic terminal, biogenic amines are endocytosed by the nerve terminals and glial cells, and are digested by the enzymes cathecol *O*-methyltranferase and monoamine oxidase. In this fashion, each release of these neurotransmitters is responsible for only a limited number of depolarizations/hyperpolarizations.

Question 5: Acetylcholine is a neurotransmitter substance localized both in the central and peripheral nervous systems. It is synthesized in the presynaptic terminal from acetyl CoA and choline by choline acetyl transferase, the rate-limiting enzyme of its synthesis. Acetylcholine has the ability to bind to both ionotropic receptors and metabotropic receptors. In skeletal muscle it is an excitatory neurotransmitter substance, binding directly to ligand-gated sodium (nicotinic receptors) as well as to potassium ion channels, and causing them to open. In cardiac muscle it is an inhibitory neurotransmitter substance, binding to G-protein-linked receptors (muscarinic receptors) that facilitate the opening of potassium ion channels.

CHAPTER 5

Question 1: The cervical and lumbar enlargements are necessary to provide space for the many neurons that are required for the innervation of the upper and lower extremities, respectively. Because the upper extremity is much more complex in humans, in that the hands and fingers possess a very rich nerve supply, the cervical enlargement is greater than the lumbar enlargement.

Question 3: White matter is composed mostly of myelinated and unmyelinated nerve fibers, which bring information into the central nervous system and transmit it to higher levels, and transmit information from higher levels to the spinal cord and to the muscles and glands. Based on the presence of sulci and fissures, the white matter is subdivided into three major columns, dorsal, lateral, and ventral funiculi. Within the funiculi the nerve fibers that have similar destinations are arranged in bundles known as tracts (fasciculi).

Question 5: The spinal cord equals the length of the vertebral canal only until the end of the first trimester of prenatal life. Thereafter the trunk elongates much faster, so that by the time of birth the conus medullaris is only at the level of the third lumbar vertebra and in the adult it extends only as far as the caudal aspect of the first lumbar vertebra. Therefore, lower levels of the spinal cord segments are displaced rostrally in relation to their corresponding vertebral levels. Because of this differential growth, the subarachnoid space caudal to the conus medullaris, known as the lumbar cistern, is devoid of spinal cord. It is this space that may be used by physicians to remove cerebrospinal fluid for diagnostic purposes without causing injury to the spinal cord.

CHAPTER 6

Question 1: They are the commissural, projection, and association fibers. Commissural fibers connect the right and left cerebral hemispheres. Projection fibers connect the cerebral cortex to lower levels, namely the corpus striatum, diencephalon, brainstem, and spinal cord; the majority of these fibers are axons of pyramidal cells and fusiform neurons. Association fibers are restricted to a single hemisphere.

Question 3: Peduncles are large fiber tracts that connect parts of the brain to the brainstem. There are two separate groups of peduncles, the cerebral and cerebellar peduncles. The cerebral peduncles are two very large, thick fiber bundles that connect the cerebral hemispheres to the brainstem. The cerebellar peduncles are three pairs of fiber bundles that connect the cerebellum to the midbrain, pons, and medulla of the brainstem.

CHAPTER 7

Question 1: The dura mater of the spinal cord differs from that of the cranial dura mater because the spinal dura is composed only of the meningeal layer. The periosteal layer is the true periosteum of the vertebral canal and is separated from the meningeal layer by a loose connective tissue and fat-filled epidural space.

Question 3: Although the brain itself may not feel pain, the dura mater possesses a very rich sensory nerve supply, derived mostly from cranial nerve V (the trigeminal nerve) but also from the first three cervical spinal nerves that serve the dura mater of the posterior cranial fossa. It is these sensory fibers that become stimulated and the patient may experience severe pain.

Question 5: Arachnoid granulations are small, mushroom-shaped evaginations of the arachnoid that protrude into the lumen of the dural sinuses. Most of the arachnoid granulations are associated with the lacunae lateralis—diverticula of the superior sagittal sinus—although some jut into the lumen of the sinus. The core of an arachnoid granulation is continuous with the subarachnoid space and is surrounded by the epithelioid layer of the arachnoid and the dura, forming a membrane that is two cell layers thick. As the arachnoid granulation evaginates into the lacuna lateralis it is invested by some cellular and collagenous elements of the meningeal dura mater, which in turn is surrounded by the endothelial lining of the blood vessel. Cerebrospinal fluid from the subarachnoid space enters into the core of the arachnoid granulation and from there penetrates, probably by osmosis, the epithelioid layers of the arachnoid granulations and the endothelial lining to escape into the lacuna lateralis. Therefore, the function of the arachnoid granulations is transporting cerebrospinal fluid manufactured by the choroid plexuses of the brain ventricles into the vascular system. It is important to note that although the arachnoid granulations protrude into the venous sinuses, they are always separated from the blood by the endothelial lining of the dural sinus/lacuna lateralis.

CHAPTER 8

Question 1: Radicular arteries are extremely important for the vascularization of the spinal cord because, with the exception of the cervical region, the anterior and posterior spinal arteries by themselves are unable to provide an adequate vascular supply to the spinal cord. Therefore, an injury to a spinal nerve damages not only the afferent and efferent fibers of a particular spinal cord level, but may also damage the segmental white and gray matter by producing ischemic conditions due to the reduction in blood supply from the radicular artery serving that region.

Question 3: The posterior communicating artery connects the cerebral portion of the internal carotid artery to the posterior cerebral branch of the basilar artery. The right and left arteries are not identical, in that one is frequently smaller than the other, and, in fact, one may be entirely absent or doubled. The main function of this vessel is to ensure a viable blood supply to the brain in case the internal carotid or vertebral artery becomes occluded. However, it also has central branches that pierce the region of the base of the cerebrum and serve part of the posterior limb of the internal capsule, the medial aspect of the thalamus, and the tissue forming the lateral border of the third ventricle.

Question 5: Four major vessels—the two internal carotid arteries and the two vertebral arteries—bring blood to the brain. Although numerous veins receive blood from the brain, they all deliver their contents into the venous sinuses of the meninges. The venous sinuses, in turn, deliver their blood into the superior bulb of the right and left internal jugular veins.

CHAPTER 9

Question 1: Preganglionic sympathetic soma are located in the lateral horn of the spinal cord only at levels T1 through L2, therefore the preganglionic fibers are located only in the corresponding spinal nerves. They leave the spinal nerves via the white rami communicantes to join the sympathetic chain ganglia. There they may synapse with postganglionic sympathetic soma at various levels along the sympathetic trunk. Postganglionic sympathetic fibers of these soma re-enter the spinal nerve (through gray rami communicantes) at the level that leads to the region of their destination. Since there are 31 pairs of spinal nerves there has to be a corresponding gray rami communicantes for each spinal nerve.

Question 3: The autonomic nervous system is designed in such a fashion that preganglionic fibers can synapse only with their own postganglionic soma, therefore a preganglionic parasympathetic fiber cannot synapse with a postganglionic sympathetic soma. The postganglionic soma can thus only be stimulated by its own preganglionic neuron. However, a target cell, such as the conducting system of the heart, may be innervated by both postganglionic sympathetic and parasympathetic fibers and the target cell has to know whether it is responding to a sympathetic or a parasympathetic message.

Question 5: As feces accumulate, the sigmoid colon distends and the individual becomes conscious of the need to defecate, but the feces are retained in the colon by the two sphincter muscles, the internal smooth muscle sphincter and the external skeletal muscle sphincter. The former is supplied by postganglionic sympathetic fibers from the hypogastric plexus as well as by postganglionic parasympathetic fibers located in Auerbach's plexus (whose preganglionic fibers arise from the sacral spinal cord). The external sphincter is supplied by the somatic nervous system, namely the inferior rectal nerve. Thus, when the sigmoid colon becomes distended, the internal sphincter muscle relaxes (due to the parasympathetic nerve supply) and at the same time the external sphincter muscle contracts, preventing the feces from exiting the bowel. While the individual is asleep, this contraction of the external sphincter muscle is a reflex response. When the individual is awake, the contraction of the external sphincter is a voluntary response.

CHAPTER 10

Question 1: Some receptors respond quickly and maximally at the onset of the stimulus, but stop responding even if the stimulus continues; these are known as rapidly adapting (phasic) receptors. They are essential in responding to changes but they ignore ongoing processes, such as when one wears a wristwatch and ignores its presence and continuous pressure on the skin of the wrist. However, there are other receptors, slowly adapting (tonic) receptors, that continue to respond as long as the stimulus is present.

Question 3: It is the degree of stretching that is proportional to the load placed on the muscle. The larger the load, the more strongly the spindles are depolarized and the more extrafusal muscle fibers are in turn activated.

Question 5: Pain perception is not only processed in the primary somatosensory cortex, but also in the anterior cingulate and anterior insular cortices. Recent studies support the finding that pain sensation persists following a lesion to the primary somatosensory cortex as a result of these additional cortical representations of pain.

CHAPTER 11

Question 1: By alpha and gamma motoneuron coactivation. When the gross muscle contracts (following stimulation by alpha motoneurons), the contractile portions of the intrafusal fibers undergo a simultaneous corresponding contraction (following stimulation by gamma motoneurons), stretching their central noncontractile portion. The muscle spindles are then ready to detect muscle stretch when the muscle becomes stretched from the contracted state or from any length. Therefore, when the gross muscle begins to stretch from the contracted state, the intrafusal fibers will be immediately stretched and their afferent (sensory) fibers will fire, informing the central nervous system that muscle stretching is occurring.

Question 3: Although the upper motoneurons arising from the primary motor cortex may be damaged, the tectospinal, reticulospinal, and vestibulospinal tracts and the upper motoneurons contributed by the secondary motor cortex provide a motor input to the interneurons and lower motoneurons innervating the skeletal muscles.

Question 5: The cortical group, which includes the lateral corticospinal tract.

CHAPTER 12

Question 1: The limbic system consists of a group of cortical and subcortical structures that are involved in the processing of emotions. Via its connections to the basal ganglia, the limbic system can influence the underlying motivational aspects of behavior or movement. Here is an example of the role played by the limbic system in movement. The pleasant aroma of freshly brewed coffee and baked cinnamon rolls are enough to motivate anyone of us to walk toward the coffee and cinnamon rolls and taste them by lifting the coffee cup and roll to take a sip and a few bites. Tasting the cinnamon roll may elicit certain facial expressions that may indicate to those looking at us that we are enjoying the delicious tasting cinnamon roll. Furthermore, the warm cinnamon aroma may evoke fond memories of the first time we tasted a cinnamon roll. In this example, the olfactory system (mediating the sense of smell), the limbic system (processing emotions and memory), and the basal ganglia involved in movement are all interconnected.

Question 3: Normally, the subthalamic nucleus projects glutaminergic (excitatory) fibers to the two output nuclei of the basal ganglia, the medial segment of the globus pallidus and the substantia nigra pars reticulata, which in turn send inhibitory projections to the thalamus. Thalamocortical fibers that are excitatory project to the motor cortex. Projections up to this point are ipsilateral; however, the upper motoneurons arising from the cortex decussate in the pyramids, thus affecting the opposite side of the body. A lesion in the subthalamic nucleus would result in disinhibition (excitation) of the thalamus, which in turn becomes overactive, overstimulating the motor cortex, which in turn results in hyperkinetic symptoms in the opposite side of the body.

Question 5: If excessive L-DOPA is administered to an individual with Parkinson's disease, the individual will manifest choreic movements. L-DOPA administered to a patient with Huntington's disease will intensify the choreic movements.

CHAPTER 13

Question 1: The cerebellar efferents and the descending motor pathways (i.e., the corticospinal and rubrospinal tracts) are crossed. Thus a lesion in the right cerebellar hemisphere via its efferents (which decussate) affects the left side of the brain. As the left corticospinal tract descends to the pyramids, most of its fibers cross to the opposite (right) side as the lateral corticospinal tract, terminating in the right spinal cord, and synapsing with lower motoneurons that innervate the muscles on the right side of the body. The corticorubral fibers arising from the left side of the brain descend to the left red nucleus, which in turn gives rise to the rubrospinal tract whose fibers cross to the right side in the midbrain. The right rubrospinal tract will descend to terminate on lower motoneurons in the right spinal cord that innervate muscles on the right side of the body.

Question 3: The hemispheric (lateral) zone of the cerebellum. It is interesting to note that although both motor and cognitive functions are affected by the consumption of alcohol, the cells of the cerebellum are very susceptible to the effects of alcohol. This becomes apparent by the awkward, ataxic, uncoordinated execution of movements by the intoxicated individual, especially when the eyes are closed.

Question 5: A decrease in resistance to passive manipulation resulting in excess movement of the limbs (referred to as "rag-doll appearance") is caused by the absence of cerebellar influence on the stretch reflex.

CHAPTER 14

Question 1: Nociceptive input from the body is transmitted to the spinal cord dorsal horn by first order pseudounipolar neurons whose cell bodies are located in the dorsal root ganglia. Second order neurons, whose cell bodies are located in the dorsal horn of the spinal cord, give rise to axons that ascend as the spinothalamic or spinoreticular tracts. The spinothalamic tract terminates in the ventral posterior lateral nucleus of the thalamus, but also sends collaterals to the brainstem reticular formation. The spinoreticular tract terminates in the reticular formation, and also sends collateral to the thalamus.

Nociceptive input from the orofacial region is transmitted to the pons by the pseudounipolar neurons whose cell bodies are located in the trigeminal ganglion. Fibers conveying nociceptive input descend in the spinal tract of the trigeminal nerve to terminate in the subnucleus caudalis of the spinal nucleus of the trigeminal. This nucleus also receives the central processes of sensory neurons of other cranial nerves relaying nociceptive input from structures in the head. Second order neurons housed in the subnucleus caudalis cross to the opposite side of the pons, and join the ventral trigeminal lemniscus to terminate in the ventral posterior medial nucleus of the thalamus with collaterals to the reticular formation.

Question 3: Through their ascending fibers the neurons of the medial zone influence the autonomic nervous system, and the level of arousal. Via their descending fibers, which join the reticulospinal tracts, the neurons of the medial zone influence the motor control of the axial and proximal limb musculature.

Question 5: Lesions damaging the midbrain reticular formation can cause hypersomnia associated with slow respiration. When the midbrain is compressed with consequent extensive damage of the ARAS pathways, a comatose state ensues.

CHAPTER 15

Question 1: Interruption of the parasympathetic innervation of the sphincter pupillae muscle causes the pupil ipsilateral to the lesion to remain dilated (mydriasis) and to not respond (constrict) to a flash of light. This may be the first clinical sign of intracranial pressure on the general visceral efferent fibers of the oculomotor nerve. The ciliary muscle is also nonfunctional due to interruption of its parasympathetic innervation, and cannot accommodate the lens for near vision (that is, cannot focus on near objects).

Question 3: The abducens nucleus innervates a single extraocular muscle, the lateral rectus. A lesion in the abducens nucleus damages not only the general somatic efferent (GSE) motor fibers innervating the lateral rectus muscle, but also the internuclear fibers projecting to the contralateral oculomotor nucleus, that synapse with the motoneurons that innervate the medial rectus.

A lesion in the abducens nucleus that damages the GSE motor fibers innervating the lateral rectus results in paralysis of the lateral rectus muscle, which normally abducts the eye. Since the individual will be unable to move the ipsilateral eye laterally, it deviates medially as a result of the unopposed action of the medial rectus. The individual can turn the ipsilateral eye from its medial position to the center (looking straight ahead), but not beyond it. This paralysis results in medial strabismus (convergent, internal strabismus, esotropia). Since the eyes become misaligned, the individual experiences horizontal diplopia (double vision). The diplopia is greatest when looking toward the side of the lesion and is reduced by looking towards the unaffected side since the visual axes become parallel. The individual realizes that the diplopia is minimized by turning his head slightly so that the chin is pointing toward the side of the lesion. Bilateral abducent nerve lesion results in the individual becoming "cross-eyed."

A lesion involving the abducens nucleus damaging the internuclear neurons results in the inability to turn the opposite eye medially as the individual attempts to gaze toward the side of the lesion. This condition is referred to as lateral gaze paralysis.

Question 5: A lesion in the vicinity of the abducens nucleus that involves the entire ipsilateral abducens nucleus as well as the decussating medial longitudinal fasciculus fibers arising from the contralateral abducens nucleus, results in a rare condition referred to as "one-and-a-half."

If, for example, a lesion is present in the vicinity of the left abducens nucleus the following will occur.

1 The GSE motoneurons whose axons form the left abducent nerve innervating the left lateral rectus are damaged. Therefore that lateral rectus muscle is paralyzed.
2 The internuclear neurons housed in the left abducens nucleus are also damaged. Therefore their crossing fibers do not form excitatory synapses with the motoneurons of the contralateral oculomotor nucleus that innervate the right medial rectus muscle.
3 The crossing fibers of the internuclear neurons arising from the contralateral (right) abducens nucleus are also damaged. Thus they do not form excitatory synapses with the motoneurons of the left oculomotor nucleus that innervate the left medial rectus.

Therefore, when attempting to gaze to the left, the left eye will not abduct and the right eye will not adduct during conjugate horizontal gaze to the left. When attempting to gaze to the right, the right eye responds normally, that is it is able to abduct, whereas the left eye will not be able to adduct during conjugate horizontal gaze to the right.

It is important to note that the innervation to all the extraocular muscles of both eyes is intact, except to one—the left lateral rectus. If you ask this individual to look at a near object placed directly in front of his face, both eyes will converge since both medial recti and their innervation (branches of the oculomotor nerve) are intact. This type of lesion becomes apparent only during conjugate horizontal eye movement.

Question 7: The first cranial nerve that is likely to be damaged from a growing pituitary tumor is the optic nerve. The decussating axons at the optic chiasma will be compressed, followed by the nondecussating fibers. If the tumor becomes very large, the cranial nerves located on the medial wall of the cavernous sinus (namely the oculomotor, trochlear, and ophthalmic division of the trigeminal and the abducent nerves) will likely be compressed and cause deficits in the structures that these nerves innervate.

CHAPTER 16

Question 1: Although light travels from the inner to the outer layers of the retina (internal limiting membrane → pigment epithelium), visual electrical signals are transmitted in the opposite direction from the outer to the inner layers of the retina (rod and cone layer → optic nerve fiber layer).

Question 3: When the right eye was illuminated, only the consensual (left) papillary light reflex was elicited. This indicates that a lesion may be present in the efferent limb of the pupillary light reflex arc of the right side. When the left eye was illuminated, again, only the left eye responded, which indicates that the lesion may be present in the efferent limb of the pupillary light reflex arc on the right side.

Question 5: The patient had a lesion affecting the ganglion cell axons arising from the nasal half of each retina, which cross at the optic chiasma over the body of the sphenoid bone. The crossing fibers may be damaged due to compression by a tumor of the pituitary gland.

CHAPTER 17

Queston 1: The middle ear functions in the transmission and transduction of tympanic membrane vibrations to the inner ear (from an air to a fluid medium). The oval window and the round window both serve necessary functions in these processes.

Question 3: The basilar membrane is an elastic structure exhibiting a gradual increase in width, and a decrease in stiffness from the oval window (at the cochlear base) to the helicotrema (at the cochlear apex). The gradual decrease in stiffness permits this membrane to be sensitive to high frequency vibrations near the cochlear base, and low frequency vibrations near its apex, at the helicotrema.

Question 5: The olivocochlear bundle has an inhibitory effect on cochlear nerve activity, modulating and sharpening auditory transmission.

CHAPTER 18

Question 1: Sensory input from the visual, vestibular, and proprioceptive systems, is integrated by the nervous system, especially the cerebellum, to generate motor responses. These motor responses maintain equilibrium, posture, and muscle tone, as well as reflex movements of the eyes, all of which are carried out at the subconscious level.

Question 3: The neuroepithelia of the cristae ampullares, macula utriculi, and macula sacculi are covered with a gelatinous glycoprotein membrane. The stereocilia and kinocilia are embedded in this membrane. In the utricle and saccule, the gelatinous glycoprotein membranes overlying their macula have, on their free surface, otoconia (G., "ear dust")—also referred to as otoliths (G., "ear stones")—which are crystals consisting of calcium carbonate. Since the gelatinous glycoprotein membrane of the utricle and saccule has otoliths, it is referred to as the otolithic membrane, and the utricle and saccule are referred to as otolithic organs. The otoliths have a specific gravity that is greater than that of the endolymph which surrounds them, and they are consequently pulled by gravity. Gravity applies a continuous linear acceleration on the head, and thus deflects the gelatinous membrane, which in turn stimulates the hair cells.

The glycoprotein membrane of the cristae ampullares is dome-shaped and is called the cupula; it is devoid of crystals. The cupula increases resistance to the flow of endolymph and, unlike the otolithic membrane, is not influenced by gravitational forces. Instead, it responds to endolymphatic flow. The cupula is a mechanical structure that narrows the lumen of the canal and so increases resistance to flow. The three cristae ampullares are enclosed in the semicircular duct ampullae (one crista in each ampulla) and detect angular acceleration or deceleration (rotational movement) of the head (as in turning or tilting the head). The receptors in the utricle and saccule (the macula utriculi and macula sacculi within the utricle and saccule, respectively) detect spatial orientation of the head in space relative to gravity and linear acceleration or deceleration forces.

Question 5: The vestibular nerve is unique since it is the only cranial nerve that sends some of its first order afferent fibers relaying sensory input directly from the peripheral receptors to the cerebellar cortex. The vestibular nuclei and the cerebellum serve as the first relay centers of the vestibular pathway.

Question 7: When an individual fixes his gaze on ("stares at") an object and then begins to turn his head, for example to the right, the eyes will reflexly (via medial longitudinal fasciculus vestibular connections to the extraocular nuclei) "turn" to the left (as the head is moving), which is opposite to the direction of head movement. This turning of the eyes (dictated by vestibular reflex connections) compensates for shifting of the head position in order to maintain visual fixation on an object. Without this vestibular reflex mechanism coupling head and eye movements, as the erect head moves from a certain position (to the right or to the left) the eyes would remain still, perceiving a changing visual field during the head movement.

CHAPTER 19

Question 1: Olfactory receptor cells, the first order bipolar neurons of the olfactory pathway, reside in a peripheral structure, the olfactory epithelium (instead of being housed in a sensory ganglion). They are the only neurons that are in direct contact with the environment and they give rise to unmyelinated axons, the slowest impulse-conducting axons of the central nervous system. They serve the functions of: (i) sensory receptors (chemoreceptors that become

activated by chemical stimuli in their surroundings); (ii) transducers (generate graded potentials); and (iii) first order neurons (relaying olfactory sensation centrally to the olfactory bulbs).

Question 3: Odorant-receptor molecules (transmembrane G-protein-coupled receptors) are embedded in the plasmalemma of the ciliary membrane of the olfactory receptor cells.

Question 5: The binding of an odorous substance to the odorant-receptor protein molecules (on the ciliary membrane of the olfactory receptor cell), stimulates the initiation of a second messenger pathway associated with an olfactory-specific G-protein, which subsequently stimulates adenyl cyclase, which generates cAMP. The cAMP elevation unlocks a cyclic nucleotide-gated cation channel embedded in the ciliary membrane, permitting sodium and calcium cations to pass into the cell. This stimulates the chemosensitive cilia of the olfactory receptor cells, and a wave of depolarization (generator potential) is propagated from the dendrites to the cell body of the olfactory receptor cell. A high enough depolarization triggers a nerve impulse that is propagated along the axon of the olfactory receptor cell, centrally to the olfactory bulb.

CHAPTER 20

Question 1: The limbic lobe consists of the subcallosal, cingulate, and parahippocampal gyri, as well as the hippocampal formation, all of which collectively form a cortical perimeter around the corpus callosum. The limbic lobe is considered to be a component of the more extensive limbic system.

The limbic system includes all the structures of the limbic lobe as well as the amygdaloid body, septal area, and some nuclei of the thalamus and hypothalamus. The two main structures of the limbic system are the hippocampal formation (which includes the hippocampus proper, dentate gyrus, and the subiculum) and the amygdala.

Question 3: The dentate gyrus gets its name from its tooth-like configuration, created by numerous blood vessels that pierce the ventricular surface of the hippocampus and then the dentate gyrus, imparting a notched appearance.

Question 5: The entorhinal cortex. Widespread areas of the association cortex relay input to the entorhinal cortex and it is via the entorhinal cortex that these cortical association areas have access to the hippocampus and play a role in memory consolidation.

Question 7: The hypothalamus mediates autonomic nervous system (visceral) responses that accompany the expression of emotions.

Question 9: The perforant pathway from the entorhinal cortex.

CHAPTER 21

Question 1: The nuclei of this zone include the periventricular, suprachiasmatic, and arcuate nuclei. The periventricular and arcuate nuclei control the functions of the anterior pituitary gland (adenohypophysis), which synthesizes and releases various endocrine hormones into the bloodstream. The suprachiasmatic nucleus functions in the control of circadian rhythms, and is referred to as the "master clock" of the body.

Question 3: The lateral zone of the hypothalamus includes the following nuclei: the lateral preoptic nucleus anteriorly, the lateral tuberal nuclei in the tuberal region, and the lateral hypothalamic nucleus, which extends throughout the anteroposterior extent of the lateral zone. The lateral zone receives input from the limbic system and plays an important role in the behavioral expression of emotions.

Question 5: The supraoptic region contains nuclei that function in the control of circadian rhythms, temperature regulation, and the control of water balance.

Question 7: The mammillary region includes the prominent mammillary nuclei and the posterior hypothalamic nucleus. The mammillary nuclei are associated with emotions, whereas the posterior hypothalamic nucleus serves as a "thermostat" and regulates body temperature.

Question 9: In addition to the neural input, the hypothalamus also receives non-neural input from the vascular system. Hypothalamic neurons serve as receptors that are sensitive to rapid changes in the temperature, osmotic pressure, and hormone levels of the circulating blood. These receptors are referred to as circumventricular organs (CVOs). They consist of hypothalamic neurons that are embedded in the wall of the third ventricle, and are sensitive to alterations in the chemical composition of the cerebrospinal fluid. One of these structures is associated with the lamina terminalis, and is referred to as the organum vasculosum of the lamina terminalis (OVLT). The OVLT is a chemosensory structure that detects and responds to peptides and macromolecules present in the bloodstream. The other CVO is the subfornical organ located inferior to the fornix, near the interventricular foramen. The subfornical organ serves in the regulation of body fluids. The fenestrated capillaries supplying these receptors do not have a blood–brain barrier, thus they permit substances present in the bloodstream to pass through and enter the extracellular space surrounding the receptor cells.

Question 11: The fornix.

Question 13: The ascending reticular activating system relays nociceptive input to the hypothalamus, which mediates the autonomic and reflex responses to nociception.

Question 15: The tuberohypophyseal tract carries fibers from the arcuate and periventricular nuclei to the infundibular stalk (posterior pituitary). The axon terminals of the tuberohypophyseal tract release "releasing hormones" or "release-inhibiting hormones" in the hypophyseal portal system, which carries them to the anterior lobe of the pituitary gland, where they regulate the synthesis and release of anterior pituitary hormones. The tuberohypophyseal tract and the hypophyseal portal system serve as a connection between the hypothalamus and anterior pituitary gland.

Question 17: There are two main problems that might cause this condition: (i) a blockage of the superior hypophyseal artery, thus depriving the anterior pituitary of nutrition; or (ii) a lesion in the periventricular zone of the hypothalamus.

CHAPTER 22

Question 1: The anterior nuclear group, a relay nucleus of the Papez circuit of emotion, has extensive connections with the limbic system. It receives afferent fibers relaying information from the mammillary body and the hippocampal formation. It in turn projects to the cingulate gyrus of the limbic association cortex. Due to its limbic connections, the anterior nuclear group functions in the expression of emotions and, due to its considerable connections with the hippocampal formation, this nuclear group is also believed to be associated with learning and memory processes.

The lateral dorsal nucleus (of the lateral group of thalamic nuclei) is the caudal continuation of the anterior thalamic nuclear group and may play a role in the expression of emotions. Like the anterior thalamic nuclear group, it receives inputs from the mammillary body and in turn projects to the cingulate and parahippocampal gyri of the limbic system.

The dorsomedial nucleus (of the medial group of thalamic nuclei) also functions in the processing of information related to emotion via its connections to the limbic system components such as the amygdala and the orbitofrontal cortex.

Question 3: The posterior portion of the ventral lateral (VLp) nucleus receives prominent projections arising from the deep cerebellar nuclei (mainly from the dentate nucleus) of the opposite side, via the dentatothalamic tract. The VLp then relays the information to the premotor and primary motor cortex (Brodmann's areas 6 and 4, respectively).

Question 5: The nonspecific nuclei of the thalamus, which includes the intralaminar and reticular thalamic nuclei.

CHAPTER 23

Question 1: Most of the cerebral cortex consists of association cortex, which is classified into unimodal association cortex and multimodal (heteromodal) association cortex. Unimodal association areas are located next to, near, or around the primary sensory cortices that expand on the functions of the respective primary areas. As an example, the primary visual cortex (Brodmann's area 17) projects to the visual association cortex (Brodmann's areas 18, 19, 20, 21, and 37), and only processes a single modality, in this case vision, and is thus referred to as a unimodal association cortex. In contrast, the multimodal association cortical areas receive inputs from multiple sensory modalities; they then integrate the information and, via their higher order cognitive functions, formulate a composite experience. The multimodal association cortex is associated with imagination, judgement, decision making, and making long-range plans.

Question 3: Studies of patients who had their corpus callosum sectioned showed the following. When patients were asked to read words that were presented in their right visual field, they were able see and to read the words. However, when words were presented in their left visual field, they could not read them, since they were not even aware that the words were there. One explanation is as follows. Visual information in the right visual field is relayed to the left cerebral hemisphere (via the visual pathway, which was not affected when the corpus callosum was sectioned), which is the dominant hemisphere in the processing of language in most individuals. Thus the patients were able to see and read the words. In contrast, visual input from the left visual field is relayed to the right cerebral hemisphere (again, via the visual pathway, which was not affected when the corpus callosum was sectioned), the nondominant hemisphere for language. As a result of the bisection of the corpus callosum, the visual input relayed to the right cerebral hemisphere has no way of also reaching the left hemisphere containing the language areas. Consequently, patients could not see or read the words —as if they had a left homonymous hemianopia. These individuals are *not* blind. When they were asked to select with their hand an object that corresponds to the object that was presented in their left visual field, they selected the matching object. This showed that the visual system is functioning properly, and that it is the language function that is not.

Question 5: Broca's and Wernicke's areas are supplied by the middle cerebral artery. This vessel has an extensive distribution and supplies parts of the frontal, parietal, temporal, and occipital lobes. If only the cortical branches of the middle cerebral artery supplying Broca's area are occluded, the cerebral cortex of Broca's area becomes infarcted, resulting in Broca's aphasia. If the proximal segment of the middle cerebral artery is occluded, the cerebral cortex of the insula and subcortical white matter will also become infarcted, and a severe form of Broca's aphasia results, which is accompanied by motor deficits in the contralateral lower face, tongue, and upper limb.

If only the cortical branches of the middle cerebral artery supplying Wernicke's area are occluded, the cerebral cortex of Wernicke's area becomes infarcted, resulting in Wernicke's aphasia. If the subcortical white matter and geniculocalcarine tract (optic radiations) are also involved, visual deficits will also be present.

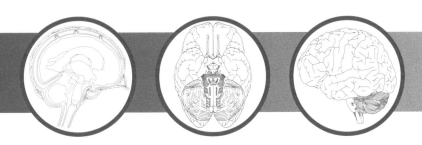

Index

Note: Page numbers in *italic* refer to figures and/or tables